Theory & Practice of
THERAPEUTIC MASSAGE

Theory & Practice of
THERAPEUTIC MASSAGE

4th Edition

Mark F. Beck

Photography by Yanik Chauvin

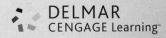
DELMAR
CENGAGE Learning™

Australia • Brazil • Japan • Korea • Mexico • Singapore • Spain • United Kingdom • United States

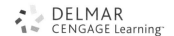
DELMAR
CENGAGE Learning™

Theory and Practice of Therapeutic Massage, 4th Edition
Mark F. Beck

Vice President, Health Care Business Unit:
  William Brottmiller

Editorial Director: Matthew Kane

Acquisitions Editor: Kalen Conerly

Developmental Editor: Juliet Steiner

Editorial Assistant: Molly Belmont

Marketing Director: Jennifer McAvey

Marketing Coordinator: Christopher Manion

Production Director: Carolyn Miller

Production Manager: Barbara A. Bullock

Production Editor: John Mickelbank

Project Editor: Ruth Fisher

Art and Design Specialist: Robert Plante

Cover design and Photograph: Yanik
  Chauvin, www.yanikchauvin.com

For product information and technology assista nce, contact us at
Cengage Learning Customer & Sales Support, 1-800-354-9706
For permission to use material from this text or product,
submit all requests online at **cengage.com/permissions**
Further permissions questions can be emailed to
permissionrequest@cengage.com

ExamView® and ExamView Pro® are registered trademarks of FSCreations, Inc. Windows is a registered trademark of the Microsoft Corporation used herein under license. Macintosh and Power Macintosh are registered trademarks of Apple Computer, Inc. Used herein under license.

Library of Congress Control Number: 2005054851

Hard cover   ISBN-13: 978-1-4018-8029-3
              ISBN-10: 1-4018-8029-0

Soft cover   ISBN-13: 978-1-4018-8030-9
              ISBN-10: 1-4018-8030-4

Delmar
Executive Woods
5 Maxwell Drive
Clifton Park, NY 12065
USA

Cengage Learning is a leading provider of customized learning solutions with office locations around the globe, including Singapore, the United Kingdom, Australia, Mexico, Brazil, and Japan. Locate your local office at:
international.cengage.com/region

Cengage Learning products are represented in Canada by Nelson Education, Ltd.

For your lifelong learning solutions, visit **delmar.cengage.com**

Visit our corporate website at **www.cengage.com**

Notice to the Reader

Publisher does not warrant or guarantee any of the products described herein or perform any independent analysis in connection with any of the product information contained herein. Publisher does not assume, and expressly disclaims, any obligation to obtain and include information other than that provided to it by the manufacturer. The reader is expressly warned to consider and adopt all safety precautions that might be indicated by the activities described herein and to avoid all potential hazards. By following the instructions contained herein, the reader willingly assumes all risks in connection with such instructions. The publisher makes no representations or warranties of any kind, including but not limited to, the warranties of fitness for particular purpose or merchantability, nor are any such representations implied with respect to the material set forth herein, and the publisher takes no responsibility with respect to such material. The publisher shall not be liable for any special, consequential, or exemplary damages resulting, in whole or part, from the readers' use of, or reliance upon, this material.

Printed in the United States of America
4 5 6 7 8 9 10 09 08

CONTENTS

PART I
The History and Advancement of Therapeutic Massage

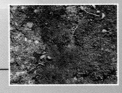

PART II
Human Anatomy and Physiology

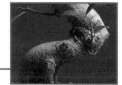

PART III
Massage Practice

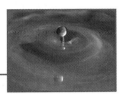

PART IV
Massage Business Administration

PREFACE

Welcome to the new *Theory and Practice of Therapeutic Massage*, 4th Edition. It is very exciting to present the new edition of this classic text containing all of the vital material of the past editions that you have come to trust plus new information essential to today's student of massage. The text is primarily written for massage students in 500- to 1,200-hour massage programs and their instructors. This comprehensive text is also an important reference for massage therapists who want to refresh and expand their knowledge of the massage profession. *Theory and Practice of Therapeutic Massage,* 4th Edition, is a basic textbook and starting point for students entering the massage profession. It contains the essential knowledge base for a massage therapist in an easily accessible form, as well as a treasure trove of vital information for a number of possible career paths within the massage profession.

As more states regulate massage, massage education is becoming more standardized and organized, with a core body of knowledge reflected in licensing requirements and the National Certification Exam. Although the majority of massage training takes place in one of many private massage schools, more massage programs are being offered in junior colleges and business/career schools. All of these programs depend on solid core curriculum materials augmented with ancillary products. *Theory and Practice of Therapeutic Massage* and its ancillary products fit perfectly with these programs, providing instructors and students with easily accessible materials that contain the fundamental knowledge base needed to become a successful massage practitioner.

Most massage education in the United States begins with a 500- to 1,000-hour program that lasts 6 months to a year. Programs include instruction in anatomy, physiology, kinesiology, ethics, sanitation, business practices, and the application of massage technique; most include clinical practice. Many schools include instruction in some specialty techniques. Most of these programs provide a good foundation for a student to begin the journey as a massage professional. *Theory and Practice of Therapeutic Massage* is an excellent core textbook for these programs because it contains the vital information about these basic subjects all in one text.

Graduating from massage school is a first and important step in becoming a successful massage professional. The journey continues as the new professional gains experience by doing massages and exchanging with other therapists while expanding their knowledge base through continuing education and personal study. In the massage profession, there are many paths and a wide variety of techniques. While *Theory and Practice of Therapeutic Massage* provides the strong foundation a student requires for entering the massage field, the text also provides introductions into several areas within the profession, with chapters devoted to spa massage, sports massage, and massage in medicine. The therapeutic modalities chapter has been augmented with expanded discussions of lymphatic massage, trigger-point therapies, muscle energy technique, and position release, as well as introductions into Oriental touch therapies, reflexology, and chair massage. Entire books have been written on these subjects. However, this book provides enough of an overview of these modalities for the student to get a sense as to whether he or she may want to pursue further study of a particular specialty. There is a lifetime of learning condensed into this text, and it is only a beginning of what is possible. There is always more to learn.

HISTORY OF *THEORY & PRACTICE OF THERAPEUTIC MASSAGE*

Frank Nichols, who I am led to believe was a pen name for a consortium of contributing writers, was the author of the 1948 publication of *Theory and Practice of Body Massage.* The first edition of *Theory and Practice of Therapeutic Massage,* initiated in 1984, was a revision of the Nichols book and a collaborative effort of several writers under the editorial direction of Bobbi Ray Madry of Milady Publications when Milady was a small, stand-alone publisher. It was not until the text was ready to go to the printer that I was asked for permission to use my name as the author because I was the largest contributor and they could not use Frank Nichols' name. Little did I know that I would become the author of *Theory and Practice of Therapeutic Massage* and still be working on the project more than 20 years later.

I am honored to be involved in the continuing evolution of *Theory and Practice of Therapeutic Massage.* As an insatiable student of massage, my yearning to learn was only whetted by the 1,000-hour massage apprenticeship program I completed in 1974. Reading numerous books on topics such as anatomy and natural healing techniques and accumulating hundreds of hours of continuing education while working with a steadily growing clientele created more questions than answers. More schooling in a holistic practitioner program increased my skills. I started teaching massage in 1978 and became a massage school owner and director in 1980. As school director for over 15 years, I developed curricula, taught classes, and continued a part-time clinical practice. I served on the

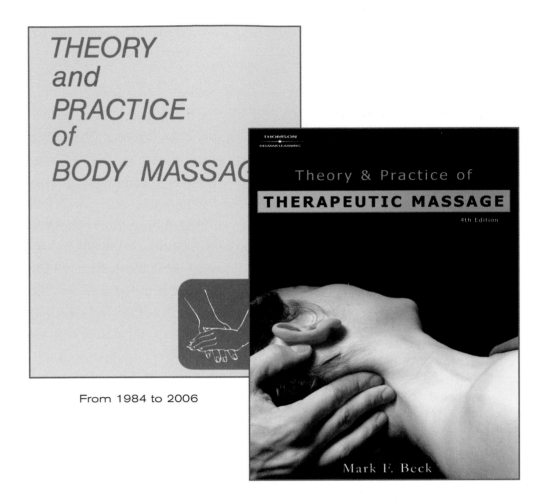

THEORY
and
PRACTICE
of
BODY MASSAG...

THOMSON
DELMAR LEARNING

Theory & Practice of
THERAPEUTIC MASSAGE
4th Edition

Mark F. Beck

From 1984 to 2006

boards of a state and a national massage organization in different capacities, including secretary of education, secretary of certification, and president. In 1992, I returned to school and earned a bachelor's degree in vocational education with an emphasis on massage therapy. When Milady Publishing invited me to be a consultant for the revision of Frank Nichols' *Theory and Practice of Body Massage* in 1984, I saw it as an opportunity to participate in the creation of a much-needed textbook for the emerging massage therapy profession. In 1988, *Theory and Practice of Therapeutic Massage* was introduced as the first comprehensive massage therapy textbook on the market. Since then, each new edition has been expanded and updated in response to the emerging trends and needs of the fastest-growing profession in the United States, including this newest 4th edition.

The 1st edition provided the industry with a much needed textbook for massage education. The 2nd edition was updated to contain the vital knowledge and concepts needed by the student to enter the massage profession. The 3rd edition added important features so the instructor had all the elements to assist the student in gaining the skills and knowledge to become a massage practitioner. The 4th edition strengthens key subjects, including ethics and therapeutic application of massage, and has added important chapters to help students choose a career path as they move into the massage profession.

NEW TO THE 4TH EDITION

The new 4th edition builds on the solid content of the former editions. The text maintains an easily readable style. Revisions have been made throughout the text to reflect the latest industry standards and research. The ethics chapter has been expanded. Pathologies, along with indications and contraindications, have been included with each system in the anatomy chapter. Beyond the basic information for Western/Swedish massage and skills focusing on wellness and relaxation massage, several new chapters have been added. A new chapter is devoted to therapeutic procedures, with an emphasis on assessment, planning, and treatment of soft tissue dysfunction. Two new chapters have been added to explore the current trends in the profession. The new chapter "Massage in the Spa Setting" examines the knowledge requirements and expectations for a massage therapist working in the bourgeoning spa industry. The new medical massage chapter examines the historical and current aspects of the massage professional working within the medical community. The athletic/sports massage chapter has been updated to reflect the latest procedures. There is also expanded material on prenatal massage, lymph massage, trigger-point therapy, muscle energy technique, and position release. Finally, an important new appendix on basic pharmacology for massage therapists has been added that responds to new content knowledge requirements for individuals seeking to take the national certification exam.

Theory and Practice of Therapeutic Massage is chock full of invaluable knowledge and fundamental concepts for learning massage. While the text provides excellent information, instruction from a competent instructor and guided practice are required to become proficient at using the techniques described in the text. Hands-on classroom instruction, along with literally hundreds of hours of practice and application of skills in a clinical setting on real clientele, is required to master the techniques.

ORGANIZATION

The text is organized into sections that can be studied sequentially, or better yet, simultaneously.

Part I (Chapters 1 through 3) gives a general introduction to therapeutic massage. Chapter 1 is an overview of the history of massage, which has been practiced in some form since prehistoric times. Chapter 2 discusses the legal and educational requirements to practice massage. Chapter 3 is concerned with professional standards and contains an expanded discussion of ethical considerations in the practice of therapeutic massage.

Part II (Chapters 4 and 5) is a richly detailed presentation of anatomy, physiology, and pathology, the study of which is a foundation for the understanding and practice of therapeutic massage. Full-color illustrations enhance descriptions in the text of structure and function, especially of the skeletal, muscular, circulatory, and nervous systems, as well as the other systems of the body.

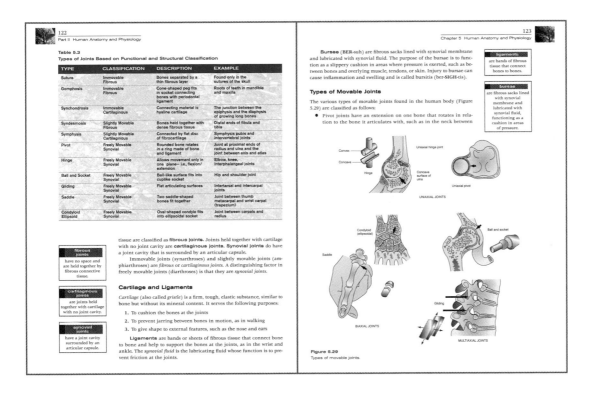

Part III (Chapters 6 through 18) combines theory with the practice of massage. Chapter 6 covers benefits, indications, and contraindications of massage. Chapter 7 discusses equipment and supplies. Chapter 8 addresses hygiene, sanitation, and safety practices. Chapter 9 covers the preliminary consultation, communication skills, and charting for basic wellness massage. Chapters 10 through 12 define the classification of massage movements and describe the application of massage technique and the procedure for a general full-body relaxation massage.

Chapter 13 takes the application of massage to the therapeutic level in which each client is considered for the specific conditions he or she brings to the session. New techniques are introduced to determine the client's needs and the specific soft tissues involved, and modalities are described to address soft tissue dysfunction.

The remaining chapters in Part III provide fundamental information to enhance and expand the student's skills in several specialty areas. Chapter 14 introduces the student to the therapeutic uses of water and hydrotherapy. Chapter 15 expands upon the content of the hydrotherapy chapter and provides insight into the expectations and requirements of spa massage and working in the fast-growing spa industry. Chapter 16, "Athletic/Sports Massage," introduces students to the fundamentals of sports massage, working with athletes, and the various applications of specialized massage in the sports world. Chapter 17 explores medical massage, both historically and the current use of therapeutic massage as it integrates with modern medicine. Chapter 18 introduces several therapeutic touch modalities, including lymphatic, neuromuscular, prenatal, Oriental, and chair massage, along with several others. Only a brief glimpse is given of many of these techniques to whet the student's curiosity because entire books have been written about each of these topics.

Part IV is devoted to the business side of a massage practice. What workplace setting appeals to you—sports clinic, day spa, chiropractor's office, your home? Should you start your own business or work for someone else? Learn about licensing, setup costs, bookkeeping, advertising, office management, and other aspects of running a successful business.

The instructor might design the curriculum so that the student is studying several different sections of the text at the same time. For example, early in the program, the student may study the history of massage, begin the study of anatomy and physiology, and begin learning the classification of massage movements all at the same time. As the program continues, the curriculum may cover legal requirements and ethics at the same time as benefits, indications, and contraindications while the study of anatomy and massage techniques continues. When the student has progressed to the point of doing full-body massages, the consultation is covered as the study of anatomy and kinesiology continues. Advanced and specialty applications of massage follow at the same time as business practices and more anatomy, physiology, and pathology.

SPECIAL FEATURES

The textbook is organized and designed in such a way as to make retention easier and learning more enjoyable. Pages xxviii–xxix provide some additional information on the features highlighted below.

- *Clear, step-by-step instructions* augmented by hundreds of dynamic photos guide the student through basic and advanced massage techniques.

- *Learning Objectives* at the beginning of each chapter focus student learning and are excellent tools for study and review.

- *Margin glossary terms.* Important terms are highlighted, with definitions conveniently displayed in the page margin for easy referral and study; plus, a comprehensive glossary at the back of the book gives students immediate access to definitions.

- *Charts and tables* emphasize crucial concepts. An extensive table in Chapter 5 illustrates the insertion, origin, and action of skeletal muscles, knowledge essential to the effective practice of therapeutic massage. More than 40 full-color illustrations help the student identify and locate all the major muscle groups.

- *Informational text boxes* and *bulleted lists* throughout the text highlight important content for easy reading and enhanced review.

- *Review of specialized massage applications.* In addition to a strong foundation in basic massage, explore the therapeutic application of massage, sports massage, spa massage, massage in a medical setting, lymph massage, soft tissue manipulation, chair massage, reflexology, and more.

- *Questions for discussion and review.* At the end of each chapter, test your comprehension and identify what areas need to be reviewed by answering questions covering material in the chapter. The answers are located in Appendix II of the textbook.

EXTENSIVE TEACHING AND LEARNING PACKAGE

A number of ancillary materials accompany *Theory and Practice of Therapeutic Massage,* 4th Edition. These materials are designed to support student learning and to provide massage instructors with everything they need to successfully teach the concepts in the core textbook.

THEORY AND PRACTICE OF THERAPEUTIC MASSAGE 4TH EDITION WORKBOOK

The *Theory and Practice of Therapeutic Massage 4th Edition Workbook* is made up of questions that directly correspond to each chapter of the textbook. Questions are in the form of fill-in-the-blank, matching, word reviews, and labeling illustrations. An exam review in a multiple-

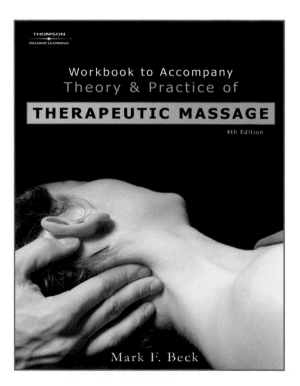

choice format supplements the workbook questions. Together the workbook and the exam review help the student prepare for certification and licensing exams.

THEORY AND PRACTICE OF THERAPEUTIC MASSAGE INSTRUCTOR'S MANUAL

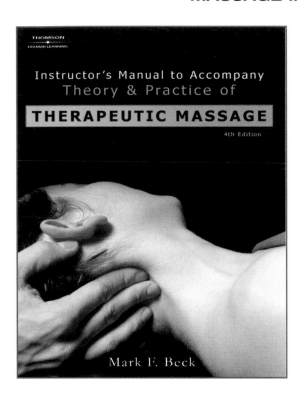

The *Theory and Practice of Therapeutic Massage Instructor's Manual* is a comprehensive teaching aid that contains:

- lesson plans, each keyed to a section of the text and the student workbook
- an outline of topics to cover in both the theory and practical sessions of each class
- time allotments for each activity
- suggested projects, resources, and assignments
- teaching tips to help instructors successfully engage and instruct students
- skills checklists that can be used to gauge and track student mastery of specific massage skills
- additional resources and sources for information
- answer key for the student workbook

The *Instructor's Manual* is designed to help massage educators by simplifying and organizing classroom preparation and presentation. Teaching becomes more efficient, more effective, and more enjoyable.

THEORY AND PRACTICE
OF THERAPEUTIC MASSAGE
ELECTRONIC CLASSROOM MANAGER

Theory and Practice of Therapeutic Massage Electronic Classroom Manager is an innovative instructor resource to support customized instruction. This CD-ROM for instructors contains excellent tools, including:

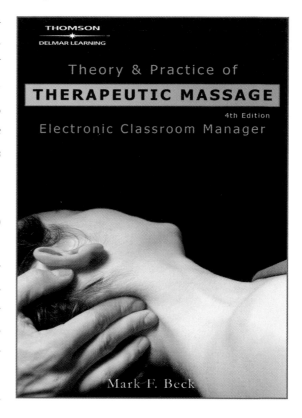

- A *Computerized Test Bank* of over 1,100 questions in multiple-choice, matching, and short-answer format, as well as the accompanying answers, organized by chapter, that can be used to generate quizzes and tests.

- A searchable *Image Library* containing over 225 color drawings and figures from *Theory and Practice of Therapeutic Massage,* 4th Edition, to incorporate into lectures, electronic presentations, assignments, testing, and handouts.

- A *PowerPoint Presentation* of approximately 750 slides that can be used in classroom lectures. Slides in each chapter reinforce the main information from the chapter, including figures and animations to enliven the presentation. Where appropriate, there are teaching tips in the comments section that give instructors additional information to use during lectures.

- *Student Skills Proficiency Checklists* in both ready-to-use PDF and customizable MS Word formats.

- A *Customizable Syllabus* instructors can tailor to meet individual teaching styles and course objectives, complete with course schedules, assignments, grading options, paper topics, and more.

The *Electronic Classroom Manager* is an incredibly powerful resource that instructors can customize to fit their individual instructional goals.

ACKNOWLEDGMENTS

The author and Delmar Cengage Learning wish to express our deep appreciation to the many professional people who have contributed their valuable time and counsel during the preparation of this text. Massage therapy has developed over hundreds of years. There is actually very little information that is unique, original, or new in this text, although each edition has been refined and expanded to contain the fundamental and vital concepts needed for today's serious student of therapeutic massage. There have been literally hundreds of people involved in both the production and the content of this text throughout its history and development. The 4th edition would not be possible without the three editions that preceded it and all of the work and talent of the many individuals that went into those editions. We are indebted to and appreciative of every contributor.

We especially want to thank the following people for their contributions in their special areas of expertise:

Richard Van Why for his unceasing research into the history of massage and the information provided in the history chapter.

Jack Meagher and Pat Archer for the material they provided in the sports massage chapter.

Gay Koopman for her expertise and help in the revision of the sports massage chapter.

Leslie Grow for her help with the initial photos in the lymph massage and sports massage portions of the text.

David Palmer, founder and director of TouchPro Institute in San Francisco, for contributing the section on chair massage.

Cherie Sohnen-Moe for her valuable contributions to the massage profession and especially to the business and ethics chapters of this text.

Steve Capellini for the valuable addition of the spa chapter and his expert help during the photo shoot.

Yanik Chauvin for the incredible photography in this 4th edition.

Dan Cronin of the Center for Natural Wellness School of Massage Therapy, Albany, New York, for inviting us to hold the photo shoot at his beautiful facility and providing us unlimited access to the school's resources.

All the models in the photos, each one a licensed massage therapist or a student on the road to a massage career, with special thanks to Dale Perry, LMT, CLT, NSMT, for sharing his expertise in lymph massage.

Faye Schenkman for lending her expertise on pharmacology, herbology, and nutritional supplements as they relate to the practice of massage therapy in the new appendix.

The author also expresses a special appreciation to the following individuals:

Bobbi Ray Madry, editor of the original *Theory and Practice of Therapeutic Massage,* for her encouragement of my involvement in this project and her gift of the authorship of the text.

Bob Rogers for the training that began my journey into the marvelous and rewarding profession of massage.

My mentors, teachers, students, and many clients who have provided me the knowledge and skills that were the foundation of my own practice and the curriculum at the massage schools I directed and taught.

The creation of this magnificent 4th edition would not have been possible without the expertise and dedication of the entire production team and Delmar Cengage Learning, including:

Kalen Conerly—Acquisitions Editor

Juliet Steiner—Developmental Editor

Molly Belmont—Editorial Assistant

Bob Plante—Art & Design Specialist

John Mickelbank—Production Editor

Ruth Fisher—Project Editor

The many reviewers for their assistance, comments, and expertise in reviewing the developing text.

I want to acknowledge Frank Nichols, author of the original *Theory and Practice of Body Massage* (1948), for the original work from which *Theory and Practice of Therapeutic Massage* evolved.

Finally, Natasha, wherever you are, thank you for my first real massage and the advice, "Whenever your back hurts like that, find someone who knows how to do massage."

ABOUT THE AUTHOR

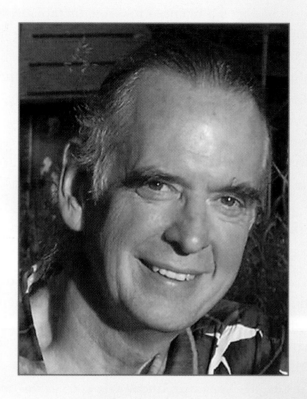

Mark Beck began his massage career in 1974 (more than 30 years ago) after completing a massage apprenticeship under the guidance of Bob Rogers. One of the main things he gained in his training was the knowledge of how expansive the world of massage is and an insatiable appetite to learn more. He has been the director of two massage schools and has been active in state and national professional massage organizations. He holds a bachelor's degree in vocational education with an emphasis in massage therapy from the University of Idaho. Mark developed the Structural Muscular Balancing Seminars and is coauthor of the *Structural Muscular Balancing Manual*.

Because of a spinal cord injury in 1990, Mark retired from the practice of massage therapy but continues to be an advocate for excellence in massage education. He has also become an ambassador of disability advocacy.

CONTRIBUTORS TO *THEORY AND PRACTICE OF THERAPEUTIC MASSAGE*, 4TH EDITION

Steve Capellini

Steve Capellini has been a licensed massage therapist since 1984. He has worked in the spa industry for over 20 years as a therapist, supervisor, trainer, manager, and consultant. He has written many articles for industry publications and was a spa columnist for *Massage Today* for 4 years. His books include *The Royal Treatment, Massage Career Guide for Hands-On Success,* and *Massage for Dummies.* He teaches workshops for therapists who plan to integrate spa services into their practices and is currently writing a textbook to complement spa training curricula in massage schools.

Yanik Chauvin

Yanik Chauvin is the administrative director of a leading massage therapy school in Gatineau, Quebec, Canada. He's also a professional photographer selling massage therapy images through his Web site www.touchphotography.com and offering his photography services to various organizations through www.yanikchauvin.com. He specializes in corporate and health-oriented imagery and has been working closely with Delmar Cengage Learning since early 2005 as the designer and photographer of the book covers for the complete massage therapy line.

Faye N. Schenkman

Faye Schenkman is a licensed massage therapist in New York and holds a master's degree in Chinese history. She is a diplomate of Asian bodywork therapy and Chinese herbal medicine and the National Certification Commission for Acupuncture and Oriental Medicine (NCCAOM). She is a charter member and certified instructor of the American Organization of Bodywork Therapies of Asia (AOBTA). She is a former faculty member of The University of Illinois Oriental Studies Department and a teacher of Chinese in some New York City high schools. Faye currently is an instructor of Integrative Therapies, Graduate School of Nursing at Columbia University. She is a former Board of Trustees member of the New York College for Wholistic Health Education and Research, and she was director of the Wholistic Health Center at the college for over 10 years. Faye was also the chair of the Massage Therapy School at New York College, as well as the dean of the Advanced Amma program, where she taught Advanced Amma Therapeutic Massage, Chinese and Western herbal medicine, Eastern nutrition, and Oriental sciences. Faye has been an advanced practitioner of Amma Therapeutic Massage for over 20 years. She is a co-founder, with her partner Kim Rosado, of Wholistic Healing Arts, LLC, in Huntington, New York, where patients are treated for a wide range of physical illnesses using Amma, acupuncture, herbal medicine, wholistic nutrition, craniosacral therapy, uterine massage, and Qi Gong. Faye and Kim conduct workshops throughout the United States.

REVIEWERS OF *THEORY AND PRACTICE OF THERAPEUTIC MASSAGE*, 4TH EDITION

Bernice Bicknase
Ivy State Technical College

Constance Jakubcin
Southeastern Career College

Jennifer Britt
Intellitec Medical Institute

Brian Klucinec
University of Pittsburgh

Lonnie Catlin
Community College of Denver

Scott LaSalle
Florida Career College

Mary Alice Farina
Sandhills Community College

James Mizner
Applied Career Training

Ramona Moody French
Desert Resort School of Somatherapy

Bernadette Della Bitta Nicholson
Springfield Technical Community College

Nan Gillett
El Paso Community College

Carolyn Talley-Porter
Greenville Technical College

Barbara Harwell
Stark State College of Technology

Paul David Tuff
Monterey Peninsula College

HOW TO USE *THEORY AND PRACTICE OF THERAPEUTIC MASSAGE*, 4TH EDITION

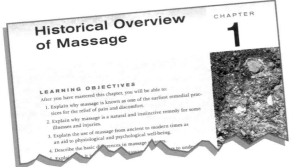

Learning Objectives

Before beginning a chapter, review the Learning Objectives for a "road map" of what the chapter will cover. These Learning Objectives cover the main points of each chapter and are also an excellent tool for review and study.

Introduction

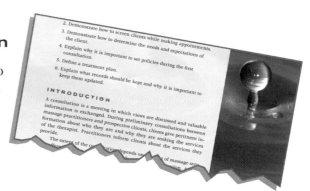

Each chapter begins with a "big picture" introduction to the information that follows. These introductions provide a solid framework for understanding the concepts covered in the chapter. They are the springboard from which the reader can delve into the depths of each chapter.

Key Terms and Margin Definitions

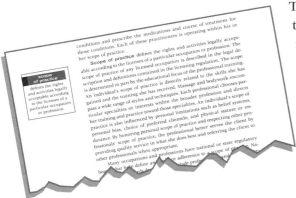

The amount of new terminology faced by the massage therapy student can be overwhelming. To help the reader quickly and easily master important terms, new words are bolded in color in the text on their first use. This key term is then defined in the margin, providing immediate access to the definition. All terms bolded and defined in the margin are also included in the text's main glossary, found at the back of the book. Readers are encouraged to use the margin glossary terms while studying and reviewing.

Informative Boxes

Throughout the book there are special boxes of additional information to enhance the information in the main text. These boxes highlight important concepts and provide a deeper perspective into the material.

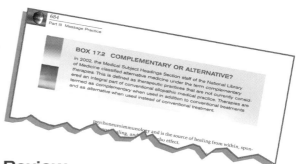

Chapter 5 Section Review

Some of the densest and most challenging information may be found in the comprehensive Chapter 5: "Human Anatomy and Physiology." This lengthy chapter is broken into sections on the different body systems. Each section provides review questions to help gauge mastery of this important material. Review questions include matching, true/false questions, and questions for discussion and review. Answers to these questions can be found at the back of the book to support independent study.

Procedure Photos

Brand-new photos in dramatic black and white demonstrate with technical accuracy and beauty the massage therapy techniques discussed throughout. Step-by-step procedures provide detailed instructions in the figure captions to walk the reader through each series in preparation for hands-on work.

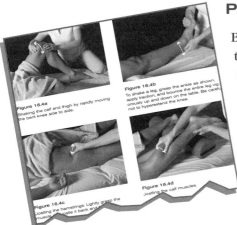

Questions for Discussion and Review

At the conclusion of each chapter are questions to help focus learning and spark thoughtful discussion. These are an excellent review tool and can be done independently or as part of an organized assignment. While the answers to all the questions can be found in the chapter itself, they are also provided at the back of the book for easy reference.

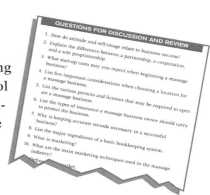

Bibliography

For readers looking for more information on therapeutic massage and the specific topics covered in this text, the author has provided a bibliography of additional sources. Although the bibliography is updated with current titles and new editions, there is also a good selection of classic and foundational works that readers may be interested in.

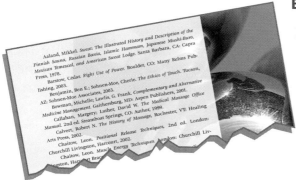

Appendix I: Basic Pharmacology for Massage Therapists

Increasingly, massage therapists are expected to have a basic understanding of pharmacology for certification and licensure. This new appendix on Basic Pharmacology for Massage Therapists is a general introduction to this important information. Covering basics of pharmacology as well as drugs, vitamins and minerals, and herbs, this is an excellent resource.

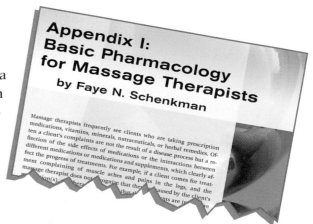

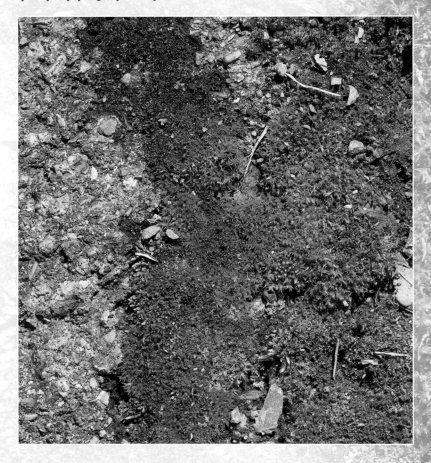

PART I

The History and Advancement of Therapeutic Massage

Historical Overview of Massage

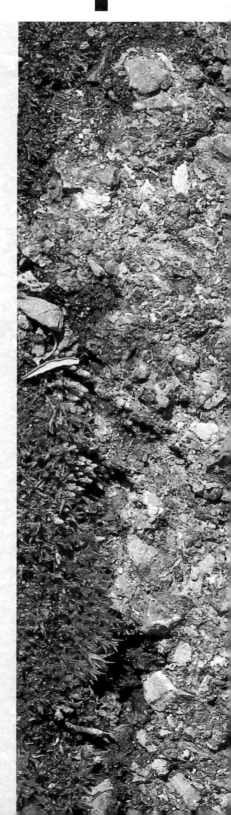

LEARNING OBJECTIVES

After you have mastered this chapter, you will be able to:

1. Explain why massage is known as one of the earliest remedial practices for the relief of pain and discomfort.

2. Explain why massage is a natural and instinctive remedy for some illnesses and injuries.

3. Explain the use of massage from ancient to modern times as an aid to physiological and psychological well-being.

4. Describe the basic differences in massage systems.

5. Explain why it is important for massage practitioners to understand massage history.

INTRODUCTION

Massage (muh-**SAHZH**) is defined as the systematic manual or mechanical manipulations of the soft tissues of the body by such movements as rubbing, kneading, pressing, rolling, slapping, and tapping, for therapeutic purposes such as promoting circulation of the blood and lymph, relaxation of muscles, relief from pain, restoration of metabolic balance, and other benefits both physical and mental.

The massage practitioner has been referred to as a massage technician or massotherapist. In the past, a male massage practitioner may have been called a masseur (ma-**SUR**), and a female practitioner a masseuse (ma-**SOOS**). Today, most professionally trained men and women prefer to be called *massage practitioners* or *massage therapists*. For practical purposes, massage practitioner or massage therapist are the terms used throughout this book.

The origin of the word *massage* can be traced to at least five sources:

- The Greek root *masso,* or *massein,* means to touch or to handle but also means to knead or to squeeze.

- The Latin root *massa* comes directly from the Greek *masso* and means the same.

- The Arabic root *mass'h,* or *mass,* means to press softly.

- The Sanskrit word *makeh* also means to press softly.

> **massage**
>
> is the systematic manual or mechanical manipulations of the soft tissues of the body for therapeutic purposes.

- The modern use of the term *massage* to denote using the hands to apply manipulations of the soft tissues is of fairly recent origin. The term was first used in American and European literature around 1875. In America, the use of the word *massage* was popularized by Douglas Graham from Massachusetts. The term *massage,* as well as the common names for the strokes (effleurage, petrissage, tapotement) and frictions, is generally attributed to a Dutchman, Johann Georg Mezger.

MASSAGE IN ANCIENT TIMES

Even though the term *massage* is fairly new, the practice of various techniques can be traced back to antiquity. Massage is one of the earliest remedial practices of humankind and is the most natural and instinctive means of relieving pain and discomfort. When a person has sore, aching muscles, abdominal pains, a bruise, or wound, it is a natural and instinctive impulse to touch, press, and rub that part of the body to obtain relief.

Artifacts have been found in many countries to support the belief that in prehistoric times men and women massaged their muscles and rubbed herbs, oils, and various substances on their bodies as healing and protective agents. In many ancient cultures some form of touch or massage was practiced. In many groups a special person such as a healer, spiritual leader, or doctor was selected to administer healing power. Some ancient civilizations used therapeutic massage not only as a pain reliever but also to improve their sense of well-being and physical appearance.

Massage has been a major part of medicine for at least 5,000 years and important in Western medical traditions for at least 3,000 years. Massage was the first and most important of the medical arts and was practiced, developed, and taught primarily by physicians. It has been written about extensively in medical books since 500 B.C. and was a major topic in the first medical texts printed after the discovery of the printing press.

Chinese Anmo Techniques

In the British Museum, records reveal that as early as 3000 B.C., massage was practiced by the Chinese. *The Cong Fou* of Tao-Tse was one of the ancient Chinese books that described the use of medicinal plants, exercises, and a system of massage for the treatment of disease and the maintenance of health. The Chinese continued to improve their massage techniques through a special procedure they called *anmo.* This massage technique was developed over many years of experience in finding the points on the body where various movements such as rubbing, pressing, and manipulations were most effective. Today, the use of massage is an integral part of the Chinese health system and is practiced in China's medical clinics and hospitals. A more modern term for Chinese massage is *tui-na,* which literally means "push-pull."

Japanese Tsubo and Shiatsu

The practice of the anmo method of massage entered Japan around the sixth century A.D. The points of stimulation remained much the same as the Chinese points but were called **tsubo.** These points are pressed to effect the circulation of fluids and *Ki* (life force energy) and stimulate nerves in a finger pressure technique the Japanese called **shiatsu.** This massage method has become quite popular in recent years. Early records show that a book on massage, *The San-Tsai-Tou-Hoei,* was published by the Japanese in the sixteenth century and listed both passive and active massage procedures.

> **tsubo**
> are points on the body that are sensitive to pressure applied during shiatsu.

> **shiatsu**
> is a massage technique from Japan in which points of stimulation are pressed to effect the circulation of fluids and *ki* (life force energy).

Indian and Hindu Practices

Massage has been practiced on the Indian subcontinent for over 3,000 years. Knowledge of massage came to India from the Chinese and was an important part of the Hindu tradition. The *Ayur-Veda (Art of Life),* a sacred book of the Hindus written around 1800 B.C., included massage treatments among its hygienic principles. In writings dating back to 300 B.C., *The Laws of Manu,* or *The Laws of Man,* defined the duties of everyday life. These included diet, bathing, exercise, and **tschanpua,** or massage at the bath. *Tschanpua* included kneading the extremities, tapotement, frictioning, anointing with perfumes, and cracking the joints of the fingers, toes, and neck.

> **tschanpua**
> is a Hindu technique of massage in the bath.

Greek Massage and Gymnastics

From the East, the practice of massage spread to Europe and is believed to have flourished well before 300 B.C. The Greeks made gymnastics and the regular use of massage part of their physical fitness rituals. Homer, the Greek poet who wrote the *Iliad* and the *Odyssey* (the story of the Trojan war and its aftermath) in the ninth century B.C., spoke of the use of nutritious foods, exercise, and massage for war heroes to promote healing and relaxation.

The Greek priest-physician Aesculapius, who lived in the seventh century B.C., was the first in a long line of physicians and was later worshipped as the god of medicine. He is said to have combined exercise and massage to create gymnastics and founded the first **gymnasium** to treat disease and promote health. The gymnasium and baths became important centers where philosophers and athletes gathered to exercise and discuss ideas. It was a place where the young were educated, soldiers trained, the sick healed. The staff of Aesculapius with its serpents remains today as the symbol of medicine and pharmacy.

> **gymnasium**
> is a center where exercise and massage are combined to treat disease and promote health.

Greek women participated in gymnastics and dancing, and used massage as part of their health and beauty regimens. The Greeks referred to exercise as *ascesis,* based on their belief that an **ascete** was a person who exercised his or her body and mind. This was the same principle as today's holistic health concept of the cultivation of total health of body and mind.

> **ascete**
> is a person who exercises body and mind.

The Greek physician Herodicus of the fifth century B.C. prolonged the lives of many of his patients with diet, exercise, and massage using beneficial herbs and oils. Herodotus, the Greek historian of the time, wrote of the benefits of massage. Hippocrates (460–380 B.C.), a pupil of Herodicus and a descendant in the lineage of Aesculapius, later became known as the father of medicine. His code of ethics for physicians, the **Hippocratic Oath,** is still in use today. This oath, which incorporates a code of ethics for physicians and those about to receive medical degrees, binds physicians to honor their teachers, do their best to maintain the health of their patients, honor their patients' secrets, and prescribe no harmful treatment or drug. The Hippocratic Oath can be found in its entirety in most medical dictionaries.

That Hippocrates understood the effects of massage is revealed in one of his descriptions of massage movements. He said, "Hard rubbing binds, much rubbing causes parts to waste, and moderate rubbing makes them grow." This has been interpreted to mean that rubbing can help to bind a joint that is too loose or loosen a joint that is too tight. Vigorous rubbing can tighten and firm; moderate rubbing tends to build muscle. In his writings, Hippocrates used the word **anatripsis,** which means the art of rubbing a part upward, not downward. He stated that it is necessary to rub the shoulder following reduction of a dislocated shoulder. The advice Hippocrates gave still serves as a valuable guideline for modern practitioners. Hippocrates believed that all physicians should be trained in massage as a method of healing.

Roman Art of Massage and Therapeutic Bathing

The Romans acquired the practice of therapeutic bathing and massage from the Greeks. The Romans built public baths that were available to rich and poor alike. A brisk rubdown with fragrant oils could be enjoyed following the bath. The art of massage was also highly respected as a treatment for weak and diseased conditions and as an aid in removing stiffness and soreness from muscles.

The Romans, as the Greeks before them, used massage as part of their gymnastics. Celsus, who lived during the reign of Emperor Tiberius (about 42 B.C. to A.D. 37), was considered to be one of the most eminent of Roman physicians. He wrote extensively on many subjects, including medicine. *De Medicina* deals extensively with prevention and therapeutics using massage, exercise, and bathing. He recommended rubbing the head to relieve headaches and rubbing the limbs to strengthen muscles and to combat paralysis. Massage was used to improve sluggish circulation and internal disorders and to reduce edema. Although circulation of the blood was not completely understood, physicians of the time followed the teaching of Hippocrates and believed that rubbing upward was more effective than rubbing downward.

The Greek physician Claudius Galen (A.D. 130–200), who became physician to the Roman emperor Marcus Aurelius, is said to have

---

| Hippocratic Oath |
| is a code of ethics for physicians. |

| anatripsis |
| is the art of rubbing a body part upward. |

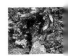

discovered that arteries and veins contain blood; however, William Harvey (1578–1657), an English physician, is credited with discovering the circulation of the blood in 1628. Galen was a prolific writer, and his medical texts were the principal ones in use for more than a thousand years. As a physician to gladiators, Galen gained great knowledge of anatomy. His books on hygienic health, exercise, and massage stressed specific exercises for various physical disorders. Greek and Roman philosophers, statesmen, and historians such as Cicero, Pliny, Plutarch, and Plato wrote of the importance of massage and passive and active exercise to the maintenance of a healthy body and mind. Even Julius Gaius Caesar, Roman general and Emperor of Rome (100–44 B.C.), is said to have demanded his daily massage for the relief of neuralgia and prevention of epileptic attacks. Both the Bible and the Koran mention the use of oils and aromatics to lubricate and anoint the skin.

The Decline of Arts and Sciences in the West

With the decline of the Roman Empire, beginning around A.D. 180, the popularity of bathing and massage also declined. According to Richard van Why, "The Roman emperor Constantine (A.D. 228–337) who converted to Christianity, abolished and destroyed the baths and gymnasiums because of widespread abuses of a sexual nature." Oribasius, Antyllus, Caelius Aurelianus, Aetius of Amida, and Paul of Aegina are some of the few medical writers and physicians who lived during the decline of the Roman Empire. They all wrote favorably of the use of massage, exercise, and bathing as therapeutic and conditioning agents.

There is little recorded history of health practices during the Middle Ages (the Dark Ages). This was the period between classical antiquity and the European Renaissance, extending from the downfall of Rome in about 476 to about 1450. The sciences and arts suffered severe setbacks during the Dark Ages. Few medical or historical books were written during this time, and much recorded history was lost. This decline was due in part to wars and to religious superstitions that caused people to fear placing too much importance on the physical self. In Europe in the Middle Ages, the medical institutions abandoned massage in favor of other remedies. Massage was practiced sporadically by laypeople, folk healers, and midwives and was occasionally the object of persecution as a magic cure and the work of Satan.

The Arabic Empire and the Rise of Islam

Beginning in the seventh century, the spread of Islam throughout North Africa, Asia Minor, Mesopotamia, and Persia actually served to preserve much of the Greco-Roman culture. As the Greco-Roman culture fell into decay in the Middle Ages, many of the important teachings of the great physicians and philosophers were carried on by the Persians. The Islamic Persian philosopher/physician *Rhazes*, or *Razi* (A.D. 860–932), was a follower of Hippocrates and Galen and a prolific writer. He wrote several books, the most important of which was an encyclopedia of Arabic, Roman, and Greek medical practices that esteemed the use of exercise, diet, and massage in the treatment of disease and the preservation of health. Another prominent Persian philosopher/physician, Avicenna (A.D. 980–1037), authored what is considered to be the most important single book in medical history. He was an ardent follower of Galen, and the *Canon of Medicine* made numerous references to the use of massage, exercise, and bathing. Eventually these volumes paved the way for the Renaissance as these writings returned to the West by way of trade and conquest.

The Renaissance Revives Interest in Health Practices

The Renaissance (rebirth, 1450–1600) revived interest in the arts and sciences. After a long intellectual slumber, the classical writings of the ancient Greek, Roman, and Persian masters were revived and studied as a basis from which to develop new ideas. Once again, people became interested in the improvement of physical health and appearance. By the second half of the fifteenth century, the printing press had been invented, which led to the publication of many scholarly writings in the arts and sciences. The advancement in the distribution of printed materials also helped stimulate interest in better health practices.

The Growth and Acceptance of Massage as a Healing Aid

By the sixteenth century, medical practitioners began to reinvent and employ massage as part of their healing treatments. Ambroise Pare (1517–1590), a French barber-surgeon, one of the founders of modern surgery and inventor of the ligation of arteries, described in one of his publications the positive effects of massage in the healing process. He classified massage movements as gentle, medium, and vigorous frictions and employed flexion, extension, and circumduction of joints. His concepts were passed down to other French physicians who believed in the value of physical therapeutics. During his lifetime, Pare served as personal physician to four of France's kings. He is credited with restoring the health of Mary, Queen of Scots (1542–1587) by use of massage. Mercurialis (1530–1606), a professor of medicine at the University of Padua, Italy, published a book, *De Arte Gymnastica,* in 1569 on gymnastics and the benefits of massage when integrated into treatments for the body and mind.

The sixteenth, seventeenth, and eighteenth centuries witnessed an expansion in all fields of knowledge. Emergent literature from English, French, German, and Italian authors re-established massage as a preferred scientific practice for the maintenance of health and the treatment of disease.

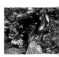

Frictions, manipulations, anointing, bathing, and exercise were regarded as important tools in the medical armament. These subjects were taught in institutions of higher learning to physicians and other practitioners of the healing practices and were based in the sciences of anatomy, physiology, and pathology as they were known in that day and age.

Throughout history, a kind of massage or hands-on healing has been practiced by laypeople or commoners. It was often practiced by folk healers and midwives and was passed on as an art and a gift. A body of knowledge was never established, so techniques were lost and rediscovered through the ages.

THE DEVELOPMENT OF MODERN MASSAGE TECHNIQUES

In the early part of the nineteenth century, John Grosvenor (1742–1823), a well-respected English surgeon and a practitioner of **chirurgy** (healing with the hands), stressed to his colleagues the value of friction in the relief of stiff joints, gout, and rheumatism. His efforts helped further the belief in massage as an aid to healing.

Per Henrik Ling (1776–1839) of Smaaland, Sweden, a physiologist and fencing master, is known as the father of physical therapy. He systemized and developed movements he found to be beneficial in improving his own physical condition. He called the system of movements **medical gymnastics.** He based this system on the developing science of physiology. The Ling System's primary focus was on gymnastics applied to the treatment of disease and consisted of movements classified as active, duplicated, and passive. *Active movements* were performed by the patient and could be referred to as exercise. *Duplicated movements* were performed by the patient in cooperation with the therapist. These correspond to modern-day resistive or assistive exercises. *Passive movements* were performed by the therapist to the patient and would be considered range of motion and massage. In 1813, Ling established the Royal Swedish Central Institute of Gymnastics, which was chartered and financed by the Swedish government. Ling died in 1839, but his students published his works posthumously. The Ling System, more commonly called Swedish Movements or the Movement Cure, spread throughout Europe and Russia. By 1851, there were 38 institutions for education in the Swedish Movements in Europe, most of them located in Germany. These schools were generally open to learned men. The programs were as long as three years, with classes lasting six to eight hours a day.

Mathias Roth, an English physician, studied under Ling at the Royal Central Institute and in 1851 published the first book in English on the Swedish Movements. He established the first institute in England to teach Swedish Movement Gymnastics and gave private instruction to Charles Fayette Taylor, a New York physician, who in 1858 introduced the methods to the United States. In the United States, the technique became known as *The Swedish Movement Cure.* Charles's brother, George

| **chirugy** |
| is healing with the hands. |

| **medical gymnastics** |
| gymnastics applied to the treatment of disease, consists of active, duplicated, and passive movements. |

Henry, in the meantime attended the Dr. Sotherberg Institute in Stockholm and completed full training in the Swedish Movements. They both returned to the United States and started an orthopedic practice in New York, where they specialized in the Swedish Movements. Within a year they dissolved their joint practice, but they both continued to practice and write about the Swedish Movement Cure. George Henry published the first American textbook on the Swedish Movement Cure in 1860 and established the Improved Movement Cure Institute in New York City. Charles Fayette wrote many articles and published a textbook introducing the Swedish Movements in 1861. Both brothers practiced and taught the cure until their deaths in 1899. Thus it was the competitive Taylor brothers who introduced the Swedish Movement Cure to the United States and brought massage more into public and medical acceptance.

Modern Massage Terminology

Modern massage terminology is credited to Dr. Johann Mezger (1839–1909) of Holland, who established the practice and art of massage as a scientific subject for physicians in the remedial treatment of disease. He was acknowledged by many of the authors of his day as the founder of scientific massage. Through Dr. Mezger's efforts, massage became recognized as fundamental to rehabilitation in physical therapy. Mezger's preference for the French terminology has remained an influence to this day (thus the use of the terms **effleurage**, **petrissage**, **tapotement**, and even *massage*). The word *massage* was not seen or used in the United States until 1874, when Douglas Graham from Boston and Benjamin Lee and Charles Mills from Philadelphia published articles using Mezger's terminology. Dr. Douglas O. Graham was a practitioner and a historian of massage who wrote extensively about the subject for 50 years from 1874 to 1925. He was a founding member of the American Physical Education Association.

By the early part of the nineteenth century, physicians in medical schools in Germany and Scandinavia were including massage in their teachings as a dignified and beneficial asset in the medical field. In 1900, the distinguished German physician Albert J. Hoffa published *Technik Der Massage*. The publication remains one of the most basic books in the field and contains many of the techniques used in Swedish massage.

Throughout Germany, Denmark, Norway, and Sweden, therapeutic exercises, massage, and baths were recommended by physicians for the restoration and maintenance of health. These physicians believed that massage helped the body rid itself of toxins, relieved such ailments as rheumatism, and promoted the healthy functioning of all body systems.

In England in 1894, a group of women formed the Society of Trained Masseuses. By 1920, this society had grown in members and prestige. Later, the society became known as the Chartered Society of Massage and Medical Gymnastics; it was registered in 1964 as the Chartered Society of Physiotherapy.

effleurage

is a succession of strokes applied by gliding the hand over an extended portion of the body.

petrissage

lifts, squeezes, and presses the tissues.

tapotement

movements include tapping, slapping, hacking, cupping, and beating.

THE DECLINE OF MASSAGE IN THE TWENTIETH CENTURY

The beginning of the twentieth century brought with it a decline in the scientific and medical use of massage. There were several reasons for this decline. The increasing popularity of massage in the nineteenth century precipitated an increase in not only qualified practitioners and schools but also lay practitioners and unscrupulous schools and practitioners.

A special inquiry by the British Medical Association in 1894 revealed numerous abuses in the education and practice of massage practitioners, which dealt a severe blow to the reputation of the profession. The inquiry found many schools using unscrupulous recruitment practices and offering inadequate training. As a result, graduates were unqualified or incompetent and in debt to the school. To repay that debt, students and graduates would work in clinics that would offer poor massage and often became no more than houses of prostitution. Other abuses included false certification and deceptive advertising, in which exorbitant claims were made that were totally unfounded and untrue. The reputation of massage was scandalized among physicians and the general public alike.

Technical innovations also had a detrimental affect on massage. The invention of electricity and various electrical apparatuses, such as the vibrator, greatly affected the use of hands-on therapy in favor of these new electrical modalities. This trend continues to this day.

Technical and intellectual advances in medicine developed new treatment strategies based more on pharmacology and surgical procedures. The old ideas of treating disease through diet, exercise, and bathing gave way to the more sophisticated practices of modern medicine. Physicians no longer learned massage as a part of their training, nor did they employ trained therapists. Massage's place in nursing eroded to no more than the administering of a back rub.

CONTEMPORARY DEVELOPMENTS IN MASSAGE

A number of important developments during the second quarter of the twentieth century continue to influence modern massage.

An Austrian named Emil Vodder developed a method of gentle rhythmical massage along the superficial lymphatics that accelerates the functioning of the lymphatic system and effectively treats chronic lymphedema (limf-e-**DEE**-muh) and other diseases of venous or lymph circulation. Today this system is widely known and taught as **Dr. Vodder's Manual Lymph Drainage.**

In the 1940s, a German, Elizabeth Dicke, developed *Bindegewebsmassage,* or **Connective Tissue Massage,** which was later popularized in England by Maria Ebner. *Bindegewebsmassage* is directed toward the subcutaneous connective tissue and is believed to affect vascular and visceral reflexes related to a variety of pathologies and disabilities. This

---

Dr. Vodder's Manual Lymph Drainage

is a method of gentle, rhythmical massage along the superficial lymphatics that aids in lymphatic system functioning and treats chronic lymphedema.

Connective Tissue Massage

is massage directed toward the subcutaneous connective tissue believed to affect vascular and visceral reflexes related to a variety of pathologies and disabilities.

method continues to be widely employed in many countries for pathologic conditions of circulation or visceral disease.

Dr. James H. Cyriax, an English orthopedic physician, is credited with popularizing **Deep Transverse Friction Massage**. This method broadens the fibrous tissues of muscles, tendons, or ligaments, breaking down unwanted fibrous adhesions and thereby restoring mobility to muscles in a way that cannot be achieved by passive stretching or active exercise. Transverse Friction Massage retains its popularity today in physical therapy and massage therapy regimes as an effective treatment in restoration and rehabilitation of muscle and soft tissue injuries.

Two American physical therapists who have had a major impact on massage therapy in the United States are Gertrude Beard and Frances Tappan. Both devoted much of their lives to promoting massage as an important part of the health care system. Tappan's book, *Healing Massage Techniques*, and *Beard's Massage* remain as standards in the massage industry.

Massage did play an important role immediately following World War I (1914–1918), when it proved beneficial as a restorative treatment in the rehabilitation of injuries. Again in World War II (1939–1945), massage was employed on an even larger scale in the hospitals of the Armed Forces. However, in the years following World War II, manual massage played a secondary role in physical therapy as more mechanical and electrical means of stimulation and rehabilitation gained popularity. During the postwar recovery, massage was directed more toward relaxation and athletics and less toward rehabilitation. Most practitioners were employed in athletic clubs or YMCAs or as trainers for athletic teams.

A MASSAGE RENAISSANCE IN THE UNITED STATES

Beginning around 1960, another massage renaissance began to take place in the United States, and it continues to this day. With the decline of the use of massage in traditional medicine, a surge of interest in the use and value of massage developed in the paraprofessional and lay public. Several factors precipitated this trend. Increased awareness of physical and mental fitness as well as the increasing cost of traditional medicine opened the way for viable alternatives in health care. The development of the wellness model, which placed more emphasis on prevention and recognized the importance of controlling stress, advocated the value of massage. The psychological benefits of touch and its proven use in the treatment of pain returned massage to a place of prominence in the health care system.

During this time, chiropractic began to receive more recognition. Chiropractic developed in the West when Dr. Daniel David Palmer began teaching techniques of directed manual pressure against the bony processes to manipulate the vertebrae of the spine and other articulations of the body. Today, chiropractors often employ massage practitioners as assistants.

> **Deep Transverse Friction Massage**
>
> is massage that broadens the fibrous tissues of muscles, tendons, or ligaments, breaking down unwanted adhesions and restoring mobility to muscles.

During the 1970s and 1980s, a significant rise in the popularity of massage as well as a number of other forms of bodywork occurred in the United States. Several professional associations and numerous schools emerged to teach and promote a variety of massage disciplines.

The American Massage Therapy Association (AMTA), which began in 1943, is the largest and oldest professional massage association. Its popular publication, *The Massage Therapy Journal,* carries a variety of articles that are of interest to the massage professional. The Association of Bodywork Professionals (ABMP) and the International Massage Association (IMA) were both created in the 1980s, essentially to offer an alternative for massage professionals to obtain professional liability insurance. The ABMP also publishes *Massage and Bodywork Quarterly Magazine. The Massage Magazine* began publication in 1985 as an independent trade magazine to bring the science, art, and business of massage to the general public. *Massage Today* started publication in 2000 as a no-cost subscription available to anyone in the massage industry with news of current events as well as articles from industry leaders.

Articles about massage appeared in a wide variety of news magazines, including *Time, Life,* and *Newsweek.* Newspapers would run common interest stories about massage or massage practitioners. Most of these articles were about the practitioners and the positive effects and benefits of massage. Massage therapists in communities would give presentations at club meetings and gatherings about the positive aspects of massage. As the public became more aware of the effects and benefits of therapeutic massage, the association between massage and prostitution dissipated.

The growing popularity of massage continued during the 1970s and 1980s in terms of more people receiving massage and more people choosing to learn massage, either for personal satisfaction or to become massage practitioners. Massage training programs varied widely in content and length with classic Swedish or Western massage being at the core of a majority of the curriculums. Early programs were as short as 100 hours for an introductory course. Adult education programs at community colleges or universities would sometimes have "Friends and Family" massage classes that may be as short as a weekend or a few evening classes. Training for those wishing to practice massage tended to be somewhat longer, with length and content often determined by local or state licensing requirements. The establishment of the National Certification Exam in 1990 required an applicant to have a minimum of 500 hours of training from a state-recognized school. Massage school curriculums tended to be between 500 and 600 class hours consisting of anatomy, physiology, business practices, and massage techniques. A few schools offered longer, more comprehensive programs of up to 1,000 to 1,200 class hours. Massage training was done largely at private massage schools or through apprenticeships. A vast majority of private massage schools were established after 1970 with well over 1,000 schools in the United States by the year 2000. With the growing popularity of massage and massage education, along with the increase in states regulating massage, private business schools and public community colleges began offering accredited massage training programs.

Massage was consistently becoming more visible, accessible, and popular with the American public. Massage of athletes became more commonplace. Athletes at organized runs, marathons, and triathlons would line up after the event to receive their post-event massage at the **sports massage** tent. Sports massage services were made available to the athletes at the 1984 Summer Olympics for the first time. Since that time, athletic massage has been part of every Summer and Winter Olympics. Many professional and even semipro athletic teams including baseball, football, basketball, hockey, and tennis either employed or provided for the services of sport massage therapists. Serious athletes from a variety of sports would seek out the services of a skilled massage therapist to help them maintain the highest level of performance while addressing myriad physical and sometimes emotional conditions that accompany the sport.

Sports massage teams at sporting events provided relief to athletes from the rigors of the race. Another type of massage team began appearing at the sites of disasters. Specially trained emergency response massage teams coordinated with the Red Cross to provide the relief of massage to firefighters, emergency workers, and sometimes the victims in disaster locations such as floods, wildfires, or earthquakes. Team members set up massage tables or chairs in relief areas where emergency workers could take much needed breaks from the long, intense hours at the scene and enjoy a few minutes of caring, rejuvenating massage before heading back out to the front lines.

Seated massage, or **chair massage,** was a great innovation that helped demystify massage and make it more accessible to a wider audience. Chair massage, introduced in 1985 by David Palmer, is performed with the client clothed and seated on a special massage chair. This innovative massage application brought massage out of the studio and into the public arena. Massage no longer required a table, sheets, lubricants, or the removal of clothing. Suddenly, massage could be practiced in corporate offices, teacher's lounges, shopping malls, airports, health fairs, state legislatures, and on the street. Massage was less of a mystery, less threatening, safer. In the 1990s, corporate massage became more popular, and therapists started taking their massage chairs into offices, schools, hospitals, or other workplace settings to offer 15-minute massage breaks. Massage was coming out!

In the late 1980s, efforts to return massage and bodywork to the mainstream of health and wellness care prompted members from the various disciplines to come together and share ideas. In 1988, Robert Calvert, editor of *Massage Magazine,* created a forum called Head, Heart and Hands that had three gatherings, one in the center of the country, one on the East Coast, and one on the West Coast, in an attempt to discuss common issues and organize massage on a national level. In 1991, a Federation of Bodywork Organizations was formed to assure equitable recognition of the different forms of bodywork in the development of standards and legislation.

---

sports massage

is a method of massage designed to enhance an athlete's performance. It is achieved through specialized manipulations that stimulate circulation of the blood and lymph.

---

chair massage

takes place in a chair, which is a good choice for people not able to or not amenable to receive full-body massage on a table.

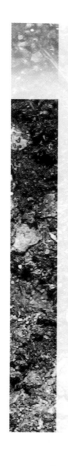

BOX 1.1 THE FEDERATION OF THERAPEUTIC MASSAGE, BODYWORK AND SOMATIC PRACTICE ORGANIZATIONS

In 1991, the Federation of Therapeutic Massage, Bodywork and Somatic Practice Organizations was formed to assure equitable recognition of all forms of bodywork in the formation of public wellness policy and practice. The Federation's vision is to promote networking, share expertise, and create programs that advance the fields of touch and movement, and to encourage coalitions in the development of appropriate legislation. Members of the federation include:

- American Massage Therapy Association® (AMTA)

- American Organization for Bodywork Therapies of Asia™ (AOBTA)

- American Polarity Therapy Association (APTA)

- American Society for the Alexander Technique (AmSAT)

- FELDENKRAIS GUILD® of North America (FGNA)

- ISMETA–International Somatic Movement Education and Therapy Association

- The Rolf Institute®

- United States Trager® Association

The trend toward massage regulation steadily progressed during the final quarter of the twentieth century. The majority of massage regulation during the 1950s through the 1970s were local ordinances initiated to control prostitution. Since the 1980s, most massage legislation has been practitioner based, focusing on educational standards, scope of practice, title protection, and protecting the public from harm. The American Massage Therapy Association in cooperation with individual state organizations actively pursued state legislatures to enact state licensing for massage therapists. In 1985, only 10 states regulated massage. By 2005, 36 states and the District of Columbia have state-wide massage licensing.

In 1988, the AMTA provided funding for the development of a National Certification for Massage Therapists. In 1990, the National Certification Board for Therapeutic Massage and Bodywork (NCBTMB) became an independent certifying entity, and the first exams were administered in 1992. The National Certification Exam (NCE) was originally designed to be a voluntary exam a practitioner could take to become recognized as being nationally certified in therapeutic massage and bodywork. Since its inception, however, several states that license massage adopted the NCE as part of their licensing requirements. As of the publication of this text, 28 of the 37 states requiring massage licensing use the successful completion of the National Certification Exam as a qualification for licensing. As a result, many massage schools design their curriculums guided by the requirements and content of the exam.

The recognition, acceptance, and growth of massage continued through the 1990s. Surveys by David Eisenberg in 1990 and 1997, published in the *New England Journal* and the *Journal of the American Medical Association* respectively, indicated that an increasing number of Americans were using complementary and alternative medicine (CAM) therapies and paying for it at a rate estimated at $27 billion in 1997, which exceeded the out-of-pocket expenditures for all U.S. hospitalizations. The same studies showed that massage was the third most common CAM modality used behind chiropractic and relaxation practices such as deep breathing and meditation.

Another phenomenon that was initiated in the 1990s and continues into the new century is the proliferation of massage research. Research, which is funded by various sources, validates the effects and benefits of massage and helps to legitimize massage in the eyes of the medical community and the public. Some of the leaders in promoting massage research include the Touch Research Institute, the Massage Therapy Foundation, and the National Institutes of Health, Center for Complementary and Alternative Medicine.

The Touch Research Institute (TRI) was founded in 1992 under the direction of Tiffany M. Fields in collaboration with the University of Miami Medical School expressly to study the effect of touch therapy on human well-being. Studies at TRI have shown that massage can induce weight gain in premature infants, alleviates depressive symptoms, reduces stress hormones, alleviates pain, and positively alters the immune system in children and adults with various medical conditions.

The AMTA Foundation was formed in 1990 as an independently governed public charity to advance the knowledge and practice of massage by supporting scientific research, education, and community service. The foundation accepts and solicits donations, then grants funds for research, community service, and educational scholarships. The foundation also provides direct consultation to the medical and research community and educates massage therapists about research methods. As of September 2004, the AMTA Foundation was renamed The Massage Therapy Foundation.

In 1998, the National Institutes of Health (NIH) established the National Center for Complementary and Alternative Medicine (NCCAM) (http://nccam.nih.gov). The NIH started providing grants for research of complementary medicine modalities to verify the effectiveness of their use. Massage research also continues to advance through other funding sources.

With the continuing research, the growing number of states requiring massage licensing, and the development of more sophisticated educational standards, massage continues to emerge as a recognized and respected allied health profession.

MASSAGE SYSTEMS

The methods of massage generally in use today descend directly from the Swedish, German, French, English, Chinese, and Japanese systems.

1. The Swedish system is based on the Western concepts of anatomy and physiology and employs the traditional manipulative techniques of effleurage, petrissage, vibration, friction, and tapotement. The Swedish system also employs movements that can be slow and gentle, vigorous or bracing, according to the results the practitioner wishes to achieve.

2. The German method combines many of the Swedish movements and emphasizes the use of various kinds of therapeutic baths.

3. The French and English systems also employ many of the Swedish massage movements for body massage.

4. Acupressure stems from the Chinese medical practice of acupuncture. It is based on the Traditional Oriental Medical principles for assessing and treating the physical and energetic body and employs various methods of stimulating acupuncture points in order to regulate *chi* (the life force energy). The aim of this method is to achieve therapeutic changes in the person being treated as well as relieve pain, discomfort, or other physiological imbalance.

5. The Japanese system, called *shiatsu,* a finger pressure method, is based on the Oriental concept that the body has a series of energy (*tsubo*) points. When pressure is properly applied to these points, circulation is improved and nerves are stimulated. This system is said to improve body metabolism and to relieve a number of physical disorders.

The following are additional systems that have gained recognition as beneficial forms of massage.

Sports massage refers to a method of massage especially designed to prepare an athlete for an upcoming event and to aid in the body's regenerative and restorative capacities following a rigorous workout or competition. This is achieved through specialized manipulations that stimulate circulation of the blood and lymph. Some sports massage movements are designed to break down lesions and adhesions or reduce fatigue. Sports massage generally follows the Swedish system, with variations of movements applied according to the judgment of the practitioner and the results he wants to achieve. Sports teams, especially those in professional baseball, football, basketball, hockey, ice skating, and swimming, often retain a professionally trained massage practitioner. Athletes, dancers, and others who must keep muscles strong and supple are often instructed in automassage (how to massage one's own muscles) and in basic massage on a partner.

Polarity therapy is a method developed by Randolph Stone (1890–1971) using massage manipulations derived from both Eastern and Western practices. Exercises and thinking practices are included to balance the body both physically and energetically.

The *Trager method* was developed by Dr. Milton Trager. This method uses movement exercises called *mentastics* along with massage-like, gentle shaking of different parts of the body to eliminate and prevent pent-up tensions.

> **polarity therapy**
> uses massage manipulations derived from Eastern and Western practices.

rolfing

aligns the major body segments through manipulation of the fascia or the connective tissue.

reflexology

stimulates particular points on the surface of the body, which in turn affects other areas or organs of the body.

Touch for Health

is a simplified form of applied kinesiology that involves techniques from both Eastern and Western origins.

neuromuscular techniques

a group of techniques that assess and address soft tissue dysfunction by affecting the neurological mechanisms that control the muscle.

craniosacral therapy

is a gentle, hands-on method of evaluating and enhancing the functioning of the craniosacral system.

Rolfing® is a systematic program developed out of the technique of structural integration by Dr. Ida Rolf. Rolfing aligns the major body segments through manipulation of the fascia (**FAH**-shuh) or the connective tissue.

The method of **reflexology** originated with the Chinese and is based on the idea that stimulation of particular points on the surface of the body has an effect on other areas or organs of the body. Dr. William Fitzgerald is credited with first demonstrating the effects of reflexology in the early 1900s. Eunice Ingham worked for Dr. Fitzgerald, and later, in the 1930s, she systemized the technique (popular today) that focuses mainly on the hands and feet.

Touch for Health is a simplified form of applied kinesiology (ki-nee-see-**AHL**-o-jee) (principles of anatomy in relation to human movement) developed by Dr. John Thie, D.C. This method involves techniques from both Eastern and Western origins. Its purpose is to relieve stress on muscles and internal organs. There are also a number of styles of bodywork and alternative health-related practices that utilize specialized kinesiology (a form of muscle testing) to derive information about the conditions of the body or how a particular substance or type of treatment might affect it.

Neuromuscular techniques originated in Europe around 1940 with the work of osteopaths Dr. Stanley Lief and Boris Chaitow. Western approaches have been developed or advanced by Paul St. John, Bonnie Prudden, Janet Travell, Lawrence Jones, Judith DeLany, and Dr. Leon Chaitow among others. Varieties include Neuromuscular Therapy, Myotherapy, Trigger Point Therapy, Muscle Energy Technique, Orthobionomy, and Strain/Counterstrain among others. Neuromuscular techniques utilize manipulations common to Swedish massage to systematically activate or sedate neuroreceptors usually located in contractile tissue. Reflex activity tends to normalize contractile tissue and brings the body more toward balance.

Craniosacral therapy has been developed by Dr. John Upledger and researchers at the Upledger Institute in Palm Beach Gardens, Florida. Craniosacral therapy is a gentle, hands-on method of evaluating and enhancing the functioning of a physiological body system called the craniosacral system. During craniosacral therapy, trained practitioners use a light touch, equivalent to a nickel's weight, to feel the rhythmic motion theoretically created by the movement of the cerebrospinal fluid within the craniosacral system. Craniosacral therapy treatment techniques are noninvasive, usually indirect approaches, intended to resolve restrictive barriers and restore symmetrical, smooth craniosacral motion. Craniosacral therapy is effective for a wide range of physiological conditions associated with pain and dysfunction and is used as a preventive health practice because of its ability to improve the function of the central nervous system and bolster the body's resistance to disease.

The foregoing is a brief list and does not include the great number and forms of massage and bodywork being practiced today. Although there are many excellent massage methods, the Swedish system is still the most widely used and is incorporated into many other procedures. Whatever method the practitioner prefers, it is essential to have a thorough knowledge of all technical movements and their effects on the various body systems. It is important for practitioners to be thoroughly trained in anatomy, physiology, pathology, medical communication, and technique in schools that are licensed or have credentials meeting the professional standards required by state boards and ethical associations. The objectives of all professional practitioners are generally the same: to provide a service that enhances the client's physical health and sense of well-being.

(For a more concise history of massage, the author recommends *The Bodywork Knowledgebase, Lectures on History of Massage* by Richard P. van Why, from which a good portion of this chapter was adapted.)

QUESTIONS FOR DISCUSSION AND REVIEW

1. Define *massage*.

2. How do we know that ancient civilizations used therapeutic massage and exercise in their social, personal, or religious practices?

3. Why is massage said to be the most natural and instinctive means of relieving pain and discomfort?

4. What did the Chinese call their early massage system?

5. Why did the Greeks and Romans place so much emphasis on exercise and massage?

6. Which Greek physician became known as the father of medicine?

7. Why were the Middle Ages also called the Dark Ages?

8. How did the Arabic Empire and the rise of Islam help preserve the practice of massage?

9. Why was the Renaissance an important turning point for the arts and sciences?

10. How did the invention of the printing press in the fifteenth century help further the practice of massage and therapeutic exercise?

11. What is the basis of Per Henrik Ling's Swedish Movement Cure?

12. Who introduced the Swedish Movement Cure to the United States?

13. What are some of the reasons for the decline of massage at the turn of the twentieth century?

14. Why did the acceptance of massage and therapeutic exercise increase during World Wars I and II?

15. Why did manual massage become a secondary treatment following World War II?

16. How has more awareness of health and personal wellness in recent years caused a renewed interest in massage?

17. What is the difference between passive and active exercise?

18. Describe the theory on which the Japanese shiatsu system of massage is based.

19. What part does proper exercise and use of massage play in athletics?

20. Of what benefit is the history of therapeutic massage to the student who wishes to pursue a career in the field?

21. Which massage system is the most widely used in general massage?

22. In what way are the Chinese and Japanese systems similar?

23. Why is massage used as a treatment in sports or athletic medicine?

Requirements for the Practice of Therapeutic Massage

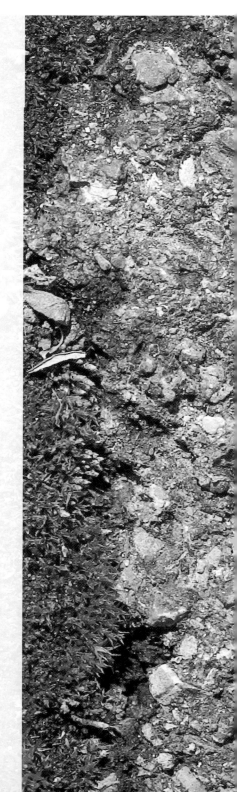

LEARNING OBJECTIVES

After you have mastered this chapter, you will be able to:

1. Explain the educational and legal aspects of scope of practice.
2. Explain how state legislation defines the scope of practice of therapeutic massage.
3. Explain why the massage practitioner must be aware of the laws, rules, regulations, restrictions, and obligations governing the practice of therapeutic massage.
4. Explain why it is necessary to obtain a license to practice therapeutic body massage.
5. Explain the difference between certifications and licenses.
6. Give reasons why a license to practice massage might be revoked, canceled, or suspended.

INTRODUCTION

Therapeutic massage is a personal health service employing various soft tissue manipulations for the improvement of the client's health and well-being; therefore, the massage practitioner has an ethical responsibility to the public and to individual clients. In addition to being technically well trained, the practitioner must understand the laws, rules, regulations, limitations, and obligations concerning the practice of massage.

SCOPE OF PRACTICE

In the world of health care, practitioners are able to perform certain duties as prescribed by their occupation, their license, and their level of training. For instance, in a health care facility, a nurse's aide can attend to a patient's comfort and care, but cannot distribute medications. In some instances, a licensed practical nurse may be able to distribute specified medications except for narcotics, injections, and IVs. A registered nurse must oversee these distributions and handle the dangerous drugs and injections. The orders for any of these must come from a physician. According to law, only doctors can diagnose illness and other medical

scope of practice
defines the rights and activities legally acceptable according to the licenses of a particular occupation or profession.

conditions and prescribe the medications and course of treatment for those conditions. Each of these practitioners is operating within his or her scope of practice.

Scope of practice defines the rights and activities legally acceptable according to the licenses of a particular occupation or profession. The scope of practice of any licensed occupation is described in the legal description and definitions contained in the licensing regulation. The scope is determined in part by the educational focus of the professional training. An individual's scope of practice is directly related to the skills she has gained and the training she has received. Massage and bodywork encompass a wide range of styles and techniques. Each professional chooses particular specialties or interests within the broader profession and directs her training and practice toward those specialties. An individual's scope of practice is also influenced by personal limitations such as belief systems, personal bias, choice of preferred clientele, and physical stature or endurance. By honoring personal scope of practice and respecting other professionals' scope of practice, the professional better serves the client by providing quality service in what she does best and referring the client to other professionals when appropriate.

Many occupations and professions have national or state regulatory boards that help define and enforce adherence to a scope of practice. National or state boards develop and upgrade professional standards and oversee testing and licensing procedures.

At the time of publication of this text, 37 of the 50 states in the United States and the District of Columbia have adopted licensing regulations governing the practice of massage. The definition of massage and the educational requirements contained in those regulations define the scope of practice of massage in those states. (See Box 2.1.) Whereas there is some basic agreement between those states regarding the need to license massage, there is a vast diversity in defining the purpose, object, procedure, or educational requirements. With more than two thirds of the states requiring licenses for massage, there is not a clearly defined scope of practice for massage therapy. Regardless of this fact, it is important for massage practitioners to recognize and practice within their legal and professional boundaries and refer clients to appropriately trained and licensed professionals when indicated.

BOX 2.1 LEGISLATIVE DEFINITIONS OF MASSAGE THERAPY

This box contains the portions of legislative documents from selected states that license massage and define "massage therapy." The educational requirements for licensing and continuing education requirements for license renewal are also listed. These states were selected to show the diversity of definition of massage therapy and the requirements to practice. Become familiar with the laws of the state where you choose to practice.

Arizona

Educational requirement:	500 hours from an approved school
Continuing education requirement:	25 hours biennial

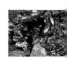

"Massage therapy" means the following that are undertaken to increase well-ness, relaxation, stress reduction, pain relief and postural improvement or provide general or specific therapeutic benefits:

(a) The manual application of compression, stretch, vibration or mobilization of the organs and tissues beneath the dermis, including the components of the musculoskeletal system, peripheral vessels of the circulatory system and fascia, when applied primarily to parts of the body other than the hands, feet and head.

(b) The manual application of compression, stretch, vibration or mobilization using the forearms, elbows, knees or feet or handheld mechanical or electrical devices.

(c) Any combination of range of motion, directed, assisted or passive movements of the joints.

(d) Hydrotherapy, including the therapeutic applications of water, heat, cold, wraps, essential oils, skin brushing, salt glows and similar applications of products to the skin.

"Practice of massage therapy" means the application of massage therapy to any person for a fee or other consideration. Practice of massage therapy does not include the diagnosis of illness or disease, medical procedures, naturopathic manipulative medicine, osteopathic manipulative medicine, chiropractic adjustive procedures, homeopathic neuromuscular integration, electrical stimulation, ultrasound, prescription of medicines or the use of modalities for which a license to practice medicine, chiropractic, nursing, physical therapy, acupuncture or podiatry is required by law.

Iowa

Educational requirement: 500 hours from an accredited school

Continuing education requirement: 12 hours biennial

"Massage therapist" means a person licensed to practice the health care service of the healing art of massage therapy under this chapter.

"Massage therapy" means performance for compensation of massage, myotherapy, massotherapy, bodywork, bodywork therapy, or therapeutic massage including hydrotherapy, superficial hot and cold applications, vibration and topical applications, or other therapy which involves manipulation of the muscle and connective tissue of the body, excluding osseous tissue, to treat the muscle tonus system for the purpose of enhancing health, muscle relaxation, increasing range of motion, reducing stress, relieving pain, or improving circulation. "Massage therapy" does not include diagnosis or service which requires a license to practice medicine or surgery, osteopathic medicine and surgery, osteopathy, chiropractic, cosmetology arts and sciences, or podiatry, and does not include service performed by athletic trainers, technicians, nurses, occupational therapists, or physical therapists who act under a professional license, certificate, or registration or under the prescription or supervision of a person licensed to practice medicine or surgery or osteopathic medicine and surgery.

continues

Maine

Educational requirement: 500 hours from an accredited school

Continuing education requirement: None

"Massage therapist" or "massage practitioner" means a person who provides or offers to provide massage therapy for a fee, monetary or otherwise.

"Massage therapy" means a scientific or skillful manipulation of soft tissue for therapeutic or remedial purposes, specifically for improving muscle tone and circulation and promoting health and physical well-being. The term includes, but is not limited to, manual and mechanical procedures for the purpose of treating soft tissue only, the use of supplementary aids such as rubbing alcohol, liniments, oils, antiseptics, powders, herbal preparations, creams or lotions, procedures such as oil rubs, salt glows and hot or cold packs or other similar procedures or preparations commonly used in this practice. This term specifically excludes manipulation of the spine or articulations and excludes sexual contact of any kind.

New Mexico

Educational requirement: 650 hours

Continuing education requirement: 16 hours biennial

"Massage Therapy" means the assessment and treatment of soft tissues and their dysfunctions for therapeutic purposes as defined in the Massage Therapy Practice Act, NMSA 1978, Section 61-12C-3.E.

(1) The treatment of soft tissues is the repetitive deformation of soft issues from more than one anatomical point by manual or mechanical means to accomplish homeostasis and/or pain relief in the tissues being deformed;

    (a) "soft tissue" includes skin, adipose, muscle and myofascial tissues;

    (b) "manual" means by use of hands or body;

    (c) "mechanical" means any tool or device that mimics or enhances the actions possible by the hands; and

    (d) "deformation" specifically prohibits the use of high velocity thrust techniques used in joint manipulations.

(2) The practice of Massage Therapy applies to Shiatsu, Tui Na, and Rolfing.

(3) The practice of Massage Therapy **does not** apply to the practice of: Craniosacral, Feldenkrais, Polarity Therapy, Reiki, Foot and Hand Reflexology (without the use of creams, oils, or mechanical tools), and Trager.

Texas

Educational requirement: 300 hours from state approved school

Continuing education requirement: 6 hours annually

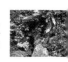

"Massage therapy" means the manipulation of soft tissue by hand or through a mechanical or electrical apparatus for the purpose of body massage and includes effleurage (stroking), petrissage (kneading), tapotement (percussion), compression, vibration, friction, nerve strokes, and Swedish gymnastics. The terms "massage," "therapeutic massage," "massage technology," "myotherapy," "body massage," "body rub," or any derivation of those terms are synonyms for "massage therapy."

Practices in massage therapy include the use of oil, salt glows, heat lamps, hot and cold packs, and tub, shower, or cabinet baths.

Massage therapy constitutes a health care service if the massage therapy is for therapeutic purposes. Massage therapy does not constitute the practice of chiropractic. The terms therapy and therapeutic when used in the context of massage therapy practice do not include (1) the diagnosis or treatment of illness or disease; or (2) a service or procedure for which a license to practice medicine, chiropractic, physical therapy, or podiatry is required by law.

Alabama

Educational requirement: 650 hours from an accredited massage school

Continuing education requirement: 16 hours biennial

"Massage Therapist" is a person licensed under this Act who practices massage therapy or touch modalities upon a patron of either gender for compensation, working to alleviate pain, reduce stress, and instigate the normalization of the soft tissue, muscles, tendons, ligaments, and connective tissue of the patron. A massage therapist shall not be designated as a "massage parlor" employee.

"Massage Therapy" is the profession in which the practitioner applies massage techniques and related touch therapy modalities with the intention of positively affecting the health and well being of the client as defined in the Act. Massage Therapy does not include diagnosis except to the extent of determining whether massage therapy is indicated. Massage Therapy may be applied in response to physician, osteopathic, chiropractic, podiatric, or other prescription by a licensed practitioner in that field acting within the scope of his or her profession.

The definitions above were attained from the Internet Web site of the various states. Those sites as of November 2004 are:

Arizona—http://MassageTherapy.AZ.Gov

Iowa—http://www.idph.state.ia.us

Maine—http://www.state.me.us

New Mexico—http://www.rld.state.nm.us

Texas—http://www.tdh.state.tx.us

Alabama—http://www.almtbd.state.al.us

LICENSES: THEY ARE THE LAW

In the United States, laws and regulations for massage may fall under the auspices of the state, the county, the municipality, or may not exist at all. Where massage laws are in effect, massage practitioners must register with the proper authorities and satisfy certain requirements to obtain a license to practice. These requirements may vary depending on the licensing agency and the original motives for instituting the legislation. Many municipalities adopt ordinances to curb unethical practices, misleading advertising, and the use of the term *massage* to conceal questionable or illegal activities, especially prostitution and illicit drug sales and distribution. This type of licensing often requires mug shots, fingerprinting, and criminal record searches and has little regard for massage proficiency. As massage becomes more recognized as a reputable and respected health care practice, most of these ordinances are being replaced with licensing laws that contain educational, technical, ethical, and sanitation requirements.

Laws and regulations vary greatly from state to state and city to city. Being licensed in one state does not guarantee that the same license will be valid or recognized in another state. If your license is from a city, it is almost guaranteed that the only place that license is valid is in the city where the license was issued. A practitioner who has a license and wishes to practice in another city or state should contact the proper agency in the area where she wishes to practice. Usually the county commissioner's office, the city attorney, city clerk, or the mayor's office will be able to provide information concerning massage regulations. If there is reciprocity between the two licensing agencies, the valid license will be honored; if not, the practitioner should provide proof of ability to meet any requirements and make applications as required.

In the United States, a growing number of states are adopting legislation that requires all massage practitioners to obtain and maintain a license. These state laws usually take precedence over city and county laws and are professional licenses wherein the applicant must satisfy an educational requirement as well as pass a written and practical examination and pay certain fees before being issued a license to practice massage. As of the latest publication of this text, in the United States 36 states and the District of Columbia license massage therapists. Each of these states has an agency or board that oversees the licensing process. Of the 37 regulated states (which includes the District of Columbia), 28 have adopted the National Certification Exam for Therapeutic Massage and Bodywork as a requirement for licensing.

Licensed physical therapists, physicians, registered nurses, osteopaths, chiropractors, athletic trainers, and podiatrists may practice massage as part of their therapeutic treatments. However, these professionals usually obtain a license specifically for the practice of massage when they wish to be known as massage practitioners.

Massage establishments must abide by local laws, rules, and regulations. Where it is required, they must be licensed and employ only

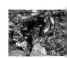

licensed practitioners. In addition to massage ordinances and licenses, local business and zoning laws must be followed when setting up a massage business. Most states require massage practitioners to display their licenses at their place of business.

EDUCATIONAL REQUIREMENTS

Educational requirements to enroll in a program of instruction at a certificate-granting school or institute of massage may differ, but generally a high school diploma or equivalency diploma is required. In some states that have massage licensing, a student actively enrolled in a qualified school of massage may work as an apprentice under the supervision of a licensed massage practitioner.

The educational requirements to practice massage or bodywork vary depending on the discipline or techniques and the licensing requirements of the city or state where the practice is located. There are many disciplines or styles of hands-on therapies being practiced. Few of these have clearly defined educational requirements. Professional organizations affiliated with these various disciplines often set educational guidelines that include the length and content of training programs and recognize schools that comply with those guidelines. The American Massage Therapy Association Council of Schools, for example, requires member schools to have a curriculum of at least 500 in-class hours, whereas the Commission for Massage Training Accreditation (COMTA) requires that schools have a minimum of 600 classroom hours of training before they will be considered for accreditation. Required subjects include:

- Anatomy, physiology, and pathology of the human body
- Knowledge of the effects of massage and bodywork techniques
- Indications, contraindications, and precautions for massage
- Application of massage therapy including assessment, planning, and performance
- Development of successful therapeutic relationships with clients

If a license is required to practice massage, an educational requirement is usually included in the licensing legislation. Without a national standard for massage therapy, educational requirements contained in licensing laws vary widely. City or municipal licenses may contain no educational requirement or may require as much as 1,000 hours of training. Of the states that license massage at the time of publication of this text, the educational requirements vary from 300 to 1,000 hours of training; some Canadian provinces require as many as 2,200 hours of schooling.

The National Certification for Therapeutic Massage and Bodywork recommends a minimum standard educational requirement, which has been established as the equivalent of 500 hours of training including the subjects of anatomy, physiology, pathology, business practices, massage technique, and ethics.

HEALTH REQUIREMENTS FOR PRACTITIONERS

Since massage is a touch or hands-on profession, the massage practitioner is expected to be physically and mentally fit and be free of any communicable diseases. Some state licensing requirements or employers may request a health certificate or written confirmation from a physician. It is the practitioner's duty to keep himself in top physical condition. Massage is hard work and requires that the practitioner have physical stamina and the ability to concentrate on giving a therapeutic massage.

REASONS LICENSE MAY BE REVOKED, SUSPENDED, OR CANCELED

Because the practice of massage deals with the health and welfare of the public and specifically that of individual clients, the profession must be regulated by the issuance of licenses only to people who have met the requirements to practice. The professional massage practitioner must have integrity, the necessary technical skills, and a willingness to comply with rigid health standards.

The following are grounds on which the practitioner's license may be revoked, canceled, or suspended:

1. Being guilty of fraud or deceit in obtaining a license
2. Having been convicted of a felony
3. Being engaged currently or previously in any act of prostitution
4. Practicing under a false or assumed name
5. Being addicted to narcotics, alcohol, or like substances that interfere with the performance of duties
6. Being willfully negligent in the practice of massage so as to endanger the health of a client
7. Prescribing drugs or medicines (unless you are a licensed physician)
8. Being guilty of fraudulent or deceptive advertising
9. Ethical or sexual misconduct with a client

CERTIFICATION VERSUS LICENSE

A license is issued from a state or municipal regulating agency as a requirement for conducting a business or practicing a trade or profession. A certification, on the other hand, is a document that is awarded in recognition of an accomplishment or achieving or maintaining some kind of

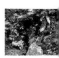

standard. A certification may be given for successfully completing a course of study or passing an examination showing a level of proficiency or ability. Certificates are awarded by schools and institutions to show the successful completion of a course of study. Professional organizations have certificates of membership to indicate that the recipient has met the qualifications to become a member. Often those organizations have testing programs that provide recognition of achievements in their chosen professions. Many professions (the massage profession included) have a national certification program whereby proficiency toward a national standard can be achieved and certified. Since 1992, the National Certification Board for Therapeutic Massage and Bodywork (NCBTMB) has administered the National Certification Exam for Therapeutic Massage and Bodywork (NCETMB). Participation in national certification is voluntary; however, several states that license massage require successful completion of the National Certification Exam to be licensed. Successful completion of the National Certification Exam earns the testee the designation of being nationally certified in therapeutic massage and bodywork. In 2005 the National Certification Board added another credentialing exam, the National Certification Exam for Therapeutic Massage (NCETM), which focuses on classic Western massage without the Asian bodywork component. These certifications do lend an air of credibility to a practitioner but do not take the place of a license where a license is required to practice.

QUESTIONS FOR DISCUSSION AND REVIEW

1. Why must the massage practitioner be concerned about the laws, rules, regulations, and obligations pertaining to the practice of therapeutic body massage?

2. What are the legal and educational aspects of scope of practice?

3. Why do laws governing the practice of massage often differ from one state to another?

4. Does having a license in one locale permit a practitioner to practice anywhere? Why?

5. What is the general educational requirement for a license to practice massage?

6. What are the reasons a person would receive a certificate?

7. What are the specific grounds on which a practitioner's license may be revoked, canceled, or suspended?

Professional Ethics for Massage Practitioners

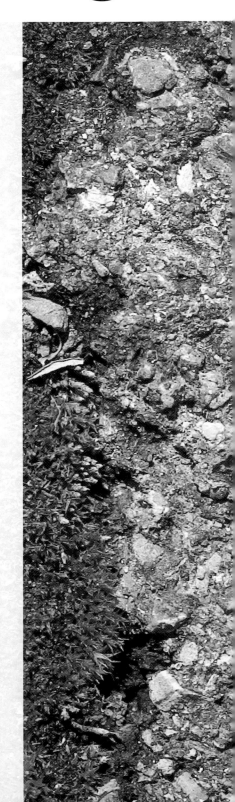

LEARNING OBJECTIVES

After you have mastered this chapter, you will be able to:

1. Define the meaning of professional ethics.

2. Explain how the practice of good ethics helps build a successful massage practice.

3. Differentiate between personal and professional boundaries.

4. Designate at least eight areas to consider when establishing professional boundaries.

5. Define a therapeutic relationship and a client-centered relationship.

6. Explain the effects of a power differential in the therapeutic relationship.

7. Explain the effects of transference, countertransference, and dual relationships in the therapeutic setting.

8. Discuss why sexual arousal may occur during a massage session and what to do if it does.

9. Discuss why and how to desexualize the massage experience.

10. Define supervision and its importance to the massage professional.

11. Discuss the importance of good health habits and professional projection.

12. Discuss the importance of human relations and success attitudes.

13. Discuss ways to build a sound business reputation.

INTRODUCTION

When massage therapy students complete the initial course of study and graduate from massage school, they enter the profession of massage. They become professionals. Being a professional is more than simply having a job. A professional has completed a course of study to gain knowledge in a specific field of practice, usually to provide a service. A profession is usually regulated, is represented by a professional association, and adheres to a **code of ethics**.

code of ethics

a set of guiding moral principles that governs a person's choice of action.

boundaries

are personal comfort zones that help an individual maintain a sense of comfort and safety. They can be professional, personal, physical, emotional, intellectual, and sexual.

Professionalism in massage not only encompasses the application of massage technique to a client but also involves clear communication, managing boundaries, and ethical business practices. Professional standards include educational requirements, scope of practice, state and local regulations, codes of ethics, and standards of practice.

Massage professionals engage in therapeutic relationships with their clients. A healthy therapeutic relationship requires an understanding and respect for personal and professional **boundaries.** Personal boundaries provide protection and a sense of self. Each person's set of boundaries is unique depending on her life experiences. Professional boundaries are the foundation of an ethical practice. Honoring personal boundaries and maintaining professional boundaries ensure that the therapeutic relationship will benefit the client and avoid ethical dilemmas.

Ethics is the study of the standards and philosophy of human conduct and is defined as a system or code of morals of an individual, a group, or a profession. To practice good ethics is to be concerned about the public welfare, the welfare of individual clients, your reputation, and the reputation of the profession you represent. Ethics are moral guidelines that are established by experienced professionals to reduce the incidence and risk of harm or injury in the professional relationship due to abuse of a position of power. A professional person is one who is engaged in an avocation or occupation requiring some advanced training to gain knowledge and skills. However, without ethics there can be no true professionalism.

Ethical conduct on the part of the practitioner gives the client confidence in the place of business, the services rendered, and the entire industry. A satisfied client is your best means of advertising because his good recommendation helps you maintain public confidence and build a sound business following. The business establishment that becomes known for its professional ethics will stay in business longer than one that makes extravagant claims and false promises or that is involved in questionable practices. (See Box 3.1 for two examples of ethics codes.)

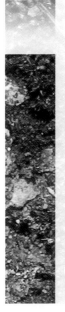

BOX 3.1 CODES OF ETHICS

Codes of ethics are adopted by professions, professional organizations, and sometimes by state regulatory agencies. This box presents the Code of Ethics of the American Massage Therapy Association and the Louisiana State Massage Therapy Board.

AMTA Code of Ethics

This Code of Ethics is a summary statement of the standards by which massage therapists agree to conduct their practices and is a declaration of the general principles of acceptable, ethical, professional behavior.

Massage therapists shall:

1. Demonstrate commitment to provide the highest quality massage therapy/bodywork to those who seek their professional service.

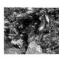

2. Acknowledge the inherent worth and individuality of each person by not discriminating or behaving in any prejudicial manner with clients and/or colleagues.

3. Demonstrate professional excellence through regular self-assessment of strengths, limitations, and effectiveness by continued education and training.

4. Acknowledge the confidential nature of the professional relationship with clients and respect each client's right to privacy.

5. Conduct all business and professional activities within their scope of practice, the law of the land, and project a professional image.

6. Refrain from engaging in any sexual conduct or sexual activities involving their clients.

7. Accept responsibility to do no harm to the physical, mental, and emotional well-being of self, clients, and associates.

State of Louisiana Massage Board Code of Ethics

A licensed massage therapist will:

1. Represent their qualifications honestly, including education and professional affiliations, and provide only those services which they are qualified to perform.

2. Accurately inform clients, other health care practitioners, and the public of the scope and limitations of their discipline.

3. Acknowledge the limitations of and contraindications for massage and bodywork and refer clients to appropriate health professionals.

4. Provide therapy only where there is reasonable expectation that it will be advantageous to the clients.

5. Consistently maintain and improve professional knowledge and competence, striving for professional excellence through regular assessment of personal and professional strengths and weaknesses and through continued education training.

6. Conduct their business and professional activities with honesty and integrity, and respect the inherent worth of all persons.

7. Refuse to unjustly discriminate against clients or other ethical health professionals.

8. Safeguard the confidentiality of all client information, unless disclosure is required by law, court order, or absolutely necessary for the protection of the public.

9. Respect the client's right to therapy with informed and voluntary consent.

10. Respect the client's right to refuse, modify, or terminate therapy regardless of prior consent given.

11. Exercise the right to refuse to treat any person or part of the body for just and reasonable cause.

12. Refrain, under all circumstances, from initiating or engaging in any romantic or sexual conduct, sexual activities, or sexualizing behavior involving a client, even if the client attempts to sexualize the relationship.

13. Respect the client's boundaries with regard to privacy, disclosure, exposure, emotional expression, beliefs, and the client's reasonable expectations of professional behavior. Practitioners will respect the clients' autonomy.

BOUNDARIES

Any discussion of ethical professional practices must include an understanding of boundaries, both personal and professional. Boundaries delineate personal comfort zones, the realm in which we operate with a sense of safety and control. Boundaries also help screen input to what is appropriate for our personal comfort. Everyone has boundaries that dictate how they act and interact with the world and other people.

Boundaries are individual, personal, and usually intangible. There are many kinds of boundaries that we establish and maintain in order to keep a sense of comfort and safety. Some of those boundaries may be classified as physical, emotional, intellectual, and sexual. They act as personal protection. A boundary is like a safety net or force field that surrounds every person. Boundaries are contextual depending on circumstances and relationships. The field shifts depending on the situation.

Personal boundaries help define who we are emotionally, intellectually, spiritually. They help determine how and with whom we choose to share our lives and beliefs. Boundaries are defined by our experiences, beliefs, and expectations. They separate us as individuals and provide a framework to safely function in the world. People with a good sense of boundaries are able to claim their own space, embrace their own emotions, be spontaneous, intake information easily, make clear decisions, and be responsive and sensitive to the needs of others.

Some determining factors in the formation of personal boundaries include family, school, or religious upbringing. Cultural and ethnic influences also shape our attitude about relationships, privacy, and touch. Boundaries are flexible, permeable, and constantly changing according to new information. Though many boundaries are established early in our lives, relationships, both good and bad, continue to influence our boundaries and comfort zones in the way we relate to others.

Personal boundaries vary widely between individuals. Relationships involve the interaction between the boundaries of individuals. Often, one person in the relationship will give in to the other's wishes or needs, thereby shifting the boundaries. People with whom we interact have different boundaries, so we must be sensitive and able to respond with understanding. In some situations we must hold strong boundaries, and at other appropriate times we must be flexible to merge or expand our experience. Dependent on the level of trust or control exhibited in the relationship, many minor boundary fluctuations occur with little negative impact. When a boundary is severely invaded or violated, this may constitute a situation of neglect or even abuse. Even in the case of minor boundary infractions, there will be a sense of discomfort or confusion.

When we move outside of our own boundaries or push beyond another's, we find ourselves in dangerous territory that may easily lead to disappointment, questionable behavior, emotional turmoil, or abuse.

Professional Boundaries

Professional boundaries are predetermined practices that protect the safety of the client and the therapist. An important aspect of a professional practice is to recognize, respect, and honor the client's personal boundaries. A new client of massage is asked to stretch his personal boundaries in several ways. He enters a facility that is unfamiliar. He discloses personal information relative to his physical condition to a practitioner whom he does not know. He disrobes and lies down on a table under a sheet. He lies on the table, rather passively, while the practitioner applies touch and manipulations that sometimes approach levels of discomfort. In each of these activities, the client may move beyond his normal comfort boundary. What allows him to do this is trust that the massage practitioner will maintain certain professional boundaries.

Professional boundaries are preliminarily outlined in policy and procedure statements that are presented to the client very early in the therapeutic relationship. These boundaries create a stable framework and a safe environment from which to practice.

Cherie Sohnen-Moe and Ben Benjamin, in their exceptional book *The Ethics of Touch,* list eight major areas to consider in establishing professional boundaries: location of service, interpersonal space, appearance, self-disclosure, language, touch, time, and money.

Location

The location refers to the therapeutic setting where the massage takes place that is professional, safe, and comfortable. Therapeutic massage can be performed in a wide variety of settings ranging from a medical office, to a cabana on the beach, to an outdoor tent at a marathon, to a client's home, to a cruise ship or a home office. Seated massage may happen just about anywhere a massage chair can be set up. Regardless of the setting, consideration must be taken to assure safety, comfort, and security for the client and a sense of professionalism from the practitioner that inspires confidence and respect.

Interpersonal Space

Interpersonal space refers to the actual space maintained between the client and practitioner during interactions before and after the actual massage. Creating an appropriate space means maintaining a physical space between the client and practitioner that makes both parties comfortable. Height variation is also considered. Carry on conversations at eye level whenever possible. Sit or stand so neither party must look up or down when discussing topics relevant to the session. Try to complete most of the important conversation before the client lies down on the table. Discussions that take place when both persons are at the same height minimize the power differential.

Appearance

Appearance refers to the way the practitioner looks and dresses when providing or promoting massage. Professional appearance includes appropriate clothing and good personal hygiene. The goal is to foster a sense of comfort, trust, and safety in the client. Avoid clothing that is too casual, revealing, or sexually provocative, or that may focus attention on the practitioner instead of the client.

Self-disclosure

Seek and provide self-disclosure appropriate to the therapeutic relationship. During the presession interview, the client will disclose personal information at the request of the practitioner. The extent and depth of that information should only cover what is relevant to the conditions presented for treatment. Avoid probing for personal information that does not pertain to the session.

In an effort to impress or get closer to the therapist, the client may expound on personal and sensitive information. The client may be unclear as to his own or the therapist's boundaries and give information in an attempt to gain psychological support or to leverage the practitioner to somehow act on the client's behalf beyond the scope of the therapy session.

The practitioner must also be aware of appropriate self-disclosure practices. Pertinent information regarding training, experience, modalities practiced, treatment plan, appointment policies, and fees are necessary to gain informed consent and confidence from the client. Beyond this the practitioner must exercise caution that any personal information she chooses to share will somehow benefit the client and the therapeutic goals of the session. Some level of sharing personal experience may actually strengthen the therapeutic relationship, whereas certain personal information will tend to direct the focus toward the practitioner rather than the client. This should be discouraged and avoided.

Language

According to Sohnen-Moe and Benjamin, "language is one of the most potent means for creating and maintaining healthy boundaries" (p. 55). The choices of words, voice intonation, and overall skills as a communicator are vital aspects of creating effective boundaries.

Touch

Touch and how it is applied can create a feeling of comfort and safety or be threatening and uncomfortable. Touch is directly related to physical boundaries both on and off of the table. Be aware of appropriate touch when greeting and saying good-bye to a client. Is a hug called for, or a hand on the shoulder, or is a handshake more appropriate?

On the treatment table, touch boundaries include what parts of the practitioner's body touch the client, what parts of the client's body are and are not touched, as well as the depth and quality of touch. In the treatment setting, only the practitioner's hands, forearms, and elbows make contact with the client. Care is taken that other body parts do not inadvertently touch the client. Only areas of the client's body that are being therapeutically treated are included in the treatments. The genitals and anus are not included in a therapeutic massage treatment. Women's breasts are only included as a part of a massage when therapeutically indicated and only after obtaining written informed consent from the client before the massage begins. Therapeutic massage does not include any kind of sexually oriented touch.

Quality and depth of touch should be discussed before the session begins and included in the informed consent. Touch that is too light or too deep may cause discomfort, violate boundaries, and be inappropriate. Avoid inflicting excessive pain on a client. Some types of deep tissue work can be quite intense; however, when the pain threshold is crossed, trust is broken that is difficult or impossible to restore. Anytime any aspect of touch might go beyond or deviate from what was discussed for the original informed consent, clear and complete disclosure must be discussed with the client so that he can, once again, give informed consent. This greatly reduces the possibility of crossing boundaries.

Time

A defining aspect of a professional relationship is time. The client comes for a massage at an appointed time and expects a treatment that lasts a predetermined amount of time. The way a practitioner manages time sets clear boundaries. Beginning and finishing sessions on time honors professional and personal boundaries. Adequate time should be scheduled to accommodate a preliminary interview, assessments, undressing, dressing, closure, and so on. Schedule enough time between appointments to complete records, return phone calls, take a break, or accommodate an unexpected late or long appointment. The client can rely on the fact that he can come for, receive, and complete a massage within a certain time frame and can schedule his day around those activities. Establishing and maintaining policies regarding session length, late arrivals, no shows, and missed appointments define boundaries, letting clients know what to expect.

Money

In a therapeutic relationship, the practitioner provides a service that is of benefit in exchange for a set fee. The fee is predetermined and adds value to the client's experience. The amount of the fee is determined based on the service provided and should directly reflect the value of the service. When establishing a fee structure, the practitioner establishes boundaries, further defining a professional practice. Fees that are too low or exorbitantly high for the services rendered are professional boundary infractions. Charging different fees to different populations for the same service should be avoided or done with extreme scrutiny. Clients challenge boundaries by not bringing money or a check to pay for a session, by writing a check with insufficient funds, or by being late paying or not paying a bill.

Be aware of and honor a client's personal boundaries. Respect a client's comfort levels with respect to room temperature, level of dress or undress, amount of pressure used during the massage, parts of the body to omit or give extra attention. Early in the therapeutic relationship, the practitioner can help the client to become more aware and responsive to his own boundary issues and at the same time reduce the chance of inadvertently invading or violating those boundaries with a statement like: "At any time while we are together, if I ask, say, or do anything that causes any discomfort at all, please let me know what it is." This empowers the client and provides the opportunity to discuss and clarify the reason for whatever was the cause of the discomfort and adjust the session to better serve the needs of the client. When applying any technique that may be in any way intrusive, such as ischemic compression on a trigger point or approaching a sensitive area on the body, a similar statement informs and empowers the client with more control over his session.

Recognizing and honoring client's boundaries and maintaining clear professional boundaries are the cornerstones for building and maintaining an ethical professional practice.

THE THERAPEUTIC RELATIONSHIP

The therapeutic relationship is a practitioner/client relationship that is client centered, where all activities are to benefit and enhance the client's well-being and maintain or promote his welfare. Therapeutic relationships directly influence people's mental, emotional, and physical well-being. Inherent in the therapeutic relationship is an implicit contract between the therapist and the client. The client will come by appointment to a prearranged location, receive an agreed upon treatment, for a specified length of time, for an agreed upon fee. The client will expect to receive treatment to address certain conditions or otherwise enhance his state of wellness in accordance to the knowledge of the therapist dependent on the therapist's skills and education. It is the responsibility of the practitioner to provide an environment that is secure and safe. The client puts his trust in the practitioner that the practitioner will always act in the best interest of the client.

A client enters a therapeutic relationship expecting to gain from the skills of the practitioner. A central goal in developing a therapeutic relationship is to create a safe environment, a place where any client is secure enough to allow healing to occur; a place that is safe enough to be vulnerable, to be open, to release, to relax, be nonthreatened; a place of trust; a safe haven in which to unwind. The client assumes that he is safe from physical, emotional, or sexual impropriety.

Confidentiality in the practitioner/client relationship is the foundation of safety, protection, trust, and respect that provides an environment for the client to relax, open, release, transform, and heal. To uphold confidentiality, the practitioner keeps all personal information regarding any client, including the fact of being a client, private except with permission of the client or in certain circumstances required by law. The client should sign a release of medical information before the practitioner confers with other health care providers concerning the client. (This is discussed on pages 376 and 700.) There is a legal requirement that the practitioner report to authorities situations of imminent or life-threatening danger by or to a client or situations of child abuse. This is known as *the duty to warn and protect*. Clients must be informed about the limits of confidentiality near the beginning of the initial interview or assessment.

In a client-based relationship, a good litmus test to determine whether an activity or procedure is appropriate is to ask "To whose benefit is the questioned activity?" If the answer is not "the client's," the decision should be not to proceed.

In the therapeutic relationship, being sensitive to, respecting, and maintaining both personal and professional boundaries are critical to avoiding potential ethical dilemmas.

Power Differential

Throughout our lifetime, we experience many kinds of relationships. Relationships include those with friends, schoolmates, siblings, parent/child, romantic partner, spouse, employer/employee, and therapist/client. Each kind of relationship involves various levels of intimacy, commitment, and responsibility, and in each there is a balance or imbalance of power. In some relationships, such as friendships or romantic couplings, the balance of power is fairly even or shifts back and forth according to what is happening at any given moment. In relationships such as parent/child, teacher/student, or employer/employee there is an evident power differential where more authority is held by the person on one side of the relationship while the other person is in a more vulnerable or submissive role. With that power comes responsibility.

Practitioner/client relationships by their very nature exhibit a power differential. The client seeks out the services of the practitioner due to the practitioner's knowledge, skill, and authority. The practitioner is in a place of power to provide actions or services to enhance the well-being of the more vulnerable client. Due to the nature of the massage session, the practitioner stands over the client who is lying unclothed (although draped) on a massage table. The client literally looks up to and submits to the ministrations of the practitioner. The client is often passive while the practitioner actively uses her hands to manipulate the client's body. There is an inherent power differential favoring the practitioner where the client is in a more vulnerable position. Because of the power differential, the client may quietly succumb to the actions of the practitioner rather than articulate any discomfort. The client may feel that the practitioner is "all knowing" and therefore may not speak up when his needs are not being met or when the practitioner does or does not do something that crosses or violates the client's boundaries.

Due to the fact that we are human, it is inevitable that boundaries will be crossed or even violated. When subtle boundary crossings occur, they may be experienced as a feeling of discomfort or unease on the part of either party due to the action of usually the other, although a signal you may have crossed your own boundary can be a feeling of personal unease. These small discomforts should be noted and articulated. When the practitioner notices signs of discomfort such as withdrawal or fidgeting during the interview or grimacing during the session, she should encourage the client to articulate his feelings. The practitioner can help balance the power differential by discussing treatment options with the client and giving him a choice on how to proceed at the beginning of the session. Establishing a policy early in the therapeutic relationship that encourages the client to speak up anytime he feels discomfort of any kind during the course of treatment empowers the client to better direct his experience and reduces the likelihood of personal boundaries being severely crossed. Clear communication is the most effective tool to both prevent and clarify boundary issues.

In the therapeutic relationship, the practitioner holds the advantage in the power differential and therefore has the responsibility to establish and maintain a safe, healthy therapeutic environment where the client's well-being, safety, and comfort are the focus of all activities. It is the role of the practitioner to ensure that the power differential is not abused to the detriment of the client. The practitioner has the responsibility to be sensitive to, to respect, and to maintain both personal and professional boundaries, even if the client initiates the questionable activity.

Transference and Countertransference

When a client seeks the services of a professional, an authority figure, someone to whom he can defer judgment, he enters a relationship where he may respond as he may have done with other authority figures in his past. There may be an unconscious tendency for the client to project onto the practitioner attributes of someone from a former relationship. The client may seek more out of the relationship than is therapeutically appropriate. Psychotherapists have been aware of this type of phenomenon since the time of Freud. When a client tries to personalize the therapeutic relationship, it is known as **transference.** Transference involves misperceptions the client may have toward the practitioner or therapist. Those misperceptions may be positive or negative. Transference may surface in any relationship where there is a power differential. This occurs quite unconsciously. Transference tends to diminish the effectiveness of the therapeutic relationship.

The therapist should be aware of the signs of transference and take necessary measures to reduce its occurrence.

Transference usually happens at an unconscious level. Some signs of transference include the following:

- The client attempts to become more personally involved with the practitioner.
- The client asks personal questions not related to the reason for the visit.

transference

happens when a client personalizes, either negatively or positively, a therapeutic relationship by unconsciously projecting characteristics of someone from a former relationship onto a therapist or practitioner.

- The client may vie for extra time during or at the end of the session.
- The client may invite the practitioner to social activities, or try to get closer physically, socially, or emotionally.
- The client brings or offers gifts or favors.
- The client proposes friendships or sexual involvement.
- The client may become more demanding of the practitioner's time and attention or even become angry, disappointed, or rejected if the practitioner does not respond.
- The client may want to adore, befriend, and please the practitioner or berate and mistrust the practitioner.

All these are signs of transference. They are not necessarily about the practitioner, but are related to the power differential and the attempts of the client to personalize the therapeutic relationship.

Ultimately, it is the responsibility of the practitioner to maintain clear professional boundaries when transference occurs in order to uphold a healthy therapeutic relationship.

Countertransference

Occasionally, transference works in the other direction—the practitioner begins to personalize or take the relationship with the client personally. When the practitioner tends to personalize the relationship, it is known as **countertransference.** Countertransference involves misperceptions of the practitioner toward the client. It is usually unconscious and always detrimental to the therapeutic process.

Signs of countertransference include:

- Strong emotional feelings toward the client, either positive or negative.
- Thinking excessively about a client between sessions.
- Dressing in a special manner when a certain client is coming.
- Making special provisions or spending extra time with a client.
- Fantasizing or having sexual feelings toward a client.
- Yawning excessively during an appointment.
- Dreading an upcoming appointment with a client.
- Negative reactions to a client, such as
  - Feeling guilty, frustrated, or angry if a client does not respond to treatment.
  - Feeling anger or disappointment if a client is late or cancels.
  - Experiencing fatigue, disappointment, depression, or even infatuation after a session.

Any strong feelings toward a client may signal countertransference. Feelings range from love, sexual attraction, and a need to rescue to avoidance, aggravation, and anger.

Many times a client's transference, when not recognized, will spawn countertransference on the part of the unwitting practitioner.

> **counter-transference**
>
> happens when a therapist or practitioner personalizes a therapeutic relationship by unconsciously projecting characteristics of someone from a former relationship onto a client. This is almost always detrimental to a therapeutic relationship.

This is nearly always a recipe for disappointment and possible disaster for the practitioner.

Transference and countertransference are natural, unconscious phenomena that occur in therapeutic relationships where there is a power differential. If not recognized and effectively diffused, the result will negatively impact the relationship, possibly emotionally harming the client and potentially devastating the professional's practice.

Maintaining healthy professional boundaries is the best defense against transference and countertransference. When boundaries are stretched or when a professional is tempted to move beyond those boundaries, it is a warning sign to assess motivations and how one is operating as a professional and seek supervision.

In a relationship where there is a power differential, it is ultimately the responsibility of the person in the more powerful role to provide a safe, secure environment. Therefore, the practitioner is responsible to recognize and assure that transference and countertransference issues are not acted out in a manner that is in any way harmful to the client or the therapeutic relationship. In some circumstances, this may require discontinuing the relationship and referring the client to another practitioner.

Dual Relationships

The therapeutic relationship is a practitioner/client relationship that is client centered, which means every activity of the relationship is directed to the benefit of the client in exchange for the predetermined fee for service.

A dual relationship is any situation that combines the therapeutic relationship with a secondary relationship that extends beyond the massage practitioner/client relationship. There is a broad spectrum of dual relationships. Dual relationships usually involve various dynamics that have complicated tendencies that affect both sides of the relationship. There is increased potential that evolving circumstances in one relationship will negatively affect the other. The numerous risks of dual relationships are generally not favorable to a healthy therapeutic relationship. Dual or multiple relationships are preferably avoided.

Awareness of dual relationships and potential pitfalls originated in the field of psychology where strong standards now exist that discourage or even prohibit dual relationships. Numerous cases of sexual impropriety stemming from dual relationships between therapists and clients in the 1960s and 1970s were documented, prompting authorities and regulators in the mental health professions to establish regulations that dissuade practitioners and therapists from engaging in dual relationships with their patients.

Dual relationships may arise when someone the practitioner knows becomes a client, such as a family member, a friend, a work associate, or someone from the practitioner's club, organization, or church. This is especially common for students who are eager for bodies to practice on or for new practitioners in the beginning stages of building their practices.

In smaller communities, the chance of a client and practitioner interacting socially increases. When encountering a client in a social setting, to uphold and honor confidentiality, it is professionally and ethically proper to engage the client only if the client initiates the contact. If the client initiates the conversation, steer clear of therapy-related topics.

In rare cases, if not exploitive or sexual, and when well-managed, the dual relationship may benefit or at least not interfere with the therapeutic relationship. The fact that someone already knows the practitioner may influence the decision to call for a massage appointment. In some cases, knowing someone's personal life circumstances may help when designing a personal care plan.

There are several factors to consider concerning dual relationships. Which came first, the therapeutic relationship or the social relationship? Who initiated the secondary relationship? What is the nature of the nontherapeutic relationship? (Relationships of a sexual or romantic nature are never appropriate.) What is the reason for or nature of the therapeutic relationship? What is the frequency or how intimate is the nontherapeutic relationship? Can the relationships be separate and independent? Remember, the best interest of the client must always be served in the therapeutic relationship.

Another type of dual relationship develops when we barter either work or services for our services. When we barter health services, for instance, we switch from the role of therapist to the role of client while the other party does the same. This has the potential to become complicated if one party does not feel that she is receiving or giving equally. Another difficulty may arise with the level of disclosure one or both parties are required to give as a part of the service that may interfere with the other's ability to provide an appropriate level of service. Work barters may become difficult if the quality of work does not meet the expectations of the therapist or hard feelings arise over the seemingly inequitable number of hours of work in exchange for a one-hour massage.

The classic dual relationship, however, and the one of more concern is when a client and practitioner take on another relationship role. The relationship begins when a prospective client makes an appointment and comes in for a session. An attraction, one for the other or mutual, results in a social or romantic relationship outside or beyond the therapeutic relationship.

If the feelings or attractions are on the part of the client, clearly state your professional boundaries and responsibility to uphold them. If the feelings are on the part of the practitioner, seek out supervision to clarify where the feelings are coming from and strengthen your boundaries, or refer the client to another practitioner for the sake of the safety of both parties.

Because of the power differential in the therapeutic relationship, it is the practitioner's responsibility to act ethically. The practitioner can pose questions such as: How will the client-centered therapeutic relationship be affected? Will the dual relationship improve or enhance the client's well-being? Choices must be made that maintain and enhance the well-being of the client. The professional is ultimately responsible for maintaining boundaries even when the client initiates the activities. It is the practitioner's responsibility to inform the client of the possible positive and negative implications of pursuing the relationship. If there is a strong mutual attraction, both parties should openly discuss the ramifications and complexities before proceeding. Carefully examine the motives of entering the nontherapeutic relationship. Mutual and equal consent is essential. Without good communication, feelings get hurt, which leads to all aspects of the relationship suffering. Before becoming involved or pursuing any social relationship, the client/practitioner relationship should end. The practitioner should seek supervision with peers or a supervisor to explore the source of the feelings. If the feelings persist and the client seeks the practitioner outside of the therapeutic setting, use extreme caution before establishing any social relationship. It is usually a good idea to wait a period of time after the professional relationship is discontinued before continuing a personal or romantic relationship. Dual relationships are a normal part of human interaction but nearly always detrimental to the therapeutic relationship.

ETHICAL TOUCH

The massage practitioner is a professional who is engaged in the business of giving appropriate, nurturing, and ethical touch. The massage or bodywork profession is unique in that human touch is the primary vehicle whereby services are performed. Whether it is relaxation, wellness massage, sports massage, Therapeutic Touch, or the specifically applied soft tissue manipulation of clinical massage, it is the beneficial human response to skillfully applied touch that is the basis for the success of the massage profession.

In *Touching: The Human Significance of the Skin,* Ashley Montague presents compelling anthropological evidence that touch is an essential element for healthy growth and development. He illustrates the importance of how, from a very early age, positive touch affects human physical and emotional health throughout our lives. This book is highly recommended for anyone entering any touch or health profession.

Multiple studies by Tiffany Fields and her colleagues at the Touch Research Institute in Miami, Florida, show that the positive touch of massage reduces stress, lowers blood levels of cortisol and norepinepherine, while increasing levels of serotonin and dopamine. Low levels of serotonin and dopamine are evident in people who suffer from depression, whereas significantly higher levels are associated with elevated moods.

The United States, however, is by and large a low-touch society. Usually infants and young children are the only ones who receive a significant amount of positive touch. By the time they enter school, children are taught to "keep their hands to themselves." Beyond the adolescent years, positive touch primarily occurs with a handshake, an occasional pat on the back or hug, in contact sports, in romantic relationships, or in touch-related therapies. For many adults, the only experience of caring touch is related to romantic relationships, happens only in the most intimate settings, and is often associated with sexual activity.

In the therapeutic setting, the practitioner is the giver, and the client is the recipient of touch. The massage professional's business is to provide caring, compassionate touch to the client. Massage therapists practice it every day and are comfortable administering touch as therapy. The client's experience of touch is personal, individual, and dependent on a multitude of factors. The way in which the client perceives and responds to touch is not only dependent on what techniques are applied but also on who the client is, his personal history, and the individual circumstances the client brings to the table. Perceptions are also influenced by ethnic, cultural, familial, or religious backgrounds as well as previous experiences involving touch, both good and bad. Every client comes with a personal reason for seeking massage. It is the practitioner's responsibility to be sensitive to the individual client's needs and boundaries.

The touch professional is unique in that the primary means in which services are rendered is through caring touch. The practitioner applies skilled touch to assess and treat the client in exchange for some kind of remuneration. Though there is some verbal communication, usually at the beginning of a therapy session, touch is the primary means of communication between the client's body and the practitioner's hands. The practitioner feels the conditions of the soft tissues of the client and applies appropriate touch to soothe and normalize the tissues. How that touch is perceived is dependent on the intension of the giver, what body part does the touching, the quality of touch (including pressure and movement), what part of the body is touched or the sequence, verbal communication that accompanies the touch, previous experience of the recipient with the giver, or similar touch modalities. The client may have different reactions to touch applied to different areas of the body. Some areas of the body, such as the anterior torso or face, are more vulnerable and must be approached with caution and sensitivity. Certain areas may trigger an emotional response due to a previous experience such as trauma, surgery, or abuse. During a full body massage, the practitioner applies massage technique to nearly every skin surface of the client's body, except the genitals and other sensitive areas. This gives the client the opportunity to literally get in touch with or become conscious of his entire body.

Generally, reactions to therapeutically applied touch are positive unless the touch is perceived as threatening or is more intimate than expected. Physical and sexual abuse is common in our society. Individuals who have been victims of abuse at one extreme perceive a touch as threatening or, on the other hand, may have great difficulty setting appropriate boundaries. Some types of therapeutic touch can be perceived as invasive, such as may be experienced in some medical procedures or settings. Touch might be classified as hostile, aggressive, casual, pleasurable, sensual, erotic, and therapeutic. Touch is considered hostile or aggressive when it is applied to do harm to or dominate the receiver. That is not appropriate in the therapeutic setting. If a practitioner harbors any ill will toward or is angry or upset with a client, it is wise to refer that client to another practitioner or at least postpone any therapy session until the difficulties are resolved. Even though the practitioner does not employ any aggressive or harmful manipulations, the intension with which touch is applied may carry elements of the hostility.

Professional massage does not include touch that is intentionally sexual or erotic, although sometimes a client may perceive touch to be erotic that is not applied with that intention. Clients may bring sexual issues into the session in the way of a history of abuse, a sexual disorder, or poor sexual boundaries. The client may project sexual issues onto the therapist, or the practitioner may have sexual feelings toward the client. Sexual feelings are normal, healthy, and pleasurable. In a therapeutic relationship, acting out those feelings is always inappropriate and detrimental to the relationship. Sexual intimacy, including seductive behavior or language, is never appropriate in a therapeutic relationship. In a therapeutic setting, touching the genitals, erotic touch, or touch with the intention of sexual arousal, is never appropriate. Touch is never used with the intent of sexually stimulating a client. Practitioners are responsible to maintain clear sexual boundaries regarding their own actions and to monitor and prohibit any sexual behavior on the part of the client.

Clear communication with a client, stating how, where, and what forms of touch will be used, informing the client of any changes in the treatment plan, and getting consent from the client will help create a safe environment. Always impress upon clients that they have the option to say no to any portion of the session.

Touch and Arousal: The Sexual Response

Massage is a sensual experience. A possible effect of touch during the massage session is sexual arousal. Sexual arousal is a natural physiological and cognitive response to a stimulation that is perceived as erotic by the body. Sexual arousal does not necessarily correspond to sexual desire or attraction. It is not usually an overt sign or a request to respond sexually to the arousal.

Conditions that may initiate sexual arousal vary. It is possible that the only previous touch experiences of the client have been sexual. The type of touch, the position of the client, the degree of undress, or the way draping is done may play a role. The same nerve plexus that controls the genitals also serves the lower abdomen, buttocks, and thighs. Slow, rhythmic massage of those areas may initiate an arousal response.

Sexual arousal is quite obvious in men in the form of a penile erection. Arousal is more difficult to recognize in women. Proper draping conceals most signs of a woman's arousal. Visual signs may include a slight flushing in the face or fidgeting. During a massage, a spontaneous erection or arousal may become uncomfortable, even fearful, for the practitioner, the client, or both.

The appropriate response to sexual arousal depends on the circumstance. If there is apparent discomfort or embarrassment on the part of the client or practitioner, immediate steps should be taken to diffuse the situation. If the practitioner has been massaging an area adjacent to the genitals, usually discontinuing the massage, redraping the area, and moving to a less vulnerable and sensitive area of the body will remedy the situation. Usually sexual arousal passes quickly when the initiating stimulus is removed. The practitioner may open a dialogue with the client acknowledging the reaction and assuring the client that it may be a natural response to touch stimulation and give the client the opportunity to respond. It may be helpful to simply have the client turn face down and continue the massage. If there are no other signs of discomfort by either party, the session may continue and the arousal may simply dissipate.

It is the practitioner's responsibility to act in a nonsexual manner, clarify to the client that there is no sexual intent or involvement in the relationship, and maintain appropriate boundaries.

In the case that the client indicates—verbally, or nonverbally—persistent sexual intent, it is the practitioner's responsibility to stop the session and reestablish clear professional boundaries wherein sexual activity is not part of the relationship. If the client agrees, the session may continue if the practitioner feels comfortable enough to resume. If the client persists with any sort of sexual intent, the session is terminated. The practitioner may state, "I no longer feel comfortable with this massage, and the session is now over."

Desexualizing Massage

In today's society, touch is often sexualized. The media predominately portray touch as either sexual or violent. Even touch involving massage in the media often has a sexual context. For many years massage was related to sexual activities in massage parlors. Therapeutic massage has made great strides since about 1970 in shedding the massage parlor persona; nervertheless, there are still those who use massage as a front for erotic and sexual endeavors. The massage profession has worked hard to separate from these practices; however, there is still the occasion when a new prospective client will call for an appointment seeking services that include sexual massage. It is usually easy to recognize these callers. Use a simple question such as "What type of massage services are you seeking?" or "What are the conditions you would like to address during the massage?" Responses to this type of question will usually reveal the caller's intentions. If they are seeking sexual services, a simple statement such as "I am a health professional and do not provide any kind of sexual services" or "I practice only therapeutic massage and do not engage in sexual practices of any kind" will either end the conversation or clarify your policy. If and when such people do come in for an appointment, they will know what to expect.

Clarity in advertising and communication greatly reduces the incidence of callers wanting illicit massage. A clear statement of your policies is usually sufficient to detour sexual advances in the office.

Occasionally a client will attempt to sexualize the therapy session. Sexual comments, overt advances, or requests for sexual favors may be prompted by physical attraction, by former experiences, or because sexual abuse has blurred the client's perception of appropriate boundaries. Because such acts may cause confusion, anger, or other emotional response, it is the responsibility of the practitioner to not succumb to the client's suggestive behavior and to redirect the therapeutic process, re-establish boundaries, and educate the client about appropriate behavior and the limits of the relationship. Professional, therapeutic massage does not include any kind of sexual practice or intentional erotic stimulation. The firm statement "I am a professional massage practitioner and I do not offer any type of sexual activity" may be all that needs to be said. If the client persists, the practitioner must end the session and the relationship. State that you are uncomfortable with the client's comments and intentions and therefore have terminated the session. Instruct the client to dress and leave, and then promptly leave the room. The practitioner should document in the session notes what took place and what actions were taken.

Supervision

When a therapist finds that she is involved in instances of transference, countertransference, or dual relationships, a common and helpful activity to pursue is supervision. Supervision also helps deal with issues of confidentiality, prejudice, guilt, intimacy, sexuality, and with many other difficulties that surface when working with clients. Supervision has been practiced in the mental health professions for decades. It has more recently become an important aspect of the wellness professions, especially for those who practice body therapy.

Supervision may take place with a counselor who is familiar with supervision, the massage profession, and issues involving transference and countertransference; with a mentor, who is more experienced, who is trusted, and who understands supervision and the pitfalls of transference and countertransference; or with a peer group, made up of other practitioners with similar backgrounds and experiences. Supervision is an opportunity to explore why transference or countertransference is happening in certain situations and gain insight as to how to respond to feelings in a positive way when they surface.

Mental health professionals often include supervision as one of their services. Psychotherapists, psychologists, and mental health counselors practice supervision within their professions and may be available as supervisors to other health care providers. A good supervisor is trained in issues of transference and countertransference, is familiar with the massage therapy profession, and is an invaluable model and support in helping to establish and maintain healthy personal and professional boundaries.

Massage practitioners new to the profession often find a more experienced therapist who may become a mentor. A mentor can be very helpful, providing insight into many aspects of developing a successful massage business or practice. A trusted mentor can also be a great asset in dealing with difficult clients, with special circumstances, or with issues of transference and countertransference.

Supervision in a peer group is done with a small group of practitioners and offers the possibility of sharing stories and scenarios with colleagues who may have similar experiences and may have ideas on how to work with difficult situations. It offers a chance to explore problematic situations in a supportive atmosphere. Supervision through a small group of practitioners who practice similar styles of therapy creates a support system where one can learn from another's experience and, in doing so, not feel as isolated and alone when dealing with difficult situations.

Peer group supervision consists of a number of individuals who practice similar forms of therapy who agree to meet regularly and consistently, using an agreed upon format in an atmosphere of honesty, warmth, respect, openness, and confidentiality. Some advantages of peer supervision are that it offers multiple perspectives on any situation, it decreases professional isolation while increasing professional support and networking opportunities, and it is generally free.

A professional clinical supervisor may initially help start the peer group and help establish a format to examine issues. After that, the supervisor may be called in to rejoin the group occasionally to delve more deeply into issues or concerns the group may have.

Regular supervision offers a way to improve therapeutic relationships with clients. Seeking supervision is not looking for someone to tell us what to do. A good supervisor will point out strong points as well as help shore up mistakes or pitfalls a practitioner might stumble into as she deals with issues of transference and countertransference in the practice of massage therapy. Rather than dictate what action a practitioner should take, a good supervisor will help the practitioner explore the internal, underlying issues related to the dilemma; define appropriate boundaries related to the client and practitioner; and help devise appropriate actions to maintain healthy therapeutic relationships (see Box 3.2).

A practitioner who uses supervision must have permission from the client to specifically discuss the client's case with a supervisor. Supervisors are sworn to the same or even more rigid rules of confidentiality as are practitioners.

When working with clients who have been sexually abused or are mentally ill (depressed, bipolar, or schizophrenic), supervision with someone familiar with these conditions is invaluable to help the practitioner understand possible reactions these clients may have to bodywork.

Supervision should offer a trusted, shame-free environment in which to sort out emotional or boundary issues that arise in the professional arena. Supervision is self-care for the practitioner.

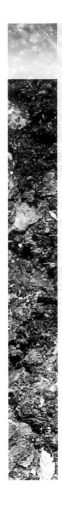

BOX 3.2 REASONS FOR SUPERVISION

Some reasons to seek supervision include the following:

- You have a client or clients who are difficult or controlling.
- Difficult or confusing situations arise in your practice.
- Clients challenge professional or personal boundaries.
- You experience feelings of exhaustion or burnout at the end of a session or day.
- You sense disappointment, depression, agitation, or ill will related to a client.
- You are working with clients who have been sexually or physically abused.
- You stretched or crossed a professional boundary with a client.
- You are attracted to a client or a client is attracted to you.
- Sexual or romantic feelings enter into a therapeutic relationship.
- You have strong feelings toward a client, either positive or negative.
- You have feelings for a client that alter the way you work with that client.
- You have feelings of infatuation, intimidation, powerlessness, anger, or frustration toward any client.
- You change your regular care protocol for a particular client.
- You have feelings for any client that come up outside of the therapy session.

ETHICAL BUSINESS PRACTICES

Ethics are the basis for standards of acceptable and professional behavior by which a person or business conducts business. The following are ethical standards of practice to which you as a massage professional should adhere:

1. Treat all clients with the same fairness, courtesy, respect, and dignity.

2. Provide the highest quality care for those who seek your professional services.

3. Have knowledge of and always stay within the limitations of your scope of practice.

4. Respect and protect client confidentiality. Solicit only that information from the client that is relevant to the therapeutic relationship. Never share a client's name, condition, or any information from conversation or written forms with anyone outside the therapy session without the client's written approval. Obtain a "Release of Medical Information" form, signed and dated by the client, before conferring with any other health care provider for the purpose of benefiting the quality of service to the client.

5. Set an example of professionalism by your conduct at all times.

6. Be respectful of the therapeutic relationship, and maintain appropriate boundaries.

7. Be aware of the effects of transference and countertransference and avoid dual relationships that may adversely affect the therapeutic relationship.

8. In no way allow or encourage any kind of sexual activity in your practice. Do not participate in any sexual relationship with a client at any time during the term of the therapeutic relationship.

9. Do not participate in the practice of massage when under the influence of drugs or alcohol.

10. Retain the right to refuse or terminate service to any client who is sexually inappropriate, abusive, or under the influence of drugs or alcohol.

11. Disclose to clients adequate information regarding your qualifications, the massage procedures, and the expected outcome and obtain an informed consent from them or their advocate (in the case they are under the age of 18 or are not competent) before providing treatment. Respect the client's right to refuse, terminate, or modify treatment regardless of prior consent.

12. Provide massage services only when there is a reasonable expectation that it will be advantageous to the client.

13. Represent your education, professional affiliations, certifications, and qualifications honestly and provide only those services you are qualified to perform.

14. Respect and cooperate with other ethical health care providers to promote health and wellness, and refer to appropriate medical personnel when indicated.

15. Maintain accurate and truthful client records and make them available to review with the client.

16. Provide adequate draping procedures so that the client feels safe, secure, comfortable, and warm at all times.

17. Provide a safe environment, employ hygienic practices, and use universal precautions.

18. Charge fair prices for all services. Disclose fee schedules and discuss any financial arrangements in advance of the session.

19. Know and obey all laws, rules, and regulations of your city, county, and state pertaining to your work.

20. Strive to improve the credibility of massage as a valuable health service by educating the public and medical community as to its benefits.

21. Be fair and honest in all advertising of services.

22. Communicate in a professional manner on the telephone, in personal conversations, and in letters.

23. Refrain from the use of improper language and any form of gossip.

24. Eliminate prejudice in the profession and do not discriminate against colleagues or clients.

25. Be well organized so that you make the most of your time.

26. Maintain your physical, mental, and emotional well-being so that you are looked on as a credit to your profession. Seek out and use supervision when indicated and appropriate.

27. Dress in a manner that is professional, modest, and clean.

28. Continue to learn about new developments in your profession by participating in local and national professional associations and pursuing continuing education and training.

29. Keep foremost in your mind that you are a professional person engaged in giving an important and beneficial personal service. Operate all aspects of your business with honesty and integrity.

30. Do your utmost to keep your place of business clean, safe, comfortable, and in alignment with all legal requirements.

Remember that people judge you by first impressions (see Box 3.3).

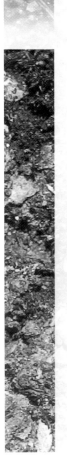

BOX 3.3 PERSONAL HYGIENE AND HEALTH HABITS

To inspire confidence and trust in your clients, you should project a well-groomed, professional appearance at all times. In a personal service business, personal health and good grooming are assets that clients admire and are essential for your protection and that of the client.

Your personal health and grooming habits should include the following:

1. Bathe or shower daily and use a deodorant as necessary.

2. Keep your teeth and gums healthy. Visit your dentist regularly.

3. Use mouthwash and avoid foods that contribute to offensive breath odor.

4. Keep your hair fresh and clean, and wear an appropriate hairstyle. Hair should be worn in a style that you do not have to touch or fuss with during a massage session. In addition, your hair must not touch the client during the session.

5. Avoid strong fragrances such as perfumes, colognes, and lotions.

6. Keep your hands free of blemishes and calluses. Use lotion to keep your hands soft and smooth.

7. Keep your nails clean and filed so that they do not extend to the tips of the fingers. Sharp nails should never come in contact with the client's skin. Never wear garish nail polish.

8. If you are a woman, wear appropriate makeup in appropriate colors for your skin tone. Be sure makeup is applied neatly.

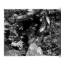

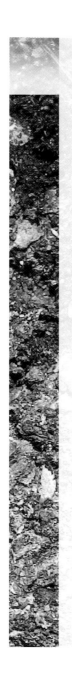

9. If you are a man, keep beard or mustache neat and well groomed. If you prefer the clean-shaven look, be sure to shave as often as necessary.

10. Avoid gum chewing or smoking in the presence of clients.

11. Keep your face clean and free of blemishes.

12. Practice all rules of sanitation for the client's and for your own protection.

13. Have a complete physical examination by a physician before beginning work as a massage practitioner. Continue to have checkups, follow your physician's advice, and do all that is possible to maintain optimum health.

14. If you perspire heavily, take precautions so that your perspiration does not drop on your client.

15. Take time for relaxation and physical fitness. Receive massages regularly. A regimen of daily exercise is recommended. This may be accomplished by participation in active sports of your choice (swimming, tennis, etc.), working out at the gym, or by devising a set of beneficial exercises you can do at home.

16. Eat a well-balanced, nutritious diet. Maintain your normal weight for your height and bone structure. You should not be extremely overweight or extremely underweight. If you have a weight problem, follow your physician's advice on how to attain your most healthful weight.

17. Be aware of good posture and proper body mechanics when walking, standing, sitting, and working. Poor posture habits such as slouching contribute to fatigue, foot problems, and strain to your back and neck.

18. Wear the appropriate clothing for your profession. Refrain from low-cut necklines and tight or sexually provocative clothing. Clothing should be loose enough to allow for optimal movement. It should be free of accessories that might catch on the massage table or touch the client when you are performing the massage (such as a long chain, necklace or tie, a wide belt, or long sleeves). Consider clothing that allows your body heat to escape. Clothing made of natural fibers such as cotton is good. Some synthetic fabrics hold the heat of your body and may be uncomfortable for the physical exertion of this profession.

COMMUNICATION SKILLS

In addition to gaining the necessary technical skills as a professional massage practitioner, you must be able to understand your client's needs. This is the basis of all good human relations. A pleasant voice, good manners, cheerfulness, patience, tact, loyalty, empathy, and interest in the client's welfare are some of the desirable traits that help build the client's confidence in you and your place of business.

It is important to be able to interact with people without becoming too familiar. Often, clients will confide their personal feelings, and they trust you not to betray their confidence. This is where the art of listening is an invaluable asset. Listen with empathy, change the subject when necessary (tactfully), and never betray the client's confidence in you.

The following rules for good human relations will help you interact successfully with people from all walks of life:

Tact: Tact is required with a client who is overly critical, finds fault, and is hard to please. It may be that he just wants attention. Tact helps you deal with this client in an impersonal but understanding manner. To be tactful is to avoid what is offensive or disturbing and to do what is most considerate for all concerned. For example, you might discover that a client needs medical care and you feel you should suggest that he see a physician. You must approach the problem with the utmost tact and diplomacy.

Cheerfulness: A cheerful attitude and a pleasant facial expression will go a long way toward putting a client at ease.

Patience: Patience is the ability to be tolerant under stressful or undesirable conditions. Your patience and understanding will be the best medicine when you work with people who are ill, agitated, or in pain. Patience helps you change negative situations to more positive ones.

Honesty: To be honest does not mean that you must be brutally frank with a client. You can answer questions in a factual but tactful manner. For example, if a client has unrealistic expectations regarding the benefits of a treatment, you can discuss what can or cannot be accomplished in a sincere, conscientious manner.

Intuition: Intuition is your ability to have insight into people's feelings. When you genuinely like people, it is easier to show sympathy and understanding for their problems. People will often confide in you when their intuition tells them you are trustworthy. In turn, your own intuition will help you avoid embarrassing situations and involving yourself in problems you cannot solve. Remember, the primary reason your clients come to you is for relaxation. Keep conversations to a minimum to allow the client maximum relaxation.

Sense of humor: It is important to have a sense of humor, especially when dealing with difficult people or situations. A good sense of humor helps you remain optimistic, courteous, and in control.

Maturity: Maturity is not so much a matter of how old you are, but what you have gained from your life experience. Maturity is the quality of being reliable, responsible, self-disciplined, and well adjusted.

Self-esteem: Self-esteem is projected by your attitudes about yourself and your profession. If you respect yourself and your profession, you will be respected by others.

Self-motivation: Self-motivation is your ability to set positive goals and put forth the energy and effort required to achieve those goals. It means making sacrifices when necessary to save time and money and to achieve your goals.

BUILDING A PROFESSIONAL IMAGE

If you want to be successful in business, you must prepare for success. Preparation, planning, and performance are the assets that help you do your job in the most professional manner. You should take every opportunity to pursue new avenues of knowledge. Attend professional seminars, read trade journals and other publications relating to your business, and become active in associations where you can exchange ideas with other dedicated people.

Your business image is important and should be built on good service and truth in advertising. A reliable reputation is particularly important in the personal service business because you are dealing with the health and well-being of individuals. Consistently high standards and good service are the foundations on which successful businesses are built. (Refer to Chapter 19, "Business Practices," for more ideas on massage business management.)

YOUR BUSINESS NAME

Using appropriate wording in your business name in advertising will help you establish a good reputation. You can see how the name "Smitty's Massage Parlour" or "Smith Massage Clinic" can totally change how your business is perceived by potential clients.

Some massage professionals, especially those entering a new community, may feel they need to state in their advertising that only therapeutic and nonsexual massage is given. Keeping regular business hours, rather than late-night hours, also improves your reputation.

Another point to remember is that using proper draping techniques to ensure your client's privacy is very important in building a good reputation. Word of mouth is the massage professional's best advertising. Satisfied clients will spread the message that you work in a professional manner.

QUESTIONS FOR DISCUSSION AND REVIEW

1. Why is it important to have a code of ethics for your business?

2. Why is a satisfied client your best means of advertising?

3. Why do successful business managers prefer employees who are concerned with personal and professional ethics?

4. What is the connection between boundaries and ethics?

5. Differentiate between personal and professional boundaries.

6. What are major areas to consider when establishing professional boundaries?

7. Who does the power differential favor in the therapeutic relationship?

8. What is the effect of a boundary being crossed?

9. What can a practitioner do to reduce the risk of crossing a client's boundary?

10. What is transference and countertransference?

11. Whose responsibility is it to manage boundary issues and instances of transference or countertransference?

12. What constitutes a dual relationship in a therapeutic setting?

13. How should a practitioner respond if a client becomes sexually aroused?

14. What is supervision?

15. Why is it necessary for the massage practitioner to have strict personal hygiene and health habits?

16. What is meant by professional projection in attitude and appearance?

17. How do you define human relations as applied to working with or serving others?

18. Why is the practice of human relations so important to the massage practitioner?

19. When building your business (practice) image, how can you be sure the public gets the right message?

PART II

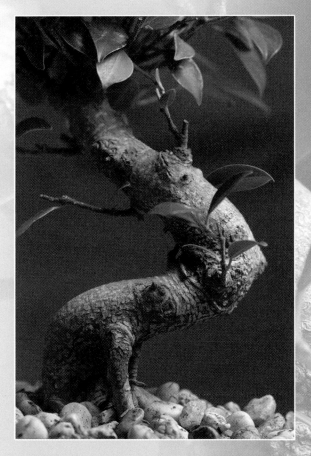

Human Anatomy and Physiology

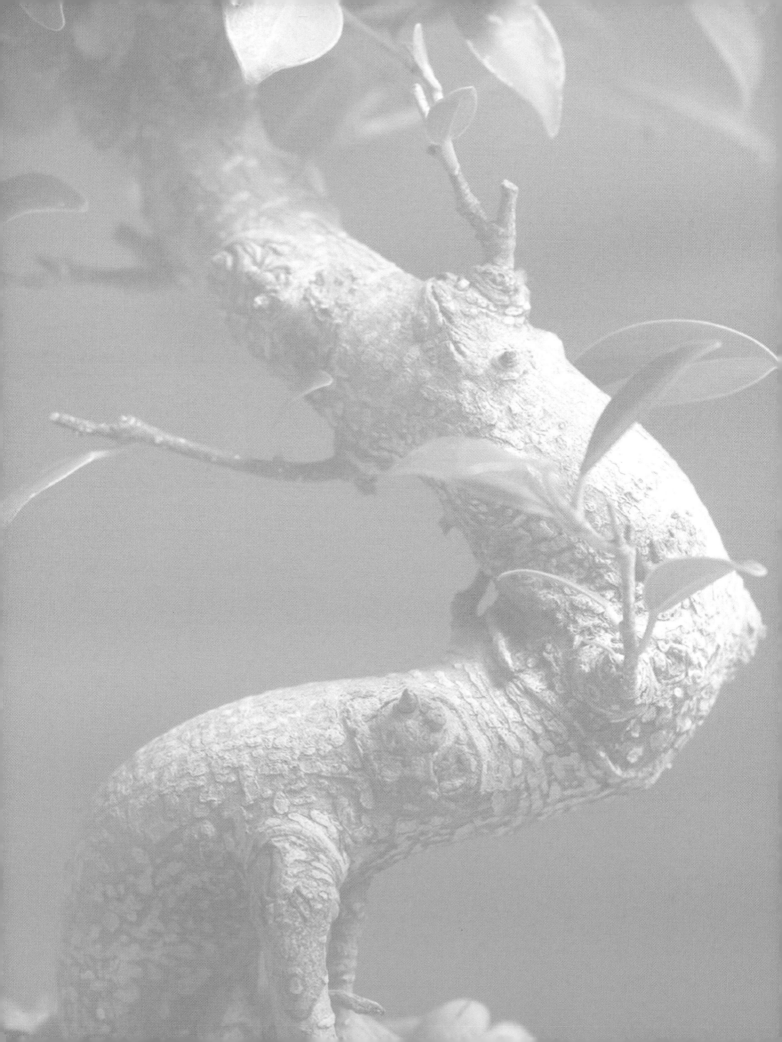

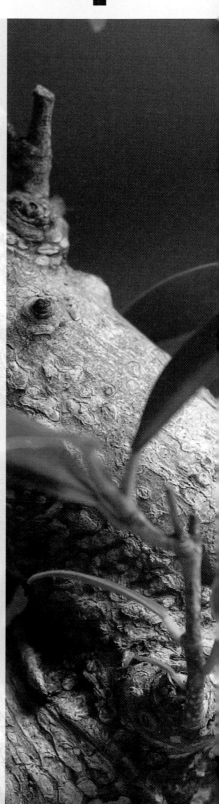

Overview

LEARNING OBJECTIVES

After you have mastered this chapter, you will be able to:

1. Explain the meanings of the important terms indicated in boldface listed in this chapter.

2. Explain why a massage therapist should have a good understanding of anatomy, physiology, and pathology.

3. Explain the physiological and psychological effects of stress and pain and the role of massage therapy in the management of stress and pain.

4. Describe the healing functions of the body in terms of inflammation and tissue repair.

5. Describe the wellness model and how massage may be a part of that model.

6. Be able to derive the meaning of medical terms by breaking the terms into their parts and defining the parts.

INTRODUCTION

A basic knowledge of **histology, anatomy, physiology, kinesiology,** and **pathology** is necessary in mastering the theory and practice of therapeutic massage. The massage practitioner should study the structures and functions of the human body in order to know when, where, and how to apply massage movements for the most beneficial results. This knowledge enables the practitioner to adjust the massage treatment to the needs of the individual and to anticipate results.

DEFINITION OF ANATOMY AND PHYSIOLOGY

Anatomy is the science of morphology or structure of an organism or body. Physiology concerns the normal functions performed by the various systems of the body. Anatomy and physiology are interrelated in that the structures are associated with their functions. Structure and function are dependent on the interaction of the organism's parts, and each part has a role in the operation of the whole.

histology is a branch of biology concerned with the microscopic structure of tissues of a living organism.

anatomy is the study of the gross structure of the body and the interrelations of its parts.

physiology is the science and study of the vital processes, mechanisms, and functions of an organ or system.

kinesiology is the scientific study of muscular activity and the anatomy, physiology, and mechanics of body movement.

pathology is the study of the structural and functional changes caused by disease.

Anatomy (uh-**NAT**-o-mee) is defined as the study of the gross structure of the body or the study of an organism and the interrelations of its parts. For example, when we describe the skeleton or other anatomic parts of the body, naming the parts and how they relate to one another, we are describing anatomy.

Physiology (fiz-ee-**AH**-lo-jee) is the science and study of the vital processes, mechanisms, and functions of an organ or system of organs. When we describe how the organs or parts of the body function and how their functions relate to one another, we are speaking of physiology.

Kinesiology (kin-ee-see-**AH**-lo-jee) is the scientific study of muscular activity and the anatomy, physiology, and mechanics of body movement.

Histology (his-**TAHL**-o-jee) is a form of microscopic anatomy. It is the branch of biology concerned with the microscopic structure of tissues of a living organism. All living structures are composed of cells and intercellular materials that are organized to form the various tissues, organs, and systems of the body.

Pathology (pa-**THAL**-o-jee) is the study of the structural and functional changes caused by disease.

RELATIONSHIP OF ANATOMY AND PHYSIOLOGY TO MASSAGE AND BODYWORK

Therapeutic massage is applied to and directly affects the structures and the functions of the human organism. It has direct effects such as increased local circulation of venous (**VEE**-nuhs) blood and lymph (**LIMF**), stretching of muscle tissue, and loosening of adhesions and scar tissue. Massage has indirect effects of increased circulation to the muscles and internal organs, reduced blood pressure, and general relaxation of tense muscles. Massage also has reflex effects such as reduced heart rate and slower, deeper breathing.

An important purpose of massage and bodywork is to promote functional improvement in the recipient's body. The more understanding therapists have of the human body and how it functions, the better they will be able to direct their treatment to produce desired effects. A working knowledge of anatomy and physiology gives therapists a basis on which they can plan effective treatments and discuss those applications with other health care professionals. A basic knowledge of pathology provides massage therapists with an understanding of disease processes in order that they can make decisions to provide massage services or refer clients to appropriate medical professionals. Through clear understanding of kinesiology and the structures involved in body movement, the massage therapist is better able to identify areas of pain and/or dysfunction when working with clients. As therapists continue to develop therapeutic skills by learning more effective methods of bodywork, a thorough knowledge and understanding of anatomy, physiology, and pathology become essential.

PHYSIOLOGICAL CHANGES DURING DISEASE

Physiologically, the body strives to maintain the delicate balance in its internal environment. Changes in the stresses posed by the external environment constantly force the body to compensate to maintain that delicate internal balance called **homeostasis** (ho-mee-o-**STAY**-sis). When the body's homeostasis is disturbed, the person may experience symptoms of disease.

homeostasis
is the internal balance of the body.

Signs and Symptoms of Disease

Disease is an abnormal and unhealthy state of all or part of the body wherein it is not capable of carrying on its normal function. Diseases generally have **symptoms** and **signs**. A symptom is caused by the disease and is perceived by the victim, such as dizziness, chills, nausea, or pain. A symptom is a clear message to the individual that something is wrong. Signs of a disease are observable indications such as abnormal pulse rate, fever, abnormal skin color, or physical irregularities. When signs and symptoms of disease appear, it is advisable to seek help from proper medical authorities. Symptoms and signs, along with medical examinations, medical histories, and laboratory tests, are the bases for proper diagnosis and treatment of most disease conditions.

There are many possible direct causes for disease, including disease-producing organisms, trauma, environmental agents, malnutrition, degenerative processes, and stress. Other conditions that may be a predisposing factor include age, working or living conditions, gender, and heredity.

disease
is an abnormal and unhealthy state of all or part of the body wherein it is not capable of carrying on its normal function.

symptom
is subjective evidence of disease or bodily disorder.

sign (of disease)
is an observable indication of disease or bodily disorder.

Stress

Stress is any psychological or physical situation or condition that causes tension or strain. Stress can be any element or situation that requires our body or mind to compensate in order to maintain our delicate internal balance and harmony. Stress may affect individuals differently. What is extremely stressful to one person may not affect another at all. However, if too many stressful conditions occur without an effective method to manage or cope with them, the health of the individual will suffer. Regardless of the source or nature of the stress, the physiological reaction of the body is essentially the same.

Stress is most notably associated with the **adrenal glands** and their secretion of the "fight or flight" hormones. The principal and most understood adrenal hormones are *adrenaline* (uh-**DREN**-uh-lin) and *cortisol* (**KAUR**-ti-zol). When we encounter high levels of stress, the adrenal secretions give us a physical and mental boost that heightens our senses, sharpens our reflexes, and prepares our muscles for maximum exertion. The adrenal glands by no means work alone. In conjunction with the *pituitary* (pi-**TOO**-i-tar-ee) and the *hypothalamus* (high-po-**THAL**-uh-muhs), they affect the function of most of the internal systems. Muscle

stress
is any psychological or physical situation or condition that causes tension or strain.

adrenal glands
situated on the top of each kidney, produce epinephrine, norepinephrine, and corticosteroids.

tone increases, blood pressure rises, and breathing deepens. Blood is directed toward the skeletal muscles and nervous system and away from the digestive organs. Digestion virtually stops. Glycogen, glucose, and oxygen-carrying red blood cells are mobilized. Blood-coagulating chemicals are added to the blood, and the kidneys retain fluids in case of injury and bleeding. Cortisol promotes the breakdown of the body's proteins to form glucose and acts as an anti-inflammatory and antiallergenic.

These biochemical effects are essential in emergency, fight or flight situations; however, if the dosage of these hormones is sustained over a long period of time, as it would be with long-term stress, the consequences can be devastating. The ongoing anti-inflammatory effect of cortisol, for example, would inhibit the natural inflammatory response to injury. The body's healing process of flooding the injured area with wound-healing leukocytes, nutrients, fibroblasts, and oxygen would be interfered with, and eventually the body's ability to resist infection of all kinds is decreased. Continued secretion of adrenaline would eventually exhaust not only the adrenal glands but, because of its effect on the sympathetic nervous system, would have the same effect on the organs as severe loss of sleep—exhaustion! Other effects of sustained levels of these hormones include gastric ulcers, high blood pressure, depressed immune system function, **atherosclerosis** (ath-eer-o-skler-**O**-sis) and, finally, death.

Stress in and of itself is not the problem. Life is inherently stressful. When effectively worked with, stress tends to strengthen our physical, mental, and emotional resolve. However, when we load ourselves with unrelenting, inescapable, and overburdening stress, it becomes unhealthy and even deadly.

Pain

Pain is one of the body's primary sensations, along with touch, pressure, heat, and cold. Its function is primarily protective in that it warns of tissue damage or destruction somewhere in the body. Pain is the result of stimulation to specialized nerve ends located near the surface of the body, in the periosteum of the bones, in the arterial and intestinal walls, and, to a lesser extent, in the deeper organs, muscles, and viscera (**VIS**-er-uh).

There are two responses to pain: psychological and physical. The physical response to pain is very similar to the body's response to stress. Blood pressure and pulse increase, and blood flow is shifted from the intestines and brain to the muscles as mental alertness intensifies, readying the body for fight or flight. The physical experience of pain also informs about the location, intensity, and duration of the ailment.

The individual's psychological and emotional reaction to pain varies depending on many factors, such as previous experience with pain, training in coping with pain, anxiety, tension, and fatigue. The fear and anxiety associated with pain can be more debilitating than the actual pain.

---

atherosclerosis

is characterized by an accumulation of fatty deposits on the inner walls of the arteries.

---

pain

has a primarily protective function in that it warns of tissue damage or destruction somewhere in the body. It is the result of stimulation of specialized nerve ends in the body.

Pain-Spasm-Pain Cycle

A painful syndrome of interest to the massage therapist is the *pain-spasm-pain cycle* associated with muscle spasms. The cycle may start with a rather minor injury such as a bruise or muscle strain that in itself has little effect on the function of the organism. The natural reflex reaction to the tissue damage and pain is a contraction of the muscles that surround the injury, which acts to support and protect the damaged tissue. The contracted muscles constrict the blood vessels and capillaries in the muscles, inhibiting blood flow to the area (a condition known as **ischemia** [is-**KEE**-mee-uh]). At the same time, the metabolic activity of the contracting muscles increases, consuming more energy. Oxygen and nutrients are burned, producing increased amounts of metabolic waste. The available oxygen is quickly burned, and the amounts of lactic acid and other toxins collect in the tissues. Soon, *ischemic pain* appears, which is often more intense than the pain from the original injury. The reflex reaction to the ischemic pain is identical to the response to the original injury. Pain causes muscle contraction and ischemia, thereby causing spasm that causes more pain. It is easy to see how this can become a vicious cycle that can perpetuate itself and continue long after the original injury heals.

ischemia
is localized tissue anemia due to obstruction of the inflow of blood.

THE ROLE OF THERAPEUTIC MASSAGE IN STRESS, PAIN, AND THE PAIN-SPASM-PAIN CYCLE

Therapeutic massage combines the power of sensitive touch with the knowledge of anatomy and physiology to become a valuable tool in relieving the psychological and physical suffering of stress and pain. Skillfully applied massage provides pleasurable stimulation that is carried to the brain on thicker, faster, more numerous nerve fibers that actually override or drown out the pain signals. Even though the diversion is temporary, it gives the individual a chance to relax and disassociate with the noxious stimulus, possibly long enough to shut down the fight or flight reaction. Psychologically, the reassuring touch of the therapist helps relieve anxiety and fear. The individual in many cases is able to regain some sense of control over the situation. Physically, as soothing, pleasant sensations flood the brain, adrenal secretions subside, breathing slows and deepens, blood pressure lowers, pulse rate slows, and the body relaxes and begins to recuperate.

In the case of the pain-spasm-pain cycle where pain is intensified because of ischemia, skillfully applied massage therapy is very effective in breaking the cycle, relieving the pain, and restoring mobility. Sensitive touch can divert some attention away from the acute intensity of the pain. By gentle palpation, the actual source of the pain can be isolated and differentiated from the contracted and ischemic areas around it. By massaging the contracted ischemic tissues, chronic spasms can be relieved and circulation restored. As oxygen and nutrients flood the area and lactic acid and other irritants are removed, the pain disappears and mobility is restored.

Even though massage is an effective tool in controlling pain, it must be remembered that pain is an indication of tissue damage or nerve irritation. Generally, the more severe the pain, the more severe the tissue

bacteria
are minute, unicellular organisms exhibiting both plant and animal characteristics and are classified as either harmless or harmful.

virus
is any class of submicroscopic pathogenic agents that transmit disease.

fungus
(pl. fungi) is a diverse group of organisms potentially capable of causing disease that thrive or grow in wet or damp areas.

parasite
is an organism that may potentially cause disease that exists and functions at the expense of a host organism without contributing to the survival of the host.

local infection
is invading organisms confined to a small area of the body.

systemic infection
is invading organisms that have spread throughout the body.

inflammation
is a protective tissue response characterized by swelling, redness, heat, and pain.

fever
is an elevated body temperature.

damage. Acute or severe pain is a warning that something is physically wrong and should be checked by a physician. If massage is used as an aid for controlling pain, the attending physician should be advised. If massage increases the overall level of pain, it should be discontinued. Please note that some massage techniques can be uncomfortable as they are being applied; however, the discomfort should not be so intense that it hurts the client or lingers beyond the direct application of the manipulation.

HEALING MECHANISMS OF THE BODY

Infection

The most common cause of disease in humans is the invasion of the body by disease-producing *microorganisms* such as **bacteria, viruses, fungi,** or **parasites.** If microorganisms enter the body in sufficient numbers to multiply and become harmful and are capable of destroying healthy tissue, the body reacts by developing an infection. If the invading organisms are confined to a small area, the condition is considered a **local infection.** If, however, the organisms spread through the body, the condition is termed a **systemic infection.**

Massage should not be applied in cases of systemic infection or to the site of local infection.

Inflammation

If invading microorganisms cause any destruction of tissue, inflammation occurs. Inflammation will also result from physical injury such as a sprain or blow, excessive heat, cold or radiation, or physical irritants such as splinters, stings, and chemical exposure where tissue is damaged.

When tissue is damaged, substances are released that cause dramatic secondary reactions that are collectively called **inflammation.** Inflammation is a protective tissue response that is characterized by swelling, redness, heat, and pain. Blood vessels in the area of the damaged tissues dilate, increasing blood flow to the area and causing redness and heat. Capillary walls become more permeable, allowing large quantities of blood plasma and white blood cells to enter the tissue spaces, resulting in swelling. The swelling puts pressure on local nerve endings, causing pain. Increased numbers of white blood cells, called leukocytes and phagocytes, flood the area to engulf and digest the invading organisms and the damaged tissue debris (phagocytosis).

Sometimes, toxic bacteria or the reaction between the invading organisms and the white blood cells release a substance into the bloodstream that affects the body's heat-regulating system. The resulting elevated body temperature is called a **fever.** Fever is a warning sign that usually accompanies infectious diseases or infected burns and cuts. In cases of sudden onset or high fever (above 102° F), a physician should be consulted. In some ways, fever, if it is not extremely high, is a natural protective device. Fever increases the metabolic rate and the production of the immune substances that battle the invading organisms. The increased temperature itself destroys certain organisms. At the same time, the discomfort and weakness that accompany fever will cause the patient to rest, thereby conserving energy to battle the infection. Extreme or prolonged fever may be dangerous or even fatal. Prolonged fever will cause dehydration, so fluids must be replaced. Fevers above 106° to 108° F may cause damage to the tissues of the kidneys, liver, or other organs or may cause irreparable brain damage, possibly resulting in death.

Massage of inflamed tissue or while fever is present is contraindicated.

Tissue Repair

The degree of tissue repair varies depending on the location and type of tissue and the nature of the damage or injury. Skin and surface tissues undergo a great deal of wear and tear and are easily and quickly repaired. Bone and ligaments repair much more slowly and may require immobilization. Muscle and tendons repair with noticeable scarring and weakness. Neurons of the central nervous system injured by trauma or infection do not repair at all.

Injury or wound healing and repair will only take place when infection-causing bacteria have been destroyed. Escaping fluid from the damaged tissues and capillaries will fill the wound and coagulate, forming a clot to seal the wound. Connective tissue cells called *fibroblasts* migrate to the area and produce connective tissue fibers that begin to span the wound, providing a structure for regenerating vascular and epithelial tissue. When the wound is healed, this formation of fibrous connective tissue is called **scar tissue.** If the wound is small, the damage is completely and quickly restored to normal. If, however, the wound is large, measures must be taken to bring the wound surfaces close together in order to prevent the formation of excessive scar tissue.

Properly applied tissue stretching and friction massage will minimize the formation of scar tissue and adhesions resulting from tissue trauma.

| **scar** |
| a dense fibrous tissue that forms as an injury, wound, burn, or sore heals. |

| **wellness** |
| is behaviors and habits that have a positive influence on health. |

THE WELLNESS MODEL

Wellness is a concept in which a person takes personal responsibility for his state of health. It is a preventive plan wherein a person makes an effort to recognize conditions, situations, and practices that may be threatening or detrimental to her health and takes steps to change or eliminate them in order to live a more healthful life. Wellness involves taking an active role in being healthy, and adopting practices that enhance health such as a low-fat, high-fiber diet, exercise, a balance between work and play, and a positive mental and spiritual attitude. Wellness also means reducing health risks and eliminating practices that add stressful dangers to our lifestyles.

Wellness takes into consideration more than our state of physical health. Wellness is often represented as an equilateral triangle with the sides depicting body, mind, and spirit or physical, psychological/mental, and attitude/emotional. When all three aspects are healthy and in balance, optimum wellness is experienced. A wellness-oriented person strives to attain a healthy balance between these three (Figure 4.1).

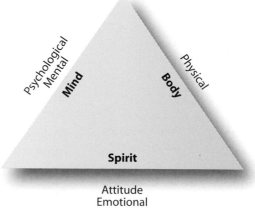

Figure 4.1

Wellness model.

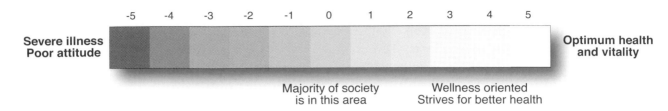

Figure 4.2
Scale of health.

Health might be gauged on a scale that ranges from −5 to 0 to 5. Minus five equates with severe illness combined with a poor attitude. Zero is okay (that is, there is no perceivable sickness). Five equates with optimum health and vitality. The great majority of our society hovers between −3 and 2. A wellness-oriented individual would strive to maintain her health rating above 3 on the scale (Figure 4.2).

MEDICAL AND ANATOMICAL TERMINOLOGY

Any profession or trade uses a language or vocabulary that is specific or peculiar to the practices, equipment, and processes of that system. Massage and bodywork is no different. Most of the terminology related to massage is derived from the health care and medical field.

Anatomical and medical terminology refers to the vocabulary or jargon commonly used by health professionals when communicating to one another concerning conditions of patients, descriptions of procedures, and anatomical structures. It is important for massage therapists to have an understanding of the body's structure and function. Therefore, becoming familiar with the related terminology is essential. By having an understanding of how medical terms are constructed, the massage therapist will be less intimidated by the long words, be better able to communicate with other health professionals, and (by speaking their language) be better respected and accepted by the medical community.

The history of medical terminology goes back nearly 2,000 years to the time when Western civilization first began systematically studying the human body. Because the languages of these first researchers were Greek and Latin, these became and remain the source languages for medical terminology.

Composition of Medical Terminology

In medical terminology, big words are compound words constructed of root words (or stems), prefixes, and suffixes. There are many terms that are constructed from relatively few word parts.

The stem, or root word, generally indicates the body part or structure involved. Occasionally, two or more stems will be combined to show relation or position (for example, cardiopulmonary pertaining to heart and lung). When stems are combined, a single-letter syllable is often used to create what is called a combining form. This is a word root plus a vowel that is used with another word root to form a compound word. A combining form is usually an "o" or an "i."

A prefix is one or more syllables added in front of the stem to further its meaning. A suffix likewise is added to the end of the word. Suffixes often denote a diagnosis, symptom, or surgical procedure or identify a word as a noun or adjective.

Anatomical terms often include more than one word. Generally, the first word acts as an adjective and will indicate the region or location of the structure. The second word is the noun and names the structure (for example, femoral artery, thoracic duct).

By breaking the terms into their parts, the logical meaning can be derived.

Table 4.1 provides a list of prefixes, suffixes, and stem words along with their meanings. As you study the following chapters, be aware of anatomical and medical terms and decipher their meaning by examining the parts. During discussions with peers and other health care practitioners, use proper terminology and make note of unfamiliar terms. Examine them and determine their meaning by breaking them apart and defining their parts. Practice and become familiar with the language. When in doubt, always keep a medical dictionary available. When a term is used that you do not understand, check your dictionary.

Table 4.1

Alphabetical Listing of Common Word Elements Used to Construct Medical Terms

PREFIXES			PREFIXES, cont'd		
Word Part	Definition	Example	Word Part	Definition	Example
a-	absent, without, away from	abacterial	hypo-	under, below	hypodermic
			in-	within, into, not, negative	internal, inept
ab-	away from	abduction	infra-	beneath	infraspinatus
ad-	to, toward	adduction	intra-	inside	intravenous
ambi-	both	ambidextrous	leuk-(o)	white	leukocyte
a-; an-	without	atypical	macr-(o)	large, long	macrophage
anti-	against	antibody, antidote	mal-	abnormal, bad	malpractice
			medi-	middle, midline	medial
ante-	before	anterior	mega-	large, extreme	megadose
bi-	two	biceps	micr-(o)	small	microscope
bio-	life	biology	mon-(o)	one, single	monolith
carcin-(o)	cancer	carcinogenic	multi-	many, multiple	multiply
circum-	around	circumvent	narc-	stupor, numbness	narcotic
co-	with, together	cooperate	ne-(o)	new	neophyte, neonatal
contra-	against, counter to	contraindicate	nutri-	nourish	nutrition
de-	down, from	descend	para-	next to, resembling, beside	paralysis, paraplegic
di-	two	dissect			
dis-	apart, away from	dislocate	path-	pertaining to disease	pathology
dors-	back	dorsal	per-	through	perforate
dys-	abnormal, impaired	dysfunction	peri-	around	periosteum
e-	out, from	emetic	poly-	many, much	polyunsaturated
ect-	outside, without	ectoplasm	post-	after, later in time	posthumous
end-(o)	inside, within	endoderm	pre-, pro-	before in time	previous
epi-	upon, over, in addition	epimysium	pseud-(o)	false	pseudonym
ex-	out of	exit, excrete	quad-	four	quadriplegic
extra-	beyond, outside of, in addition	extracellular	re-	back, again	repeat, review
flex-	bent	flexion	retro-	backward	retrofit
front-	front, forehead	frontalis	sub-	under, below	subscapularis
hemi-	half	hemiplegic	super-	above, in addition	superior
hetero-	the other	heterosexual	supra-	over, above, upper	supraspinatus
hom-	common, same	homogenous	syn-	together, along with	synergist
hydro-	denoting water	hydrotherapy	tri-	three	triceps
hyper-	above, extreme	hypertensive	uni-	single, one	unilateral

continues

Table 4.1, cont'd

Alphabetical Listing of Common Word Elements Used to Construct Medical Terms

SUFFIXES			COMMON WORD ROOTS OF STEMS, cont'd		
Word Part	Definition	Example	Word Part	Definition	Example
-al; -ar	pertaining to an area	femoral, clavicular	brachi	arm	brachialis
			cardi	heart	cardiac
-algia	painful condition	neuralgia	cephal	head	brachiocephalic
-ase	denoting an enzyme	lactase	cerebr(o)	brain	cerebrospinalis
-desis	a binding	tenodesis	cervic	neck	cervix, cervical
-ectomy	surgical removal of body part	tonsillectomy	chondr(o)	cartilage	osteochondritis
			cost	rib	intercostal
-gram	a record	sonogram	crani	skull	cranial
-graph	write, draw, record	electrocardiograph	cyt	cell	leukocyte
			dent	teeth	dentine, dental
-ia	a noun ending of a condition	leukemia	derm	skin	subdermal
			fibr	fiber	fibrositis
-ic	a noun/adjective ending	pelvic, hypodermic	gastr(o)	stomach	gastritis
			gyn	woman	gynecology
-ist	one who does	artist, antagonist	hem	blood	hematoma
			hepat	liver	hepatitis
			hist	tissue	histology
Word Part	Definition	Example	labi	lip	quadratus labii
-itis	inflammation	arthritis	my(o)	muscle	myology
-oid	resembling	styloid, lipoid	nephr(o)	kidney	nephritis
-ology	study of, science of	biology	neur(o)	nerve	neurology
-oma	tumor	carcinoma	ocul	eye	ocular
-ostomy	forming an opening	colostomy	oss, ost(e)	bone	osteoblast
-otomy	excision, cutting into	lobotomy	phleb	vein	phlebitis
-pathic	diseased	psychopathic	pneum	lung	pneumonia
-phobia	morbid fear of	claustrophobia	pod	foot	podiatrist
-tomy	surgical procedure	colostomy	psych	mind	psychologist
COMMON WORD ROOTS OF STEMS			pulmo	lung	cardiopulmonary
			therm	heat	thermometer
Word Part	Definition	Example	vas	vessel	vascular
aur	ear	auricular			
arth(ro)	joint	arthritis			

QUESTIONS FOR DISCUSSION AND REVIEW

1. What is anatomy?

2. What is physiology?

3. What is histology?

4. What is pathology?

5. Define *disease*.

6. Differentiate between a sign and a symptom of a disease.

7. What is the physiological reaction to stress?

8. What is the physical reaction of the body to pain?

9. Describe what is meant by the pain-spasm-pain cycle.

10. Describe the role of the massage therapist in breaking the pain-spasm-pain cycle.

11. Explain the difference between infection and inflammation.

12. What are the four principal signs and symptoms of inflammation?

13. What is fever?

14. When does fever become dangerous?

15. How are medical terms constructed?

16. What do the parts of a medical term generally indicate?

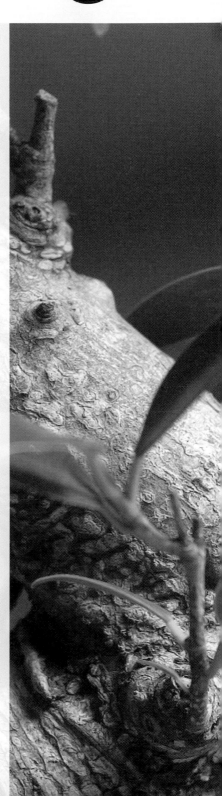

Human Anatomy and Physiology

LEARNING OBJECTIVES

After you have mastered this chapter, you will be able to:

1. Demonstrate knowledge of basic human anatomy and physiology as a requisite in mastering the theory and practice of therapeutic massage.

2. Name the anatomical planes, regions, cavities, and parts of the body.

3. Name the 10 most important body systems.

4. Explain the structures and functions of the various body systems.

INTRODUCTION

An elementary knowledge of anatomy, physiology, kinesiology, and pathology is necessary in mastering the theory and practice of therapeutic massage. To obtain the most beneficial results, the practitioner who knows the principles of anatomy, physiology, and kinesiology is better able to adjust the massage treatment to the needs of the client and to maximize desired results. An understanding of pathology is important so that the practitioner can recognize certain irregularities or conditions and make appropriate decisions to either work on a client or refer that client to a doctor for further diagnosis.

Anatomy (a-**NAT**-o-mee) is the science of **morphology** (morf-**AL**-o-jee) or structure of an organism or body. *Physiology* (fiz-ee-**OL**-o-jee) concerns the normal functions performed by the various systems of the body. *Histology* (his-**TOL**-o-jee) is a form of microscopic anatomy. It is the branch of biology concerned with the microscopic structure of tissues of a living organism. *Pathology* (path-**OL**-o-jee) is the study of disease and disease processes. *Kinesiology* (kin-ee-see-**OL**-o-jee) is the scientific study of muscular activity and the mechanics of body movement. Through clear understanding of the structures involved in body movement, the massage therapist is better able to identify the areas of pain and/or dysfunction when working with clients.

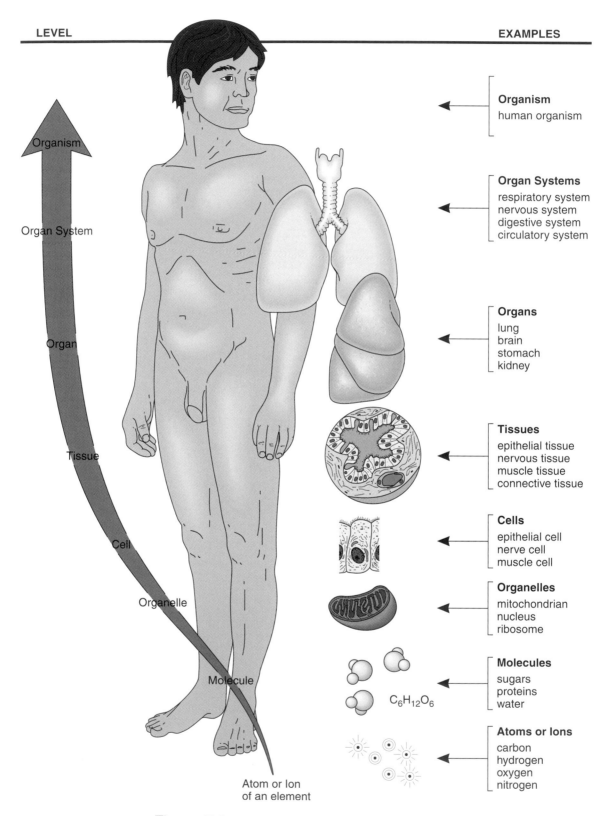

LEVEL

EXAMPLES

Organism

Organism
human organism

Organ System

Organ Systems
respiratory system
nervous system
digestive system
circulatory system

Organ

Organs
lung
brain
stomach
kidney

Tissue

Tissues
epithelial tissue
nervous tissue
muscle tissue
connective tissue

Cells
epithelial cell
nerve cell
muscle cell

Cell

Organelle

Organelles
mitochondrian
nucleus
ribosome

Molecule

Molecules
sugars
proteins
water

$C_6H_{12}O_6$

Atoms or Ions
carbon
hydrogen
oxygen
nitrogen

Atom or Ion
of an element

Figure 5.1

Levels of complexity of the human organism.

LEVELS OF COMPLEXITY OF LIVING MATTER

All substances are made of subatomic particles that form **atoms**. Atoms are arranged in specific patterns and structures called **molecules**. Molecules are arranged in such a way as to produce compounds and matter. Within the human organism, the basic unit of structure and function is the **cell**. Cells are organized into layers or groups called **tissues**. Groups of tissues form complex structures that perform certain functions. These structures, called **organs,** are arranged in **organ systems**. Organ systems are arranged to form an organism. The human body is the organism we study in relation to therapeutic massage (Figure 5.1).

CELLS

All living matter is composed of **protoplasm** (**PRO**-to-plazm), a colorless, jelly-like substance in which food elements, such as protein, fats, carbohydrates, mineral salts, and water, are present. Cells are the basic functional units of all living matter of animals, plants, and bacteria. Living cells differ from one another in size, shape, structure, and function. In the human body, cells are highly specialized to perform such vital functions as movement, digestion, thought, and reproduction.

The principal parts of a cell are the **cytoplasm** (**SIGH**-to-plazm), **nucleus,** and **cell membrane.** A thin cell membrane or wall separates one cell from another and permits soluble substances such as nutrients and waste products to enter and leave the cytoplasm. Near the center of the cell is a nucleus (dense protoplasm). Outside the nucleus is the cytoplasm (less dense protoplasm).

The cytoplasm contains a network of various membranes that mark off several distinct parts called **cytoplasmic organelles** (Figure 5.2). Organelles perform specific functions necessary for cell survival. (See Table 5.1.) The centrosome and nucleus control cell reproduction. As long as the cell receives an adequate supply of food, oxygen, and water, eliminates waste products, and is surrounded by a favorable environment (proper temperature and the absence of waste products, toxins, and pressure), it will continue to grow and function. When these requirements are not provided, the cell will stop growing and will eventually die.

Cell Division

The human body is composed of more than 100 trillion cells, which develop from a single cell, the fertilized ovum (egg). During the early developmental stages, the repeated division of the ovum results in many specialized cells that differ from one another in composition and function. This process is **differentiation** (dif-er-en-shee-A-shun).

After the tissues and organs of the organism have developed, growth and maintenance of the various tissues are carried on through cell division. As a cell matures and is nourished, it grows in size and eventually

| **morphology** |
| is the structure of an organism or body. |

| **atoms** |
| consist of subatomic particles that all substances are composed of. |

| **molecules** |
| are specific arrangements of atoms. |

| **cells** |
| are basic functional units of all living matter. |

| **tissues** |
| are collections of similar cells that carry out specific bodily functions. |

| **organs** |
| a combination of tissues and cells that form a complex structure to perform a certain function within the system. |

| **organ system** |
| is a number of organs working together to perform a bodily function. |

| **protoplasm** |
| is a colorless, jelly-like substance in which food elements, such as protein, fats, carbohydrates, mineral salts, and water, are present. |

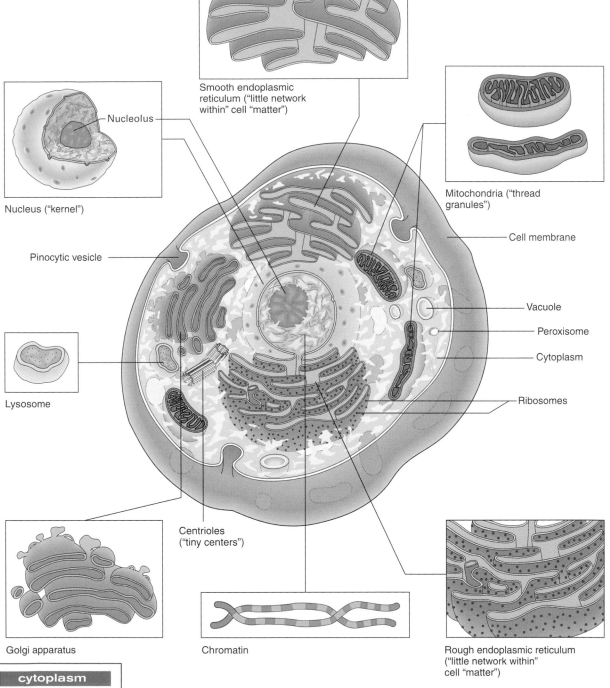

Smooth endoplasmic reticulum ("little network within" cell "matter")

Nucleolus

Nucleus ("kernel")

Pinocytic vesicle

Lysosome

Mitochondria ("thread granules")

Cell membrane

Vacuole

Peroxisome

Cytoplasm

Ribosomes

Golgi apparatus

Centrioles ("tiny centers")

Chromatin

Rough endoplasmic reticulum ("little network within" cell "matter")

cytoplasm

all of the substance within the cell wall other than the nucleus.

nucleus

the main central body of living cells that contains the genetic information for continuing life.

Figure 5.2

Structure of a typical animal cell.

divides into two smaller daughter/like) cells. This form of cell division, called **mitosis** (migh-**TO**-sis), produces new cells.

In the human body, some cells reproduce continually, some occasionally, and some not at all. For example, skin and intestinal lining cells are exposed to continuous wear and tear and reproduce continually throughout life. Most body cells are capable of growth and self-repair during their life cycle. However, delicate nerve cells in the cen-

Table 5.1
Structure and Function of Cellular Organelles

An organelle is a discrete structure within a cell, having specialized functions, identifying molecular structures, and a distinctive chemical composition.

ORGANELLE	STRUCTURE	FUNCTION
Cell membrane	A thin covering of the outer surface of the cytoplasm composed of protein and lipid molecules	Transports materials between the outside and inside of the cell, helps to control cell activity and contains cellular material
Centrosome	A nonmembranous structure near the nucleus composed of two rod-shaped centrioles	Divides into two parts during mitosis and moves to the opposite poles of the dividing cell; helps to distribute the chromosomes into the daughter cells
Chromatin	Network of fibers composed of protein and DNA that form the chromosomes	Contains the genes by which hereditary characteristics are transmitted and determined
Endoplasmic reticulum	Network of sacs and canals connected to the cell membrane, the nuclear membrane, and other organelles	There are two varieties: a smooth type that produce lipid and a rough type that has ribosomes attached to its surface; provides for the transportation of materials withn the cell
Fibrils and microtubules	Minute rods and tubules	Support the cytoplasm and contribute to movement of substances within the cytoplasm
Golgi apparatus	Composed of flattened membranes and small vesicles	Collects the products of cell synthesis, synthesizes carbohydrates, holds protein molecules for secretion
Lysosome	Membranous structure containing hydrolytic enzymes	Digests proteins, carbohydrates, and other foreign substances that enter the cell
Mitochondria	Shape varies according to function, but all exhibit a double membrane with the inner membrane lifted into folds	Contains enzymes for releasing energy and converting it to useful forms for cell operation; in the form of adenosine triphosphate (ATP)
Nuclear membrane	The covering structure of the nucleus that separates the nucleus and the cytoplasm	Controls passage of substances between the nucleus and the cytoplasm
Nucleolus	A dense body composed mainly of protein with some RNA molecules, and found in the nucleus of most cells	Forms ribosomes
Nucleus	Protein-coated heredity material (DNA) containing chromosomes that transmit heredity	Supervises all cell activity
Ribosome	Minute particle or granule composed of RNA and protein molecules	Synthesizes proteins
Vacuole	Membrane-lined containers	Involved in rapid ejection of fluids or introduction of substances

tral nervous system are incapable of self-repair after injury or destruction and disease.

From the time the cell forms until it reproduces is the life cycle of a cell. In the human body, when a cell reaches maturity, reproduction takes place by indirect division or *mitosis,* in which a series of changes occurs in the nucleus before the entire cell divides in half.

Mitosis is accomplished in five stages: interphase, prophase, metaphase, anaphase, and telophase.

cell membrane
permits soluble substances to enter and leave the protoplasm.

cytoplasmic organelles

a discrete structure within a cell, having specialized functions, identifying molecular structures, and a distinctive chemical composition.

differentiation

is the repeated division of the ovum during early developmental stages, resulting in specialized cells that differ from one another.

mitosis

is the process of cell division in which a cell divides into two cells identical to the parent cell.

amitosis

is a process of cell division in which the nucleus and cytoplasm split in two.

1. *Interphase:* This is a normal state of the cell during which most of the cellular work and growth are done. During interphase, chromosomes exist in thin threads. It is during mitosis that the chromosomes assume the twin helical (rodlike) structure.

2. *Prophase:* Prophase occurs when the chromosomes, composed of DNA (deoxyribonucleic acid), which houses the genes, become larger and more defined. They can be seen within the cell duplicated in two coiled strands called *chromatids* (**KRO**-muh-tids). During the last part of prophase, the nuclear membrane disappears.

3. *Metaphase:* During metaphase, the chromosomes arrange themselves in a plane called the equatorial plane. The nuclear membrane and the nucleolus are absent.

4. *Anaphase:* During anaphase, the chromatids are separated and are again called chromosomes.

5. *Telophase:* This is the stage when the chromosomes reach the centrioles (small bodies) and begin to uncoil. The cytoplasm divides into two parts or two cells (Figure 5.3).

Direct division of a cell, **amitosis** (a-mi-**TO**-sis), is the method of reproduction in which the nucleus and cytoplasm divide by simple construction without the duplicating of chromosomes.

Cellular Activity

The activity of cells may be divided into three categories: vegetative, growth and reproduction, and specialized.

1. *Vegetative:* Vegetative activities include maintenance of the cell such as absorption, assimilation, and excretion of waste products.

2. *Growth and reproduction:* Growth involves the development of additional structural materials. Reproduction is the process of mitosis or indirect division of cells. The centriole and nucleus play important roles in this process.

3. *Specialized activities:* Because of cell differentiation (see Figure 5.4), different cells perform different functions. For example, muscle cells exhibit contractility. Epithelial cells secrete and absorb. Nerve cells transmit nerve impulses. The cell is usually in the vegetative state, and then as time passes it either grows and reproduces or undergoes regression (atrophy) and finally dies.

metabolism

is the process taking place in living organisms whereby the cells are nourished and carry out their activities.

Metabolism

As the basic units of life, cells perform individually much like small factories. All chemical reactions within a cell that transform food for cell growth and operation are broadly termed *cellular metabolism.* **Metabolism** is the complex chemical and physical process that takes place in living

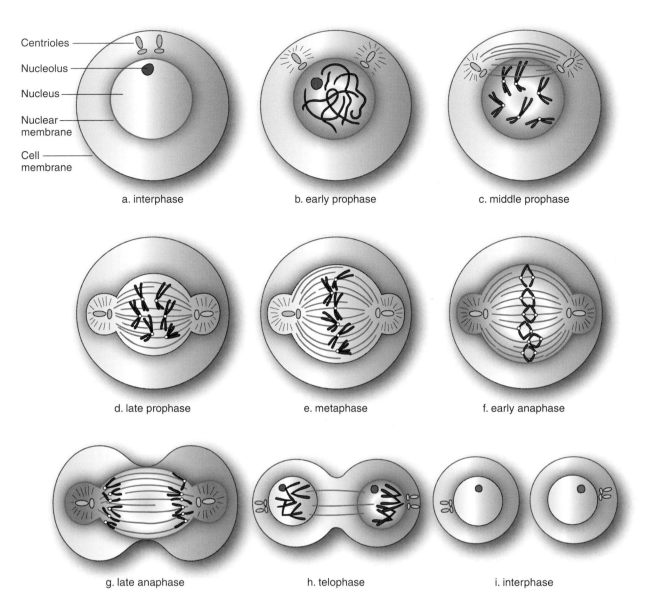

Figure 5.3

Stages of mitosis in animal cells.

a. Interphase
b. Early prophase
c. Middle prophase
d. Late prophase
e. Metaphase
f. Early anaphase
g. Late anaphase
h. Telophase
i. Interphase

organisms whereby the cells are nourished and carry out their various activities. Different kinds of cells perform specialized metabolic processes; however, all cells perform basic reactions that include the building up or breaking down of proteins, carbohydrates, fats, and other nutrients. There are two phases of metabolism: anabolism and catabolism. **Anabolism** (a-NAB-o-lizm) is the process of building up of larger molecules from smaller ones. This process requires energy because it is the constructive phase of cellular metabolism during which substances needed for cell growth and repair are manufactured. **Catabolism** (ka-TAB-o-lizm) is the breaking down of larger substances or molecules into

anabolism

is the process of building up of larger molecules from smaller ones.

catabolism

is the breaking down of larger substances into smaller ones.

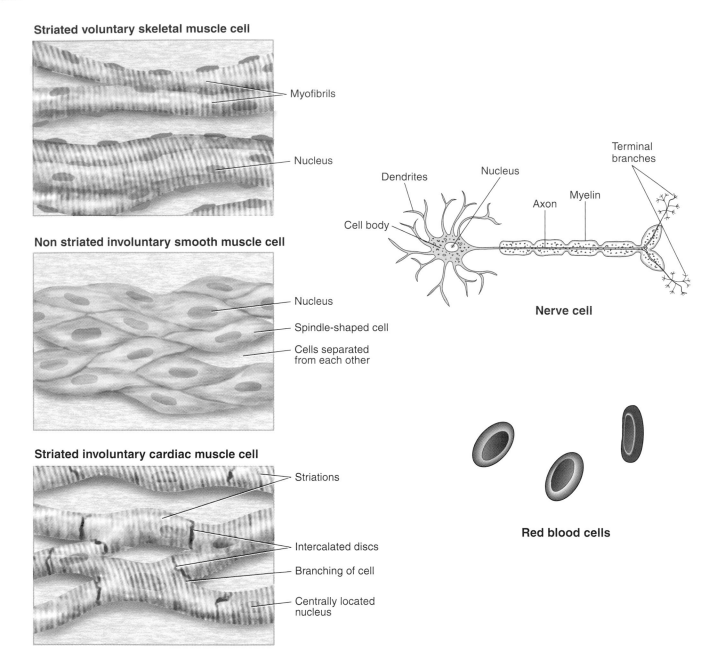

Figure 5.4
Variations in specialized cells.

smaller ones. This process releases energy that may be stored by special molecules to be used for other reactions, such as muscle contraction or heat production.

Anabolism and catabolism are carried out simultaneously and continuously in the cells. Their activities are closely regulated so that the breaking-down or energy-releasing reactions are balanced with building-up or energy-using reactions. Therefore, homeostasis (the maintenance of normal, internal stability in an organism) is maintained.

ENZYMES

Enzymes are protein substances that act as organic catalysts to initiate, accelerate, or control specific chemical reactions in the metabolic process while the enzymes themselves remain unchanged. The reaction promoted by a particular enzyme is very specific. Because cellular metabolism includes hundreds of different chemical reactions, there are hundreds of different kinds of enzymes.

Enzymes are involved in the process of releasing energy from nutrients, principally from carbohydrates, fats, and proteins. Energy is the capacity to produce change in matter or to do work. During the digestive process, carbohydrates are broken down into simple sugars (glucose), fats are split into fatty acids, and proteins are converted into amino acids. These materials are absorbed by the blood and transported to the cells of the body, where they become the fuel for cell metabolism. As they are further broken down into other compounds, energy is released. Some of this energy is in the form of heat, while some is used to carry on the various cellular functions or to promote further cellular metabolism. Some energy may be stored in a special molecule called **adenosine** (a-**DEN**-o-seen) **triphosphate (ATP)**. ATP stores the energy until it is needed for muscular and other cellular activity.

> **enzymes**
> are proteins that act as catalysts for chemical reactions in metabolism while remaining unchanged themselves.

> **adenosine triphosphate (ATP)**
> a molecule that stores energy in the body and releases it when it breaks down into ADP.

TISSUES

The basic unit of tissue is the cell. Tissues are collections of similar cells that carry out specific functions of the body. Tissues comprise all body organs and are subdivided into five main categories:

1. Epithelial tissue

2. Connective tissue

3. Muscular tissue

4. Nervous tissue

5. Liquid tissue

The human body develops from a single cell. By the second week of growth of a human fetus (the embryonic stage), distinct layers of cells develop. The innermost layer of cells is called the **endoderm,** the middle layer is the **mesoderm,** and the outermost layer is called the **ectoderm.** These layers form the primary germ layer, which in turn forms all tissues and organs of the body.

The endodermal (inner layer) cells produce the epithelial linings of the respiratory and digestive tracts as well as linings of the urethra and urinary bladder. The mesodermal (middle layer) cells develop into all types of muscle, bone, blood, blood vessel tissues, various connective tissues, lymph, and the linings of all body cavities as well as the kidneys and the reproductive organs. The ectodermal (outer layer) cells form the glands of the skin, linings of the mouth, the anal canal, the epidermis, hair, nails, and the nervous system.

> **endoderm**
> is the innermost layer of cells of the zygote.

> **mesoderm**
> is the middle layer of cells of the zygote.

> **ectoderm**
> is the outermost layer of cells of the zygote.

Epithelial Tissue

> **epithelial tissue**
>
> is a protective layer that functions in the processes of absorption, excretion, secretion, and protection.

Epithelial tissue is a thin protective layer or covering that functions in the process of absorption, excretion, secretion, and protection. There are various classifications of epithelial tissue named according to the shape or number of layers of cells. Epithelial cells are classified by shape as *squamous* (**SKWA**-muhs) (flat), *cuboidal* (small cube shape), and *columnar* (tall or rectangular). These cells are also classified according to arrangement. For example, a simple squamous arrangement is one cell thick, the stratified squamous arrangement is several cells thick, and the transitional squamous is an arrangement of several layers of cells that are flat and closely packed (Figure 5.5).

Epithelial tissue covers all the surfaces of the body both inside and out. It forms the skin, the covering of the organs, and the inner lining of all the hollow organs. It also makes up the major tissue of the glands. Because epithelial tissue acts as a surface covering or a lining, it always has a free surface that is exposed to outside influences, whereas the other surface is well anchored in the connective tissue from which it derives nourishment.

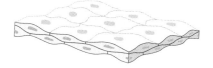

Simple squamous

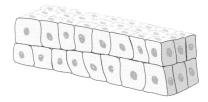

Cuboidal

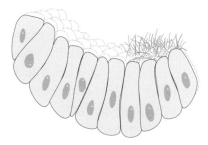

Simple columnar

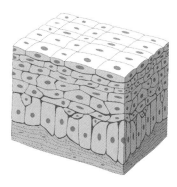

Stratified squamous

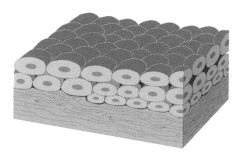

Transitional squamous

Figure 5.5
Types of epithelial tissue.

Membranes

Membranes are structures closely associated with epithelial tissue. There are two main categories of membranes: epithelial membranes and fibrous connective tissue membranes. *Epithelial membranes* have their outer surface faced with epithelium. They are further divided into two main subgroups: mucous membranes and serous membranes. *Mucous membranes* produce mucous, a thick, sticky substance that acts as a protectant and lubricant. Mucous membranes line the surfaces of the digestive and upper respiratory tracts. In some instances their secretions contain a high number of enzymes that perform specific actions, such as digestion.

Serous membranes produce serous fluid, a watery substance that also acts as a lubricant. Serous membranes line the body cavities and sometimes form the outermost surface of the organs contained in those cavities. The covering of the serous membranes in the body cavities is a special epithelial tissue called the *mesothelium* (mez-o-THEE-lee-um). This is a smooth covering that allows the movements of the organs to take place with little or no friction. Three major serous membranes are the pleura that encase the lungs, the pericardium around the heart, and peritoneum that lines the abdominal cavity.

Skeletal membrane covers bones and cartilage. The membrane covering bone is the **periosteum** (per-ee-**OS**-tee-um). The membrane covering cartilage is the **perichondrium** (per-i-**KON**-dree-um). Cavities and capsules in and around joints are lined with a connective tissue membrane called **synovial membrane,** which secretes synovium, or synovial fluid, an agent that acts as a lubricant between the ends of bones in the joint cavity and in spaces of great activity and friction. There are many other membranes in the body. All can be classified as either epithelial or connective.

Connective Tissue

Connective tissue binds structures together, provides support and protection, and serves as a framework. There is an abundance of intercellular substance (matrix) in connective tissue, consisting of fibers and thick, gel-like fluid.

The loose connective tissue, or **areolar** (a-**REE**-o-lar) **tissue,** binds the skin to the underlying tissues and fills the spaces between the muscles. This is the tissue that lies beneath most layers of epithelium and is also known as **superficial fascia.** It is rich in blood vessels and provides nourishment to the epithelial tissues. **Adipose tissue** is areolar tissue that has an abundance of fat-containing cells. Adipose tissue acts as a protection against heat loss and stores energy in the form of fat molecules. It is found in abundance in certain abdominal membranes, and around the surface of the heart, between the muscles, around the kidneys, and just beneath the skin.

---

skeletal membrane
covers bone and cartilage.

periosteum
is a fibrous membrane that functions to protect the bone and serves as an attachment of tendons and ligaments.

perichondrium
is the membrane covering cartilage.

synovial membrane
is a connective tissue membrane lining cavities and capsules in and around joints.

areolar tissue
is loose connective tissue that binds the skin to the underlying tissues and fills the spaces between the muscles.

superficial fascia
refers to the connecting layer between the skin and those structures underlying the skin.

adipose tissue
is areolar tissue with an abundance of fat cells.

reticular tissue
is composed of fibers that form the framework of the liver and lymphoid organs.

fibrous connective tissue
is composed of collagen and elastin fibers that are closely arranged to form tendons and ligaments.

tendons
are bands that attach muscle to bone.

ligaments
are bands of fibrous tissue that connect bones to bones.

fascia
fibrous connective tissue that forms a network throughout the body, surrounding every structure to support, separate, and give shape to the body.

deep fascia
refers to fibrous tissue sheaths that penetrate deep into the body, separating muscle groups.

fibrocartilage
is found between the vertebrae and pubic symphysis.

Reticular tissue resembles fine fibers when viewed under a microscope. These fibers form the framework of the liver and lymphoid organs. **Fibrous connective tissue** is composed of collagen (albuminoid substance) and elastic fibers that are closely arranged to form tendons and ligaments. **Tendons** or *sinews* are white, glistening cords or bands that serve to attach muscle to bone. **Ligaments** are tough, fibrous bands that connect bones to bones or support viscera.

Fascia

Fascia is a type of connective tissue that forms a fibrous network under the skin from the top of the skull to the tips of the toes and throughout the body. It is a continuous membranous envelope that glistens with a sticky lubricating fluid, surrounding every organ, every blood vessel, every nerve, every bone, and every muscle. Fascia is composed of collagen and elastin fibers in viscous, gel-like ground substance. It envelops, supports, separates, and gives shape to the body and its component parts. Fascia provides form and cohesiveness and at the same time allows movement between different structures without irritation. It has different names according to its location. Around the brain and spinal cord it is the meninges. Around the heart, it is the pericardium. In the abdominal cavity, it is the peritoneum. The layer just under the skin is the superficial fascia, whereas **deep fascia** envelops and permeates the skeletal muscles. Deep fascia covers each muscle fiber (endomysium), the muscle fascicles (perimysium), the whole muscle (epimysium), and groups of muscles (investing fascia). Each layer of deep fascia is invested into the next. Fascia in muscles organize and separate the muscle fibers, allowing them to move independently while at the same time directing the muscle contraction into the muscle attachments, thereby creating movement. Muscles and fascia are anatomically inseparable. Without fascia, muscle would be without form or functionality. Fascia also provide support and pathways for nerves, blood, and lymph vessels. All fascia throughout the body is continuous (Figure 5.6).

Cartilage

Fibrocartilage

Fibrocartilage is found between the vertebrae and in the pubic symphysis where strong support and minimal range of movement are required. In dense fibrous connective tissue, repair to damaged tissue is slower due to low vascularity.

Hyaline (**HIGH**-a-lin) is a type of cartilage that contains little fibrous tissue and is made up of cells embedded in a somewhat translucent matrix, as found in the nose and trachea and on the end of bones and in movable joints.

Elastic cartilage is the most resilient of cartilages and is found in the external ear, the larynx, and like structures.

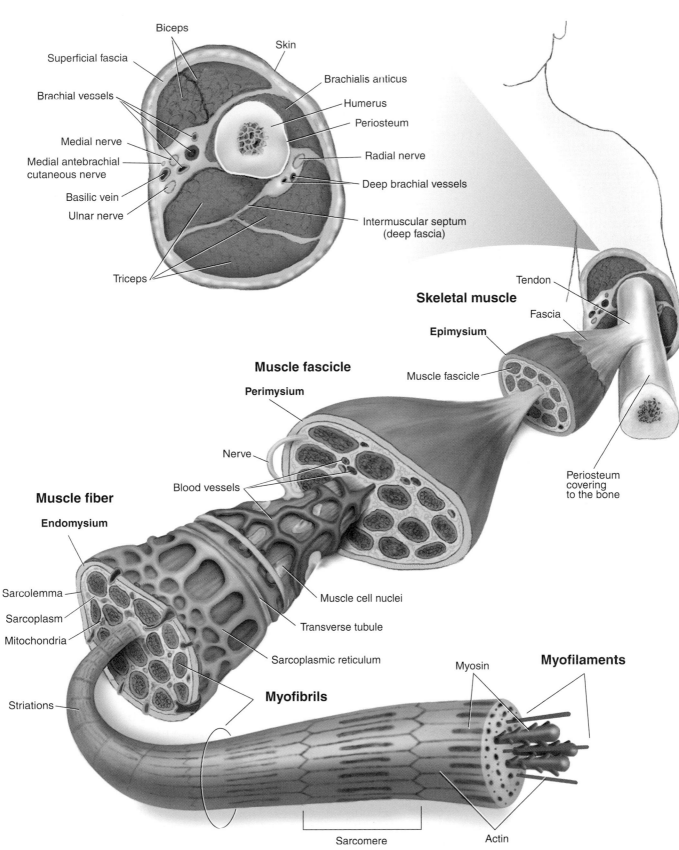

Figure 5.6

Planes of fascia form compartments—cross section of the arm.

bone tissue
is connective tissue in which the intercellular substance is rendered hard by mineral salts, chiefly calcium carbonate and calcium phosphate.

Bone Tissue

Bone or osseous (bonelike) tissue is connective tissue in which the intercellular substance is rendered hard by being impregnated with mineral salts, chiefly calcium phosphate and calcium carbonate. Compact, dense material forms the dense, outer layer of a long bone; cancellous (porous) material forms the bone's inner tissue. Dentine, the substance beneath the enamel of the teeth, closely resembles bone but is harder and denser. Unlike bone, dentine contains no distinct cells or blood vessels.

Muscle Tissue

The main function of muscle tissue fibers is to contract their elongated cells, which pulls attached ends closer together, causing a body part to move. The three types of muscle tissue are skeletal muscle tissue, smooth muscle tissue, and cardiac muscle tissue (Figure 5.7).

Skeletal muscles are usually attached to bone or other muscle by way of tendons and can be controlled by conscious effort. These are called **voluntary muscles**. Skeletal muscles are responsible for moving the limbs of the body, facial expression, speaking, and other voluntary movements. Voluntary muscle cells appear long and threadlike under a microscope and have alternating light and dark cross-markings called *striations* (strigh-A-shuns). Muscles containing striations are called *striated muscles*.

Smooth muscle tissue lacks striations (nonstriated) and cannot usually be stimulated to contract by conscious effort. Smooth muscle contractions generally result from involuntary nerve or gland activity. Smooth muscle tissue is found in the hollow organs of the stomach, small intestine, colon, bladder, and the blood vessels. Nonstriated muscle is responsible for the movement of food through the digestive tract, the constriction of blood vessels, and the emptying of the bladder.

Cardiac muscle tissue occurs only in the heart. It is controlled involuntarily and can continue to function without being directly stimulated by

Striated voluntary skeletal muscle cell

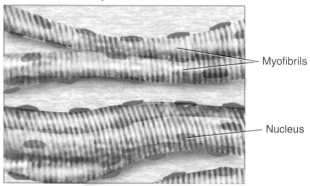

— Myofibrils

— Nucleus

Non-striated involuntary smooth muscle cell

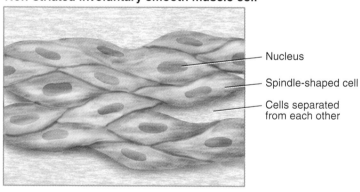

— Nucleus

— Spindle-shaped cell

— Cells separated from each other

Striated involuntary cardial muscle cell

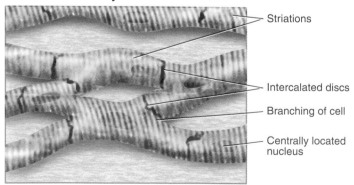

— Striations

— Intercalated discs

— Branching of cell

— Centrally located nucleus

Figure 5.7

Types of muscle tissue.

nerve impulses. Cardiac tissue is responsible for pumping blood through the heart into the blood vessels.

Nerve Tissue

Nervous or **nerve tissue** is composed of **neurons** (**NOOR**-ons) (nerve cells) and is found in the brain, spinal cord, and associated nerves. Nerves are sensitive to specific types of stimuli from their environment and are able to transmit impulses through specialized extensions of their cell bodies to other nerves, the brain, and muscles. Nerves act as channels for the transmission of messages to and from the brain and various parts of the body, such as sensory nerves in the skin and organs of hearing, taste, smell, and sight. Nervous tissue initiates, controls, and coordinates the body's adaptation to its surroundings. Neurons (nerve cells) are linked together to form nerve pathways.

Liquid Tissue

Liquid tissue is connective tissue represented by blood and lymph. Blood is a fluid tissue that circulates throughout the body and from which the body cells obtain nutrients and by which waste products are removed. Lymph is derived from the blood and tissue fluid and is collected into the lymphatic vessels along with metabolic waste and toxins. Lymphoid tissue found in the lymph nodes (small, compact, knotlike structures) and in the adenoids, thymus, tonsils, and spleen is important in the production of antibodies.

Specialized Types of Tissue

1. *Nervous tissue proper:* Neurons consisting of the cell body and nerve fibers

2. *Neuroglia:* Supportive tissue of the central nervous system

3. *Dentine:* Hard, dense, calcareous tissue forming the body of a tooth beneath the enamel

4. *Hemopoietic:* Tissue found in bone marrow and the vascular system

5. *Bone:* Tissue found in all bones of the skeleton

6. *Lymphoid:* Tissue found in lymph nodes and other compact structures such as the tonsils and adenoids

Loose Connective Tissue

1. Areolar: Fibroelastic tissue

2. Adipose: Tissue containing fat cells

3. Reticular: Provides framework of liver and other lymphoid organs (Figure 5.8)

---

skeletal muscles
are attached to bone by tendons and are responsible for moving the limbs, facial expression, speaking, and other voluntary movements.

voluntary muscles
are skeletal muscles that can be activated by conscious effort.

Smooth muscle tissue
lacks striations and cannot be stimulated to contract by conscious effort.

Cardiac muscle tissue
occurs only in the heart and is responsible for pumping blood through the heart into the blood vessels.

nervous tissue
is composed of neurons and initiates, controls, and coordinates the body's adaptation to its surroundings.

neuron
is the structural unit of the nervous system.

Liquid tissue
is represented by blood and lymph.

Cartilage

1. Hyaline: Fundamental type of cartilage consisting of fine white fibers

2. Fibrous: Characterized by collagenous fiber in the matrix

3. Elastic: Characterized by elastic fibers in the matrix (Figure 5.9)

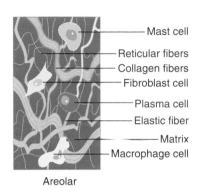

Mast cell
Reticular fibers
Collagen fibers
Fibroblast cell
Plasma cell
Elastic fiber
Matrix
Macrophage cell

Areolar

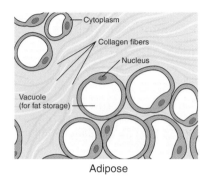

Cytoplasm
Collagen fibers
Nucleus
Vacuole
(for fat storage)

Adipose

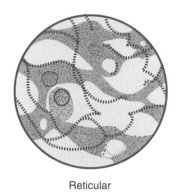

Reticular

Figure 5.8
Loose connective tissue.

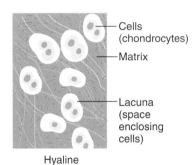

Cells
(chondrocytes)
Matrix
Lacuna
(space
enclosing
cells)

Hyaline

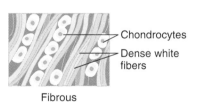

Chondrocytes
Dense white
fibers

Fibrous

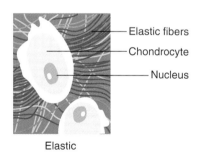

Elastic fibers
Chondrocyte
Nucleus

Elastic

Figure 5.9
Cartilage.

SECTION QUESTIONS FOR DISCUSSION AND REVIEW

1. Why is the cell called the basic unit of all living matter?

2. Name the four principal parts of a cell.

3. Which parts of the cell control reproduction?

4. What conditions are required for a cell to grow and function?

5. By what process does cell reproduction occur in human tissue?

6. Name the five phases of cell mitosis.

7. Name the two phases of metabolism.

8. Explain anabolism.

9. Explain catabolism.

10. What are enzymes and what is their function?

11. Of what substances are tissues composed?

12. Name the five main categories of tissues.

13. What do the terms *endoderm, mesoderm,* and *ectoderm* refer to?

14. Where is epithelial tissue found and what is its function?

15. Name the two main types of membranes.

16. What is the main function of connective tissue?

17. What is the main function of areolar (loose) tissue?

18. What is adipose tissue?

19. Name the three types of cartilage.

20. What makes bone tissue hard?

21. What is dentine?

22. Name the three types of muscle tissue.

23. What is the difference between striated and smooth muscle tissue?

24. In what part of the body is cardiac muscle tissue found?

25. What is the main function of nervous tissue proper?

26. Where is liquid tissue found?

THE ANATOMICAL POSITION OF THE BODY

When studying anatomy, it is helpful to know the anatomical terms that designate specific regions of the body. These terms refer to the body as seen in the **anatomic position,** which shows a figure standing upright with the palms of the hands facing forward.

Anatomists divide the body with three imaginary planes called the sagittal (vertical), the coronal (frontal), and the transverse (horizontal) planes. (See Figure 5.10.)

1. The **sagittal (SAJ-i-tal) plane** divides the body into left and right parts by an imaginary line running vertically down the body. *Mid-sagittal* refers to the plane that divides the body or an organ into right and left halves.

2. The **coronal (KOR-on-al) plane** is an imaginary line that divides the body into the anterior (front) or ventral half of the body and the posterior (back) or dorsal half of the body.

3. The **transverse plane** is an imaginary line that divides the body horizontally into upper and lower portions. A transverse section cuts through a body part perpendicular to the long axis of the body part.

anatomic position
standing with feet shoulder width apart, arms at the side, with the palms of the hands facing forward.

sagittal plane
divides the body into left and right parts.

coronal plane
divides the body into the front and back.

transverse plane
divides the body horizontally into an upper and lower portion.

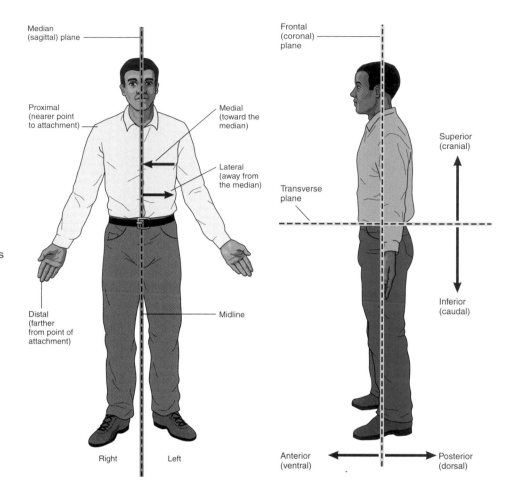

Figure 5.10

Planes of the body in terms of location and position.

ANATOMICAL TERMS AND MEANINGS

The following chart presents anatomical terms and their meaning:

TERM	MEANING
1. Cranial or superior aspect	Situated toward the crown of the head
2. Caudal or inferior aspect	Situated toward the feet
3. Anterior or ventral aspect	Situated before or in front of
4. Posterior or dorsal aspect	Situated behind or in back of
5. Transverse plane	Division of the body into an upper and lower half. Transverse section refers to a plane through a body part perpendicular to the axis, which is the vertical center line around which the body part is arranged.
6. Sagittal plane	Pertaining to the sagittal suture of the cranium. Vertical plane or section dividing the body into right and left sides. A midsagittal section divides the body into equal left and right halves.
7. Coronal plane	Pertaining to the coronal suture of the cranium. The frontal plane or section passes through the long axis of the body, dividing it into front and back halves.
8. Medial aspect	Pertaining to the middle or center, nearer to the midline
9. Lateral aspect	On the side, farther from the midline or center
10. Distal aspect	Farthest point from the origin of a structure or point of attachment. Relatively farther from the median, trunk, or center.
11. Proximal	Nearest the origin of a structure or point of attachment. Relatively nearer to the trunk or median.

BODY CAVITIES AND ORGANS

Once you know the body planes, it is easier to remember where body cavities and organs are located. There are two groups of body cavities: the dorsal or posterior cavities and the ventral or anterior cavities. The *dorsal cavities* contain the brain and spinal cord, with the skull forming the *cranial cavity* and the vertebrae forming the *vertebral* or *spinal cavity*. The *ventral cavities* are the *thoracic cavity* and *abdominopelvic cavities*. The thoracic cavity is subdivided into the pericardial cavity, which contains the heart, and the pleural cavities, which contain the lungs. The abdominal cavity is situated below the diaphragm and contains the liver, stomach, spleen, pancreas, small and large intestines. The *pelvic cavity* is the lower third of the abdominopelvic cavity and contains the bladder, rectum, and some of the reproductive organs (Figure 5.11).

Body Cavities

1. Cranial cavity (dorsal)

2. Spinal cavity (dorsal)

3. Thoracic cavity (ventral)

4. Abdominal cavity (ventral)

5. Pelvic cavity (ventral)

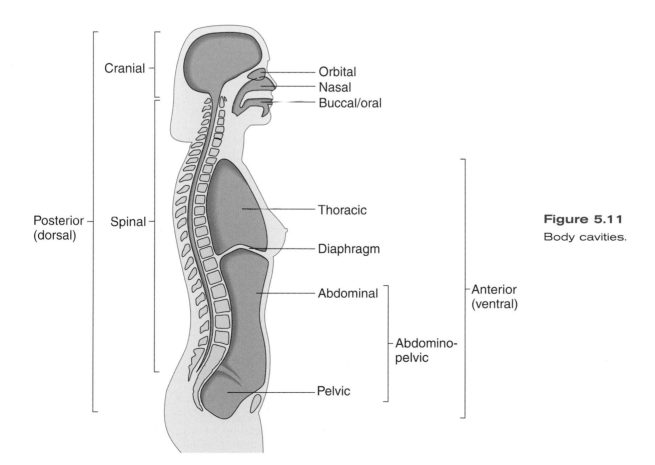

Figure 5.11
Body cavities.

THE REGIONS OF THE HUMAN BODY

Knowing the regions of the body helps us pinpoint a particular area of the body. For example, the pectoral muscle is located in the pectoral or chest region. The brachial nerve is located in the brachial region. The lower back is the lumbar region. Study the illustrations of regions of the body until you can locate each region and name the parts of the body associated with each region.

Anterior View of the Human Body Regions

1. *Frontal:* Region of the head

2. *Temporal:* Region of the temples

3. *Cervical:* Region of the neck

4. *Deltoid:* Region of the shoulder joint and deltoid muscle

5. *Axillary:* Region of the armpit

6. *Brachial:* Region between the elbow and shoulder

7. *Hypochondrium:* Region of the abdomen lateral to the epigastric region

8. *Umbilical:* Region of the navel (umbilicus); the middle of the three median abdominal regions, below the epigastric region and above the pubic region

9. *Hypogastric:* Region under the stomach and inferior to the umbilical region

10. *Patellar:* Region of the knees and kneecap

11. *Femoral:* Region of the femur or thigh

12. *Inguinal:* Region of the groin

13. *Epigastric:* Region of the abdomen

14. *Pectoral:* Region of the breast and chest (Figure 5.12)

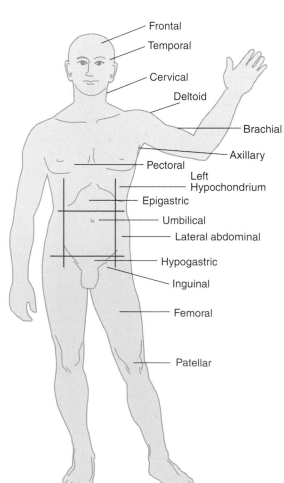

Frontal
Temporal
Cervical
Deltoid
Brachial
Axillary
Pectoral
Left Hypochondrium
Epigastric
Umbilical
Lateral abdominal
Hypogastric
Inguinal
Femoral
Patellar

Figure 5.12

Regions of the body, anterior view. Areas or regions of the body have been identified and named to aid in locating and describing the location of anatomical structures and conditions.

Figure 5.13
Regions of the body, posterior view. Regions of the body are generally named for underlying bones, joints, muscles, or other anatomical structures in the immediate area.

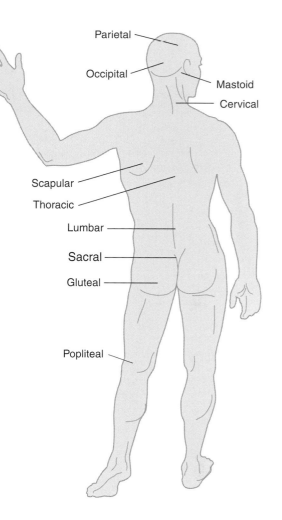

Posterior View of the Human Body Regions

1. *Occipital:* Region of the back of the head

2. *Parietal:* Region of the head, posterior to the frontal region and anterior to the occipital region

3. *Mastoid:* Region of the temporal bone behind the ear

4. *Cervical:* Region of the neck

5. *Scapular:* Region of the back of the shoulder or shoulder blade

6. *Lumbar:* Region of the lower back

7. *Sacral:* Region over the sacrum, below the low back and between the gluteals

8. *Gluteal:* Region of muscles of the buttocks

9. *Popliteal:* A diamond-shaped area behind the knee joint (Figure 5.13)

THE STRUCTURE OF THE HUMAN BODY

The main anatomical parts of the body are the following:

1. The head

2. The spine

3. The trunk

4. The extremities

The head is subdivided into

- *The cranium:* The upper portion of the head housing the brain.

- *The face:* The front and lower part of the skull including the eyes, nose, and mouth.

The spine is a column of bones that supports the head and trunk of the body and protects the spinal cord.

The trunk is subdivided into

- *The thorax or chest:* The upper part of the trunk containing the ribs, lungs, heart, esophagus (food tube), and part of the trachea or windpipe.

- *The abdomen:* Situated below the diaphragm, containing the stomach, intestines, liver, and kidneys. The diaphragm is a muscular partition located between the thoracic cavity and the *abdominal cavity*. It is the main muscle associated with breathing. The *pelvic cavity* is located below the abdomen and contains the bladder, reproductive organs, lower bowel, and rectum.

  The extremities include

- *The upper limbs:* The shoulder, arm, wrist, and hand.
- *The lower limbs:* The hip, thigh, leg, ankle, and foot.

Body Organs

Body organs are structures containing two or more major different tissues that combine to accomplish a definite function. Among the major organs of the body are the brain, heart, lungs, kidneys, liver, sense organs, organs of digestion, and the organs of reproduction.

Organ Systems

When a number of organs work together to perform a bodily function, they comprise an organ system. Systems carry on specific functions but are not independent units. All the body organ systems cooperate for a common purpose, namely the maintenance or function of the entire organism.

The human body is composed of the following 10 important organ systems (see Table 5.2):

1. Integumentary system (skin)
2. Skeletal system
3. Muscular system
4. Circulatory system (blood-vascular and lymph-vascular)
5. Nervous system
6. Endocrine system
7. Digestive system
8. Respiratory system
9. Excretory system (including urinary system)
10. Reproductive system

The Integumentary System

> **integumentary system**
>
> is composed of the skin, hair, and nails. See also Skin.

The skin is the largest organ of the body. It is often referred to as the outer covering or the **integumentary** (in-teg-you-**MEN**-ta-ree) **system.** The skin's functions include protection, heat regulation, secretion and excretion, sensation, absorption, and respiration.

The Skeletal System

The skeletal system is the structure and hard framework on which the other body systems depend for support and protection. The skeletal system is the physical foundation of the body. It is composed of differently shaped bones united by movable and immovable joints. The main function of the skeletal system is to serve as a means of protection, support, and attachment for muscles of locomotion.

The Muscular System

The muscular system is made up of voluntary and involuntary muscles that are necessary for movement of the parts of the body. The muscular system covers and shapes the skeleton. Practically every contraction and movement of the body is due to the action of the muscles. The obvious movements of the arms and hands, the contraction of the heart and stomach, and the changes in facial expression are the direct result of muscular activity.

The Circulatory System (Blood-Vascular and Lymph-Vascular)

The circulatory (vascular) system controls the circulation of blood and lymph throughout the body. It consists of two divisions: the blood-vascular system and the lymph-vascular system. The blood-vascular system includes the heart and blood vessels (arteries, veins, and capillaries). The pumping action of the heart distributes the vital fluids through the blood vessels to all parts of the body. The blood acts as a two-way carrier of supplies, bringing oxygen and food materials to the cells and taking away waste products and secretions from the tissues.

The lymph (a clear, yellow fluid) bathes all cells and assists in the exchange of supplies required by the cells and carries waste and impurities away from the cells. The lymph-vascular system consists of lymph, lymph nodes, and lymph vessels (lymphatics) through which the lymph circulates. The lymph system also includes the spleen, thymus, tonsils, and adenoids.

The Nervous System

The nervous or neurological system controls and coordinates all the body systems, helping them to work efficiently and harmoniously. The neurological system includes all the nerves of the body, spinal cord, and the brain. It is a highly developed and sensitive organization of nerve tissues. Through the nervous system, the individual is made aware of his existence and relationship to the outside world. Nerves, branching out from the brain and spinal cord, coordinate all voluntary and involuntary functions of the body.

The Endocrine System

The endocrine system represents a group of specialized organs or glands capable of manufacturing secretions called hormones that affect many functions of the body including growth, reproduction, and health. The endocrine glands, such as the pituitary and thyroid, secrete hormones into the blood to regulate the processes of growth and metabolism. Reproduction is made possible by the sex glands and their secretions.

Table 5.2

Organ Systems

SYSTEM	ORGANS IN THE SYSTEM	FUNCTIONS
Integumentary System	Epidermis, dermis, hair, sudoriferous and sebaceous glands	Protects, regulates temperature, secretion, excretion, sensation, absorption, respiration
Skeletal System	Approximately 206 bones united by movable and immovable joints attached by ligaments	Protects organs, supports body structure, and serves as attachments for the muscles of locomotion
Muscular System	Voluntary and involuntary muscles	Supports body structure; produces heat and motion, contractions of the heart, peristalsis of digestion, facial expression, locomotion, and other body movement
Circulatory System	Heart, blood vessels, capillaries, blood, lymph vessels, lymph nodes, and lymph	Controls the movement of blood and lymph throughout the body
Nervous System	Brain, spinal cord, and nerves	Controls and coordinates all the voluntary and involuntary functions of the body's systems
Endocrine System	Pituitary, pineal, thyroid, parathyroid, thymus, adrenals, pancreas, ovaries, testes	Manufactures and secretes various hormones that regulate or affect numerous body functions
Digestive System	Mouth, stomach, intestines, gastric and salivary glands, plus the accessory organs; liver, gallbladder, and pancreas	Breaks down complex food substances to be absorbed into the lymph and blood to be used by body cells
Respiratory System	Lungs and the air passages that lead to the lungs, including the nose, mouth, pharynx, trachea, and bronchial tubes	Absorbs oxygen into and releases carbon dioxide from the blood
Excretory System including the Urinary System	Kidneys, bladder, ureters, urethra, liver, large intestines, skin and lungs	Eliminates waste products from the body
Reproductive System	Female: ovaries, fallopian tubes, uterus, vagina, vulva Male: testes, vas deferens, seminal vesicles, prostate, penis	Provides for reproduction, thereby ensuring the continuation of the species

The Digestive System

The digestive system consists of all the structures involved in the process of digestion including the mouth, stomach, intestines, and salivary and gastric glands. The intestines are part of a continuous tube about 30 feet in length. The function of digestion is to break down complex food substances into simple materials fit to be absorbed and used by the body cells. Various digestive glands including the salivary glands, pancreas, and liver, along with glands in the stomach and small intestine, form and discharge enzymes that act on food in the process of digestion.

The Respiratory System

The respiratory system includes the lungs, air passages, nose, mouth, pharynx, trachea, and bronchial tubes, which lead to the lungs. The blood, as it passes through the lungs, is purified by the removal of carbon dioxide and the intake of oxygen.

The Excretory System

The excretory system includes the skin, kidneys, bladder, liver, lungs, and large intestines, which eliminate waste products from the body. The skin (integumentary system) gives off perspiration. The lungs exhale carbon dioxide gas, the kidneys excrete urine by way of the bladder, and the large intestine discharges digestive refuse from the body. The liver produces bile and urea, which contains certain waste products.

The Reproductive System

The reproductive system is the system whose function it is to ensure continuance of the species by the reproduction of other human beings. In the female, the ovaries discharge an ovum or egg cell that appears prior to menstruation. The testes in the male manufacture sperm cells. The union of the ovum with sperm results in fertilization and conception.

In the following sections of this chapter, each organ system will be discussed in more detail.

SECTION QUESTIONS FOR DISCUSSION AND REVIEW

1. What is anatomic position?

2. What are three anatomical planes of the body?

3. Why is it important to know the anatomical position and the planes and regions of the human body?

4. Name the subdivisions of the ventral and dorsal cavities and the major organs found in each.

5. What are the four main anatomical parts of the body and the structures found in each?

6. Name the 10 important organ systems of the body.

REVIEW

I. Match each term in the left column with the correct definition in the right column.

_____	1. superior	a. farthest from center
_____	2. inferior	b. pertaining to the middle
_____	3. anterior	c. dividing front and back
_____	4. posterior	d. toward the side
_____	5. transverse plane	e. dividing left and right
_____	6. sagittal plane	f. closer to the origin
_____	7. coronal plane	g. toward the top
_____	8. medial	h. dividing upper and lower
_____	9. lateral	i. toward the front
_____	10. distal	j. toward the feet
_____	11. proximal	k. toward the back

II. Match each term in the left column with the correct definition in the right column.

_____	1. cervical	a. region of the groin
_____	2. axillary	b. side of the cranium
_____	3. femoral	c. region of the armpit
_____	4. lumbar	d. behind the knee
_____	5. inguinal	e. inferior to the umbilical region
_____	6. popliteal	f. region of the neck
_____	7. gluteal	g. region of the lower back
_____	8. parietal	h. between the shoulder and elbow
_____	9. hypogastric	i. region of the thigh
_____	10. brachial	j. region of the buttocks

1 THE INTEGUMENTARY SYSTEM—THE SKIN

The word *integument* means covering or skin. The skin is the largest organ of the body and serves as an interface with the environment and protection for the body.

The principal functions of the skin are the following:

1. *Protection:* The skin protects the body from injury and bacterial invasion.

2. *Heat regulation:* The healthy body maintains a constant internal temperature of about 98.6°F (37°C). As changes occur in the outside temperature, the blood and sweat glands of the skin make the necessary adjustments in their functions.

3. *Secretion and excretion:* By means of its sweat (sudoriferous) and oil (sebaceous) glands, the skin acts both as a secretory and an excretory organ. The sudoriferous (sweat) glands excrete (eliminate) perspiration, which is mostly water with a small amount of waste matter. The sebaceous (oil) glands secrete (produce and release) sebum, which is a lubricant. The skin is about 50 to 70 percent moisture. Sebum (oil) coats the surface of the skin and helps to maintain its moisture level. The sebum level slows down evaporation of moisture and keeps excess water from penetrating the skin.

4. *Sensation:* The papillary layer of the dermis provides the body with a sense of touch. Nerves supplying the skin register basic types of sensations, such as heat, cold, pain, pressure, and touch. Nerve endings are most abundant in the fingertips. Complex sensations, such as the feelings of vibration, seem to depend on a combination of these nerve endings.

5. *Absorption:* The skin has limited powers of absorption through its pores. Some cosmetics, chemicals, and drugs can be absorbed in small amounts.

6. *Respiration:* The skin breathes through its pores much as the body breathes through its lungs, but on a much smaller scale. Oxygen is taken in and carbon dioxide is discharged.

The Structure of the Skin

The structure of the skin contains two clearly defined divisions: the **epidermis** (cuticle or scarf), which is the outermost layer, and the **dermis** (corium or true skin), which is the deeper layer that extends to form the subcutaneous tissue.

    Although the epidermis comprises almost a solid sheet of cells, the dermis is a more semisolid mixture of fibers, water, and a gel substance called "ground." There are three kinds of fibers that intermingle with the cells of the dermis: collagen, reticulum, and elastin. Collagen makes up about 70 percent of the dry weight of the skin and gives it strength, form, and flexibility. Reticulum fibers form a fine branching pattern in connective tissue that helps to link the bundles of collagen fibers. Collagen contains a protein called elastin that has elastic properties and helps to give the skin its resiliency. The dermis contains an elastic network of cells through which are distributed nerves, blood and lymph vessels, and sweat and oil glands (Figure 5.14 and Figure 5.15).

The Dermis

The *papillary layer* of the skin (directly beneath the epidermis) contains the papillae, the conelike projections made of fine strands of elastic tissue that extend upward into the epidermis. Some of the papillae contain

epidermis
is the outermost layer of the skin.

dermis
is the deeper layer of the skin that extends to form the subcutaneous tissue.

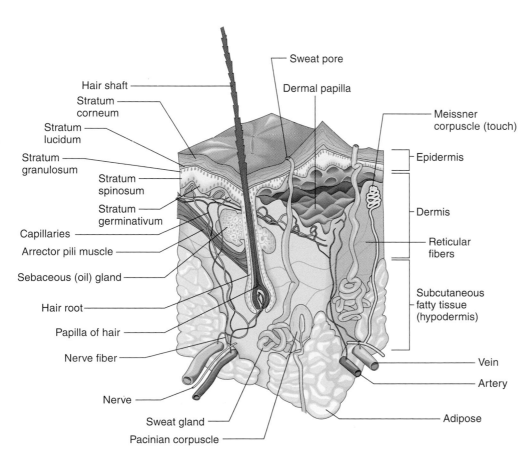

Figure 5.14

The integumentary system (showing skin and hair).

Figure 5.15
Structures in the skin.

15 sebaceous glands

1 yard of blood vessels

10 hairs

700 sweat glands

3,000,000 cells

3000 sensory cells at the end of nerve fibers

1 square centimeter of skin contains:

12 sensory apparatuses for heat

4 yards of nerves

2 sensory apparatuses for cold

25 pressure apparatus for the perception of tactile stimuli

200 nerve endings to record pain

looped capillaries; others contain terminations of nerve fibers called *tactile corpuscles*.

The *reticular layer* of the skin contains fat cells, blood and lymph vessels, sweat and oil glands, hair follicles, and nerve endings.

The **subcutaneous** (sub-kyou-**TAY**-nee-us) **tissue** (subcutis) is regarded as a continuation of the dermis. The subcutaneous tissue is continuous with the superficial fascia, which connects the skin with the underlying structures. It varies in thickness according to the age, sex, and general health of the individual. Fatty (adipose) tissue gives smoothness and contour to the body, provides a reservoir for fuel and energy, and serves as a protective cushion for the upper skin layers.

subcutaneous tissue
is regarded as a continuation of the dermis.

The Epidermis

The epidermis forms a protective layer over every part of the body and varies in thickness, being thickest on the palms of the hands and soles of the feet and thinnest on the inner sides of the limbs. It consists of a number of variable layers of cells.

The *stratum corneum* is the outermost layer. The protoplasm of the cells change into a protein substance called keratin and form a waterproof covering. Next is a layer of clear cells called the *stratum lucidum*.

The *stratum granulosum* (gran-you-**LO**-sum) (granular layer of the skin) consists of cells that look like granules. These cells are almost dead and undergo a change into cells of the more superficial layers.

The *stratum spinosum* (also called stratum mucosum) is of variable thickness and consists of irregularly shaped cells containing *melanin* (**MEL**-a-nin) (coloring matter) of the skin. Melanin helps to protect the sensitive cells from the action of strong solar rays.

The *stratum germinativum* (jer-mi-na-**TEE**-vum) is the deepest layer of the epidermis, comprising a single layer of cells that are well nourished by the dermis. These cells undergo mitosis, pushing other cells closer to the body surface. This layer also contains melanocytes that produce the pigment melanin.

Nutrition and the Skin

Blood and lymph supply nutrients to the skin. As much as one half of the total blood supply of the body is distributed to the skin. Blood and lymph, as they circulate through the skin, contribute certain materials for growth, nourishment, and repair of skin, hair, and nails. In the subcutaneous tissue are found networks of arteries and lymphatics, which send their smaller branches to hair papillae, hair follicles, and the glands of the skin. Capillaries are quite numerous in the skin.

Aging Skin

As people age, the collagen network of the skin tends to lose its elasticity, causing the skin to become less firm and supple. With age, the deeper or dermal layer of the skin undergoes changes. The skin may become thinner, drier, and more prone to growths. It may become lined and crepey. Swelling (edema) of tissues may appear around and under the eyes. Pliability of the skin depends on elasticity of the fibers of the dermis. For example, after expansion healthy skin will regain its former shape almost immediately.

Structural Changes of the Skin

Because the skin is the covering of the entire body, its condition must be taken into consideration before massage treatment is given. The skin may be sensitive to touch, or it may show signs of damage due to disease or injury. The massage practitioner must be aware of any skin condition that may require the attention of the client's physician. Freckles, birthmarks (port-wine stains), and the like present no problem; however, a lesion or any discontinuity of tissue should be reported to the client and referred to a physician before the client receives a massage.

Healthy skin is slightly moist, soft, flexible, and slightly acidic. The texture of skin, revealed by feel and appearance, should be smooth and fine grained. The color of the skin depends partly on the blood supply but more on the coloring matter called melanin. Skin pigment varies in different people and is determined by genetics. Regardless of native pigmentation, healthy skin is of good color. An overly pale, ashy, reddish, or yellow cast to the skin may indicate health problems.

Massage benefits the skin by improving circulation of the blood, which carries nutrients to the cells.

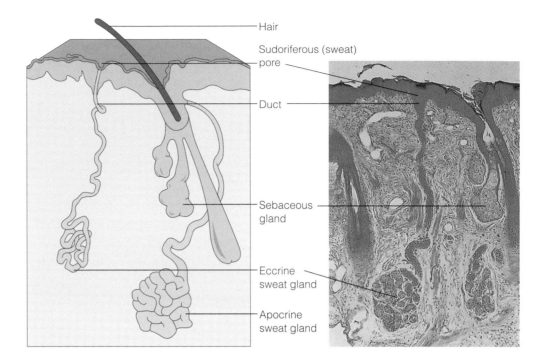

Figure 5.16

Sebaceous and sudoriferous glands.

The Appendages Associated with the Skin

Glands of the Skin

The skin contains two types of duct glands (exocrine glands) that extract materials from the blood to form new substances. These are the *sudoriferous* (soo-du-**RIF**-er-us) (sweat) glands and *sebaceous* (see-**BAY**-shus) (oil) glands. Sweat glands are under the control of the autonomic nervous system and are located in the dermis. They consist of a coiled base or fundas and a tubelike duct that terminates at the surface of the skin to form a sweat pore. Practically all parts of the body are supplied with sweat glands, but they are more abundant in the armpits, soles of the feet, palms of the hands, and forehead. The activity of the sweat glands is greatly increased by heat, exercise, and mental excitement (Figure 5.16).

The sudoriferous glands respond to elevated body temperatures resulting from environmental conditions or physical activity. The tubular extensions of these glands open at the body surface as a pore. Fluid secreted by the *eccrine* glands is mostly water and contains some bodily wastes, such as urea and uric acid. Therefore, the skin acts in some degree as an organ of excretion.

The Hair and Nails

Hair and nails are appendages of the skin. They are composed of hard keratin, a protein that in its soft form is found in skin. Hard keratin, as found in hair, has a sulfur content of 4 to 8 percent and a lower moisture and fat content than soft keratin and is a particularly tough, elastic material. It forms continuous sheets (fingernails) or long fibers (hair). Soft keratin contains about 2 percent sulfur, 50 percent moisture, and a small percentage of fats. In the epidermis, keratin occurs as flattened cells or dry scales (Figure 5.17 and Figure 5.18).

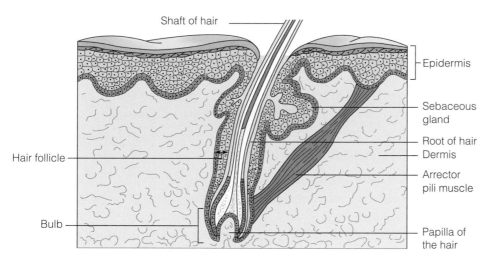

Figure 5.17
Hair follicle.

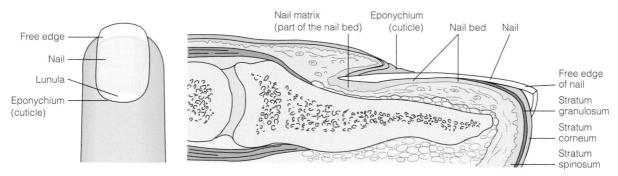

Figure 5.18
Fingernail.

Hair grows over the entire body, with the exception of the palms of the hands, soles of the feet, some areas of the genitalia, the mucous membranes of the lips, the nipples, the navel, and the eyelids. The heavier concentration of hair is on the head, under the armpits, on and around the genitals, and on the arms and legs. An individual's genes strongly influence the distribution of hair, its thickness, quality, color, and rate of growth, and whether it is curly or straight.

Each hair develops from a tubelike depression (hair follicle) that extends through the epidermis, into and through the dermis, and into the subcutaneous layer. As epidermal cells at the base of the follicle are nourished by the blood supply, they divide and push up through the hair follicle, die, and keratinize, becoming a shaft of hair.

Associated with hair follicles are sebaceous (oil) glands and arrector pili (a-**REK**-tor **PIGH**-ligh) muscles. The arrector pili muscles are fanlike muscles connected with the base of the follicle and positioned in such a way that they contract in reaction to cold or emotional stimuli. This reaction often results in a condition called *goose bumps* because the skin appears bumpy, like that of a plucked goose.

Lesions of the Skin

A lesion is a structural change in the tissues caused by injury or disease. There are three types: primary, secondary, and tertiary. Knowing how to identify the principal skin lesions helps the practitioner to avoid affected areas. The client should be advised to seek medical attention.

Definitions Pertaining to Primary Lesions (Figure 5.19a)

Bulla: A blister containing a watery fluid, similar to a vesicle, but larger (example: contact dermititis, large second-degree burns, bulbous impetigo, or pemphigus)

Macule: A small, discolored spot or patch on the surface of the skin, neither raised nor sunken, as freckles

Papule: A small, elevated pimple in the skin, containing fluid, but which may develop pus (examples: warts or elevated nevi)

Pustule: An elevation of the skin having an inflamed base, containing pus (examples: acne, impetigo, furuncles, carbuncles, or folliculitis)

Tubercle: A solid lump larger than a papule. It projects above the surface or lies within or under the skin. It varies in size from a pea to a hickory nut (examples: lipoma, erythema, nodosum, or cyst).

Tumor: An external swelling, varying in size, shape, and color such as carcinoma

Vesicle: A blister with clear fluid in it, vesicles lie within or just beneath the epidermis (example: poison ivy, herpes, or chickenpox)

Wheal: An itchy, swollen lesion that lasts only a few hours (examples: hives, or the bite of an insect, such as a mosquito)

Definitions Pertaining to Secondary Lesions

The secondary skin lesions are those in the skin that develop in the later stages of disease (Figure 5.19b).

Crust: An accumulation of serum and pus, mixed perhaps with epidermal material (example: the scab on a sore)

Excoriation: A skin sore or abrasion produced by scratching or scraping (example: a raw surface due to the loss of the superficial skin after an injury)

Fissure: A crack in the skin penetrating into the derma, as in the case of chapped hands or lips

Scale: An accumulation of epidermal flakes, dry or greasy (example: abnormal or excessive dandruff)

Scar (cicatrix) (**SICK**-ay-trix): Likely to form after the healing of an injury or skin condition that has penetrated the dermal layer

Stain: An abnormal discoloration remaining after the disappearance of moles, freckles, or liver spots, sometimes apparent after certain diseases

Ulcer: An open lesion on the skin or mucous membrane of the body, accompanied by pus and loss of skin depth

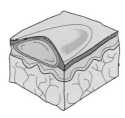

Bulla:
Same as a vesicle only greater than 0.5 cm
Example:
Contact dermatitis, large second-degree burns, bulbous impetigo, pemphigus

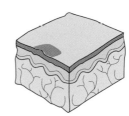

Macule:
Localized changes in skin color of less than 1 cm in diameter
Example:
Freckle

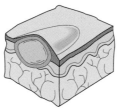

Tubercle:
Solid and elevated; however, it extends deeper than papules into the dermis or subcutaneous tissues, 0.5-2 cm
Example:
Lipoma, erythema, nodosum, cyst

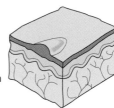

Papule:
Solid, elevated lesion less than 0.5 cm in diameter
Example:
Warts, elevated nevi

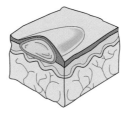

Pustule:
Vesicles or bullae that become filled with pus, usually described as less than 0.5 cm in diameter
Example:
Acne, impetigo, furuncles, carbuncles, folliculitis

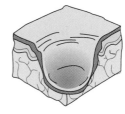

Ulcer:
A depressed lesion of the epidermis and upper papillary layer of the dermis
Example:
Stage 2 pressure ulcer

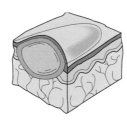

Tumor:
The same as a nodule only greater than 2 cm

Example:
Carcinoma (such as advanced breast carcinoma); **not** basal cell or squamous cell of the skin

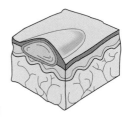

Vesicle:
Accumulation of fluid between the upper layers of the skin; elevated mass containing serous fluid; less than 0.5 cm
Example:
Herpes simplex, herpes zoster, chickenpox

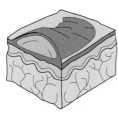

Wheal:
Localized edema in the epidermis causing irregular elevation that may be red or pale
Example:
Insect bite or a hive

Figure 5.19a
Skin lesions (primary).

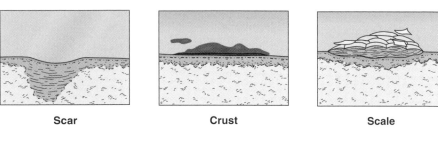

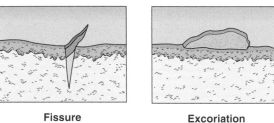

Figure 5.19b

Skin lesions (secondary).

Disorders of the Skin

Problem, Blemished Skin

It is outside the scope of practice of a massage therapist to diagnose or treat skin disorders, but he should be able to recognize some of the more common conditions in order to explain to the client why massage should or should not be given. The practitioner can suggest or recommend that the client see a dermatologist for skin conditions that are contraindications for massage.

Blackheads (comedones) are small masses of hardened, discolored sebum that appear most frequently on the face, shoulders, chest, and back. Blackheads are often accompanied by pimples during adolescence and are primarily due to overstimulated sebaceous glands. Proper cleansing of the skin will help to reduce the skin's oiliness. Any case of excessive pimples or blackheads should be treated by a dermatologist.

Massage can be given to someone who has blackheads; however, massage should not be given over areas where these skin conditions are more severe. Stimulation of blood circulation is beneficial and massage, exercise, and proper diet will, in most cases, improve these conditions.

A client may have a condition of the skin known as *staphylodermatitis,* an inflammation caused by staphylococci, bacteria that are generally found in milk and other dairy products. Massage should not be given when the skin is inflamed. The client should have the condition diagnosed by a physician.

A *bruise* is a superficial injury (contusion) generally caused by a blow or impact with some object; though not breaking the skin, it causes a reddish-blue or purple discoloration. Massage may be done above and below a bruise or contusion, but not directly over the injured area.

Acne is a chronic inflammatory disorder of the skin, usually related to hormonal changes and overactive sebaceous glands during adolescence. Common acne is also known as *acne simplex* or *acne vulgaris*. Although acne generally starts at the onset of puberty, it also afflicts adult men and women.

Modern studies show that acne is often due to heredity, but the condition can be aggravated by emotional stress and environmental factors. A well-balanced diet, drinking plenty of water, and developing healthful personal hygiene are recommended. Acne may be present on the back, chest, and shoulders. Acne may be accompanied by blackheads, pustules, and pimples that are red, swollen, and contain pus. In more advanced cases of acne, cysts (which are red, swollen lumps beneath the surface of the skin) may appear. Massage should be avoided when severe acne is present.

Seborrhea (seb-o-**REE**-uh) is a skin condition caused by overactivity and excessive secretion of the sebaceous glands. An oily or shiny condition of the nose, forehead, or scalp indicates the presence of seborrhea. It is readily detected on the scalp by the unusual amount of oil on the hair. Seborrhea is often the basis of an acne condition. Massage should not be given over infected areas.

Rosacea (ro-**ZAY**-shee-uh) is associated with excessive oiliness of the skin and a chronic inflammatory condition of the cheeks and nose. It is characterized by redness owing to dilation of blood vessels and the formation of papules and pustules. The skin becomes coarse, and the pores enlarged. Rosacea is usually caused by an inability to digest certain foods and an intolerance to strong beverages. It may also be caused by overexposure to extreme climate, faulty elimination, and hyperacidity. Massage is not given over affected areas.

A *steatoma* (stee-uh-**TOE**-muh) or sebaceous cyst is a subcutaneous tumor of the sebaceous glands that contains sebum. It usually appears as a small growth on the scalp, neck, or back. A steatoma is sometimes called a *wen*. Massage is not given over the affected area.

Asteatosis (as-tee-uh-**TOE**-sis) is a condition of dry, scaly skin, characterized by absolute or partial deficiency of sebum, usually due to aging or bodily disorders. In local conditions, such as scaling of the hands, it may be caused by alkalis in soaps and similar products. When the skin is unbroken, a mild lubricant may be massaged into the skin.

Impetigo is an acute, highly contagious, bacterial skin infection that is most common in children. It begins as an itchy, reddish discoloration that develops into pustules that form into a yellowish crust. Massage is contraindicated, and the client should be referred to a doctor for treatment.

A *furuncle* (**FYOU**-rung-kl), or boil, is caused by bacteria that enter the skin through the hair follicles. It is a subcutaneous abscess that fills with pus. A boil can be painful if neglected and should be treated by a physician.

A *carbuncle* is a mass of connected boils. Massage on the area is avoided, and the client should be referred to a doctor.

Warts are caused by the papilloma virus and are classified as common, plantar, and venereal. *Common warts* have a raised, rough surface and are generally found on the hands. *Plantar warts,* generally found on the soles of the feet, grow inward and are often painful and hard to remove. All warts are contagious. Avoid touching them, and wash your hands after making any contact.

Corns are cone-shaped areas on or between the toes caused by pressure or friction. They are not contagious but may be painful to touch or pressure.

A *keratoma* (ker-a-**TOE**-muh), or callus, is a superficial, thickened patch of epidermis caused by friction on the hands and feet. This condition is usually treated by a podiatrist.

Fungal conditions such as *ringworm* and *athlete's foot* thrive in moist environments but respond well to antifungal preparations. Avoid using lubricants near the infected area, and wash hands thoroughly because the fungus can be transmitted by contact.

Decubitus ulcers, pressure sores or bedsores, are caused by a persistent pressure against the skin usually in the area of a bony projection. The pressure causes a lack of circulation to the skin and underlying tissues. The lack of blood supply, oxygen, and nutrition causes tissue necrosis, the cells die, and an ulcer forms. Pressure sores are a concern for people who are bedridden who do not turn enough, people who use wheelchairs and do not shift their weight enough, and people who must wear casts or braces that do not fit properly. Degrees of pressure sores vary from a persistent red spot to crusted or broken skin to an open wound that may penetrate clear to the bone. Massage is contraindicated over open decubitus ulcers; however, massage to increase circulation over areas that are prone to pressure sores may help to prevent them from ever forming.

decubitus ulcers
are bedsores.

Skin Cancers and Tumors

The massage practitioner should not attempt to diagnose any kind of bump, lesion, ulceration, or discoloration as skin cancer but should be able to recognize serious skin disorders and suggest that the client seek medical attention without delay. As a massage therapist, you have the best opportunity for a close-up inspection of a client's skin. If you notice a change in appearance or behavior of an existing skin blemish or suspect the appearance of a new one, bring it to the attention of the client and/or refer the client to a doctor.

There are three kinds of skin cancer. The least malignant and most common is called **basal cell carcinoma.** This type of cancer begins as a small raised nodule that develops a crusty plaque with a slightly elevated, whitish border. Another variety of basal cell carcinoma apears on the body as a flat sore that does not heal properly. The sore may develop a crust, shed that crust, then form another. It is most common on light-skinned people over age 40 who have had excessive exposure to the sun. Basal cell carcinoma develops slowly and is successfully treated with minor surgery or local applications of freezing. Massage is locally contraindicated on or near the lesion. If the lesions are located on the client's body, the massage therapist may be the first to notice them. The client should be referred to a dermatologist or other physician for diagnosis and treatment before any other massage is performed.

basal cell carcinoma
is a type of skin cancer.

Squamous cell carcinoma is different in appearance from the basal type; it consists of scaly, red papules. Blood vessels are not visible. This cancer is more serious than the basal cell carcinoma because it can metastasize into deeper tissues and the lymph system and tends to spread more quickly than basal cell carcinomas. It can occur anywhere on the skin but is more common on the lips, ears, hands, and sun-exposed areas where the skin has had to repeatedly repair irritated tissue. As with basal cell carcinoma, squamous cell carcinoma is characterized by a sore or lesion that repeatedly crusts over but docs not heal. Squamous cell carcinoma is usually successfully treated by freezing the lesions or with local surgical removal.

Massage is contraindicated for persons with squamous cell carcinoma. If a massage practitioner discovers a suspicious lesion, the client must be referred to a dermatologist immediately. A client who has been recently treated for squamous cell carcinoma should obtain an approval or release from his physician before receiving massage.

The most serious and least common skin cancer is the **malignant melanoma.** This cancer is characterized by dark (brown, black, or discolored) patches on the skin. Early diagnosis of malignant melanoma is essential because it can metastasize quickly and can be fatal. Malignant melanoma often arises from an existing mole and may appear on any part of the body, so it is important to recognize the signs or the A-B-C-D-E warning of this disease:

> **malignant melanoma**
> is the most serious form of skin cancer.

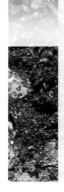

BOX 5.1   A-B-C-D-E WARNING FOR MALIGNANT MELANOMA

Asymmetry of any pigmented lesion

Borders that are irregular, notched, or indistinct

Color that is widely variable (black, brown, red, blue, or white)

Diameter larger than a pencil eraser

Elevation or partial elevation from the skin level

Malignant melanoma is a result of cumulative damage to melanocytes in the dermis from repeated exposure to the UV rays of the sun. Because melanoma tends to be so aggressive, the treatment is usually radical including surgery, radiation, and removal of local lymph nodes. Survival is dependent on the successful removal of all cancerous cells before they spread to other organs or tissues through the lymph system. Because melanoma metastasizes through the lymph system, massage is contraindicated except in cases where the patient is terminally ill and chooses to have massage for comfort and palliative care.

A **tumor** is an abnormal growth of swollen tissue that can be located on any part of the body. Some tumors are benign (mild in character) and

> **tumor**
> is an abnormal growth of swollen tissue that can be located on any part of the body.

are not likely to recur after removal, which means they are not harmful. These include moles, skintags, and sebaceous cysts. Unless these begin to change shape or color, they are harmless. If they seem irritated, change color, or begin to grow, they should be checked by a doctor. Some tumors are malignant and are more serious, as they can recur after removal. Tumors are removed by surgery, X-ray, or chemical treatments.

Venereal Diseases

venereal diseases

are associated with the sexual organs and are characterized by sores and rashes on the skin.

Venereal diseases, or sexually transmitted infections, are those diseases associated with the sexual organs and are characterized by sores and rashes on the skin. Venereal diseases can become latent and appear at a later time. This can be dangerous because the affected person may not seek treatment. Venereal diseases can also affect unborn children.

syphilis

is a serious disease that is transmitted by sexual contact with an infected person.

Syphilis (**SIF**-i-lis) is a serious disease that is transmitted by sexual contact with an infected person. When a sore first appears, especially one that is hard and ulcerated (with a hole in the center), a physician should be consulted. Without treatment the sore may go away only to appear later in the form of a rash. This is called *secondary syphilis,* which can cause degeneration of various parts of the body, ultimately causing death.

gonorrhea

is a venereal disease characterized by a discharge and burning sensation when urinating.

Gonorrhea (gon-o-**REE**-uh) is a more common disease than syphilis and is characterized by a discharge and burning sensation when urinating. Women may show no symptoms. If left untreated, harmful bacteria can enter the bloodstream.

Herpes

herpes

is a virus that affects the mouth, skin, and other facial parts, commonly called cold sores and fever blisters.

Herpes simplex is a recurrent viral infection that is highly contagious and tends to lie dormant in its carrier until stress or a depressed immune system creates an outbreak. The acute phase of the infection is usually a tingling or burning sensation followed by an outbreak of an oozing blister or blisters that scab over after a few days. An outbreak may last two to three weeks between the first signs and healing of the blisters. There are several strains of the herpes virus. *Type I* generally affects the face, around and sometimes inside the mouth with what are commonly called *cold sores* or *fever blisters.*

Herpes Simplex Type II or genital herpes outbreaks generally occur on genitals, buttocks, or inner thigh. *Herpes Whitlow* is a rarer variety with the outbreaks occurring around the nailbeds of the fingers. The virus is transmitted from the site of the outbreak via skin-to-skin contact. Each of these forms of herpes is very contagious in its acute phase and is at least a local contraindication for massage. The virus is quite virulent and can exist outside of its host, therefore linens used with clients who have an acute outbreak of herpes should be isolated and washed in hot water with a cup of bleach added to the wash. Face rests must be sanitized between clients if there is any sign of herpes to prevent infecting other clients. Practitioners with active fever blisters must take extra precaution to ensure that no client is at risk. This may mean refraining from practicing massage during the acute phase of the outbreak, and thorough hand washing and not touching the infected area during the subacute phase. When herpes is in its latent state, with no symptoms, massage is not contraindicated.

Herpes zoster, or **shingles,** is a very painful viral infection of the nervous system that is caused by the chickenpox virus. Shingles is characterized by pain in a particular dermatome, usually of the intercostal nerves, followed and accompanied by watery blisters. The pain and blisters are usually isolated to a portion of the affected dermatome and only on one side of the body. Unlike herpes simplex, herpes zoster does not seem to be particularly contagious. Generally, a person with this painful condition will not seek massage. In milder cases, massage is locally contraindicated depending on the tolerance of the client. When the pain has subsided and the blisters have healed, massage is appropriate.

> **shingles**
> is an acute inflammation of a nerve trunk by the herpes varicella-zoster virus.

Allergies

An *allergy* is a sensitivity that certain persons develop to normally harmless substances. Contact with certain types of cosmetics, medicines, and hair preparations or consumption of certain foods may bring about an itching skin eruption, accompanied by redness, swelling, blisters, oozing, and scaling. Many allergies are accompanied by headaches, congestion, or emotional inconsistency.

Millions of people suffer from various forms of allergies. Allergic dermatitis (eczema), one of the more common allergies, can be caused by a number of different factors: food, substances in the air, or materials the individual uses. Many objects, including necklaces, rings, hairpins, and bracelets, contain metals (such as nickel) that cause dermatitis. Hair dyes, makeup, and chemicals are a few of the substances to which some people are allergic.

Dermatitis (der-ma-**TIE**-tis) is an inflammatory condition of the skin. The lesions come in various forms, such as scales, vesicles, or papules.

Eczema (**EG**-ze-muh), an inflammation of the skin, either acute or chronic in nature, can appear in many forms of dry or moist lesions. The term *eczema* is applied to any number of surface lesions. It is usually a red, blistered, oozing area that itches painfully. Eczema may be the result of some type of allergy or internal disorder and the client should be referred to a physician for treatment.

Contact dermatitis refers to abnormal conditions resulting from contact with chemicals or other exterior agents. Some individuals may develop allergies to ingredients in some substances with which they work—for instance, when a cosmetologist is allergic to hair tints.

The appropriateness of massage in cases of dermatitis and eczema is dependent on the causes and extent of the inflammation. If blisters or other skin lesions are present, massage is locally contraindicated. Skin that is irritated, hot, red, and puffy contraindicates massage until the inflammation has subsided. However, if the irritation is minor and isolated, questioning the client may indicate the cause, and general massage may be appropriate.

Psoriasis (so-**RYE**-a-sis) is a common chronic, inflammatory skin disease whose cause is unknown. It is usually found on the scalp, elbows, knees, chest, and lower back, but rarely on the face. The lesions are round dry patches covered with coarse, silvery scales. If irritated, bleeding points may occur. Although not contagious, psoriasis can be spread by irritation. Massage over such a condition should be avoided.

Urticaria (hives) are red, raised lesions or weals accompanied by severe itching caused by an allergic reaction or emotional reaction. The condition is not contagious, but the area should be avoided when doing massage.

Pigmentations of the Skin

Changes in skin color may be observed in various skin disorders and in many systemic disorders. Certain drugs taken internally can affect pigmentation. Foods eaten in excess can affect the skin. The carotene in carrots is an example. A suntan is an example of external changes in the pigmentation of the skin. The fairer the skin, the easier it is to sunburn and the more difficult it may be to acquire an even suntan.

Generally, a skin that tans easily will not be sensitive to massage. However, when skin has been overexposed, it may become sensitive. When there is sunburn or peeling due to sunburn, massage may be painful.

Lentigines (len-**TIJ**-i-neez), or freckles, are small yellowish to brownish color spots on parts exposed to sunlight and air.

Stains are abnormal brown skin patches, having circular and irregular shape. Their permanent color is due to the presence of blood pigment. They occur during aging, after certain diseases, and after the disappearance of moles, freckles, and liver spots. The cause of these stains is unknown.

Chloasma (klo-**AZ**-muh) is characterized by increased deposits of pigment in the skin. It is found mainly on the forehead, nose, and cheeks. Chloasma is also called *moth patches* or *liver spots*.

A *naevus* is commonly known as a birthmark. It is a small or large discoloration of the skin due to pigmentation or dilated capillaries and is present on the skin at birth. Generally, such colored spots or areas are not affected by massage.

Leucoderma (loo-ko-**DER**-muh) are abnormal light patches of skin, due to congenital defective pigmentations. *Vitiligo* (vit-i-**LYE**-go) is an acquired condition of leucoderma that affects skin or hair.

Albinism (**AL**-bin-izm) is a congenital absence of melanin pigment in the body that affects the color of the skin, hair, and eyes. In albinos the hair is silky and white, and the skin is pinkish white and will not tan.

Color changes of the skin, such as a crack on the skin, a type of thickening, or any discoloration ranging from shades of red to brown and purple to almost black, may be danger signals and should be examined by a dermatologist.

SECTION QUESTIONS FOR DISCUSSION AND REVIEW

1. Define skin as the integumentary system.

2. Name the major functions of the skin.

3. Name the two main layers of the skin.

4. Name the layers of the epidermis.

5. Name two forms of keratin and where they are found in most abundance.

6. What is subcutaneous tissue?

7. How does the skin receive its color?

8. Name the layers of the dermis.

9. What is a gland?

10. Name the two major glands found in the skin and give the function of each.

11. Define the following: sebum, duct.

12. Name the appendages of the skin.

13. What is a lesion?

14. What kind of skin condition is contact dermatitis?

15. Why is it important for the massage practitioner to observe a client's skin condition?

2 THE SKELETAL SYSTEM

The skeletal system is the bony framework of the body. It is composed of bones, cartilage, and ligaments. The skeletal system has five main functions:

1. To offer a framework that supports body structures and gives shape to the body

2. To protect delicate internal organs and tissues

3. To provide attachments for muscles and act as levers in conjunction with muscles to produce movement

4. To manufacture blood cells in the red bone marrow

5. To store minerals such as calcium phosphate, calcium carbonate, magnesium, and sodium

Composition of Bones

Other than dentine—the dense hard tissue that forms the body of a tooth—bone is the hardest structure of the body. Despite its solid and inert appearance, bone is a complex and ever-changing organ. Bone is composed of about one third animal matter and two thirds mineral or earthy matter. The animal (organic) matter consists of bone cells (osteocytes),

| **epiphysis** |
| is an enlarged area on the ends of long bones that articulates with other bones. |

| **articular cartilage** |
| is a layer of hyaline cartilage covering the end surface of the epiphysis. |

| **diaphysis** |
| is the bone shaft between the epiphyses. |

| **periosteum** |
| is a fibrous membrane that functions to protect the bone and serves as an attachment of tendons and ligaments. |

blood vessels, connective tissues, and marrow. The mineral (inorganic) matter consists mainly of calcium phosphate and calcium carbonate.

Bone Forms or Shapes

There are several forms or shapes of bones found in the human body (Figure 5.20), namely:

- Flat bones, such as those in the skull, pelvis, and ribs (costals)
- Long bones, such as those in the legs, arms, fingers, and toes
- Short bones, such as those in the carpals and tarsals
- Irregular bones, such as the vertebrae (spine)

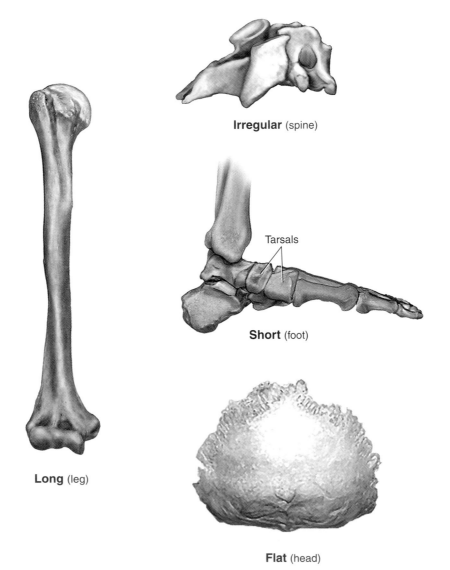

Irregular (spine)

Tarsals

Short (foot)

Long (leg)

Flat (head)

Figure 5.20
Bone shapes.

Characteristics of Long Bones

A typical long bone (see Figure 5.21) has enlarged areas on the ends, called the **epiphysis** (e-**PIF**-i-sis), which articulate with other bones. The end surface of the epiphysis is covered with a layer of hyaline cartilage called **articular cartilage.** The articular cartilage provides a smooth shock-absorbing surface where two bones meet to form a joint. The shaft of the bone between the epiphysis is the **diaphysis** (die-**AF**-i-sis).

Except for articular cartilage, the bone is covered by the **periosteum** (per-ee-**OS**-tee-um). The periosteum is a fibrous membrane whose function is to protect the bone and serve as an attachment for tendons and ligaments. It contains an abundance of nerves, blood, and lymph vessels and is essential to bone nutrition and repair. Beneath the periosteum the walls of the diaphysis are composed of **compact bone tissue.** Compact bone tissue forms the hard bone found in the shafts of long bones and along the outside of flat bones. This bone tissue is strong and rigid.

The inner portion of the bone is made up mostly of **spongy bone,** which consists of irregularly shaped spaces, collect trabeculae, defined by thin, bony plates. This provides a lightweight yet surprisingly strong interior structure to the bones. The spongy bone tissue in the flat bones and at the ends of the long bones is filled with red bone marrow and is the site of production for blood cells. The **medullary cavity** is a hollow chamber formed in the shaft of long bones that is filled with yellow bone marrow.

Marrow is the connective tissue filling the cavities of bones. Its function is largely concerned with the formation of red and white blood cells. There are two types of bone marrow, *red* and *yellow* marrow. Red bone marrow functions in the production of red and white blood cells and platelets. It occupies nearly all the bone cavities of the newborn; however, in the adult it is found in the bone spaces of the skull, ribs, sternum, vertebrae, and pelvis. Yellow marrow is the result of inactive blood-producing cells filling with fatty material and is located in the medullary cavity of the long bones.

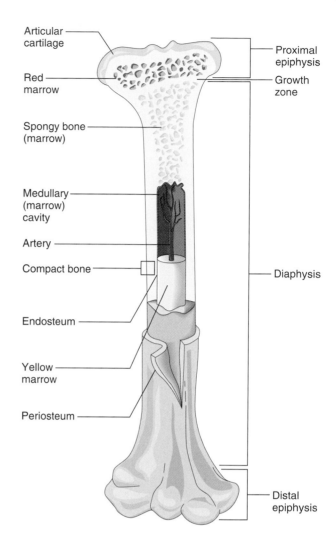

Figure 5.21
Structure of long bone.

compact bone tissue
forms the hard bone found in the shafts of long bones and along the outside of flat bones.

spongy bone
located inside long bones, consists of irregularly shaped spaces defined by thin, bony plates.

medullary cavity
is a hollow chamber formed in the shaft of long bones that is filled with yellow bone marrow.

marrow
is the connective tissue filling in the cavities of bones that forms red and white blood cells.

Bone Nutrition

Bone receives its nourishment through a highly organized system of blood vessels (capillaries) that make their way through the periosteum into the interior of bones. Bone marrow also aids in the nutrition of bone. For proper growth and hardening of bony structures, the diet should contain an adequate amount of calcium, phosphorous, and vitamin D.

THE SKELETON AS A WHOLE

The skeleton is divided into two main parts: the **axial skeleton** and the **appendicular skeleton.** The cranial and facial bones of the skull, thorax, vertebral column, and the hyoid bone comprise the axial skeleton (Figure 5.22). The appendicular skeleton is made up of bones of the shoulder, upper extremities, hips, and lower extremities. The name *appendicular* identifies these parts as appendages or extensions of the axis or axial skeleton.

In the human adult, the skeleton consists of 206 bones, distributed as follows (numbers in parentheses indicate number of bones):

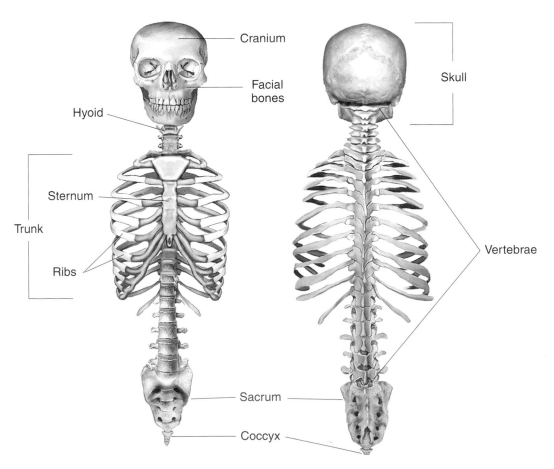

Figure 5.22
Axial skeleton.

The Axial Skeleton

- **Cranium** (8)—forms a protective structure for the brain:

   frontal (1), parietal (2), occipital (1), temporal (2), sphenoid (1), ethmoid (1)

- **Face** (14)—forms the structure of the eyes, nose, cheeks, mouth, and jaws:

   maxilla (2), palatine (2), zygomatic (2), lacrimal (2), nasal (2), vomer (1), inferior nasal concha (2), mandible (1)

- **Ear** (6)—forms the internal structure of the ears:
   malleus (2), incus (2), stapes (2)

- **Hyoid bone** (1)—supports the base of the tongue

- **Vertebral column** (26)—forms the spinal column, which supports the head, supports the trunk, protects the spinal cord, and provides attachment for the ribs:

   cervical vertebrae (7), thoracic vertebrae (12), lumbar vertebrae (5), sacrum (1), coccyx (1)

- **Thoracic cage** (25):

   ribs (costals) (24)—forms a protective cage for the lungs and heart

   sternum (1)—serves as an attachment for the ribs at the front of the chest

The Appendicular Skeleton

- **Upper extremities** (64):

   clavicle (2), scapula (2), humerus (2), ulna (2), radius (2), carpals (16), metacarpals (10), phalanges (28)

- **Lower extremities** (66):

   pelvic (fusion of three bones) (2), femur (2), patella (2), tibia (2), fibula (2), tarsals (14), metatarsals (10), phalanges (28)

The form or outline of the bones must be carefully followed and the limitations of the range of movements be considered when practicing massage therapy. Knowing the names of bones serves as a guide in recalling the names of related structures connected with the body part being massaged (Figures 5.23 to 5.27).

> **axial skeleton**
>
> is made up of bones of the skull, thorax, vertebral column, and the hyoid bone.

> **appendicular skeleton**
>
> is made up of bones of the shoulder, upper extremities, hips, and lower extremities.

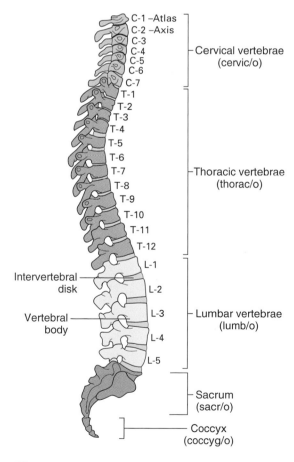

Figure 5.23

Vertebral column.

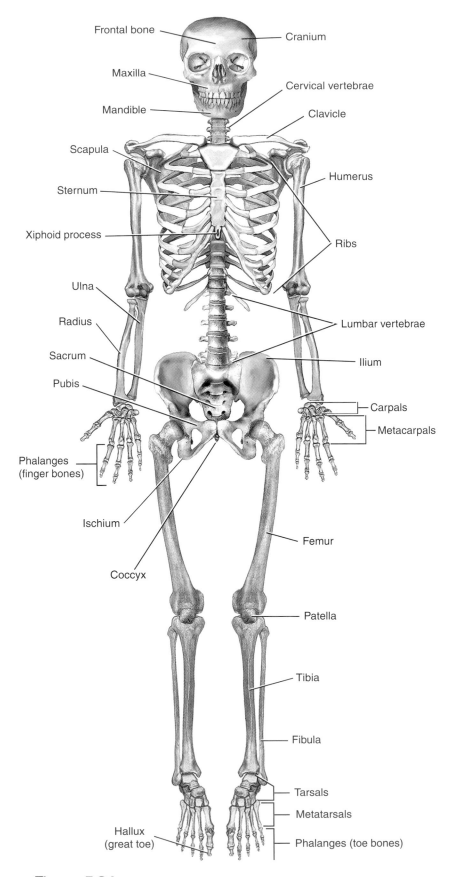

Frontal bone

Cranium

Maxilla

Mandible

Cervical vertebrae

Clavicle

Scapula

Humerus

Sternum

Xiphoid process

Ribs

Ulna

Radius

Lumbar vertebrae

Sacrum

Ilium

Pubis

Carpals

Metacarpals

Phalanges
(finger bones)

Ischium

Femur

Coccyx

Patella

Tibia

Fibula

Tarsals

Metatarsals

Hallux
(great toe)

Phalanges (toe bones)

Figure 5.24

Skeletal system, anterior view.

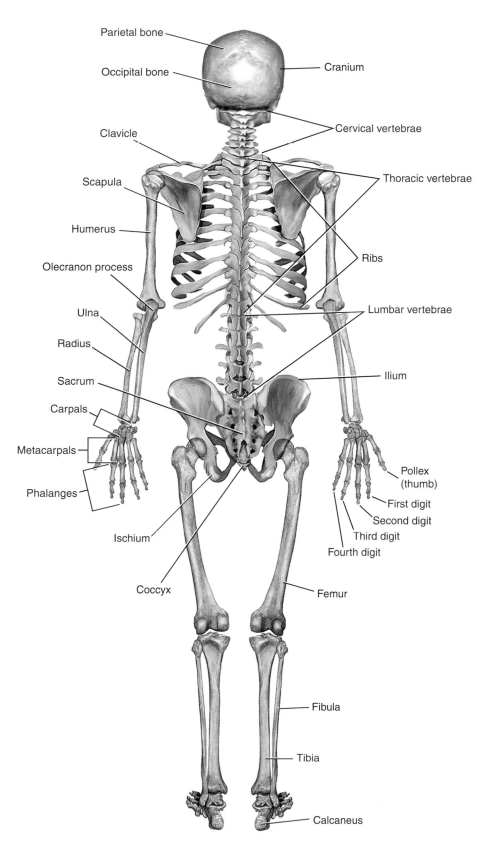

Figure 5.25

Skeletal system, posterior view.

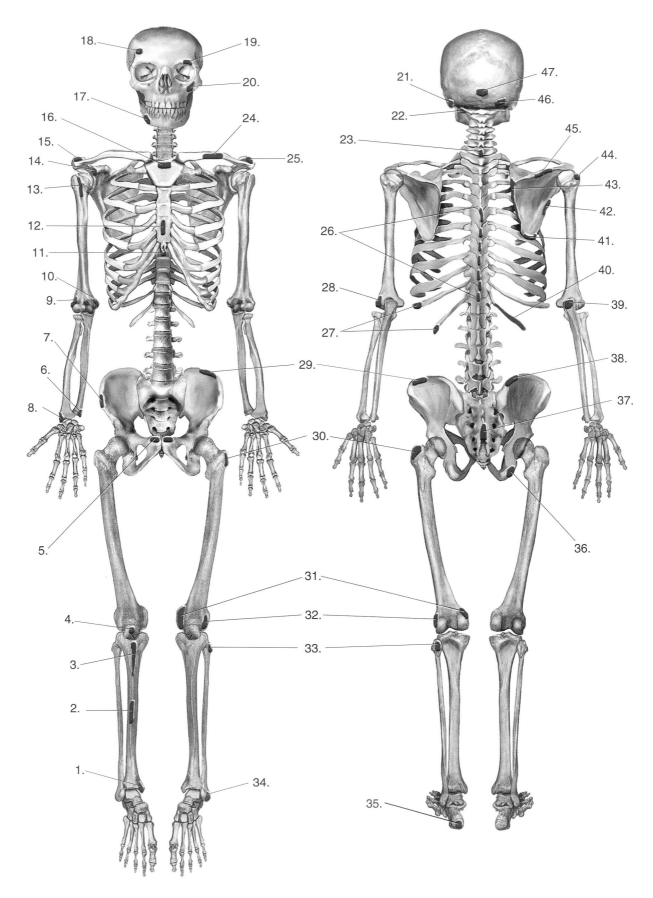

Figure 5.26

Major bony landmarks on the body.

Labels for Bony Landmarks (Figure 5.26)

1. Medial malleolus; inside or medial "ankle bone."
2. Shaft of the tibia; "shin bone."
3. Tuberosity of the tibia; prominent bump interior to the patella.
4. Patella; "kneecap."
5. Pubic arch; the middle is the pubic symphysis, the lateral portion (about one and one-half inch to each side of the symphysis) is the ramus of the pubic bone.
6. Pisiform bone; first prominent bone in the heel of the hand.
7. ASIS: Anterior Superior Iliac Spine; pointed bone at the front of the hip.
8. Styloid process of the radius; lateral process at the distal end of the radius.
9. Lateral epicondyle of the humerus; bump on outside of the elbow at the end of the humerus. Attachment of many of the wrist extensor muscles.
10. Medial epicondyle of the humerus; bump on inside of elbow at the end of the humerus. Attachment of many of the wrist flexor muscles.
11. Xiphoid process; point at the inferior end of the sternum.
12. Sternum; breastbone, between ribs on the front of the chest.
13. Bicipital groove; groove between the greater and lesser tuberosity of the humerus, location of the tendon of the long head of the biceps muscle.
14. Coracoid process.
15. A.C. joint; joint between the acromion process of the scapula and the clavicle.
16. Sternal notch; hollow just superior to the sternum and between the heads of the clavicles.
17. Ramus of the mandible; point at the angle of the jawbone.
18. Frontal eminence; slight rise between the eyebrow and hairline.
19. Supraorbital ridge; upper part of eye socket, under the eyebrow.
20. Zygomatic bone; "cheekbone."
21. Mastoid process; bony point behind lower portion of the ear.
22. Transverse process of first cervical vertebra; just below and deeper than mastoid process.

23. Spinous process of the seventh cervical vertebra; topmost of the palpable spinous processes.
24. Clavicle; collarbone.
25. Acromion process; lateral point of the spine of the scapula.
26. Spinous processes of the vertebra.
27. Ends of the floating ribs.
28. Lateral epicondyle of the humerus; refer to #9.
29. Crest of the ilium; the "hip bone," also called the iliac crest.
30. Greater trochanter of the femur; bony knob at the top of the leg bone.
31. Medial epicondyle of the femur; bony enlargement on the inside of the knee.
32. Lateral epicondyle of the femur; bony enlargement of the outside of the knee.
33. Head of the fibula; bump on the outside of the leg just below the knee.
34. Lateral malleolus; outside or lateral ankle bone, distal end of the fibula.
35. Calcaneus; "heel bone."
36. Ischial tuberosity; "sit bone."
37. Distal end of sacrum; prominent bone at upper end of gluteal crease. (Coccyx or tailbone is located deep between the buttocks.)
38. Posterior superior iliac spine (PSIS); bony prominence of the low back at the posterior end of the iliac crest.
39. Olecranon process; point of the elbow at the proximal end of the ulna.
40. Twelfth rib; last rib.
41. Inferior angle of the scapula; lower tip of the scapula.
42. Axillary border of the scapula; lateral edge of the scapula from the interior angle to the "armpit."
43. Vertebral border of the scapula; medial edge of the scapula nearest the spine.
44. Greater tuberosity of the humerus; proximal prominence of the humerus.
45. Spine of the scapula; bony ridge on the posterior scapula.
46. Occipital ridge; lowest palpable bony ridge on the posterior skull.
47. Occipital protuberance; small bump on the posterior skull.

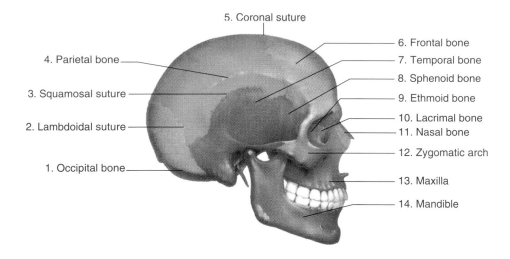

5. Coronal suture
4. Parietal bone
3. Squamosal suture
2. Lambdoidal suture
1. Occipital bone
6. Frontal bone
7. Temporal bone
8. Sphenoid bone
9. Ethmoid bone
10. Lacrimal bone
11. Nasal bone
12. Zygomatic arch
13. Maxilla
14. Mandible

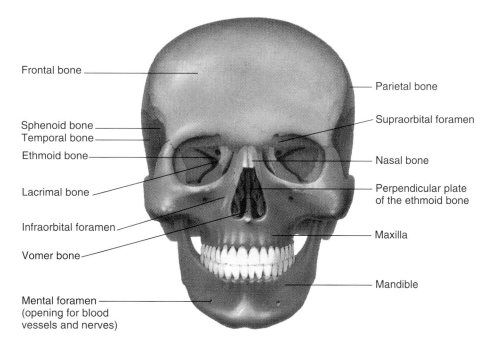

Frontal bone
Sphenoid bone
Temporal bone
Ethmoid bone
Lacrimal bone
Infraorbital foramen
Vomer bone
Mental foramen
(opening for blood
vessels and nerves)
Parietal bone
Supraorbital foramen
Nasal bone
Perpendicular plate
of the ethmoid bone
Maxilla
Mandible

Figure 5.27
Cranium, neck, and face bones.

Joints

The bones of the skeleton are connected at different parts of their surfaces. Such connections are called *joints* or *articulations*.

Joints are classified according to the amount of motion they permit.

Synarthrotic (**SIN**-ar-thro-tic) *joints*, such as those in the skull, are immovable.

Amphiarthrotic (**AM**-fee-ar-thro-tic) *joints* have limited motion. Examples are the symphysis pubis and sacroiliac joints.

Diarthrotic (**DIE**-ar-thro-tic) *joints* are freely movable. The articulating ends of the bones that meet at these joints are covered with hyaline cartilage called *articular cartilage*. A strong fibrous joint capsule surrounds the joint and is firmly attached to both bones. The outside of the capsule is constructed of ligaments that attach the bones; the inner surface or the lining of the capsule consists of **synovial membrane,** which secretes *synovial fluid* that lubricates the joint surfaces. Diarthrotic joints have a variety of shapes and are capable of several kinds of movements: pivot movement, as in turning the head; saddle movement, as in the thumb; ball and socket movement, as in the hip; and hinge movement, as in the knees (Figure 5.28).

Besides the functional classification of joints as discussed, joints are also classified according to their structure. (See Table 5.3.) The structural classification of joints is based on the type of fibrous tissue that holds the joint together and the amount and quality of space between the articulating bones. Joints with no space that are held together by fibrous connective

> **synovial membrane**
>
> is a connective tissue membrane lining cavities and capsules in and around joints.

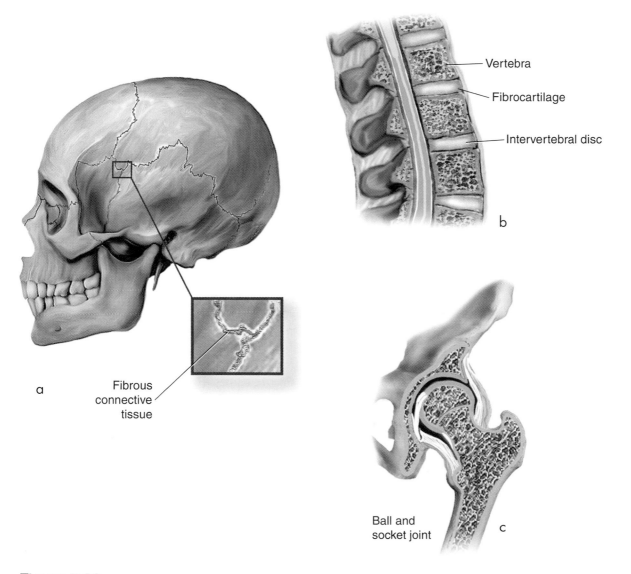

Figure 5.28

Classification of joints: a. synarthrosis or immovable joint; b. amphiarthrosis or slightly movable joint; c. diarthrosis or freely movable joint.

Table 5.3

Types of Joints Based on Functional and Structural Classification

TYPE	CLASSIFICATION	DESCRIPTION	EXAMPLE
Suture	Immovable Fibrous	Bones separated by a thin fibrous layer	Found only in the sutures of the skull
Gomphosis	Immovable Fibrous	Cone-shaped peg fits in socket connecting bones with periodontal ligament	Roots of teeth in mandible and maxilla
Synchondrosis	Immovable Cartilaginous	Connecting material is hyaline cartilage	The junction between the epiphysis and the diaphysis of growing long bones
Syndesmosis	Slightly Movable Fibrous	Bones held together with dense fibrous tissue	Distal ends of fibula and tibia
Symphysis	Slightly Movable Cartilaginous	Connected by flat disc of fibrocartilage	Symphysis pubis and intervertebral joints
Pivot	Freely Movable Synovial	Rounded bone rotates in a ring made of bone and ligament	Joint at proximal ends of radius and ulna and the joint between axis and atlas
Hinge	Freely Movable Synovial	Allows movement only in one plane— i.e., flexion/extension	Elbow, knee, interphalangeal joints
Ball and Socket	Freely Movable Synovial	Ball-like surface fits into cuplike socket	Hip and shoulder joint
Gliding	Freely Movable Synovial	Flat articulating surfaces	Intertarsal and intercarpal joints
Saddle	Freely Movable Synovial	Two saddle-shaped bones fit together	Joint between thumb metacarpal and wrist carpal (trapezium)
Condyloid Ellipsoid	Freely Movable Synovial	Oval-shaped condyle fits into ellipsoidal socket	Joint between carpals and radius

> **fibrous joints**
>
> have no space and are held together by fibrous connective tissue.

> **cartilaginous joints**
>
> are joints held together with cartilage with no joint cavity.

> **synovial joints**
>
> have a joint cavity surrounded by an articular capsule.

tissue are classified as **fibrous joints.** Joints held together with cartilage with no joint cavity are **cartilaginous joints. Synovial joints** do have a joint cavity that is surrounded by an articular capsule.

Immovable joints (synarthroses) and slightly movable joints (amphiarthroses) are *fibrous or cartilaginous joints.* A distinguishing factor in freely movable joints (diarthroses) is that they are *synovial joints.*

Cartilage and Ligaments

Cartilage (also called *gristle*) is a firm, tough, elastic substance, similar to bone but without its mineral content. It serves the following purposes:

1. To cushion the bones at the joints

2. To prevent jarring between bones in motion, as in walking

3. To give shape to external features, such as the nose and ears

Ligaments are bands or sheets of fibrous tissue that connect bone to bone and help to support the bones at the joints, as in the wrist and ankle. The *synovial fluid* is the lubricating fluid whose function is to prevent friction at the joints.

Bursae (**BER**-suh) are fibrous sacks lined with synovial membrane and lubricated with synovial fluid. The purpose of the bursae is to function as a slippery cushion in areas where pressure is exerted, such as between bones and overlying muscle, tendons, or skin. Injury to bursae can cause inflammation and swelling and is called bursitis (ber-**SIGH**-tis).

Types of Movable Joints

The various types of movable joints found in the human body (Figure 5.29) are classified as follows:

- Pivot joints have an extension on one bone that rotates in relation to the bone it articulates with, such as in the neck between

> ### ligaments
> are bands of fibrous tissue that connect bones to bones.

> ### bursae
> are fibrous sacks lined with synovial membrane and lubricated with synovial fluid, functioning as a cushion in areas of pressure.

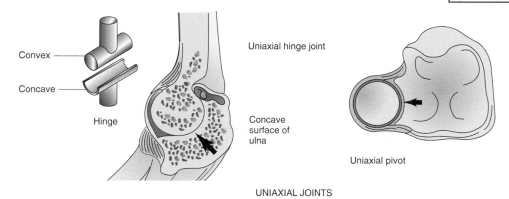

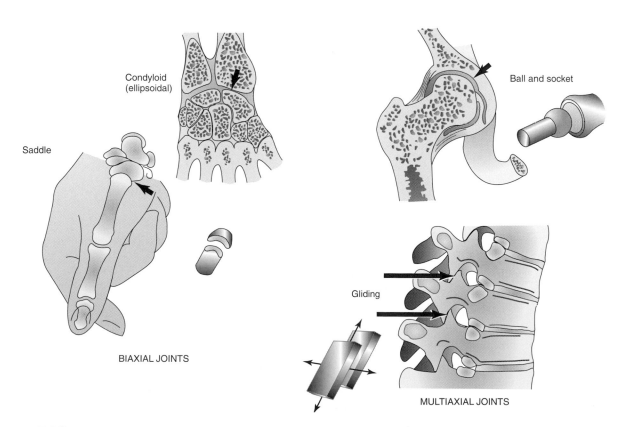

Figure 5.29

Types of movable joints.

the atlas and the axis or between the radius and ulna just distal to the elbow.

- Hinge joints only move through one plane such as in the elbow, knees, and two distal joints of the fingers.

- Ball-and-socket joints permit the greatest range of movement. A bone with a ball-shaped head articulates in a socket-shaped depression such as in the hips and shoulders.

- Gliding joints have nearly flat surfaces that glide across one another, such as in the spine or carpal and tarsal.

- Saddle joints involve bones with concave articulating surfaces such as in the thumb.

- Condyloid or ellipsoid joints have an oval-shaped end of one bone that articulates with an ellipsoid basin of another such as between the distal end of the radius and the trapezium at the wrist.

Words That Describe Bone Structures

Condyle (**KON**-dil)	A rounded knuckle-like prominence, usually at a point of articulation
Crest	A ridge
Foramen (**FO**-ray-mun)	A hole
Fossa (**FOS**-uh)	A depression or hollow
Head	A rounded articulating process at the end of a bone
Line	A less prominent ridge of a bone than a crest
Meatus (**MEE**-ay-tus)	A tubelike passage
Process	A bone prominence or projection
Sinus or antrum	A cavity within a bone
Spine	A sharp, slender projection
Trochanter (**TRO**-kan-tur)	A large process for muscle attachment
Tubercle (**TEW**-bur-kul)	A small, rounded process
Tuberosity	A large, rounded process

Skeletal and Joint Disorders

Fractures

A fracture is a break or rupture in a bone. There are several types of fractures classified according to the severity of the injury: simple or closed, compound or open, greenstick, comminuted, and spiral (Figure 5.30). Fractures are relatively easy to identify. They are usually the result of a traumatic event, are painful, and limit the function of the associated joint. A decisive diagnosis is verified by an X-ray or MRI. Fractured bones

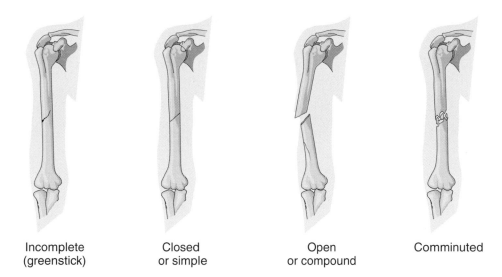

| Incomplete (greenstick) | Closed or simple | Open or compound | Comminuted |

Figure 5.30
Types of fractures.

usually heal completely after being immobilized with either a cast or surgically implanted pins, plates, and screws.

Massage is contraindicated for acute fractures that have not been set and immobilized. Massage is appropriate in the subacute stage around fractures that have been stabilized to encourage circulation and reduce edema. Massage may also help balance the developing compensation patterns that accompany the restricted movement due to the fracture.

Dislocation

A dislocation occurs when a bone is displaced within a joint. This is usually due to a traumatic injury that stretches or tears the ligaments and other soft tissues around the joint and requires reduction (realigning the bones) and rest while the ligaments heal. Massage is contraindicated during the acute phase. During the subacute stage, massage can be used to reduce scar tissue and address splinting or spasmed muscles related to the formerly dislocated joint.

Herniated Disk

A **herniated disk** is a weakening of the intervertebral disk that results in a protrusion of the nucleus pulposis or the annulus fibrosis of the disk into the vertebral canal, potentially compressing the spinal nerve root or the spinal cord. Herniated disks usually occur in the lumbar or cervical spine. Symptoms include neck or back pain, numbness, and tingling or pain down the limb of the impinged nerves.

A client with a suspected herniated disk should be referred to a physician for a definitive diagnosis via X-ray, myelogram, and MRI because similar symptoms may be exhibited by other conditions such as ligament damage, spondylosis, or bone cancer that require very different treatments.

Successful treatment for herniated disks involves reducing the protrusion, preferably by reabsorption of the nucleus pulposis into the disk

> **herniated disk**
> is a weakening of the intervertebral disc resulting in a protrusion into the vertebral canal, potentially compressing the spinal cord.

and healing of the annulus fibrosis. This may be accomplished with therapies such as chiropractic or osteopathic manipulations, traction, strict bedrest, physical therapy, or special exercises done with the intention of creating more space for the disk to heal. If these are unsuccessful or if the disk is putting severe pressure on the spinal cord or spinal nerve, surgical intervention may be required.

Massage is not recommended during an acute episode of a herniated disk. After a definitive diagnosis, initial treatment, and as part of a team approach, massage may be helpful to address the muscle spasms, referred pain, and compensation patterns that accompany the condition.

Sprain

sprain
is an injury to a joint resulting in stretching or tearing of the ligaments.

A **sprain** is an injury to a joint that results in the stretching or tearing of the ligaments but is not severe enough to cause a dislocation. Sprains are classified according to their severity.

Class I sprain: There is a stretch in the ligament, some discomfort, and minimal loss of function.

Class II sprain: The ligament is torn with some loss of function. There may or may not be a discoloration due to tissue damage and bleeding.

Class III sprain: This is the most severe, where the ligaments are torn, and there is internal bleeding and severe loss of function.

All classes of sprain cause swelling and require rest and support while the tissues heal.

Sprains cause inflammation (pain, heat, redness, and swelling) as a result of tissue damage plus a painful loss of function in the associated joint. Passive movement of the joint that stretches the sprained ligament causes pain. Massage is contraindicated during the acute stage of a sprain when signs of inflammation are present. Massage is appropriate during the subacute and healing stages to help reduce adhesions, edema, and stiffness while enhancing circulation and flexibility.

Arthritis

Arthritis is an inflammatory condition of the joints often accompanied by pain and changes of bone structure. There are many kinds of arthritis; the most common are rheumatoid arthritis, osteoarthritis, and gouty arthritis.

Rheumatoid arthritis is a chronic, systemic, autoimmune inflammatory disease and is the most serious and crippling form of arthritis. It is a systemic disease, often involving a number of joints, that first affects the synovial membrane that lines the joints. The joints become swollen, hot, and red. The inflammation causes the articular cartilage to erode and the joints to calcify and eventually become immovable. Its cause is unknown, but treatments are available to slow the progress and reduce the discomfort. Massage is contraindicated in the acute stage because it will aggravate the condition. In the remission stage, gentle massage and joint movement well within pain tolerance may be beneficial.

Osteoarthritis is a chronic disease that accompanies aging. It usually affects synovial joints that have experienced a great deal of wear and tear or trauma. The knees, hips, and spine are common sites for this degenerative disease, which erodes the articular cartilage and results in abnormal bone thickening and progressive joint immobility. Arthritic pain may come and go and range from mild to unbearable. In the acute, inflammatory stage, the affected joint may be swollen, hot, and painful. In the subacute stage, the pain in the joint may subside somewhat, but there will be noticeable stiffness. There is no cure for osteoarthritis, but medication, exercise, and massage help to relieve pain and maintain mobility. Surgery is sometimes indicated to remove *spurs* or replace affected joints. Massage is contraindicated during the inflammatory, acute stages of osteoarthritis, but it is indicated during the subacute stages to help relax related muscle tension, reduce pain, and maintain flexibility.

Spondylosis is osteoarthritis of the spine that can affect the cervical, lumbar, or thoracic vertebrae. It is characterized by the degeneration of the intervertebral disks and the formation of bony growths on the vertebra called osteophytes or bone spurs. Spondylosis is a slow-progressing, degenerative condition that affects middle-aged to elderly people. There may be no symptoms until the osteophytes grow enough to put pressure on a spinal nerve, the spinal cord, or begin to limit movement between vertebrae. Gentle exercise and movement help to slow the progression of the disease. Massage may be appropriate with caution and in cooperation with the primary care provider.

spondylosis
a degenerative arthritic condition affecting the vertebrae.

Acute gouty arthritis, also referred to as *gout,* is caused by a high concentration of uric acid in the blood that precipitates out into the interstitial and synovial spaces in the form of sharp, needlelike crystals. Uric acid is a metabolic by-product of purine and is normally excreted from the body via the kidneys. High blood levels of uric acid (*hyperuremia*) may result from eating foods high in purine such as shellfish, red meat, organ meats, and lentils or consuming high amounts of alcohol, which interferes with the kidney's ability to eliminate uric acid, or because of low functioning kidneys. The most common place for the crystals to settle is in the metaphalangeal joint of the large toe where an immune system response to the presence of the uric acid crystals causes the classic inflammatory symptoms of pain, swelling, heat, and redness. Other joints that may be affected by gout include the ankle, knee, fingers, wrist, and elbow. Attacks usually last a few days and subside on their own. Over time, attacks may become more frequent and severe. Uric acid crystals may also cause kidney stones. Gout may be an indicator of other medical conditions. Before proceeding with massage, a client with symptoms of gout should receive medical clearance. Gout, in the acute stage, is a systemic contraindication for massage; in a subacute stage or remission, it is a local contraindication.

Ankylosing spondylitis is a type of inflammatory arthritis that targets the sacroiliac joint and the spinal articulations, including the ribs, although it may also affect other areas of the body such as the shoulders, hips, and small joints of the hands and feet. Sometimes the eyes can become involved, and—rarely—the lungs and heart can be affected. It is a genetic autoimmune disease that primarily affects men between the ages of 15 and 35. Chronic ankylosing spondylitis begins with stiffness and pain in the low back and hips, then progresses up the back and neck. In severe cases, bone formation leads to spinal and vertebral-costal fusion with the body in a forward-stooping posture and the rib cage frozen, which compromises breathing. Currently there is no cure, but medications and proper treatment help slow the progression and reduce symptoms. Anti-inflammatory drugs and proper exercise are essential to reduce pain and maintain posture and flexibility.

As with other inflammatory conditions, massage is contraindicated during the acute stages of ankylosing spondylitis. The appropriateness of massage during the subacute and remission stages has not been determined and must be decided on a case-by-case basis in close cooperation with the client's physician.

Bursitis

Bursitis is an inflammation of the small fluid-filled sacs (bursae) located near the joints that reduce the friction of overlying structures during movement. There are over 150 bursae in the body located between moving structures such as bones, muscles, skin, and tendons. The bursae act as a cushion to allow smooth gliding between these structures. Bursitis is a painful condition that results from repeated irritation or trauma. The most common site of bursitis is the subdeltoid bursae of the shoulder, but it can develop at any joint. Pain from an acute case of bursitis drastically limits joint mobility. After the inflammation subsides, mobility remains limited because of pain and contracted muscles. Massage is locally contraindicated during the acute stage of bursitis; however, in the subacute stage mild exercise, range of motion, and massage are very effective for restoring mobility.

Osteoporosis

Osteoporosis (**OS**-tee-o-pour-**O**-sis) literally means increased porosity of the bones. Osteoporosis affects four times as many women as men, and its prevalence increases with age. Until around the age of 35, the body is building bone density by storing various minerals, mostly calcium. After that, it begins to slowly demineralize, increasing the risk of osteoporosis. Other risk factors, besides aging, that play a part in the development of osteoporosis are genetics, having a small bone structure, cigarette smoking, alcohol abuse, and a sedentary lifestyle.

Osteoporosis is a silent disease because there are no apparent symptoms. Often, the first indicator is a fracture after a minor accident. A definitive diagnosis is done with a bone mineral density test and X-ray. The best treatment for osteoporosis is prevention through good nutrition with ample amounts of calcium and vitamin D and regular weight-bearing exercise throughout life. Increased reabsorption of calcium into the bloodstream causes a thinning of bone tissue, leaving it more fragile and prone to fracture (especially where bones are weight bearing, such as in the spine and pelvis). When severe osteoporosis is present, the massage therapist must be very cautious and avoid any deep pressure or forceful joint movements that could lead to the possibility of fractures of the delicate bones.

Spinal Curvature

The healthy adult spine has a double S curve. The cervical and lumbar portions of the spine are concave and have a normal lordodic (lor-dot-ick) curve. The thoracic portion of the spine is convex and has a normal kyphotic (kye-fah-tick) curve. These curvatures help to position the head over the pelvis and provide flexibility, strength, shock absorption, and balance. Sometimes, abnormal curvatures develop in the spine.

In many instances abnormal curvatures of the spine (see Figure 5.31) begin as functional conditions of posture or soft tissues pulling the spine out of alignment. If left untreated, the constant pull of the soft tissues or gravity will cause the vertebra and other skeletal structures to change shape and become more of a structural dysfunction.

Scoliosis is a lateral curvature of the spine that involves a rotation of the vertebra.

Lordosis is an exaggerated lordodic or concave curve most commonly found in the lumbar spine creating a condition commonly known as swayback.

Kyphosis is an abnormally exaggerated kyphotic or convex curve of the thoracic spine. This condition is also termed hyper-kyphosis. *Postural kyphosis* usually becomes apparent during adolescence and is associated with slouching. *Scheuermann's kyphosis* is a genetic condition that also becomes apparent during the early teen years but tends to be more sever with irregularly formed vertebra and disks (Figure 5.31).

These abnormal curves may develop because of a congenital defect, habitually poor body mechanics, or aging. Regardless of their origin, these abnormal conditions cause tremendous biomechanical stress on the body. Massage and exercise, though not offering a cure for these conditions, are very effective in counteracting the stress and pain associated with these abnormalities.

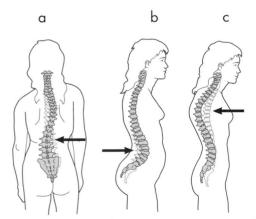

Figure 5.31
Abnormal curvature of the spine: (a) scoliosis, b) lordosis, (c) kyphosis.

SECTION QUESTIONS FOR DISCUSSION AND REVIEW

1. What structures make up the skeletal system?

2. Name five functions of bones.

3. Name the organic and inorganic matter found in bones.

4. Name two types of bone tissue and indicate where they are found.

5. Which covering protects the bone?

6. How are the bones nourished?

7. Name the various shapes of bones found in the body. Give an example of each.

8. Name two kinds of marrow and where each is found.

9. What is the function of red bone marrow?

10. What are the two main parts of the skeleton?

11. Name three classifications of joints and differentiate between them.

12. Which structure cushions the bones at the joints?

13. Which structure connects and supports the bones at the joints?

14. Which fluid lubricates the joints?

15. About how many bones are found in the human body?

16. Why must the skeletal system be considered in the practice of massage therapy?

17. List five types of movable joints and give an example of each.

18. What is a fracture?

19. What is a sprain? Describe the difference between the three classes of sprains.

20. What is arthritis? What are the three most common types of arthritis?

21. What is osteoporosis? What precautions must be observed when massaging a person with osteoporosis?

22. Describe three abnormal curves of the spine.

REVIEW

Matching Test I

Insert the letter of the proper term in front of each definition.

_____	**1.** upper arm	a. femur
_____	**2.** wrist bones	b. tarsus
_____	**3.** ankle bones	c. scapula
_____	**4.** toe or finger bones	d. tibia
_____	**5.** palm bones	e. phalanges
_____	**6.** spinal column	f. vertebrae
_____	**7.** collarbone	g. carpals
_____	**8.** shoulder blade	h. metacarpals
_____	**9.** thigh bone	i. humerus
_____	**10.** shin bone	j. clavicle

True or False Test

Carefully read each statement and decide if it is true or false; draw a circle around the letter T or F.

1.	T	F	The hyoid bone supports the base of the ear.
2.	T	F	The metatarsals and metacarpals are different bones.
3.	T	F	The patella forms the front of the knee joint.
4.	T	F	The upper limbs are attached to the pelvis.
5.	T	F	The clavicle and scapula serve as an attachment for the lower limbs.
6.	T	F	The femur is found in the thigh.
7.	T	F	The ulna and radius are found in the forearm.
8.	T	F	The lungs and heart are found in the thorax.
9.	T	F	The vertebrae provide an attachment for the ribs.
10.	T	F	The pelvis is known as the kneecap.

Matching II

Match the definition in the right column with the correct word in the left column.

_____	**1.** crest	a. rounded prominence at a joint
_____	**2.** head	b. a hole
_____	**3.** spine	c. a ridge
_____	**4.** tuberosity	d. a hollow or depression
_____	**5.** foramen	e. articulating end of a bone
_____	**6.** condyle	f. less prominent ridge on a bone
_____	**7.** fossa	g. bony prominence
_____	**8.** trochanter	h. sharp, slender projection
_____	**9.** line	i. larger process for muscle attachment
_____	**10.** process	j. large rounded process

3 THE MUSCULAR SYSTEM

Muscle is the main organ of the muscular system. Muscle is made of specialized cells or fibers that have the unique ability to change their length. The action of muscle cells produce nearly all the movement of the body. Muscle movement is responsible for locomotion and all motor functions. It is responsible for breathing, moving fluids such as blood and urine, as well as moving food through the digestive system. By their action on the fascia, tendons, ligaments, and bones, muscles also provide the stability to support the body in an erect and weight-bearing posture.

The muscular system shapes and supports the skeleton. Depending on a person's physical development, muscles comprise approximately 40 to 60 percent of the total body weight. The skeletal muscular system consists of over 600 muscles, large and small.

Metabolically, muscles use the majority of food and oxygen we consume to produce energy for movement and heat that our body uses for heat regulation. The muscular system relies on the skeletal, nervous, digestive, and respiratory systems for its activities.

Our stiff, sore, achy, tired, tense, injured, and overworked muscles benefit immensely from massage. Massage has a profound effect not only on the common soft tissue dysfunctions of muscles such as strains and spasms, but also on the activity of the blood, lymph, and nerves associated with the muscles of the body. The effects and benefits of massage on muscles and other systems will be addressed in Chapter 6.

Types of Muscles

There are three types of muscular tissue (Figure 5.32):

1. Voluntary, striated, or skeletal muscles are controlled by the will.

2. Involuntary or nonstriated muscles function without the action of the will.

3. Heart or cardiac muscle is found only in the heart, and it is not duplicated anywhere else in the body.

Skeletal (striated) muscles or *voluntary* muscles are put into action by conscious will. They are governed by the central nervous system and appear striated or striped under the microscope. They make up the fleshy areas of the body, are attached to the skeleton, and are in turn fastened to the bones, skin, or other muscles.

Smooth (visceral or involuntary) muscles function without the action of the will. They are controlled by the autonomic nervous system. Smooth muscle consists of spindle-shaped nonstriated cells that overlap at the ends, often forming fibrous bands, such as those found in the walls of the stomach, intestines, and blood vessels. Smooth muscle does not attach to bone, is rather slow acting, can maintain a contraction for a long time, and does not fatigue easily.

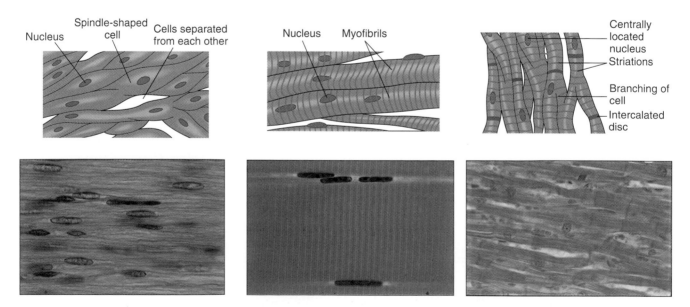

Figure 5.32

Types of muscle.

Cardiac (heart) muscle is found in the heart. It is composed of cells that are as distinctly striated as the cells of skeletal muscle. Cardiac muscle cells are quadrangular, joined end to end, and grouped in bundles supported by a framework of connective tissue.

Characteristics of Muscles

The characteristics that enable muscles to perform their functions of contraction and movement are irritability, contractility, and elasticity. **Irritability** or excitability is the capacity of muscles to receive and react to stimuli, whether mechanical (massage), electrical (currents), thermal (heat), chemical (acid or salt), or impulses of nervous origin.

Muscle also has **contractility,** which is the ability to contract or shorten and thereby exert force. When cardiac muscle contracts, it reduces the area in the chambers of the heart, causing a pumping action. Likewise, when smooth muscle contracts, the diameter of the related organ decreases. If a skeletal muscle is attached to a pair of articulating bones, when the muscle contracts the attachments are drawn closer together, resulting in movement of the bones.

Muscle has **elasticity,** which is the ability to return to its original shape after being stretched. **Extensibility** is the ability of the muscle to stretch.

Structure of Skeletal Muscles

Massage primarily is performed on and affects the skeletal muscles. Therefore, the remainder of this chapter will focus on skeletal muscles.

Skeletal muscles contain several tissues, including muscle tissue, blood and other fluids, nerve tissue, and a variety of connective tissues. The structure of skeletal muscle is unique with its arrangement of contractile fibers aligned and supported in such a way that by contracting, they exert a force on the bony levers of the skeleton, producing movement.

Muscle Tissue

Muscle tissue consists of contractile fibrous tissue arranged in separate parallel bundles (fascicles), which in turn consist of a number of parallel muscle fibers that are held in place by an extensive and intricate connective tissue system. The connective tissue supports the muscle fibers in such a way that when the fibers contract, a force is exerted on whatever structure the muscle is attached to, causing movement.

Muscle tissue is also supplied with a vast network of blood and lymph vessels and capillaries and nerve fibers. The blood supplies the oxygen and nutrients that are essential to carry on the intense metabolic activity as well as carry away the wastes and by-products of muscle activity. The nerves not only provide the motor impulses to the muscles from the central nervous system (CNS) but also supply the CNS with a variety of sensory information from sensory nerve ends located in the skin, muscles, tendons, and joints.

irritability
or excitability, is the capacity of muscles to receive and react to stimuli.

contractility
is the ability of a muscle to contract or shorten and thereby exert force.

elasticity
refers to the tissue's ability to return to normal resting length when a stress that has been placed on it is removed.

extensibility
is the ability of a muscle to stretch.

Connective Tissue

Connective tissues form a continuous netlike framework throughout the body. Connective tissue consists largely of a fluid matrix (ground substance) and collagen fibers that support, bind, and connect the wide range of body structures. Depending on its consistency and the varying proportions of fluid to fibers, a wide array of connective tissues are formed. Some examples are the fluid intercellular environment, the superficial connective tissue just below the skin, the fascia of the muscles, the tendons and ligaments, the tough cartilage, and even bone.

The muscular system is a highly organized system of compartmentalized contractile fibrous tissues that work together to produce movement. The contractile tissue is organized and supported by an intricate network of connective tissue. Connective tissue organizes muscles into functional groups, surrounds each individual muscle, extends inward throughout the muscle creating muscle bundles, and eventually surrounds each muscle fiber. Connective tissue creates a supporting structure for the intricate network of blood vessels and nerves. The connective tissue projects beyond the ends of the muscle to become tendons or flat tendonous sheaths (aponeuroses) that connect the muscles to other structures. Aponeuroses may attach muscles to other muscles or the skin; tendons intertwine with the fibrous coverings of bones (periosteum). Other connective tissue binds and supports the organs and structures in their proper place and forms anchors for lymph and blood vessels and nerves, holding them in their proper place among the organs, muscles, and bones.

The superficial fascia is situated just below the skin and covers the entire muscular system. The fascia penetrates to the bone (deep fascia), separating muscle groups and covering individual muscles, holding them in their relative positions and at the same time allowing them to move somewhat independently. The layer of connective tissue that closely covers an individual muscle is the *epimysium* (ep-i-**MI**-see-um). The *perimysium* (**PAR**-a-**MI**-see-um) extends inward from the epimysium and separates the muscle into bundles of muscle fibers or *fascicles* (**FAS**-i-kls). Within the fascicle, each muscle fiber has a delicate connective tissue covering called the *endomysium*.

The connective tissue organizes the muscle fibers and connects the muscle to tendons, tendons to bones, and even bones to bones. Without this complicated system of connecting sheets, hinges, and ropes that transfers the action of the muscle fibers to the levers of the skeleton, motion and postural stability would not be possible (Figure 5.33).

Muscle Cells or Fibers

The *muscle fiber* or muscle cell is the functional contractile unit of muscle tissue. The muscle cells are long, cylindrical, wormlike structures that usually extend the entire length of the muscle. Muscle cells are multinucleated. A single muscle cell may have hundreds of nuclei distributed just beneath the cell membrane. These nuclei produce the enzymes and proteins necessary in muscle contractions. Multiple nuclei all along the cell

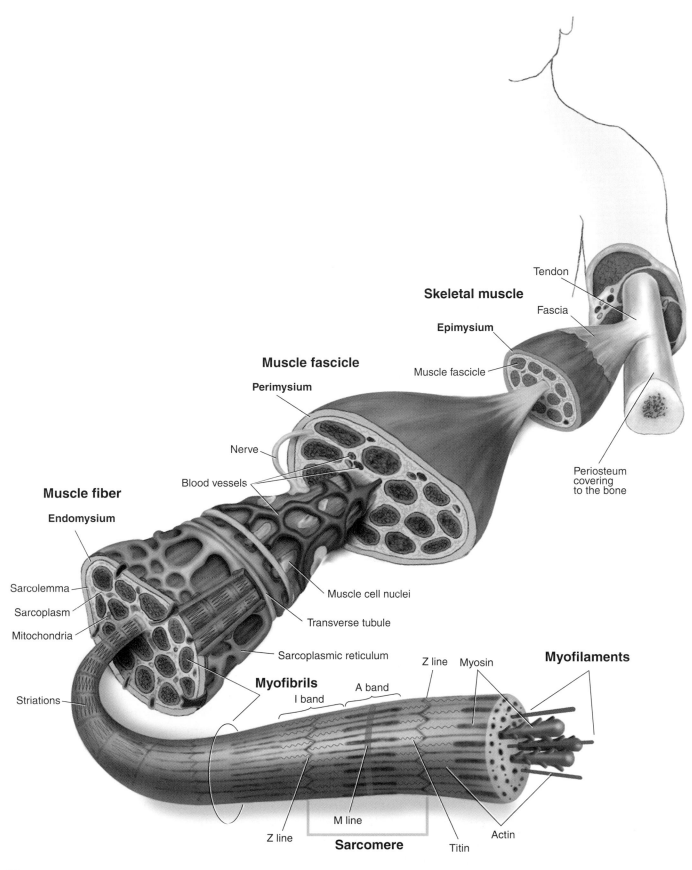

Figure 5.33

Structure of skeletal muscle.

speed up the process. The muscle cell has a connective tissue covering (endomysium [**EN**-do-**MI**-see-um]) that maintains its parallel position with other cells. Toward the end of the muscle fiber, the collagen fibers of the endomysium combine with the fibers of the perimysium and the epimysium to become tendons or the broad sheath of the aponeurosis. The tendon fibers in turn attach usually to bone where the fibers mesh into the periosteum and the bone matrix, providing a firm connection. As a result, the contraction of the muscle fiber is translated into a pull on the tendon and a movement of the bone.

Beneath the layer of connective tissue is a cell membrane (sarcolemma). Within the **sarcolemma** (**SAR**-ko-**LEM**-uh) the muscle cell is highly organized. Each muscle fiber may contain from several hundred to several thousand parallel *myofibrils* (my-o-**FYE**-brils), depending on the size of the muscle fiber.

A myofibril is as long as its muscle fiber and may consist of as many as 10,000 **sarcomeres** arranged end to end. The sarcomere is the smallest functional unit of the muscle fiber. Within every sarcomere is an arrangement of protein filaments that are made up largely of **myosin** or **actin**. The thicker filaments are composed of mostly myosin, and the thinner filaments are composed of mostly actin. The manner in which the actin and myosin filaments are arranged in the sarcomeres gives the skeletal muscle the striped or striated appearance for which it is named. Under magnification, myofibrils appear to have darker A bands and lighter I bands. All the myofibrils in a muscle cell are aligned side-by-side so that the A and I bands appear consistent across the fiber, creating the striated appearance of skeletal muscles (Figure 5.34).

The A band is in the middle of the sarcomere and is caused by the thicker myosin filament. The width of the A band is equal to the length of the myosin filament. Within the A band are the M line, the H zone or band, and the zone of overlap. The M line is the midpoint of the sarcomere where the myosin filaments seem to connect with one another to stabilize their position in the cell. The H zone represents the portion of the myosin filament that is not overlapped by the thinner actin filament. The H zone is wider in a sarcomere at rest and narrower in a cell that is in a contracted position. The zone of overlap contains both myosin and actin filaments. This is the area where the activities of contraction take place.

The I band contains only the thin actin filaments. The I band extends from the edge of the A band in one sarcomere to the edge of the A band in the next sarcomere. In the middle of the I band is the Z line, which acts as the anchor of the actin filaments and is the boundary between sarcomeres. Also anchored to the Z lines are the protein strands of titan, which extend from the ends of the myosin filaments. The titan strands seem to help keep the actin and myosin in proper alignment.

The interaction between the actin and myosin filaments in the sarcomere give muscle its unique contractile ability. When a muscle contracts, the zone of overlap becomes wider, the I band becomes narrower

---

sarcolemma

is the cell wall of the muscle cell.

---

sarcomere

the smallest functional unit of the muscle cell containing the actin and myosin filaments.

---

myosin

a protein that forms filaments that make up nearly 50% of muscle tissue and are involved in muscle contraction.

---

actin

a protein in muscle tissue that forms filaments that interact with myosin filaments to cause muscle contractions.

Figure 5.34
Structure of muscle fibers.

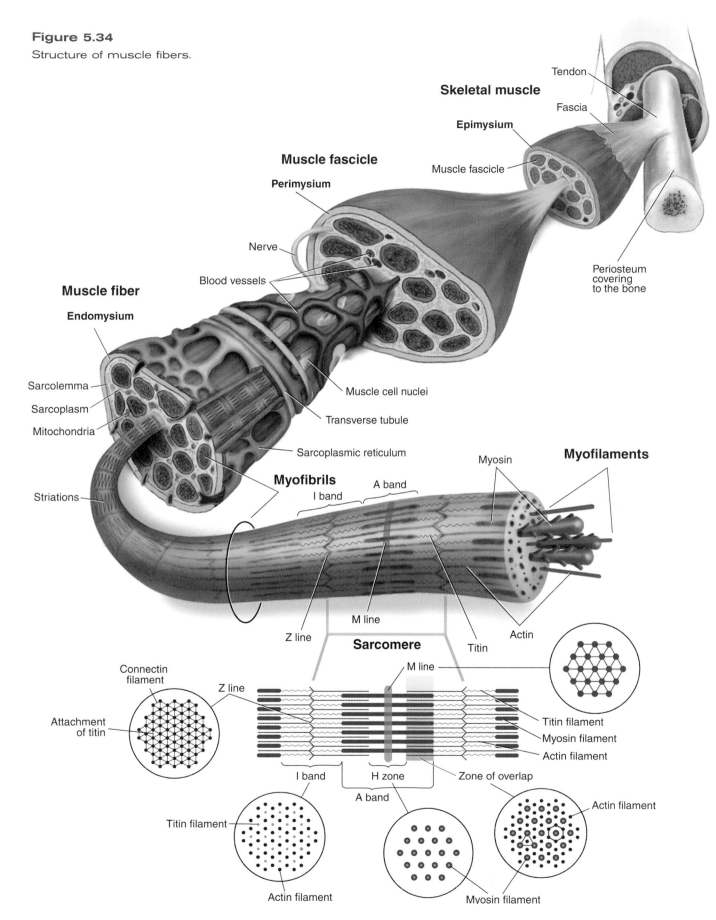

transverse tubules
a system of channels within the muscle cell containing extracellular fluid that helps transmit nerve impulses throughout the cell.

sarcoplasmic reticulum
is a network of membranous channels within the muscle cell that release calcium ions, causing muscle contraction.

myoneural junction
the connection point of the motor nerve and the muscle cell.

spindle cells
located in the belly of muscle, alert the CNS as to the length and stretch and speed of the muscle.

motor unit
consists of a motor neuron and all the muscle fibers it controls.

and the Z lines come closer together. The contraction continues until the I band is nearly eliminated, indicating that the actin filaments slide across the thicker myosin filaments toward the M line as the end of the myosin filaments are drawn toward the Z line. This is known as the *sliding filament theory.*

Extending inward from the cell membrane in the area of the transverse Z lines that anchor the actin filaments is an intricate system of **transverse tubules** that encircle each myofibril and contain extracellular fluid. These tubules play an important role in the transmission of the stimulus of muscle contraction. The **sarcoplasmic reticulum** is a network of membranous channels within the muscle cell that surrounds each myofibril and is closely associated with the transverse tubules. When an impulse is transmitted through the cell membrane and transverse tubules, the sarcoplasmic reticulum releases calcium ions. In the high concentrations of calcium ions in the sarcoplasm (intercellular fluid of the muscle cells) the actin filaments are drawn across the myosin filaments, resulting in the shortening of the cell and contraction of the muscle (Figure 5.34 and Figure 5.35).

Neuromuscular Connection

Every skeletal muscle fiber is connected to a branch of a motor neuron. The site where the muscle fiber and nerve fiber meet is called the *neuromuscular junction* or **myoneural junction.** There are a few specialized muscle cells called **spindle cells** that have both sensory and motor functions and are essential for muscle control and coordination. (More about these later in this chapter.) Although a muscle fiber has only one nerve fiber connection, a motor nerve may have many branches and therefore connect to several muscle fibers. A motor neuron and all the muscle fibers that it controls constitute a **motor unit.** When a motor nerve transmits a stimulus, ALL the muscle fibers connected by its many branches contract simultaneously. Generally, in small muscles that provide intricate movements (e.g., muscles that control speech or eye movement) the motor units may include as few as 6 to 12 muscle fibers, whereas larger muscles that provide less intricate movements (e.g., the vastus muscles or gastrocnemeus) may have several hundred muscle fibers in a single motor unit. Motor units tend to overlap with the muscle fibers of adjacent motor units interspersed among one another. This allows muscle units to support each other and provides for smooth, integrated movements (Figure 5.36).

Skeletal Muscle Contraction

Muscle has the unique ability to change chemical energy into mechanical energy or movement. When a nerve impulse travels from the brain or spinal cord through the motor neuron and reaches the end of the nerve fiber, a chemical *neurotransmitter* called *acetylcholine* (as-e-til-**KOE**-leen) is released and bridges the gap between the nerve end and muscle fiber. The acetylcholine affects the muscle fiber membrane and causes an action potential much like a nerve impulse that immediately travels the length of and throughout the muscle fiber. The impulse is transmitted through the transverse tubules of the muscle fiber, where it contacts the sarcoplasmic reticulum, causing it to release a flood of calcium ions. The calcium ions bond to the actin filaments, which opens active sites on the actin where heads of the myosin molecules attach, pivot, detach, and repeat the process as long as calcium ions and ATP are available. This bridging action causes the actin and myosin filaments to merge, shortening the fiber and contracting the muscle. The sliding mechanism between the actin and myosin filaments involves complex chemical, mechanical, and molecular activity that is beyond the scope of this text. All this mechanical activity requires energy.

The Energy Source for Muscle Activity

The energy for muscle contraction comes from the breakdown of the *adenosine triphosphate (ATP)* molecule. When a muscle contracts, an enzyme causes one of the phosphates to split from the ATP molecule, releasing energy and forming *adenosine diphosphate (ADP)*. There is only enough ATP stored in the muscle cells to sustain a contraction for a few seconds. Fortunately, within a fraction of a second, ADP is reconstituted into ATP in one of several ways.

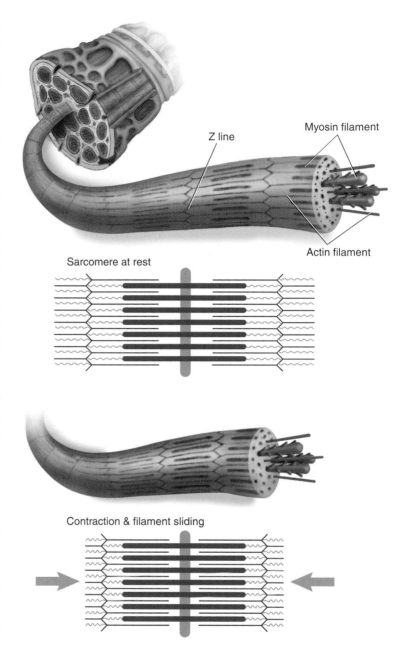

Figure 5.35

Model of muscle contraction. As actin filaments are pulled across myosin filaments, the Z lines are pulled closer together and the overall length of the cell shortens.

Another cellular substance that has a high-energy phosphate bond is *creatine phosphate*. Even though the energy stored in creatine phosphate cannot be used directly by the muscle, when it contacts ADP, the energy causes the rebonding of the phosphate ion, producing ATP. Unfortunately, the combined amounts of creatine phosphate and ATP available in the cell are still sufficient to sustain a contraction for only a few seconds.

Most of the energy to reconstitute ADP is the result of cellular respiration. **Aerobic cellular respiration** takes place in the cells'

> **aerobic cellular respiration**
>
> makes energy for reconstituting ADP in cell mitochondrion.

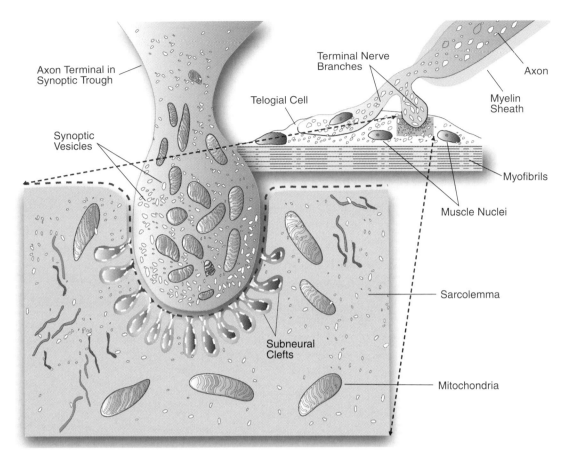

Figure 5.36
Myoneural junction.

mitochondria. Aerobic respiration is responsible for the majority of the sustained energy supply for the constant replenishing of ATP. Most of the food we eat, by the time it goes through the digestive process and is transported to the cells, has been converted to glucose. As the glucose is transported through the cell to the mitochondria, it is converted to pyruvic acid. In the mitochondria, a complex metabolic process known as the Krebs cycle or the citric acid cycle takes place, resulting in the production of carbon dioxide, water, and energy in the form of heat and the synthesis of ATP.

The oxygen required to carry on aerobic respiration is carried to the cells from the lungs in the blood by the red blood cells. The amount of oxygen taken in and the rate at which it can be delivered to the mitochondria of the cells determines how much ATP can be reconstituted and therefore how much a muscle can do.

When the oxygen available for aerobic respiration is depleted, anaerobic respiration takes place. In **anaerobic respiration** (in the absence of oxygen), glucose is broken down, releasing enough energy to synthesize some ATP and produce pyruvic acid, which is converted to lactic acid. The lactic acid is carried by the bloodstream to the liver, where it is converted back to glucose (ATP is required for this conversion).

anaerobic respiration

is a process in which glucose is broken down in the absence of oxygen.

During light or moderate activity, the lungs and circulatory system are able to supply the skeletal muscles adequate amounts of oxygen to carry on aerobic respiration. However, after just a few minutes of strenuous output, the pulse and respiration rate increase. As the strenuous activity continues, the circulatory and respiratory systems cannot supply enough oxygen to the muscles, which forces them to rely on the less efficient anaerobic respiration. Anaerobic respiration produces pyruvic and then lactic acid. As lactic acid accumulates, the person develops *oxygen debt.* After the strenuous activity ceases, the heavy breathing and accelerated heart rate continue until the oxygen debt is paid off, and then normal breathing and pulse resume.

Muscle Fatigue

If rapid or prolonged muscle contractions continue to the point that oxygen debt becomes extreme, the muscle will cease to respond. This condition is **muscle fatigue.** Muscle fatigue results either because the circulation of blood cannot keep pace with the demand for oxygen or because the waste products accumulate faster than they can be removed, affecting the muscle's ability to respond to nerve impulses.

Muscle Tone

Muscle tone is a type of muscle contraction that is present in healthy muscles even when they are at rest. A muscle possesses tone if it is firm and responds promptly to stimulation under normal conditions. Lack of tone is evidenced by a condition of flaccidness. Exercise and massage help to improve muscle tone.

Muscle Fiber Types

Muscle fiber structure varies according to function. There are two distinctive types of muscle fibers: Type I, slow twitch fibers, and Type II, fast twitch fibers. Type II fibers are subdivided into Type IIa and Type IIb.

Type I, slow twitch fibers, have a relatively slower contraction time and a high resistance to fatigue. They contain a high number of mitochondria, large amounts of myoglobin, and have an ample capillary supply. Myoglobin is a form of hemoglobin in the muscle tissue that stores oxygen and gives muscle its red color. The rich blood supply and numerous mitochondria give the fibers a high capacity to generate ATP and sustain low-level contractions for a long period of time while resisting fatigue. Type I fibers are found in large quantities in postural muscles.

Type IIb, fast twitch fibers, produce powerful, high velocity contractions for short periods of time. The contraction velocity is 5 to 10 times faster than Type I fibers. They contain few mitochondria, low myoglobin content, and few capillaries, which give them a lighter, whitish color. They depend on glycogen and creatine phosphate for ATP generation, and they fatigue easily. Type II fibers are more prevalent in the arms, shoulders, and legs.

Type IIa fibers are rarely found in humans. It seems that through extensive endurance training, Type IIb fibers take on characteristics of Type I

> **muscle fatigue**
> is a condition in which the muscle ceases to respond due to oxygen debt from rapid or prolonged muscle contractions.

> **muscle tone**
> is a type of muscle contraction present in healthy muscles even when at rest.

Table 5.4
Muscle Fiber Characteristics

MUSCLE FIBER TYPE	TYPE I	TYPE IIA	TYPE IIB
Contraction velocity	Slow	Fast	Fast
Fiber color	Red	Red	White
Fatigue time	Slow	Intermediate	Fast
Myoglobin content	High	High	Low
Capillary density	High	High	Low
Mitochondria density	High	High	Low

fibers with better blood supply, higher concentrations of mitochondria, and more myoglobin to give muscle more endurance while maintaining explosive speed and strength. Table 5.4 presents an overview of muscle fiber characteristics.

Chicken provides a graphic example of muscle types. The white breast meat is made of Type II fibers; the darker leg and thigh is Type I muscle. The legs are continuously used for walking and consist of high-endurance Type I fibers. The breast muscles are used for very occasional short bursts of flying and therefore consist of Type II fibers.

Type I muscle is slow to fatigue due to an ample blood supply and numerous mitochondria available to generate adequate amounts of ATP via aerobic respiration to sustain low to moderate muscle activity. Ninety-five percent of the muscle's ATP production takes place in the cell's mitochondria. The aerobic respiration of Type I fibers uses oxygen and glucose supplied from the blood to produce ATP to energize the muscle contraction with by-products of carbon dioxide and water, which is carried away by the bloodstream.

Type IIb muscle fibers provide on-demand, powerful, explosive contractions. These fibers tend to be larger with more actin/myosin filaments but fewer mitochondria and less blood supply. Without the rich supply of blood and oxygen, ATP generation for Type IIb muscle contraction is supplied more by creatine phosphate and the anaerobic metabolism of glycogen, both of which are stored in the muscle. The muscle converts glycogen to glucose and then in the absence of oxygen (anaerobic) metabolizes ATP with lactic acid as a by-product. The depletion of stored creatine phosphate and glycogen and the buildup of lactic acid cause the Type IIb cell to fatigue rather quickly. Rest periods between bursts of activity allow circulation to remove lactic acid and restore the oxygen debt in fast twitch muscle fibers.

Most muscles contain both fiber types. The proportion of fast and slow twitch fibers depends on the primary function of the muscle and on genetics. Postural muscles contain a higher proportion of Type I fibers. Phasic muscles—those used for quick, infrequent, powerful movement—contain a higher proportion of Type II fibers. Postural muscles are stabilizers, and phasic muscles are movers. Different muscle fibers in a particular muscle may be called upon for different functions. For example, if only slight muscle contractions are needed for a task, such as a gentle stroll down a lane, only Type I fibers in the legs are active. However, if stronger contractions are needed, say to chase after a dog that has stolen your favorite hat, Type IIb fibers would be activated. Each type of muscle fiber is energized by separate motor neurons. A single motor neuron may activate as few as 2 and as many as 2,000 muscle fibers. A single muscle may have hundreds of thousands of muscle fibers. A motor unit will only contain fibers of one type and will activate with a frequency conducive to those fibers. If the demand is light, slow twitch fibers will be stimulated. When more intense movement is called for, Type IIb fibers activate. Type I fibers have lower activation threshold than Type IIb fibers. The activation of the various motor units is controlled in the spinal cord and brain (see Box 5.2).

BOX 5.2   MAJOR PHASIC AND POSTURAL MUSCLES

Phasic Muscles

- Respond to dysfunction and stress by hypotonicity and weakening
- Anterior neck flexors
- Scalenii
- Deltoid
- Lower pectorals
- Middle and lower trapezius
- Rhomboids
- Serratus anterior
- Rectus abdominis
- Gluteals
- Hamstrings
- Vastus muscles
- Peroneals
- Arm extensors

Postural Muscles

- Respond to dysfunction and stress with hypertonicity and shortening
- Upper trapezius
- Levator scapulae
- Sternocleidomastoid
- Upper pectoralis major
- Pectoralis minor
- Latissimus dorsi
- Sacrospinalis
- Lumbar erector spinae
- Quadratus lumborum
- Iliopsoas
- Piriformis
- Oblique abdominals
- Adductor longus and magnus
- Tensor fascia lata
- Rectus femoris
- Medial hamstrings
- Soleus
- Gastrocnemius
- Tibialis posterior

Postural muscles support the body against gravity and are made up of a higher proportion of Type I fibers. They are slower to respond to stimulation and slower to fatigue. They respond to undue or sustained stress and strain by shortening, becoming hypertonic, developing trigger points and fibrosis. Under continuous strain, the connective tissue of postural muscle thickens to support the structure.

Phasic muscles move the body by responding quickly and forcefully when stimulated. They consist of a higher proportion of Type IIb fibers. As postural muscles tend to tighten and shorten when stressed, associated phasic muscles tend to be inhibited and weaken. This is important to note when working with clients with postural concerns. Because phasic muscles contract quickly and forcefully, common problems include muscle strains, tendonitis, and microtrauma at the musculotendinous and tendonoperiosteal junctions.

Muscle Insertion and Origin

As explained earlier, the connective tissue surrounding the muscle fibers extends beyond the ends of the fibers to become the fibrous, rather inelastic, tendons that anchor the ends of the muscle to the bones. The arrangement of muscle fibers and tendons varies according to muscle function and location. Some muscles, such as the biceps, form cordlike tendons at either end of the muscle belly. Other muscles, such as the deltoid and trapezius, have their attachments spread over a broad area.

The structures to which the tendons attach determine the action that the contracting muscles produce. Skeletal muscles, as their name implies, have at least one end of the muscle that is attached to bone. The end of the muscle is anchored to a relatively immovable section of the skeleton called the **origin of the muscle.** The *origin* of a muscle is generally located more proximal or nearer the center of the body.

The other end of the muscle attaches either to a bone, the deeper structures of the skin, or other muscles and creates the action of the structure. The term applied to the more mobile attachment is the **insertion of the muscle.** The *insertion* of a muscle is generally attached to the more distal aspect of an appendage. In some movements, the roles of insertion and origin of a muscle can be reversed. The action of a muscle contraction can be derived from the knowledge of its insertion and origin (Figure 5.37).

Isometric and Isotonic Contractions

When a muscle contracts and the ends of the muscle do not move or the body part that the muscle affects does not move, the contraction is an **isometric contraction.** When a person strains to move a heavy object that does not budge, the muscle effort is isometric. In the muscles that stabilize our bodies in an upright posture, most contractions are continuous and isometric.

---

origin of a muscle

is the point where the end of a muscle is anchored to an immovable section of the skeleton.

insertion of a muscle

is the more mobile attachment of a muscle to bone.

isometric contraction

occurs when a muscle contracts and the ends of the muscle do not move.

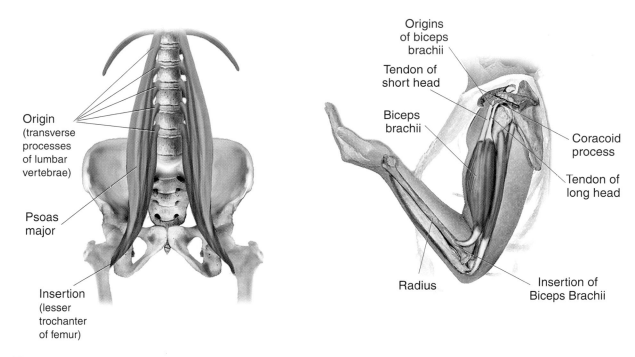

Figure 5.37
Muscle insertion and origin.

When a muscle contracts and the distance between the ends of the muscle changes, it is an **isotonic contraction.** When the distance between the ends of a contracting muscle decreases, the isotonic contraction is said to be *concentric.* When the distance between the ends of a contracting muscle increases, the isotonic contraction is said to be **eccentric.** When you do a push-up, as you push up, the loaded muscles are shortening and the contraction is concentric. As you lower yourself to the floor, the loaded muscles are getting longer and the contraction is eccentric. In both directions, the contractions are isotonic.

isotonic contraction
occurs when a muscle contracts and the distance between the ends of the muscle changes.

eccentric contraction
occurs when a muscle contracts while the ends of the muscle move farther apart.

Muscle Interaction

In some ways, the muscular system could be considered one continuous muscle that covers the entire body and is divided into various chambers by an intricate system of connective tissue. This muscle is controlled by a vast network of neuromuscular units that coordinate their activities through the central nervous system to produce smooth, coordinated, graceful movements.

The classic approach has been to study the effect of the individual muscles on joint action. But this is not physiologic. Normal muscle action is the patterned response of groups of muscles. Muscles have anatomic individuality, but they do not have functional individuality. (See K. Little, "Toward More Effective Manipulative Management of Chronic Myofascial Strain and Stress Syndromes," in *The Journal of the American Osteopathic Association,* 68:675, 685, March 1969.)

prime mover
the primary muscle responsible for a specific movement.

agonist
a prime mover.

antagonist
the muscle that performs the opposite movement of the agonist.

synergists
muscles that assist the agonist.

fixator
muscles that act to stabilize a body part so another muscle can act on an adjacent limb or body part.

Individual muscles, because of their specific attachments when contracted, generate a specific action. However, muscles never work alone. When an isolated and specific action occurs, the muscle responsible for that action is the **prime mover** (sometimes referred to as the **agonist**). When the prime mover contracts, there is a muscle that causes the opposite action. That opposing muscle is referred to as the **antagonist.** For instance, when the elbow is flexed with the hand in the supine position, the prime mover is the biceps. The opposite action would be to extend the arm. The muscle responsible for arm extension is the triceps, so the antagonist of the biceps is the triceps. It is clear from this example that when the prime mover contracts and shortens, the antagonist must extend. Most movement, however, is not that simple, and even when considering only one joint, several muscles may be involved. Muscles that assist the prime mover are called **synergists** (SIN-er-jists). **Fixator** or stabilizer muscles stabilize more proximal joints in order that more distal limbs can perform weight-bearing functions.

In observing the dynamics of movement, there are three components of motion: flexion/extension, abduction/adduction, and rotation. Most joints in the body function in at least two of these components, and many articulations involve all three. A muscle that acts across a joint will have a primary function in one of the three components of motion, but the same muscle may have a secondary or even a tertiary action depending on the mobility of the joint. For instance, in Figure 5.38, the primary function of the biceps is to flex the elbow; however, a secondary function of the biceps is to assist in supination of the forearm and a minor, tertiary function of the short head of the biceps is to flex the shoulder (Figure 5.38 to Figure 5.42).

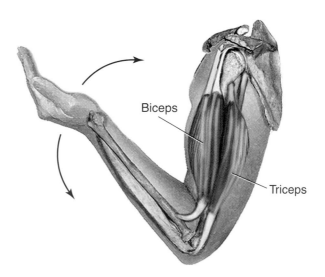

Figure 5.38
Muscle interaction.

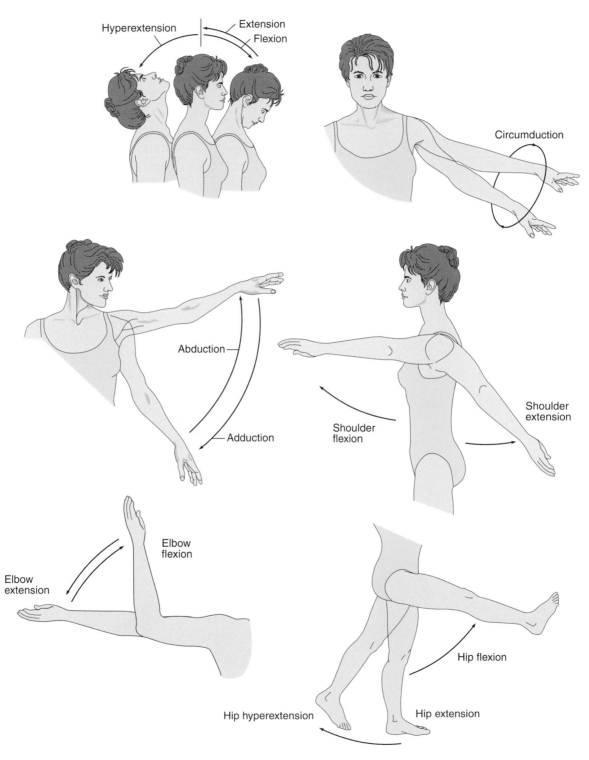

Figure 5.39

Motion in diarthrotic joints.

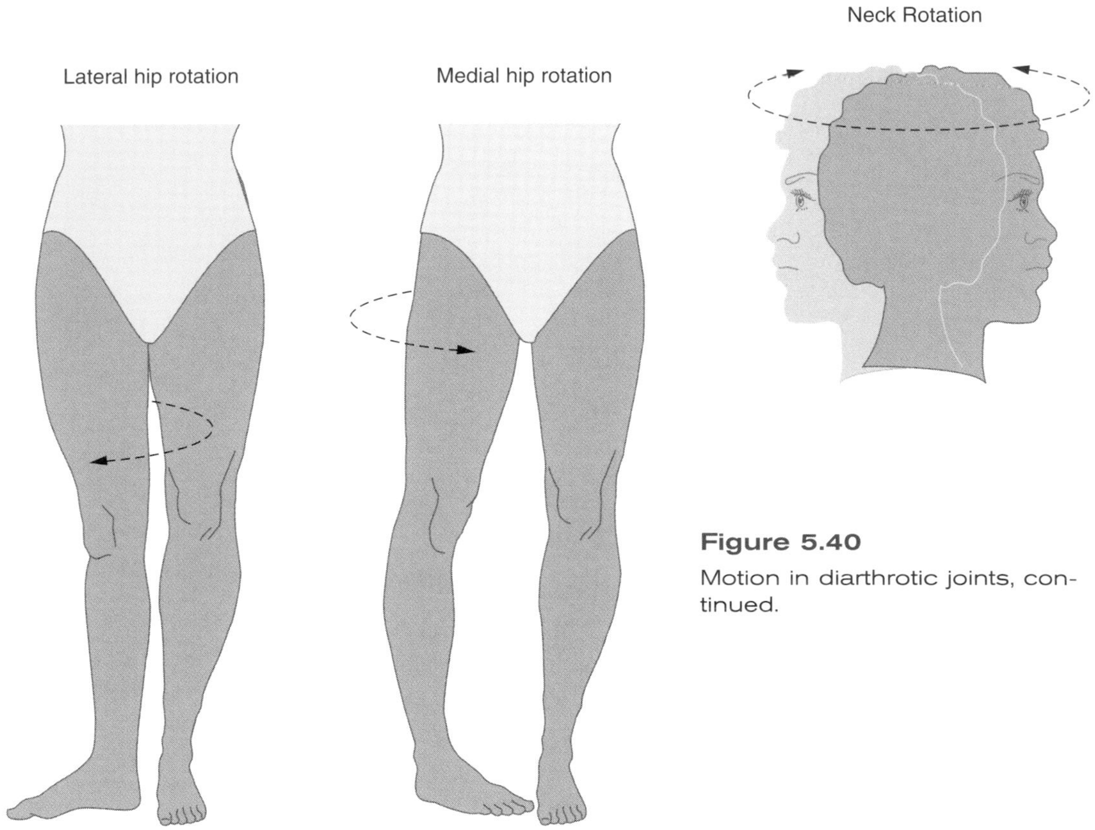

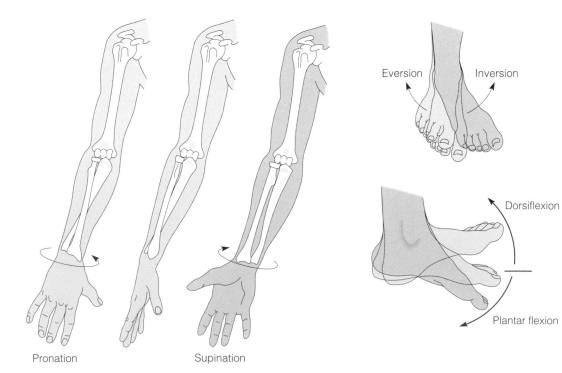

Lateral hip rotation

Medial hip rotation

Neck Rotation

Figure 5.40
Motion in diarthrotic joints, continued.

Eversion

Inversion

Dorsiflexion

Plantar flexion

Pronation

Supination

Figure 5.41
Motion in diarthrotic joints, continued.

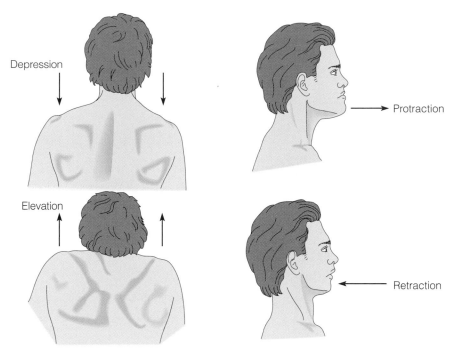

Figure 5.42
Motion in diarthrotic joints, continued.

Table 5.5, pages 155 to 196, gives a comprehensive presentation of the location and action of muscles.

Terms to Remember

A review of the words shown below will be helpful in understanding the meaning of technical terms when studying the muscular system (Figure 5.43 and Figure 5.44).

Anterior: before, or in front of

Posterior: behind, or in back of

Superior: situated above

Inferior: situated lower

Oblique or anguli: at an angle

Levator: that which lifts

Dorsal: behind, or in back of

Medial: pertaining to the middle or center

Dilator: that which expands or enlarges

Depressor: that which presses or draws down

Proximal: nearer to the center or medial line

Distal: farther from the center or medial line

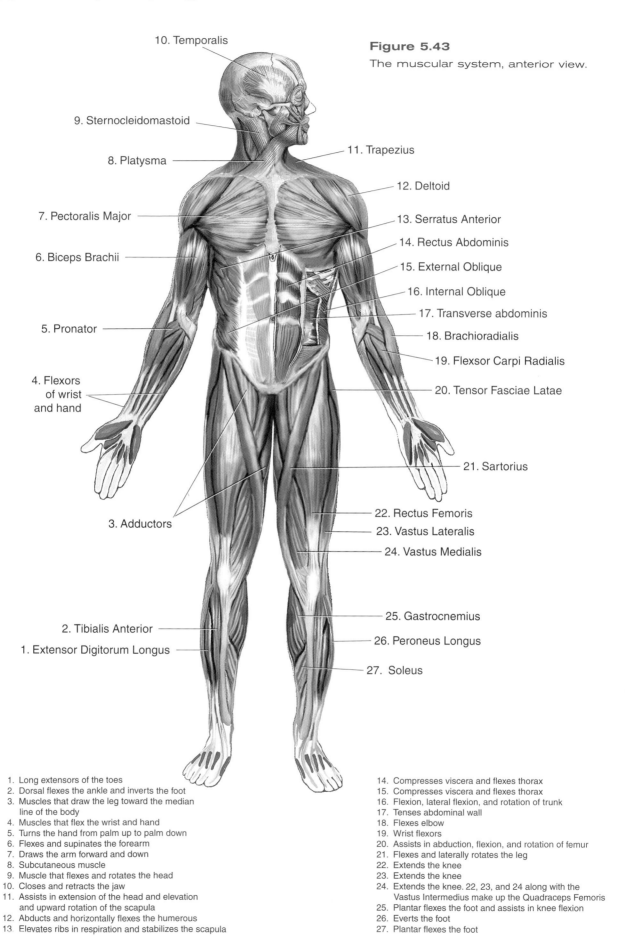

Figure 5.43

The muscular system, anterior view.

10. Temporalis

9. Sternocleidomastoid

8. Platysma

7. Pectoralis Major

6. Biceps Brachii

5. Pronator

4. Flexors of wrist and hand

3. Adductors

2. Tibialis Anterior

1. Extensor Digitorum Longus

11. Trapezius

12. Deltoid

13. Serratus Anterior

14. Rectus Abdominis

15. External Oblique

16. Internal Oblique

17. Transverse abdominis

18. Brachioradialis

19. Flexsor Carpi Radialis

20. Tensor Fasciae Latae

21. Sartorius

22. Rectus Femoris

23. Vastus Lateralis

24. Vastus Medialis

25. Gastrocnemius

26. Peroneus Longus

27. Soleus

1. Long extensors of the toes
2. Dorsal flexes the ankle and inverts the foot
3. Muscles that draw the leg toward the median line of the body
4. Muscles that flex the wrist and hand
5. Turns the hand from palm up to palm down
6. Flexes and supinates the forearm
7. Draws the arm forward and down
8. Subcutaneous muscle
9. Muscle that flexes and rotates the head
10. Closes and retracts the jaw
11. Assists in extension of the head and elevation and upward rotation of the scapula
12. Abducts and horizontally flexes the humerous
13. Elevates ribs in respiration and stabilizes the scapula

14. Compresses viscera and flexes thorax
15. Compresses viscera and flexes thorax
16. Flexion, lateral flexion, and rotation of trunk
17. Tenses abdominal wall
18. Flexes elbow
19. Wrist flexors
20. Assists in abduction, flexion, and rotation of femur
21. Flexes and laterally rotates the leg
22. Extends the knee
23. Extends the knee
24. Extends the knee. 22, 23, and 24 along with the Vastus Intermedius make up the Quadraceps Femoris
25. Plantar flexes the foot and assists in knee flexion
26. Everts the foot
27. Plantar flexes the foot

Figure 5.44

The muscular system, posterior view.

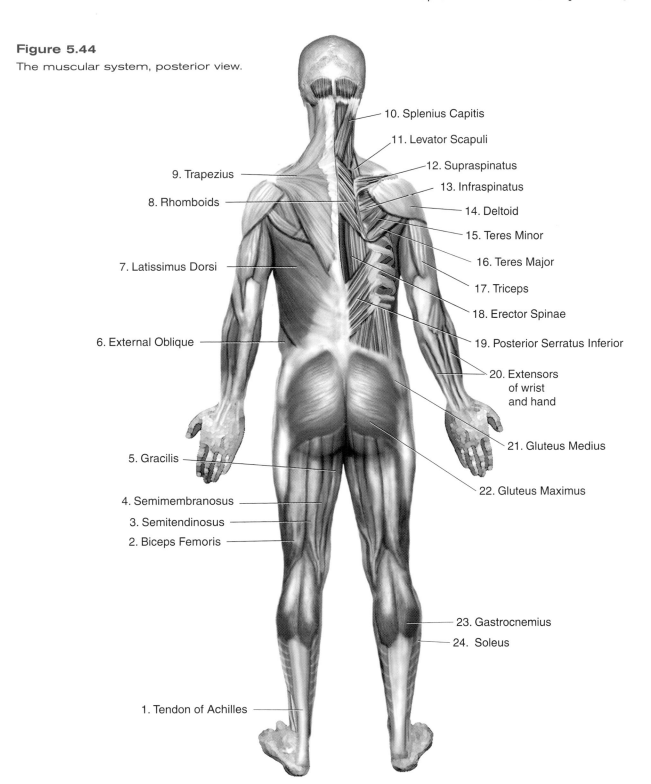

10. Splenius Capitis

11. Levator Scapuli

12. Supraspinatus

9. Trapezius

13. Infraspinatus

8. Rhomboids

14. Deltoid

15. Teres Minor

16. Teres Major

7. Latissimus Dorsi

17. Triceps

18. Erector Spinae

6. External Oblique

19. Posterior Serratus Inferior

20. Extensors of wrist and hand

21. Gluteus Medius

5. Gracilis

22. Gluteus Maximus

4. Semimembranosus

3. Semitendinosus

2. Biceps Femoris

23. Gastrocnemius

24. Soleus

1. Tendon of Achilles

1. Attaches calf muscle to heel bone
2, 3, 4. Make up the hamstrings that flex the knee and assist in extension of the hip
5. Draws leg toward the mid-line
6. Supports abdominal viscera; flexes vertebral column
7. Draws arm backward and downward: rotates arm inward
8. Draws scapula toward the spine
9. Draws scapula toward the spine; rotates scapula either upward or downward; draws head backward
10. Draws head back or rotates the head
11. Elevation and/or downward rotation of scapula
12. Abducts the arm

13. Outward rotation and extension of arm
14. Abducts and rotates humerus
15. Lateral rotation of humerus
16. Inward rotation, abduction, and extension of humerus
17. Extends the forearm
18. Extension of the spine
19. Pulls ribs outward and down; opposes diaphragm
20. Extends the wrist and hand
21. Abducts and rotates the thigh
22. Extends, abducts, and rotates the thigh outward
23. Flexes the knee and plantar flexes the foot
24. Plantar flexes the foot

Common Dysfunctions and Diseases of the Muscular System

Muscle Spasms

Muscle spasms are the most common muscle dysfunction. A spasm is a sudden involuntary contraction of a muscle or a group of muscles. Spasms vary both in duration and intensity and may affect any muscle tissue (voluntary, involuntary, or cardiac). Spasms are considered *tonic* when they are sustained or *clonic* when they alternate between contraction and relaxation. Intense, short-lived, painful spasms are often designated as *cramps*. Some common examples of muscle spasms are hiccups, tics and twitches in the face, torticollis (**TOR**-ti-koll-is), charley horses, convulsions, and muscle "splinting" associated with injuries. Spasms may occur as a result of injury, disease, or emotional stress (stuttering). Usually, spasms cease when their cause is corrected.

The appropriateness for massage depends on the nature of the spasm or cramp. Massage directly on the site of an acute cramp or charley horse is contraindicated. However, compressing from the ends of the affected muscle or resisting the contraction of the antagonist may inhibit and quiet the spasming muscle. Massage in the subacute stage or after the spasm has subsided will help restore circulation and nutrients to the muscle tissue while clearing the tissues of toxic waste and debris.

Massage on a splinting muscle that is protecting an injury site is contraindicated during the acute and even into the subacute stages of the injury. Occasionally, splinting will continue well after the injured tissue has healed, causing compensation or restricted movement. This is when massage and soft tissue interventions are appropriate to release tension and restore circulation and flexibility.

Contractures

Contractures are shortened, contracted muscles or muscle groups where the muscle atrophies and shrinks while the connective tissue thickens. Contractures are usually related to immobility or severe nerve damage and usually result in flexion rather than extension of the affected limb. Contractures are common in conditions such as cerebral palsy and spinal cord injury. Massage is of little or no benefit when addressing contractures in an advanced or chronic state. However, massage and consistent stretching exercises may help prevent or reduce the extent of a contracture if employed during the early stages of the condition before the connective tissue thickens and the muscles atrophy.

Muscle Strains

Muscle strains (also called torn or pulled muscles) are the most common injury to muscle. There are three degrees or grades of muscle strain.

Grade I is an overstretching of a few of the muscle fibers with a minimal tearing of the fibers. There is some pain but no loss of function and no palpable or visual indications.

Grade II involves a partial tear of between 10 and 50 percent of the muscle fibers. There is considerable pain and some loss of function. There is a palpable thickening of the muscle tissue, and there may be some tissue bleeding.

Grade III is the most severe injury with between 50 and 100 percent muscle tearing. There is a palpable depression and/or bunching of the muscle with severe pain and total or near total loss of muscle function.

Muscle strains may occur in different sites in the muscle. The majority of the strains (80 percent) occur in the muscle belly or at the junction between the muscle and the tendon (musculotendinous junction). Other less common sites are at the insertion or the origin or in the tendon of the muscle.

Torn fibers of a muscle strain initiate an inflammatory response, flooding the area with fluid containing white blood cells to carry away damaged debris and fibroblasts to create collagen fibers to begin to mend the injured tissues. The influx of fluid causes swelling and pain, which helps to limit movement. The preferred intervention during the acute stage of a muscle strain, which may last from 24 to 72 hours depending on the severity, is described by the acronym RICE (rest, ice, compression, and elevation). Massage is contraindicated during the acute stage of a muscle strain.

Specialized massage procedures are invaluable during the subacute stages (as the injury heals) to ensure that the newly forming scar tissue is strong and pliable, to limit the formation of adhesions between fascial sheaths, to promote circulation, and to restore range of motion. Certain massage procedures are helpful at the site of old muscle strains to reduce adhesions, improve mobility, and reduce the chance of reinjury.

Hypertrophy

Muscle hypertrophy is an enlargement of the breadth of a muscle as a result of repeated forceful muscle activity. Most of the hypertrophy is due to the increase in the size of the muscle fibers rather than an increase in the number of muscle fibers. As a result of the increased size, the power of the muscle increases as well as the metabolic support system (i.e., increased blood supply, sarcoplasm, ATP, mitochondria, etc.). It is also likely that the number of actin/myosin filaments and number of fibrils in the muscle fiber increase; however, this has not been substantiated.

Atrophy

Muscle atrophy is the reverse of hypertrophy and is the result of muscle disuse. If a muscle cannot be contracted or is only contracted very weakly, the muscle tissue will rapidly degenerate and begin to waste away. The number and size of the capillaries supplying the muscle decrease as well as the sarcoplasm and its constituents (mitochondria, sarcoplasmic reticulum, glycogen, ATP, etc.). The size of the fibrils and the actin/myosin filaments is reduced, as is the power of the muscle. If the nerve supply to the muscle is interfered with, paralysis results and muscle atrophy progresses rapidly. If atrophy continues over an extended period of time, the contractile tissue will continue to degenerate until it is replaced with connective tissue and rehabilitation becomes all but impossible.

Tendonitis and Tenosynovitis

Tendonitis is an inflammation of the tendon, often occurring at the musculotendinous or tenoperiosteal junction. Tenosynovitis is an inflammation of the tendon sheath. Both are accompanied by pain, stiffness, and often swelling. Many times, they occur simultaneously. Massage is indicated to relieve muscle tension and to assist healing in the subacute stage but should be avoided on the lesion during the acute stages.

Lupus Erythematosus

Lupus is a chronic inflammatory disease of the connective tissue that may affect many body tissues and organs. It is an autoimmune disorder that causes blood vessel inflammation (especially in the face), organ dysfunction, and arthritis. Massage may be given only under the supervision of a physician.

Fibromyalgia Syndrome

Fibromyalgia is characterized by pain, fatigue, and stiffness in the connective tissue of the muscles, tendons, and ligaments. It is associated with stress, poor sleep habits, and occupational or recreational strain and is more prevalent in women. Systemic viral or bacterial infections may be a precursor, as well as cold, damp conditions. It is often related to chronic fatigue syndrome. There are identifiable trigger points. Massage to desensitize trigger points and range-of-motion exercises are beneficial. All massage should be gentle and done with great consideration of the condition. Each person's symptoms vary, as does tolerance to the modalities and pressure applied by the practitioner. Refer to and work in conjunction with a physician.

Dystrophy

Muscular dystrophy refers to a group of related diseases that seem to be genetically inherited and that cause a progressive degeneration of the voluntary muscular system. With muscular dystrophy, the contractile fibers of the muscles are gradually replaced by fat and connective tissue until those muscles become virtually useless. All the visible effects of muscular dystrophy seem to be in the muscles. It rarely causes pain, and the intellect is not affected. Exercise and massage are helpful in prolonging muscular ability and maintaining flexibility.

Table 5.5

Location and Action of Muscles

MUSCLES OF THE UPPER EXTREMITIES					
Muscles That Act on and Support the Scapula					
MUSCLE	ORIGIN	INSERTION	ACTION	INNERVATION	PALPATION
Trapezius					
Upper	Occiput and ligamentum nuchae of cervical spine	Lateral one third of clavicle and acromion	Elevation and upward rotation of scapula	Cranial XI, Spinal Accessory	From below occiput to acromion
Middle	Spinous process C7–T5	Spine of the scapula	Pulls scapula medially	C3–4	From spinous process T1–5 to acromion
Lower	Spinous process T5–T12	Spine of the scapula	Depression and upward rotation of scapula	C3–4	From spinous process T5–12 to spine of scapula
Rhomboid					
Major	Spinous process T2–5	Lower two thirds of vertebral border of scapula	Retracts and rotates scapula downward	C5, Dorsal scapular	Under Trapezius along vertebral border of scapula
Minor	Spinous process C7–T1	Vertebral border at root of the spine of the scapula	Same as Rhomboid major	C5, Dorsal scapular	Just superior to Rhomboid major, hard to palpate
Levator Scapulae	Transverse process C1–4	Superior one third of vertebral border of scapula	Elevation of scapula and moves neck laterally	C3–5	Anterior to upper Trapezius, hard to palpate
Pectoralis Minor	Anterior ribs 3, 4, 5	Coracoid process	Forward rotation and depression of scapula	C8–T1, Medial pectoral	Under Pectoralis major in axillary space, hard to palpate
Serratus Anterior	Anterior ribs 1–8	Anterior aspect of vertebral border of scapula	Stabilization, upward rotation and protraction of the scapula	C5, 6, 7, Posterior thoracic	Lateral ribs below axilla

continues

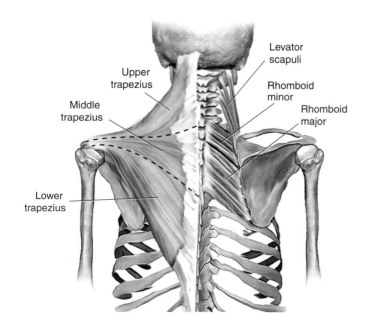

Levator scapuli

Upper trapezius

Middle trapezius

Rhomboid minor

Rhomboid major

Lower trapezius

T5–5.1

Posterior upper thorax:

Trapezius m. One side is cut away to show rhomboids and levator.

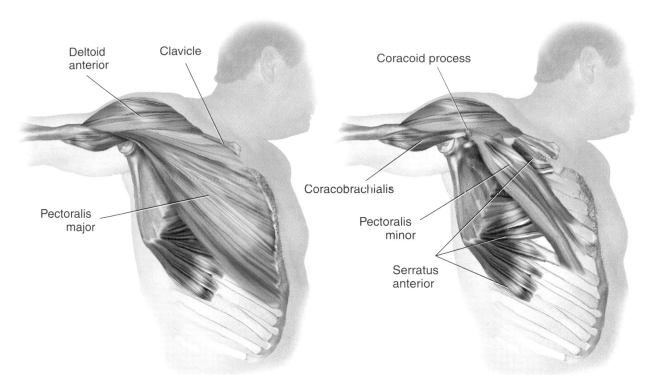

T5–5.2

Anterior lateral upper thorax (pectoralis major cut away):
serratus anterior and pectoralis minor.

Table 5.5 (continued)

MUSCLES OF THE UPPER EXTREMITIES (continued)					
Muscles That Act on the Upper Arm					
MUSCLE	**ORIGIN**	**INSERTION**	**ACTION**	**INNERVATION**	**PALPATION**
Pectoralis Major Clavicular	Medial half of clavicle, clavicular head	Lateral ridge of bicipital groove distal to pectoralis major sternal insertion	Adduction, horizontal adduction, medial rotation and flexion of humerus	C5, 6, 7, Lateral pectoral	Anterior of axilla
Sternal	Sternum, costal cartilage of ribs 1–6	Lateral ridge of bicipital groove proximal to pectoralis major clavicular insertion	Same as clavicular plus extension of humerus from flexed position	C8, T1, Lateral and medial pectoral	Anterior of axilla
Coracobrachialis	Coracoid process of scapula	Middle of medial humerus	Flexion and adduction of humerus	C6, 7, Musculocutaneous	Hard to palpate
Deltoid Anterior	Lateral one third of clavicle	Deltoid tuberosity of humerus	Flexion, horizontal rotation	C5, 6 Axillary nerve adduction, medial	This is the rounded shoulder muscle; the anterior in front, the middle lateral to and the posterior in the back of the shoulder joint
Middle	Acromion and lateral spine of the scapula	Deltoid tuberosity of humerus	Abduction to 90 degrees	C5, 6 Axillary nerve	

Table 5.5 (continued)

MUSCLES OF THE UPPER EXTREMITIES (continued) Muscles That Act on the Upper Arm (continued)					
MUSCLE	**ORIGIN**	**INSERTION**	**ACTION**	**INNERVATION**	**PALPATION**
Deltoid, cont'd					
Posterior	Lower lip of the spine of the scapula	Deltoid tuberosity of humerus	Extension, horizontal abduction, lateral rotation	C5, 6 Axillary nerve	
Supraspinatus	Supraspinous fossa of scapula	Top of greater tubercle of the humerus	Initiates abduction of the humerus	C5, Suprascapular nerve	Above spine of scapula near acromion
Infraspinatus	Infraspinous fossa of scapula	Greater tubercle of humerus	Lateral rotation of humerus	C5, 6, Suprascapular nerve	Below the spine of the scapula
Subscapularis	Anterior surface of the scapula	Lesser tubercle of the humerus	Medial rotation of humerus	C6, 7 Subscapular nerve	Hard to palpate
Teres Minor	Upper axillary border of scapula	Greater tubercle of humerus	Lateral rotation of humerus	C5, Axillary nerve	Below posterior deltoid and above teres major
Teres Major	Lateral border, inferior angle of scapula	Medial ridge of bicipital groove of humerus	Extension, adduction, medial rotation of humerus	C6, 7, Subscapular nerve	With latissimus dorsi forms posterior border of axilla
Latissimus Dorsi	Thoracolumbar aponeurosis from T7 to iliac crest, lower ribs, inferior angle of scapula	Bicipital groove of humerus	Extension, adduction, medial rotation of humerus	C6, 7, 8, Thoracodorsal nerve	Large muscle forming posterior axilla and extending down toward posterior ribs

continues

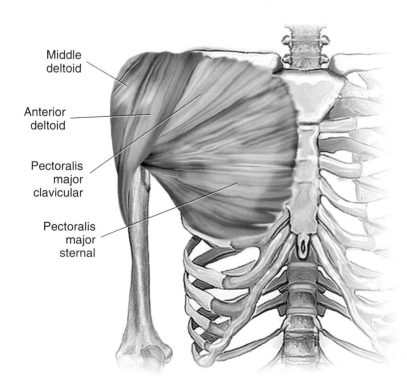

Middle deltoid

Anterior deltoid

Pectoralis major clavicular

Pectoralis major sternal

T5–5.3

Anterior shoulder; pectoralis major, anterior and middle deltoid, overlay or cut away to show coracobrachialis.

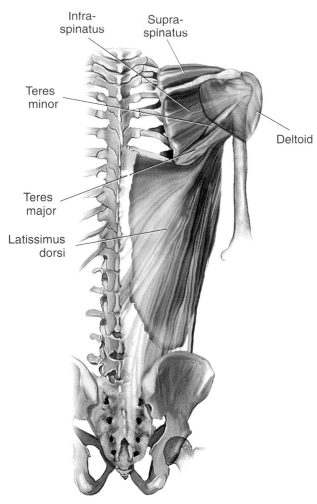

T5–5.4

Posterior shoulder; supraspinatus and infra-spinatus, posterior deltoid, teres major and minor, latissimus dorsi.

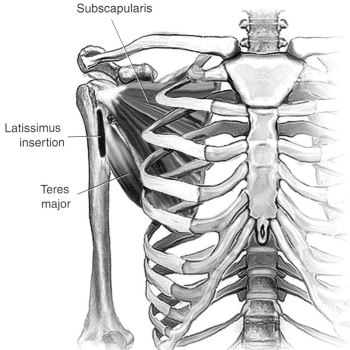

T5–5.5

Anterior shoulder cutaway shows sub-scapularis muscle and teres major and latissimus dorsi insertion.

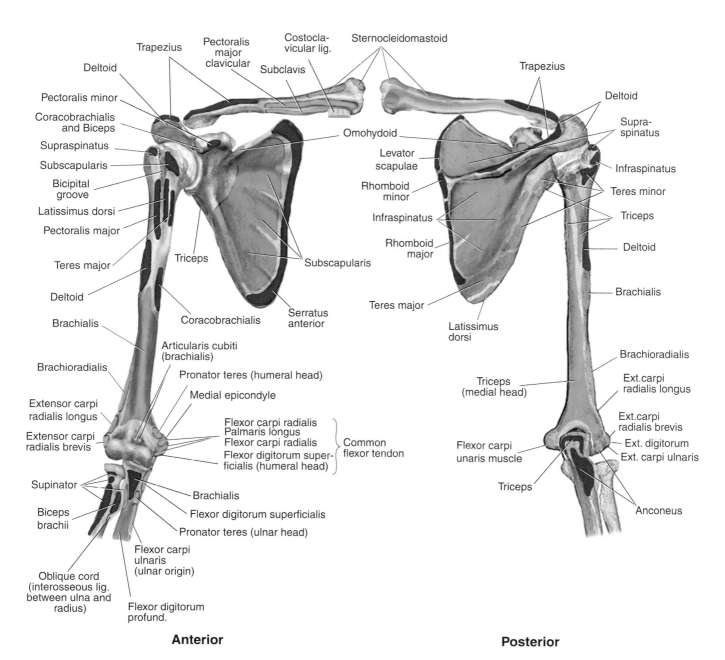

Trapezius

Deltoid

Pectoralis minor

Coracobrachialis and Biceps

Supraspinatus

Subscapularis

Bicipital groove

Latissimus dorsi

Pectoralis major

Teres major

Deltoid

Brachialis

Brachioradialis

Extensor carpi radialis longus

Extensor carpi radialis brevis

Supinator

Biceps brachii

Oblique cord (interosseous lig. between ulna and radius)

Flexor digitorum profund.

Pectoralis major clavicular

Costocla-vicular lig.

Subclavis

Sternocleidomastoid

Omohydoid

Levator scapulae

Rhomboid minor

Infraspinatus

Rhomboid major

Triceps

Subscapularis

Serratus anterior

Coracobrachialis

Articularis cubiti (brachialis)

Pronator teres (humeral head)

Medial epicondyle

Flexor carpi radialis
Palmaris longus
Flexor carpi radialis
Flexor digitorum super-ficialis (humeral head)

Common flexor tendon

Brachialis

Flexor digitorum superficialis

Pronator teres (ulnar head)

Flexor carpi ulnaris (ulnar origin)

Trapezius

Deltoid

Supra-spinatus

Infraspinatus

Teres minor

Triceps

Deltoid

Brachialis

Teres major

Latissimus dorsi

Brachioradialis

Ext.carpi radialis longus

Ext.carpi radialis brevis

Ext. digitorum

Ext. carpi ulnaris

Triceps (medial head)

Flexor carpi unaris muscle

Triceps

Anconeus

Anterior

Posterior

T5–5.6

Muscle attachments for shoulder and upper arm.

Table 5.5 (continued)

MUSCLE	ORIGIN	INSERTION	ACTION	INNERVATION	PALPATION
MUSCLES OF THE UPPER EXTREMITIES (continued) Muscles That Act on the Forearm					
Biceps Brachii Short Head	Coracoid process of the scapula	Posterior portion of the tuberosity of the radius	Flexion of arm and forearm, supinates forearm	C5, 6 Musculocutaneous	Anterior surface of humerus
Long Head	Tubercle at top of the glenoid fossa on scapula	Posterior portion of the tuberosity of the radius	Flexion of arm and forearm, supinates forearm	C5, 6, Musculocutaneous	Anterior surface of humerus
Brachialis	Distal half of anterior aspect of the humerus	Tuberosity of the ulna	Flexion of the elbow	C5, 6, Musculocutaneous and C7, 8, Radial nerve	Medial to Biceps on distal anterior humerus
Brachioradialis	Lateral supra-condylar ridge of humerus	Styloid process of radius	Flexion of the elbow	C5, 6, Radial nerve	Top of upper forearm when elbow is flexed
Triceps Brachii Long Head	Infraglenoid tuberosity of the scapula	Olecranon process of ulna	Extension of the elbow	C7, 8, Radial nerve	Posterior aspect of humerus
Lateral Head	Proximal half of posterior humerus	Olecranon process of ulna	Extension of the elbow	C7, 8, Radial nerve	Posterior aspect of humerus
Medial Head	Distal two thirds of posterior humerus	Olecranon process of ulna	Extension of the elbow	C7, 8, Radial nerve	Posterior aspect of humerus
Anconeus	Lateral epicondyle of humerus	Olecranon process of ulna	Extension of the elbow	C7, 8, Radial nerve	Hard to palpate
Pronator Teres	Just proximal to medial epicondyle of humerus	Midlateral surface of radius	Pronates the hand, assists in elbow flexion	C6, 7, Median nerve	In resisted pronation, medial anterior proximal forearm
Pronator Quadratus	Distal one fourth of anterior ulna radius	Distal one fourth of lateroanterior radius	Pronates the hand	C8, T1, Median nerve	Cannot palpate
Supinator	Lateral epicondyle, radial collateral and annular ligament and the ridge of the ulna just below the radial notch	Lateral surface of the proximal one third of radius	Assists Biceps to supinate hand and forearm	C6, Deep Radial nerve	Deep to brachioradialis on proximal forearm; hard to palpate

continues

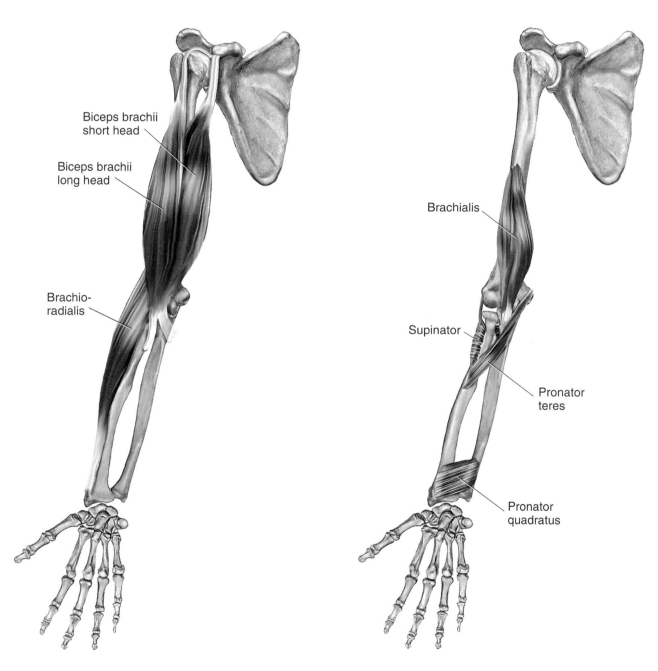

Biceps brachii
short head

Biceps brachii
long head

Brachio-
radialis

Brachialis

Supinator

Pronator
teres

Pronator
quadratus

T5–5.7
Anterior arm; biceps brachii, brachialis, brachioradialis, supinator, pronators.

T5–5.8

Posterior arm; triceps and anconeus.

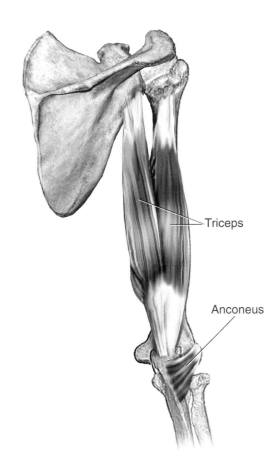

Triceps

Anconeus

Table 5.5 (continued)

MUSCLES OF THE UPPER EXTREMITIES (continued)					
Muscles That Act on the Wrist and Hand					
MUSCLE	**ORIGIN**	**INSERTION**	**ACTION**	**INNERVATION**	**PALPATION**
Flexor Carpi Radialis	Medial epicondyle of the humerus	Base of the second and third metacarpals	Flexion, abduction of wrist	C6, 7, Median	Anterior surface of forearm; tendon prominent on radial side of Palmaris longus tendon at the wrist
Flexor Carpi Ulnaris					Muscle on proximal half of medial forearm; tendon on medial anterior wrist proximal to pisiform bone
Humeral head	Medial epicondyle of humerus	Pisiform, hamate and base of fifth metacarpal	Flexion, abduction of wrist	C7, 8, T1, Ulnar	
Ulnar head	Proximal two thirds of posterior ulna and olecranon	Common insertion with Humeral head	Flexion, abduction of wrist	C7, 8, T1, Ulnar	
Palmaris Longus	Medial epicondyle of humerus	Palmar aponeurosis	Flexion of wrist	C7, 8, Median	Tendon palpated in middle of anterior wrist
Extensor Carpi Radialis Longus	Distal one third of supra-condylar ridge of humerus	Dorsal surface of base of second metacarpal	Extension, abduction of wrist	C6, 7, Radial	Next to brachioradialis on dorsal surface of forearm

Table 5.5 (continued)

MUSCLE	ORIGIN	INSERTION	ACTION	INNERVATION	PALPATION
MUSCLES OF THE UPPER EXTREMITIES (continued) **Muscles That Act on the Wrist and Hand (continued)**					
Extensor Carpi Radialis Brevis	Lateral epicondyle of humerus	Dorsal surface of base of third metacarpal	Extension of wrist	C6, 7, 8, Radial	Next to Extensor carpi radialis longus, hard to differentiate
Extensor Carpi Ulnaris	Lateral epicondyle of humerus and by aponeurosis from proximal posterior ulna	Lateral dorsal side of base of fifth metacarpal	Extension and adduction of wrist	C6, 7, 8, Deep radial	Ulnar border of dorsal forearm; tendon on dorsal wrist near ulnar styloid

continues

Flexor carpi radialis

Palmaris longus

Flexor carpi ulnaris

Extensor carpi radialis longus

Extensor carpi radialis brevis

Extensor carpi ulnaris

T5–5.9

Anterior forearm; flexor carpi radialis and ulnaris and palmaris longus.

T5–5.10

Posterior forearm; extensor carpi radialis longus and brevis, extensor carpi ulnaris.

Table 5.5 (continued)

MUSCLES OF THE UPPER EXTREMITIES (continued)					
Muscles That Act on the Fingers					
MUSCLE	**ORIGIN**	**INSERTION**	**ACTION**	**INNERVATION**	**PALPATION**
Flexor Digitorum Superficialis		By four tendons to the sides of the middle phalanges of digits 2–5	Initial action flexes middle phalanx digits 2–5; continued action flexes proximal phalanx of digits 2–5 and wrist	C7, 8, T1, Median	Muscle is hard to palpate; tendon is prominent on ulnar side of wrist between Palmaris longus and Flexor carpi ulnaris tendons
Humeral head	Medial epicondyle of humerus and ulnar collateral ligament				
Ulnar head	Medial side of coronoid process of ulna				
Radial head	Oblique line of the radius				
Flexor Digitorum Profundus	Proximal three fourths of anterior and medial ulna and interosseus membrane	By tendons to anterior bases of distal phalanges 2–5	Initially flexes distal phalanges 2–5; continued action assists flexion of middle, proximal phalanges and wrist	Digit 2–3; C8, TI, Median Digit 4–5; C7, 8, Ulnar	Muscle lies deep and is hard to palpate. Tendons pass through split tendons of Superficialis tendons and can be palpated on anterior surface of middle phalanges
Flexor Digiti Minimi	Hamate bone and flexor retinaculum	Base of proximal phalanx of little finger	Flexes metacarpophalangeal joint of little finger	C8, T1, Ulnar	Palmar surface of 5th metacarpal
Extensor Digitorum	Lateral epicondyle of humerus	By four tendons to digits 2–5. To the dorsal base of the middle and distal phalanges	Extension of MP joints and with Lumbricals and interossei extends PIP and DIP joints	C6, 7, 8, Radial	Prominent tendons on back of hand
Extensor Indicis	Distal third of posterior ulna and interosseus membrane	Extensor expansion of index finger with Extensor digitorum tendon	Extension of index finger at PIP and DIP joints with Lumbricals and interosseous and extends MP joint	C6, 7, 8, Radial	Dorsal surface of distal forearm. Tendon prominent of dorsal hand when pointing index finger
Extensor Digiti Minimi	Lateral epicondyle of humerus	Extensor expansion of little finger with Extensor digitorum tendon	Extension of MP joint and with Lumbricals and interosseous extends PIP and DIP joints	C6, 7, 8, Radial	Adjacent to Extensor digitorum; hard to palpate
Abductor Digiti Minimi	Tendon of Flexor carpi ulnaris and pisiform	Ulnar side of proximal phalanx of little finger	Abduction of little finger at MP joint	C8, T1, Ulnar	Ulnar border of fifth metacarpal
Opponens Digiti Minimi	Hook of the Hamate and flexor retinaculum	Ulnar side of fourth metacarpal	Opposition of the fifth metacarpal	C8, T1, Ulnar	Hard to palpate

Table 5.5 (continued)

MUSCLE	ORIGIN	INSERTION	ACTION	INNERVATION	PALPATION
MUSCLES OF THE UPPER EXTREMITIES (continued)					
Muscles That Act on the Fingers (continued)					
Palmar interosseous					
First	Ulnar side of first metacarpal	Ulnar side of proximal phalanx of first digit	Adducts thumb, index finger, ring finger and little finger toward axial line of hand through third finger; assists Lumbricals in MP flexion and DIP and PIP extension	C8, T1, Ulnar	Cannot palpate
Second	Ulnar side of second metacarpal	Ulnar side of proximal phalanx of second digit			
Third	Radial side of fourth metacarpal	Radial side of proximal phalanx of fourth digit			
Fourth	Radial side of fifth metacarpal	Radial side of proximal phalanx of fifth digit			

continues

Flexor digitorum superficialis

Flexor digitorum profundus

T5–5.11

Anterior forearm and hand; flexor digitorum profundus and superficialis.

Table 5.5 (continued)

MUSCLE	ORIGIN	INSERTION	ACTION	INNERVATION	PALPATION
MUSCLES OF THE UPPER EXTREMITIES (continued)					
Muscles That Act on the Fingers (continued)					
Dorsal interosseous	Adjacent surfaces of all metacarpal bones	Extensor expansion and proximal bases of digits 2, 3, and 4	Abduction of index, middle, and ring fingers. Assists lumbrical in MP flexion and DIP and PIP extension	C8, T1, Ulnar	Between metacarpals of dorsal surface of hand
Lumbricals	Flexor digitorum tendons at level of metacarpals	Radial side of extensor expansion at proximal phalanx of digits 2, 3, 4, and 5	Flexion of MP joints and extension of DIP and PIP joints	Digits 2 and 3, C6, 7, Median. Digits 4 & 5, 7 & 8, Ulnar	Hard to palpate

continues

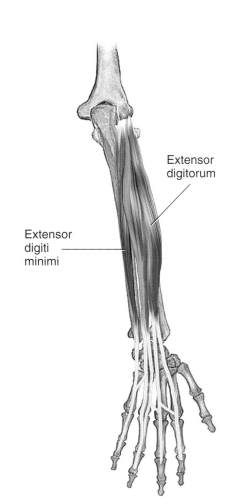

T5–5.12

Posterior forearm and hand; extensor digitorum, extensor indicus, and extensor digiti minimi.

Extensor digitorum

Extensor digiti minimi

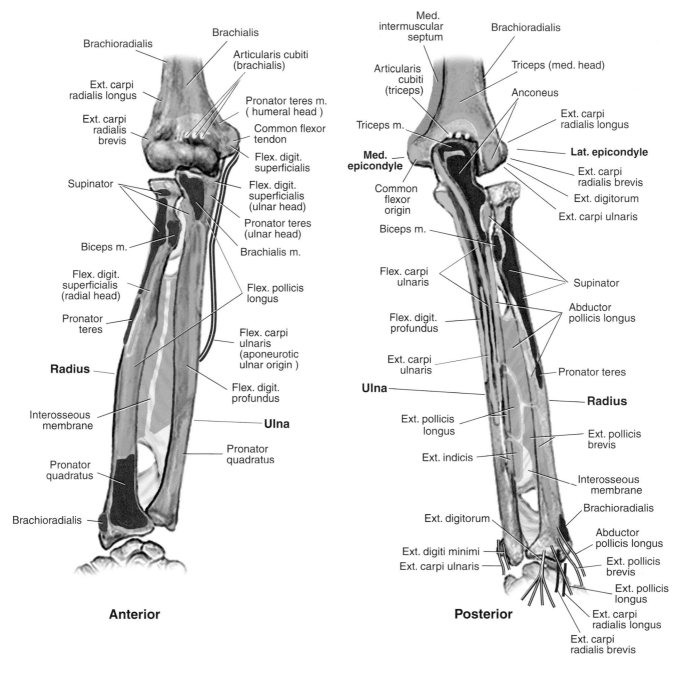

Anterior

Posterior

T5–5.13

Muscle attachments of the lower arm.

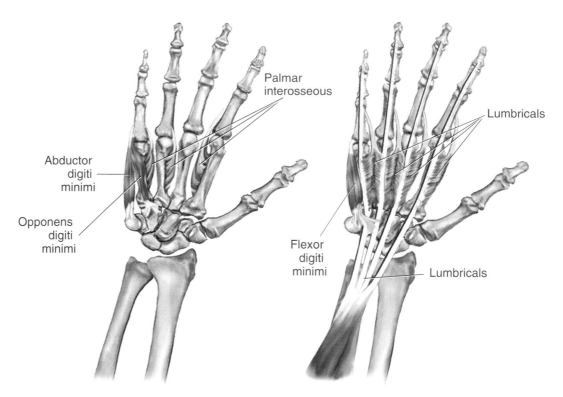

T5–5.14

Anterior hand; flexor digiti minimi, abductor digiti minimi, opponens digiti minimi, palmar interosseous, and lumbricals.

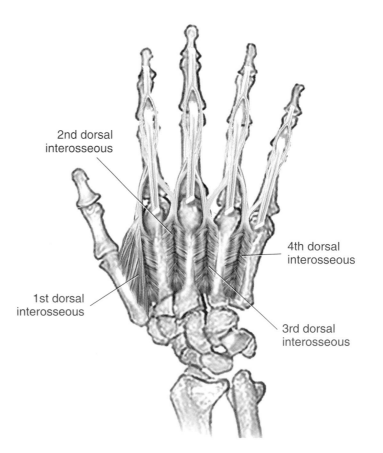

T5–5.15

Posterior hand; dorsal interosseous.

Table 5.5 (continued)

MUSCLES OF THE UPPER EXTREMITIES (continued)					
Muscles That Act on the Thumb					
MUSCLE	**ORIGIN**	**INSERTION**	**ACTION**	**INNERVATION**	**PALPATION**
Abductor Pollicis Longus	Middle third of posterior surface of ulna, radius, and interosseus	Base of radial side of first metacarpal	Abduction and extension of carpometa-carpal joint of thumb	C7, 8, Radial	Tendon palpated just anterior to Extensor pollicis longus on radial side of wrist
Abductor Pollicis Brevis	Flexor retinaculum, trapezium, and scaphoid	Radial side of proximal phalanx of thumb	Abduction of the thumb	C8, T1, Median	Radial side of palmar surface of first metacarpal
Adductor Pollicis		Ulnar side of base of the first phalanx of the thumb	Adduction of the thumb	C8, T1, Deep branch of ulnar	Palmar surface of thumb web space
Transverse Head	Palmar surface of third metacarpal				
Oblique Head	Capitate bone and base of second and third metacarpals				
Flexor Pollicis Longus	Anterior surface of middle radius and adjacent interosseus membrane	Base of palmar surface of distal phalanx of thumb	Initial action flexes distal joint of thumb; continued action assists flexion of two proximal joints	C8, T1, Palmar interosseus branch of Median nerve	Tendon palpated of radial side of anterior wrist
Flexor Pollicis Brevis		Radial side of proximal phalanx of thumb and extensor expansion	Flexion of proximal phalanx and assists with opposition of thumb	C6, 7, 8, Median	Considered to be #1 Palmar interossei muscle; along with Abductor pollicis brevis and Opponnens pollicis make up the thenar eminence
Superficial Head	Flexor Retinaculum and trapezium bone				
Deep Head	Trapezoid and capitate bones			C8, T1, Ulnar	
Extensor Pollicis Longus	Middle third of posterior surface of ulna and interosseus membrane	Base of dorsal surface of distal phalanx of thumb	Extends distal phalanx of thumb; assists extension of proximal phalanx of thumb and wrist and abduction of wrist	C7, 8, Deep radial	Tendon palpated on radial side of first metacarpal on resisted extension just posterior to Extensor pollicis brevis tendon
Extensor Pollicis Brevis	Posterior surface of radius and interosseous membrane distal to origin of Abductor pollicis longus	Dorsal surface of proximal phalanx of thumb	Extends proximal phalanx of thumb; assists in abduction of first metacarpal and wrist	C7, 8, Deep radial	Tendon palpated on radial side of first metacarpal on resisted extension just anterior to Extensor pollicis longus tendon
Opponens Pollicis	Flexor retinaculum and trapezium bone	Entire radial side of first metacarpal	Opposition of thumb	C6, 7, 8, T1, Median and Ulna	Part of thenar eminence. Along first metacarpal

continues

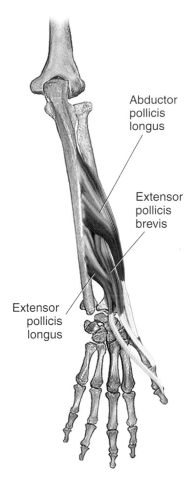

Abductor pollicis longus

Extensor pollicis brevis

Extensor pollicis longus

T5−5.16

Posterior radial hand and distal forearm; extensor pollicis longus and brevis, abductor pollicis longus and brevis.

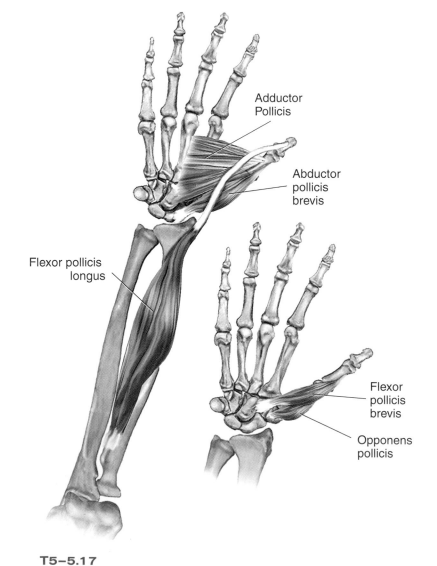

Adductor Pollicis

Abductor pollicis brevis

Flexor pollicis longus

Flexor pollicis brevis

Opponens pollicis

T5−5.17

Anterior hand and distal forearm; adductor pollicis, flexor pollicis longus and brevis, and opponens pollicis.

Table 5.5 (continued)

MUSCLES OF THE LOWER EXTREMITIES					
Muscles That Act on the Thigh					
MUSCLE	**ORIGIN**	**INSERTION**	**ACTION**	**INNERVATION**	**PALPATION**
Psoas Major	Anterior surfaces of transverse processes and sides of bodies and discs of all lumbar vertebrae	Lesser trochanter of the femur	With fixed origin: Flexes thigh; with fixed insertion, bilaterally flexes hip, unilaterally assists lateral flexion of spine	L2, 3, Lumbar plexus	Deep in abdomen and just above inguinal crease; hard to palpate
Iliacus	Superior two thirds of iliac fossa and iliac crest	With Psoas major at lesser trochanter of the femur	Same as Psoas major; assists in abduction and lateral rotation of hip	L2, 3, 4, Femoral	Difficult to palpate
Gluteus Maximus	Posterior gluteal line of ilium and adjacent iliac crest, the posterior inferior surface of the sacrum and lateral surface of coccyx	Iliotibial tract of Fascia lata and gluteal tuberosity of femur	Extends and laterally rotates thigh; supports extended knee	L5, S1, 2, Inferior gluteal	Posterior surface of buttock
Gluteus Medius	Iliac crest and external surface of ilium	Lateral surface of greater trochanter of the femur	Abducts thigh. Anterior fibers rotate hip medially	L4, 5, S1, Superior gluteal	Lateral surface of hip between greater trochanter and iliac crest
Gluteus Minimus	External surface of ilium inferior to gluteus medius muscle and margin of greater sciatic notch.	Anterior border of the greater trochanter of femur	Abducts and medially rotates hip	L4, 5, S1, Superior gluteal	Under Gluteus medius
Tensor Fascia Latae	Anterior portion of iliac spine and ASIS.	Iliotibial tract of fascia lata	Abducts and rotates thigh medially; maintains extension of knee	L4, 5, S1, Superior gluteal	Below anterior iliac spine
Pectineus	Superior ramus of anterior pubis	Between lesser tochanter and linea aspera on posterior femur	Adducts, flexes, and medially rotates thigh	L2,3,4, Femoral and obtruator	Uppermost of medial thigh muscles, just superior to Adductor longus
Adductor Brevis	Outer surface of the inferior ramus of the pubis	Proximal half of the linea aspera to the lesser trochanter on posterior femur	Adduction, flexion, and medial rotation of thigh	L3, 4, Obturator	Deep to Pectineus and Adductor longus; hard to palpate
Adductor Longus	At the crest of pubis adjacent to pubic symphysis	Middle one third of medial lip of linea aspera	Adduction, flexion, and medial rotation of thigh	L3, 4, Obturator	Groin muscle just below pubis
Adductor Magnus	Inferior pubic ramus, ischial ramus, and ischial tuberosity	The linea aspera, medial epicondylic ridge, and adductor tubercle of the medial femoral condyle	Powerful adduction; anterior fibers flexion and medial rotation, posterior fibers extension and lateral rotation	L2, 3, 4, Obturator, L4, 5, S1, Sciatic	Medial surface of thigh

continues

Table 5.5 (continued)

MUSCLES OF THE LOWER EXTREMITIES (continued)					
Muscles That Act on the Thigh & Lateral Rotaters					
MUSCLE	ORIGIN	INSERTION	ACTION	INNERVATION	PALPATION
Gracilis	Inferior half of symphysis pubis and inferior ramus of pubis	The pes anserine; medial surface of tibia inferior to medial tibial condyle	Adducts thigh, flexion and medial rotation of knee	L3, 4, Obturator	Medial thigh below pubis
Sartorius	Anterior superior iliac spine and iliac notch just inferior of spine	Proximal medial surface of tibia; pes anserine	Flexes, laterally rotates and abducts thigh; assists with flexion and medial rotation of knee	L2, 3, Femoral	Just below ASIS and diagonally across thigh
Piriformis	Anterior sacrum, greater sciatic notch and anterior portion of the sacro-tuberous ligament	Superior edge of greater trochanter of the femur	Lateral rotation of the thigh	L5, S1, Sacral plexus	Cannot palpate
Gemellus Superior	Outer surface of ischial spine	Medial surface of the posterior greater trochanter of the femur	Lateral rotation of the thigh	L5, S1, Sacral plexus	Cannot palpate

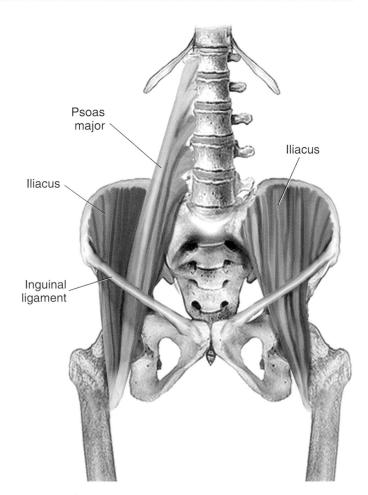

T5-5.18

Iliacus and psoas.

Table 5.5 (continued)

| MUSCLES OF THE LOWER EXTREMITIES (continued) | | | | | |
| Muscles That Act on the Thigh & Lateral Rotaters (continued) | | | | | |
MUSCLE	ORIGIN	INSERTION	ACTION	INNERVATION	PALPATION
Obturator Internus	Ramus of the ischium, inner surface of the ilium, and superior and inferior ramus of pubis	Medial surface of the posterior greater trochanter of the femur	Lateral rotation of the thigh	L5, S1, Sacral plexus	Cannot palpate
Gemellus Inferior	Ischial tuberosity	Medial surface of the posterior greater trochanter of the femur	Lateral rotation of the thigh	L5, S1, Sacral plexus	Cannot palpate
Obturator Externus	Pubis and ischium around medial side of obturator foramen	The fossa of the greater trochanter of the femur	Lateral rotation of the thigh	L3, 4, Obturator	Cannot palpate
Quadratus Femoris	Ischial tuberosity	Just distal to the greater trochantic crest	Lateral rotation of the thigh	L5, S1, Sacral plexus	Cannot palpate

continues

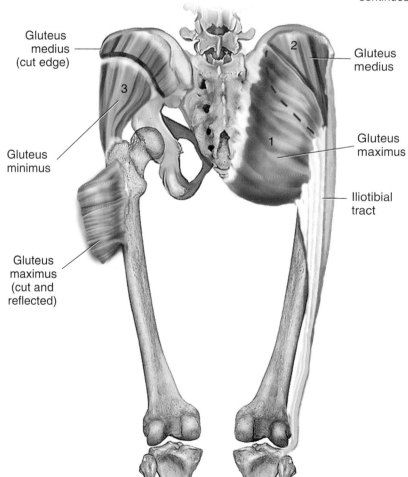

T5–5.19

Gluteus maximus, gluteus medius, and gluteus minimus.

T5–5.20

Pectineus, adductor magnus, adductor longus, adductor brevis, gracilis, sartorius.

Pectineus

Sartorius

Adductor longus

Gracilis

Adductor brevis

Adductor magnus

Obturator externus

Quadratus femoris

Piriformis

Gemellus superior

Obturator internus

Gemellus inferior

T5–5.21

Deep rotators; piriformis, gemellus superior, obturator internus, gemellus inferior, obturator externus, and quadratus femoris.

Posterior

Table 5.5 (continued)

MUSCLE	ORIGIN	INSERTION	ACTION	INNERVATION	PALPATION
MUSCLES OF THE LOWER EXTREMITIES (continued)					
Muscles That Act on the Lower Leg					
Hamstrings					
Biceps Femoris	Ischial tuberosity and sacrotuberous ligament	Lateral side of the head of the fibula and the lateral condyle of the tibia	Both heads; flex and laterally rotate the leg	L5, SI, 2, Sciatic, tibial division	Muscle on posterior surface of thigh; tendon on lateral side of posterior knee
Long Head					
Short Head	Lateral lip of the linea aspera		Long head; extends and assists in lateral rotation of the hip	L5, S1, 2, Sciatic, peroneal division	
Semi-tendinosus	Ischial tuberosity	Proximal part of medial surface of the tibia; pes anserine	Extends the thigh; flexes and medially rotates the knee	L5, S1, 2, Sciatic, tibial division	Muscle on posterior surface of thigh; tendon on medial side of posterior knee
Semi-membranosus	Ischial tuberosity	Posteromedial aspect of medial condyle of the tibia	Extends the thigh; flexes and medially rotates the knee	L5, S1, 2, Sciatic, tibial division	Muscle on posterior surface of thigh; tendon deep and hard to palpate

continues

T5–5.22

Posterior thigh; hamstrings; biceps femoris, semitendinosus, semi-membranosus.

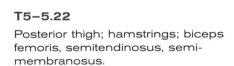

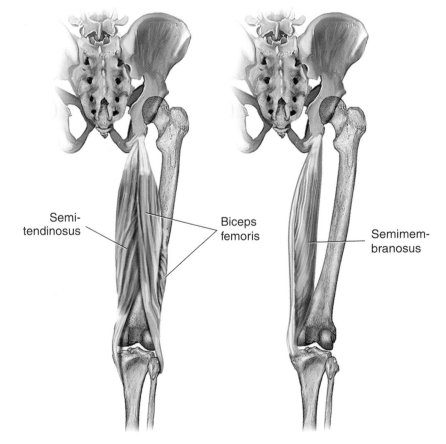

Table 5.5 (continued)

MUSCLE	ORIGIN	INSERTION	ACTION	INNERVATION	PALPATION
MUSCLES OF THE LOWER EXTREMITIES (continued) **Muscles That Act on the Lower Leg (continued)**					
Quadriceps Femoris					
Rectus Femoris	Anterior inferior iliac spine and the groove above the acetabulum	Via quadriceps expansion and patella through patellar ligament to tuberosity of tibia	Extends the leg at the knee	L2, 3, 4, Femoral	Anterior surface of thigh
Vastus Lateralis	Anterior and inferior border of greater trochanter, proximal one half of lateral linea aspera	Via quadriceps expansion and patella through patellar ligament to tuberosity of tibia	Extends the leg at the knee	L2, 3, 4, Femoral	Anterolateral surface of thigh
Vastus Intermedius	Anterior and lateral surfaces of proximal two thirds of femur	Via quadriceps expansion and patella through patellar ligament to tuberosity of tibia	Extends the leg at the knee	L2, 3, 4, Femoral	Deep to rectus femoris; hard to palpate
Vastus Medialis	Medial lip of linea aspera and posterior femur	Via quadriceps expansion and patella through patellar ligament to tuberosity of tibia	Extends the leg at the knee	L2, 3, 4, Femoral	Medial surface of distal two thirds of anterior thigh

continues

T5–5.23

Anterior thigh; quadriceps femoris: rectus femoris, vastus lateralis, vastus intermedius, vastus medialis.

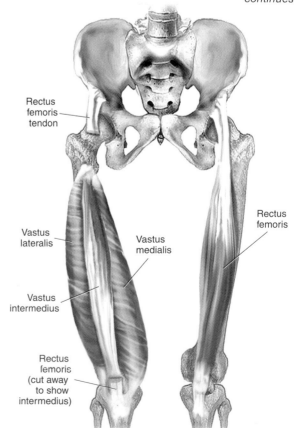

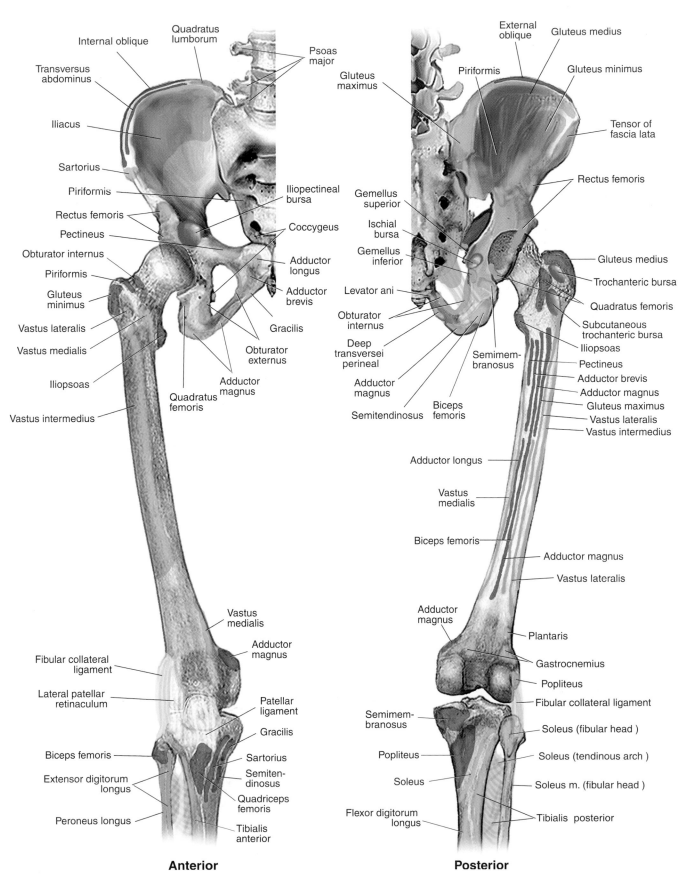

Anterior

Posterior

T5-5.24

Muscle attachments for the hip and thigh.

Table 5.5 (continued)

MUSCLES OF THE LOWER EXTREMITIES (continued)					
Muscles That Act on the Foot					
MUSCLE	**ORIGIN**	**INSERTION**	**ACTION**	**INNERVATION**	**PALPATION**
Popliteus	Lateral condyle of femur	Posterior surface of proximal tibia	Initiates leg flexion by unlocking the knee	L4, 5, S1, Tibial	Cannot palpate
Tibialis Anterior	Lateral condyle and proximal one half of tibia, interosseous membrane	Medial and plantar surface of medial cuneiform and base of first metatarsal	Dorsal flexion of ankle and inversion of foot	L4, 5, Deep Peroneal	Lateroanterior surface of tibia; tendon palpated anterior ankle medial to Extensor hallucis longus M
Peroneus Tertius	Distal one third of anterior fibula	Base of fifth metatarsal	Dorsal flexion of the ankle, eversion of foot	L4, 5, S1, Deep Peroneal	Tendon just lateral to tendon of Extensor digitorum
Extensor Digitorum Longus	Lateral condyle of tibia and proximal three fourths of the anterior fibula	By four tendons to the dorsal surfaces of the second and third phalanges of the four lateral toes	Extension of four lateral toes and dorsal flexion of ankle	L4, 5, S1, Deep Peroneal	Four tendons on dorsum of foot
Extensor Hallucis Longus	Middle two quarters of anterior fibula and interosseous membrane	Base of distal phalanx of large toe	Extends large toe, dorsal flexes ankle and inversion of foot	L4, 5, S1, Deep Peroneal	Tendon on anterior ankle and dorsum of large toe
Gastrocnemius					
Medial Head	Posterior surface of medial condyle of the femur	Middle of posterior surface of the calcaneus via Achilles' tendon	Plantar flexes the ankle or assists the flexion of the knee	S1, 2, Tibial	Major muscle of posterior calf
Lateral Head	Posterior surface of the lateral condyle of femur				
Plantaris	Distal lateral supracondylar line of the femur	Posterior surface of the calcaneus via the Achilles' tendon	Plantar flexes the ankle or assists flexion of the knee	L4, 5, S1, Tibial	Hard to palpate
Soleus	Head and proximal one third of posterior fibula and middle border and soleal line of tibia	Middle of posterior surface of the calcaneus via the Achilles' tendon	Plantar flexes the ankle	L5, S1, 2, Tibial	Lateral surface of lower leg below gastrocnemius
Flexor Digitorum Longus	Middle one third of posterior surface of tibia	By four tendons to the plantar surface of the distal phalanges of the four lateral toes	Flexes the four lateral toes; assists in plantar flexion and inversion of the foot	L5, S1, 2, Tibial	Tendon palpated posterior and inferior to medial malleolus with Posterior tibialis and Flexor digitorum longus

Table 5.5 (continued)

MUSCLE	ORIGIN	INSERTION	ACTION	INNERVATION	PALPATION
MUSCLES OF THE LOWER EXTREMITIES (continued) **Muscles That Act on the Foot (continued)**					
Flexor Hallucis Longus	Distal two thirds of posterior fibula and adjacent interosseous membrane	Base of plantar surface distal phalanx of large toes	Flexes large toe; assists plantar flexion and inversion of foot	L5, S1, 2, Tibial	Tendon palpated posterior and inferior to medial malleolus with Posterior tibialis and Flexor digitorum longus
Tibialis Posterior	Middle third of posterior tibia, proximal two thirds of medial fibula and interosseus membrane	Plantar surfaces of navicular, cuboid, second and third and fourth metatarsals	Inversion of foot; assists in plantar flexion of ankle	L5, S1, 2, Tibial	Tendon palpated posterior and inferior to medial malleolus with Flexor hallucis longus and Flexor digitorum longus

continues

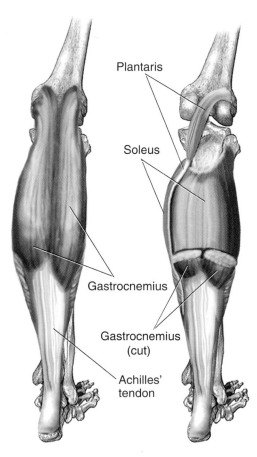

T5-5.25

Posterior leg; gastrocnemius, soleus, plantaris.

Table 5.5 (continued)

MUSCLES OF THE LOWER EXTREMITIES (continued)					
Muscles That Act on the Foot (continued)					
MUSCLE	ORIGIN	INSERTION	ACTION	INNERVATION	PALPATION
Peroneus Longus	Head and proximal two thirds of lateral surface of fibula and lateral condyle of tibia	Plantar surface of medial cuneiform and base of first metatarsal	Eversion of foot; assists plantar flexion of ankle	L4, 5, S1, Superficial Peroneal	Proximal half of lateral surface of lower leg
Peroneus Brevis	Distal two thirds of lateral surface of fibula	Lateral surface of base of fifth metatarsal	Eversion of foot; assists plantar flexion of ankle	L4, 5, S1, Superficial Peroneal	Posterior and inferior to lateral malleolus with tendon of Peroneus longus

continues

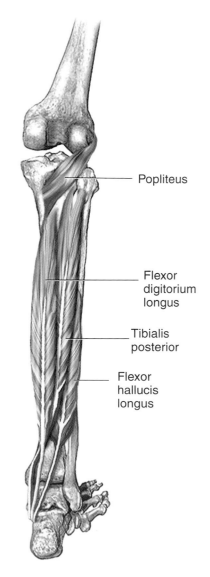

T5–5.26

Posterior leg (deep); tibialis posterior, flexor digitorum, flexor hallucis, popliteus.

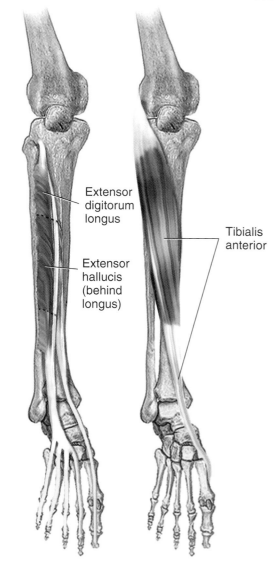

T5–5.27

Anterior leg; tibialis anterior, extensor digitorum, extensor hallucis.

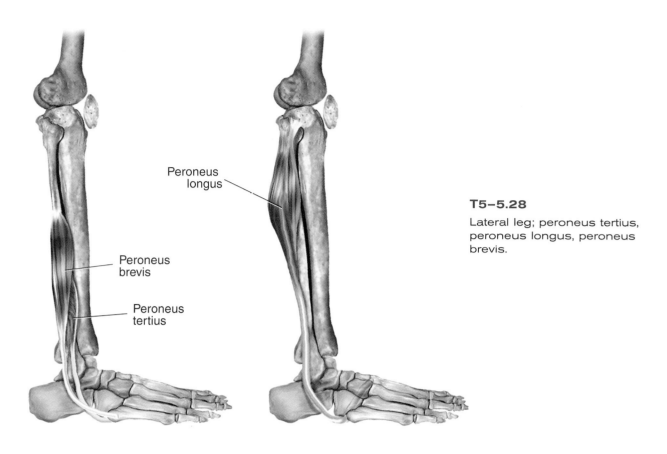

T5–5.28

Lateral leg; peroneus tertius, peroneus longus, peroneus brevis.

Peroneus longus

Peroneus brevis

Peroneus tertius

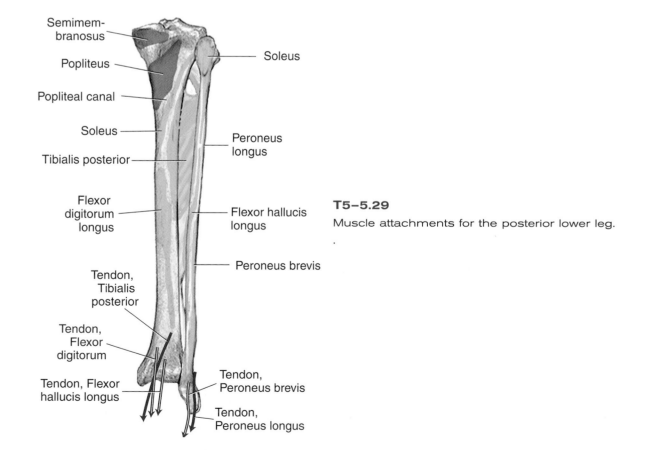

Semimem-branosus

Popliteus

Popliteal canal

Soleus

Tibialis posterior

Flexor digitorum longus

Tendon, Tibialis posterior

Tendon, Flexor digitorum

Tendon, Flexor hallucis longus

Soleus

Peroneus longus

Flexor hallucis longus

Peroneus brevis

Tendon, Peroneus brevis

Tendon, Peroneus longus

T5–5.29

Muscle attachments for the posterior lower leg.

Table 5.5 (continued)

| MUSCLES THAT ACT ON THE ABDOMEN | | | | | |
MUSCLE	ORIGIN	INSERTION	ACTION	INNERVATION	PALPATION
Rectus Abdominis	Crest of the pubis and pubic symphysis	Xiphoid process and costal cartilage of fifth, sixth, and seventh ribs	Flexion of trunk; tenses abdominal wall and compresses contents	T5–12, Intercostal, Iliohypogastric, Ilioinguinal	Anterior abdomen from pubis to sternum
External Oblique	External surface of eight lower ribs	Abdominal aponeurosis to linea alba and iliac crest	Bilaterally, same as above; unilaterally, Lateral flexion and rotation to opposite side	T8–12, Intercostal, Iliohypogastric, Ilioinguinal	Lateral surfaces of abdomen
Internal Oblique	Inguinal ligament, Iliac crest and Thoracolumbar fascia	Abdominal aponeurosis, linea alba, and costal cartilages of four lower ribs	Bilaterally, same as above; unilaterally, Lateral flexion and rotation to same side	T8–12, Intercostal, Iliohypogastric, Ilioinguinal	Deep to External Oblique Cannot palpate
Transverse Abdominis	Inguinal ligament, Iliac crest and Thoracolumbar fascia, and lower six ribs	Abdominal aponeurosis to linea alba and iliac crest	Tenses abdominal wall and compresses contents	T7–12, Intercostal, Iliohypogastric, Ilioinguinal	Cannot palpate

continues

T5–5.30

Abdominal area: external obliques, internal obliques, transverse abdominis, rectus abdominis.

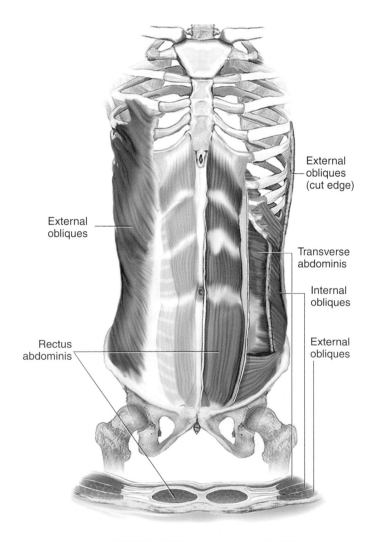

Table 5.5 (continued)

MUSCLES OF RESPIRATION					
MUSCLE	**ORIGIN**	**INSERTION**	**ACTION**	**INNERVATION**	**PALPATION**
Diaphragm	The xiphoid process, six lower ribs and costal cartilages, ligaments, bodies and transverse processes of upper lumbar vertebrae	Central tendon of the Diaphragm, a strong aponeurosis with no bony attachment	Main muscle of respiration, contracts during inspiration increasing thoracic volume; separates abdominal and thoracic cavities	C3, 4, 5, Phrenic	Cannot palpate; action can be observed on abdomen during respiration

continues

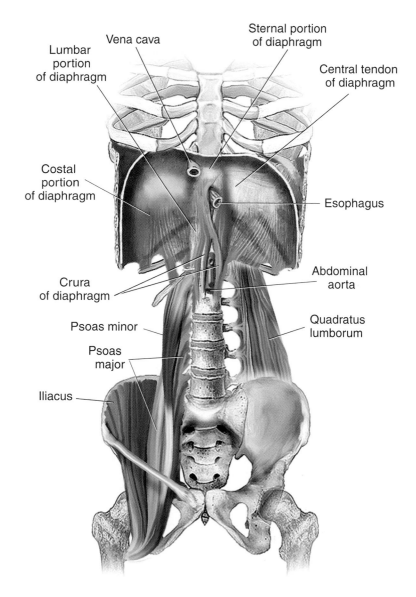

T5—5.31

Diaphragm.

Table 5.5 (continued)

MUSCLE	ORIGIN	INSERTION	ACTION	INNERVATION	PALPATION
MUSCLES OF RESPIRATION (continued)					
Intercostals					
External	Inferior margin of the rib above	Superior margin of the rib below. Fibers angle 45% lateral to medial.	Pull ribs together and elevate ribs during inhalation	T1–12, Intercostal	External palpated between ribs
Internal	Inferior margin of the rib above	Superior margin of the rib below. Fibers angle 45% medial to lateral.	Depress ribs during forced exhalation		External and internal intercostal muscles are situated perpendicular to each other, and innermost intercostals are too deep to palpate
Innermost	Sternum and inferior margin of lower ribs	Inner surface of the ventral ribs			
Serratus Posterior Superior	Spinous process C7–T2, ligamentum nuchae C6–T1 supraspinous ligament	Posterior superior surfaces of ribs 2–5	Raises ribs during deep inhalation	T1–4, Intercostal	Cannot palpate
Serratus Posterior Inferior	Spinous process T11–L3, supraspinous ligament	Inferior borders of ribs 8–12	Pulls ribs outward and down, opposes diaphragm	T9–12, Intercostal	Cannot palpate

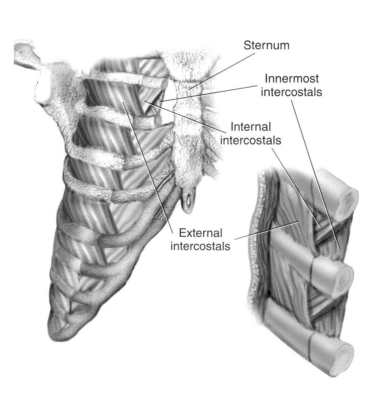

Sternum

Innermost intercostals

Internal intercostals

External intercostals

T5–5.32

Intercostals.

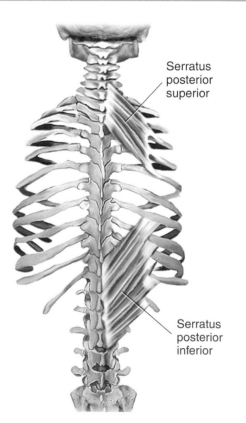

Serratus posterior superior

Serratus posterior inferior

T5–5.33

Serratus posterior superior, serratus posterior inferior.

Table 5.5 (continued)

MUSCLES THAT ACT ON THE SPINE					
MUSCLE	**ORIGIN**	**INSERTION**	**ACTION**	**INNERVATION**	**PALPATION**
Quadratus Lumborum	Posterior iliac crest	Transverse process of L1–4 and inferior border of 12th rib	Lateral flexion of spine or raises hip	T12, L1, 2, 3, Lumbar plexus	Deep to Thoracolumbar sheath; hard to palpate
Intertransversarii	Transverse processes of cervical, lumbar and T10–12 vertebra	Transverse process of vertebra directly above origin	Lateral flexion and stabilization of spine	Posterior branches of adjacent spinal nerves	Cannot palpate
Interspinales	In pairs between spinous process of cervical lumbar and T1–2 and T11–12 vertebra	Spinous process of vertebra directly above origin	Extension and stabilization of spine	Posterior branches of adjacent spinal nerves	Cannot palpate
Rotatores	Transverse process of each vertebra	Lamina of vertebra directly above	Extension, rotation to opposite side, and stabilization of spine	Posterior branches of adjacent spinal nerves	Cannot palpate
Multifidus	Transverse processes of C4–L5, PSIS, and posterior sacrum	Spans 2–4 vertebra. Inserts on spinous process.	Extension, rotation to opposite side, and stabilization of spine	Posterior branches of adjacent spinal nerves	Cannot palpate
Semispinalis			Bilaterally, Extension		
Capitis	Transverse processes C4–T7	Occipital bone between inferior and superior nuchal lines	Unilaterally, Rotation to opposite side; stabilization of spine	Posterior branches of adjacent spinal nerves	Cannot palpate
Cervicis	Transverse processes of T1–6	Spinous processes C2–5			
Thoracis	Transverse processes T6–12	Spinous processes C6–T8			
Spinalis			Bilaterally, Extension of spine	Posterior branches of adjacent spinal nerves	Cannot palpate
Capitis	Inseparable from Semispinalis	Same as Semispinalis	Unilaterally, Lateral flexion of the spine		
Cervicis	Ligamentum nuchae	Spinous processes C2–4			
Thoracis	Spinous processes T10–L2	Spinous processes T4–8	Stabilization of spine		

continues

Table 5.5 (continued)

MUSCLE	ORIGIN	INSERTION	ACTION	INNERVATION	PALPATION
MUSCLES THAT ACT ON THE SPINE (continued)					
Longissimus			Bilaterally, Extension of spine	Posterior branches of adjacent spinal nerves	Deep to Thoracolumbar fascial latissimus dorsi and trapezius muscles on either side of spine; hard to palpate
Capitis	Articular processes C4–7, Transverse processes T1–4	Posterior surface of mastoid process	Unilaterally, Lateral flexion of the spine		
Cervicis	Transverse processes T1–5	Transverse processes C2–6	Stabilization of spine		
Thoracis	Thoracolumbar fascia, transverse processes of lumbar vertebra	Transverse processes T1–12 and posterior surface of lower ten ribs			

Table 5.5 (continued)

MUSCLE	ORIGIN	INSERTION	ACTION	INNERVATION	PALPATION
MUSCLES THAT ACT ON THE NECK					
Iliocostalis Lumborum	Common origin by broad tendon arising from spinous process T12–L5, medial lip of iliac crest, and medial and lateral crest of the sacrum	Inferior borders of posterior angle of ribs 7–12	Bilaterally, extension of spine; unilaterally, Lateral flexion of the spine; stabilization of spine	Posterior branches of adjacent spinal nerves	Deep to thoracolumbar fascia, Latissimus dorsi, and Trapeszius muscles on either side of spine; hard to palpate
Thoracis	Upper borders of posterior angles of ribs 7–12	Transverse process of C7 and angles of ribs 1–6.			
Cervicis	Posterior angles of ribs 3–6	Transverse processes C4–6			
Splenius	Lower one half of ligamentum nuchae, spinous processes C7–T4	Mastoid process and lateral one third of occiput	Bilaterally, extension of neck; unilaterally, Rotation of head to same side	Posterior braches of cervical nerves	On posterior neck between Trapezius and Sternocleidomastoid; hard to to palpate
Capitis					
Cervicis	Spinous processes T3–6	Transverse processes C1–3			
Sternocleidomastoid	Sternal head: Superior aspect of manubrium. Clavicular head: Medial one third of clavicle	Mastoid process	Bilaterally, flexion of neck; unilaterally, Rotation of head to opposite side, lateral flexion	Accessory nerve and C2, 3	Anterolateral aspect of neck, diagonally from origin to insertion

Table 5.5 (continued)

MUSCLE		ORIGIN	INSERTION	ACTION	INNERVATION	PALPATION
Scalenus						
	Anterior	Anterior tubercles of transverse processes C3–6	Anterior superior aspect of first rib	Bilaterally, raise rib cage in deep inhalation, neck flexion;	C6, 7, 8	Lateral aspect of lower neck posterior to Sternocleidomastoid muscle from anterior aspect of first rib to transverse process of cervical vertebra; hard to palpate
	Medial	Posterior tubercles of transverse processes C2–7	Lateral anterior aspect of first rib	unilaterally, Lateral flexion of neck, assists in neck rotation to		
	Posterior	Posterior tubercles of transverse processes C5–7	Lateral anterior aspect of second rib	opposite side		

continues

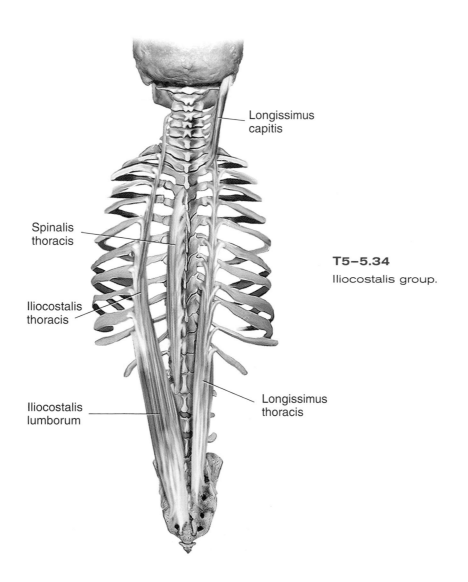

Longissimus capitis

Spinalis thoracis

Iliocostalis thoracis

Iliocostalis lumborum

Longissimus thoracis

T5–5.34
Iliocostalis group.

Table 5.5 (continued)

MUSCLES THAT ACT ON THE NECK (continued)					
MUSCLE	**ORIGIN**	**INSERTION**	**ACTION**	**INNERVATION**	**PALPATION**
Rectus Capitis					
Anterior	Anterior surface and transverse process of C1	Basal surface of occiput anterior to foramen magnum	Neck flexion, rotation to same side	Suboccipital	Cannot palapte
Lateralis	Transverse process of C1	Basil surface of occiput lateral to foramen magnum	Lateral flexion of head	C1	Cannot palpate
Posterior Minor	Posterior arch of C1 spinous process of C2	Medial segment of inferior nuchal line of occiput	Neck, head extension	Occipital	Deep to Trapezius and Semispinalis; hard to palpate.
Posterior Major	Spinous process of C2	Inferior nuchal line of occiput lateral to RCP minor attachment	Head extension, and lateral flexion	Occipital	Cannot palpate
Obliquus Capitis					
Superior	Superior aspect of transverse process of C1	Between inferior and superior nuchal lines of occiput	Head extension, rotation to same side	Occipital	Cannot palpate
Inferior	Spinous process C2	Posterior aspect of transverse process of C1	Rotation to same side	Occipital	Cannot palpate
Longus Colli	Anterior tubercles C3–5, Anterior vertebral bodies C5–T3	Anterior surface of vertebral bodies of C1–4, Anterior tubercles C5–6	Head flexion, lateral flexion and rotation to same side	C1–4	Cannot palpate
Longus Capitis	Anterior tubercles of transverse processes C3–6	Inferior surface of occiput	Flexion of head	C1–3	Cannot palpate

continues

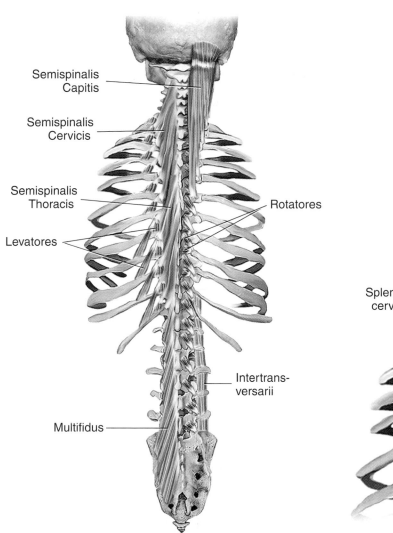

Semispinalis
Capitis

Semispinalis
Cervicis

Semispinalis
Thoracis

Rotatores

Levatores

Intertrans-
versarii

Multifidus

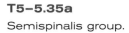

T5–5.35a
Semispinalis group.

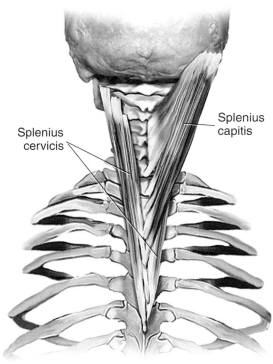

Splenius
cervicis

Splenius
capitis

T5–5.35b
Splenius group.

T5−5.36

Sternocleidomastoid.

Sternocleidomastoid

T5−5.37

Scalenus anterior, scalenus medius, and scalenus posterior.

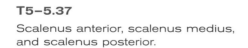

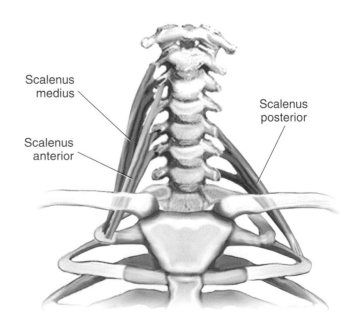

Scalenus medius

Scalenus anterior

Scalenus posterior

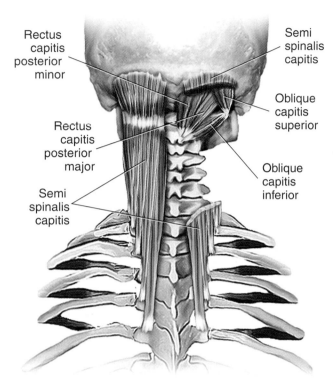

Rectus capitis posterior minor

Rectus capitis posterior major

Semi spinalis capitis

Semi spinalis capitis

Oblique capitis superior

Oblique capitis inferior

Table 5.5.38

Posterior neck; rectus capitis posterior major and minor, obliques capitis superior and inferior.

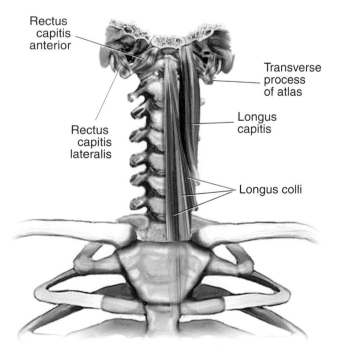

Rectus capitis anterior

Rectus capitis lateralis

Transverse process of atlas

Longus capitis

Longus colli

Table 5.5.39

Anterior neck (deep): rectus capitis anterior and rectus capitis lateralis, longus colli and longus capitis.

Table 5.5 (continued)

MUSCLE	ORIGIN	INSERTION	ACTION	INNERVATION	PALPATION
MUSCLES THAT ACT ON THE HYOID					
Infrahyoid Muscles					
Sternohyoid	Top of sternum and medial end of clavicle	Inferior body of hyoid	Depresses hyoid	C1, 2, 3	Lower anterior neck between SCM and trachea
Sternothyroid	Top of sternum and costal cartilage of first rib	Thyroid cartilage	Depresses thyroid cartilage	C1, 2, 3	Lower anterior neck between SCM and trachea
Thyrohyoid	Thyroid cartilage	Inferior body of hyoid	Depresses hyoid or raises thyroid cartilage	C1, 2, 3	Below hyoid, lateral to Sternohyoid; hard to differentiate and palpate
Omohyoid	Superior border of scapula and by tendon to clavicle	Inferior body of hyoid	Depresses hyoid		

continues

T5–5.40

Anterior neck; hyoid muscles.

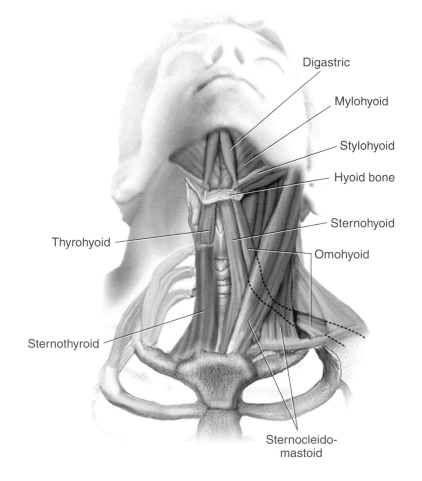

Digastric

Mylohyoid

Stylohyoid

Hyoid bone

Sternohyoid

Omohyoid

Thyrohyoid

Sternothyroid

Sternocleido-mastoid

Table 5.5 (continued)

MUSCLES THAT ACT ON THE HYOID (continued)					
MUSCLE	ORIGIN	INSERTION	ACTION	INNERVATION	PALPATION
Suprahyoid Muscles					
Geniohyoid	Mandible under chin	Body of hyoid, superior aspect	Elevates hyoid or depresses mandible	C1, 2	Deep to Mylohyoid, cannot palpate
Myohyoid	Mandible from ramus to under chin	Body of hyoid, superior aspect	Elevates hyoid or depresses mandible	Cranial V, Trigeminal	Deep muscle sheath under chin
Stylohyoid	Styloid process of temporal bone	Body of hyoid, superior aspect	Elevates hyoid or moves hyoid posteriorly	Cranial VII, Facial	Between hyoid and ramus along with Posterior digastric
Digastric					
Ant. belly	Mandible under chin	By tendon to body chin of hyoid, superior aspect	Elevates hyoid or depresses mandible	Cranial V, Trigeminal	From hyoid the point of chin between hyoid to ramus of
Post. belly	Mastoid process			Cranial VII facial	mandible along with Stylohyoid muscle

Table 5.5 (continued)

MUSCLES OF MASTICATION					
MUSCLE	ORIGIN	INSERTION	ACTION	INNERVATION	PALPATION
Masseter	Zygomatic arch	Lateral surface of ramus of the mandible	Closes jaw	Cranial V, Trigeminal	Lateral jaw, over molars
Temporalis	Temporal bone	Coronoid process and ramus of mandible	Closes and retracts jaw	Cranial V, Trigeminal	Lateral surface of temple area
Buccinator	Maxilla and mandible	Angle of mouth, blending with Obicularis oris	Holds cheeks near teeth positioning food for chewing	Cranial VII, Facial	Cheeks
Internal Pterygoid	Medial surface of pterygoid plate of sphenoid	Medial surface of ramus of the mandible	Closes jaw; unilaterally, moves jaw to opposite side	Cranial V, Trigeminal	Hard to palpate
External Pterygoid	Lateral surface of pterygoid plate of sphenoid	Anterior surface of condyle of mandible and TMJ capsule	Protrudes lower jaw	Cranial V, Trigeminal	Cannot palpate

continues

Table 5.5 (continued)

MUSCLES OF EXPRESSION					
MUSCLE	**ORIGIN**	**INSERTION**	**ACTION**	**INNERVATION**	**PALPATION**
Epicranius					
Occipitalis	Posterior occiput above occipital ridge	Epicranial aponeurosis or the Galea aponeurotica	Draws Epicranius towards posterior	Posterior auricular and small occipital	Back of head above occipital ridge
Frontalis	Blended into Procerus, corrugator and Obicularis oculi	Epicranial aponeurosis or the Galea aponeurotica	Raises eyebrow and wrinkles the forehead	Cranial VII, Facial	Forehead, above eyebrows
Corrugator	Medial aspect of supraorbital ridge	Deep surface of skin in middle of supraorbital arch	Draws eyebrows together	Cranial VII, Facial	Under medial eyebrow
Procerus	Fascia over upper nasal cartilage and lower nasal bone	Deep surface of skin between eyebrows	Draws nose up causing wrinkles across nose	Cranial VII, Facial	Bridge of nose
Orbicularis Oculi	Medial palpebral ligament to maxilla, nasal bone, nasal part of frontal bone	Fibers surround eye and blend with adjacent muscles	Closes the eye	Cranial VII, Facial	Eyelid and surrounding eye
Nasalis	Maxilla above incisors	Blends into procerus	Compresses nostrils	Cranial VII, Facial	Side of nose
Dialator Naris	Greater alar cartilage	Point of the nose	Expands opening of nostril	Cranial VII, Facial	Cannot palpate
Quadratus Labii Superioris	Lower margin of orbit, frontal process of maxilla	Blends into Obicularis oris on upper lip	Raises upper lip	Cranial VII, Facial	Above upper lip, next to nose
Zygomaticus					
Major	Zygomatic bone	Blends into Obicularis oris muscle at upper angle of mouth	Draws angle of mouth back and up	Cranial VII, Facial	Below zygomatic arch when smiling
Minor	Continuous from inferior border of Obicularis oculi	Blends into Obicularis oris on upper lip	Raises upper lip	Cranial VII, Facial	Hard to differentiate from Quadratus labii
Obicularis Oris	From numerous adjacent muscles surrounding mouth	Lips, external skin around mouth and mucous membrane adjacent to the lips inside of mouth	Closes and protrudes lips	Cranial VII, Facial	The lips
Risorius	Fascia over Masseter	Blends into Obicularis oris and skin at corner of the mouth	Draws angle of mouth back	Cranial VII, Facial	On cheek near corner of mouth; hard to palpate
Depressor Anguli Oris	Anterior inferior surface of mandible	Blends into Obicularis oris and skin at corner of the mouth	Draws angle of mouth down	Cranial VII, Facial	On chin below corner of mouth

continues

Table 5.5 (continued)

MUSCLES OF EXPRESSION (continued)					
MUSCLE	**ORIGIN**	**INSERTION**	**ACTION**	**INNERVATION**	**PALPATION**
Depressor Labii Inferioris	Anterior inferior surface of mandible	Blends into Obicularis oris and skin on lower lip of the mouth	Depresses lower lip	Cranial VII, Facial	On chin below lower lip
Mentalis	Mandible below incisors	Deep skin at point of chin	Raises chin and protrudes lower lip as if pouting	Cranial VII, Facial	The chin
Platysma	Superficial fascia of upper thorax and anterolateral aspect of neck	Blends into muscles of angle of mouth and chin	Depresses angle of mouth and wrinkles skin of neck	Cranial VII, Facial	Anterolateral aspect of neck; thin muscle and hard to palpate
Auricularis Anterior Superior Posterior	Temporal bone	Deep skin around ear	Raises and moves ear	Cranial VII, Facial	In front, above, and behind ear; small muscles, hard to palpate

continues

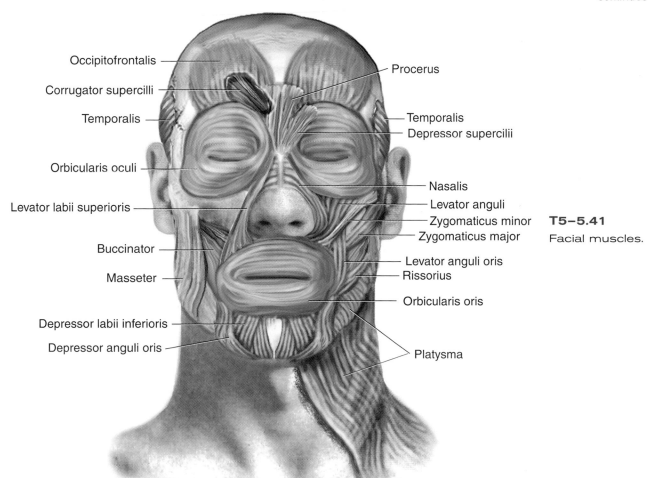

T5–5.41

Facial muscles.

Table 5.5 (continued)

MUSCLES THAT ACT ON THE EYE					
MUSCLE	**ORIGIN**	**INSERTION**	**ACTION**	**INNERVATION**	**PALPATION**
Levator Palpebrae Superioris	Common tendinous ring surrounding optic nerve near optic foramen	Upper eyelid	Opens the eye	Cranial III, Oculomotor	Cannot palpate
Superior Oblique	Common tendinous ring surrounding optic nerve via a tendon in superior orbit	Posterior lateral aspect of eyeball	Turns eye out and down	Cranial IV, Trochlear	Cannot palpate
Supetior Rectus	Common tendinous ring surrounding optic nerve near optic foramen	Anterior superior aspect of eyeball	Rotates eye up	Cranial III, Oculomotor	Cannot palpate
Lateral Rectus	Common tendinous ring surrounding optic nerve near optic foramen	Anterior lateral aspect of eyeball	Rotates eye laterally	Cranial VI, Abducens	Cannot palpate
Inferior Rectus	Common tendinous ring surrounding optic nerve near optic foramen	Anterior inferior aspect of eyeball	Rotates eye down	Cranial III, Oculomotor	Cannot palpate
Medial Rectus	Common tendinous ring surrounding optic nerve near optic foramen	Anterior medial aspect of eye	Rotates eye medially	Cranial III, Oculomotor	Cannot palpate
Inferior Oblique	Orbital surface of maxilla	Posterior lateral aspect of eyeball	Rotates eye up and out	Cranial III, Oculomotor	Cannot palpate

Table 5.5.42

Muscles of the eye.

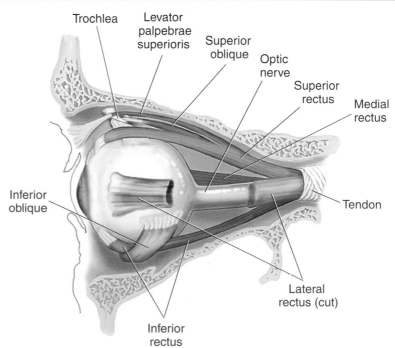

REVIEW

Muscles of the Head and Face

Matching Test I

Insert the letter of the proper term in front of each definition.

_____	1. move ears	a.	orbicularis oculi
_____	2. move scalp	b.	orbicularis oris
_____	3. opens eye	c.	auricularis
_____	4. presses lips together	d.	masseter
_____	5. raises lower jaw	e.	epicranius

True or False Test I

Carefully read each statement and decide whether it is true or false; draw a circle around the letter T or F.

1. T F Inferior oblique and superior oblique muscles do not rotate the eyeball.
2. T F Only the temporalis muscle moves the lower jaw.
3. T F The superior levator palpebrae muscle opens the eye.
4. T F The epicranius is also known as the occipitofrontalis muscle.
5. T F The corrugator muscle controls the movement of the mouth.

Muscles of the Neck and Chest

Matching Test II

Insert the letter of the proper term in front of each definition.

_____	1. rotates cranium	a.	intercostals
_____	2. draws head backward	b.	longus colli
_____	3. flexes cervical spine	c.	obliquus capitis inferior
_____	4. muscle of respiration	d.	obliquus capitis superior
_____	5. raises ribs in breathing	e.	diaphragm

True or False Test II

Carefully read each statement and decide whether it is true or false; draw a circle around the letter T or F.

1. T F Several muscles depress the jaw and raise the hyoid bone.
2. T F The sternocleidomastoid is the only muscle that bends the head forward and sideways.
3. T F The platysma muscle does not draw down the corners of the mouth.
4. T F The pectoralis major and minor muscles control the movement of the arm and shoulder.
5. T F Several groups of muscles raise the ribs in breathing.

Muscles of the Abdomen and Back

Matching Test III

Insert the letter of the proper term in front of each definition.

_____	1.	flexes trunk	a. rectus abdominis
_____	2.	keeps spine erect	b. quadratus lumborum
_____	3.	draws head backward	c. sacrospinalis
_____	4.	draws arm backward	d. trapezius
_____	5.	compresses abdomen	e. latissimus dorsi

True or False Test III

Carefully read each statement and decide whether it is true or false; draw a circle around the letter T or F.

1.   T   F   The external oblique is an external muscle of the abdomen and back.

2.   T   F   Only one muscle compresses the abdomen and bends the chest.

3.   T   F   The infraspinatus and supraspinatus muscles control the movement of the arm.

4.   T   F   The gluteus medius muscle extends the hip joint.

5.   T   F   The spine is kept erect with the aid of the sacrospinalis and multifidus muscles.

Muscles of the Arms and Hands

Matching Test IV

Insert the letter of the proper term in front of each definition.

_____	1.	flexes hand	a. brachialis
_____	2.	flexes forearm	b. triceps brachii
_____	3.	flexes arm	c. interossei
_____	4.	separates fingers	d. deltoid
_____	5.	extends forearm	e. palmaris longus

True or False Test IV

Carefully read each statement and decide whether it is true or false; draw a circle around the letter T or F.

1.   T   F   The movement of the thumb is controlled by one muscle.

2.   T   F   The biceps brachii muscle draws the palm downward.

3.   T   F   The brachioradialis muscle draws the palm upward.

4.   T   F   Quick, short movements of the fingers are produced by the lumbricales muscles.

5.   T   F   The subscapularis muscle rotates the humerus inward.

Muscles of the Legs and Feet

Matching Test V

Insert the letter of the proper term in front of each definition.

_____	1. flexes leg	a. flexor digitorum
_____	2. extends leg	b. biceps femoris
_____	3. flexes hip	c. rectus femoris
_____	4. extends foot	d. pectineus
_____	5. flexes toes	e. soleus

True or False Test V

Carefully read each statement and decide whether it is true or false; draw a circle around the letter T or F.

1. T F The sartorius muscle bends the thigh and leg.

2. T F The movement of the big toe is controlled by the extensor hallucis longus muscle.

3. T F The extensor digitorum brevis muscle does not extend the toes.

4. T F The soleus and gastrocnemius muscles both plantar flex the foot.

5. T F The gracilis adducts the femur and flexes the knee joint.

SECTION QUESTIONS FOR DISCUSSION AND REVIEW

1. What is the structure and function of muscles?

2. Approximately how many muscles are there in the human body?

3. Name three types of muscular tissue and give examples of where they are found.

4. What is the difference between voluntary and involuntary muscles?

5. Which characteristics enable muscles to produce movements?

6. What are skeletal muscles?

7. What is the functional unit of skeletal muscle?

8. What structures cause the striated appearance of skeletal muscles?

9. What tissues are found in muscle?

10. To which structures are skeletal muscles attached?

11. What is the origin of a muscle? Give an example.

12. What is the insertion of a muscle? Give an example.

13. Which structure attaches the muscle to the bone?

14. What is the function of fibrous connective tissue in muscle?

15. What is fascia?

16. Name and locate the three connective tissue layers of muscle.

17. What is meant by the term *motor unit?*

18. What is acetylcholine? Where is it found? What does it do?

19. What molecular structure provides the energy for muscle contraction?

20. What is the relationship between oxygen debt and muscle fatigue?

21. When does a muscle have tone?

22. When does a muscle lack tone?

23. Why is it important for the massage practitioner to understand how muscles function?

24. What is meant by extensibility of muscle?

25. Explain the difference between isometric and isotonic muscle contractions.

26. Explain the difference between eccentric and concentric contractions. What do they have in common?

27. To what does the term *agonist* or *prime mover* refer?

28. When flexing the elbow, would the triceps be the prime mover or the antagonist?

29. What are the three components of motion?

30. Do diarthrotic joints remain motionless or are they capable of free movement?

31. Describe three degrees of muscle strain.

32. What is muscle atrophy?

33. What joints have limited motion?

34. Are synarthrotic joints movable or immovable?

4 THE CIRCULATORY SYSTEM

The vascular or circulatory system controls the circulation of the blood and lymph throughout the body by means of the heart, blood, and lymph vessels. The primary function of the circulatory system is to supply body cells with nutrient materials and carry away waste products.

There are two divisions to the vascular system:

1. The *blood-vascular system* or **cardiovascular system** includes the blood, heart, and blood vessels (arteries, capillaries, and veins).

2. The *lymph-vascular system*, or *lymphatic system*, consists of lymph, lymph nodes, and lymphatics through which the lymph circulates.

These two systems are intimately linked with each other.

cardiovascular system

a network of structures including the heart, blood vessels, and blood that pumps and carries blood throughout the body.

The Blood-Vascular System or Cardiovascular System

The blood-vascular system is a closed-circuit system that consists of the heart, the arteries, capillaries, veins, and the blood. This system continuously circulates the blood throughout the body. Even though the blood-vascular system is considered to be a closed system, in which the blood normally does not leave the blood vessels, in the capillaries there is a constant and extensive interchange of fluids and the substances they contain.

The Heart

The *heart* is an efficient pump that keeps the blood circulating in a steady stream through a closed system of arteries, capillaries, and veins. The heart is a muscular, conical-shaped organ, about the size of a closed fist, located in the chest cavity between the lungs and behind the sternum. It is enclosed in a double-layered membrane, the **pericardium** (per-i-**KAR**-dee-um). The inner layer of the pericardium is a thin serous covering of the heart; the outer layer is a protective fibrous connective tissue sac that is attached to the diaphragm, the vertebral column, the back of the sternum, and the large blood vessels that emerge from the heart. Between these two layers is a space, the *pericardial cavity*, that contains a serous fluid so that the heart is supported in position and at the same time allowed to move frictionlessly as it continually pulsates.

The walls of the heart consist of three distinct layers. The **epicardium** is the protective outer layer that includes the inner pericardium. This layer includes and supports the nerves, blood and lymph capillaries, and fat that surround the heart. The next thick layer is the cardiac muscle or the **myocardium** and is responsible for the muscular pumping action of the heart. The thin innermost layer is the **endocardium**, which provides a smooth protective covering that lines the inner chambers of the heart and heart valves and is continuous with the linings of the blood vessels (endothelium) (Figure 5.45).

The interior of the heart contains four chambers, two on each side of a muscular wall called the **septum** (**SEP**-tum). The upper thin-walled cavities, the right and left atrium (sometimes called the auricle), receive blood into the heart from the veins. The lower thick-walled chambers, the right and left ventricle, pump the blood out of the heart into the arteries. Four valves allow the blood to flow in only one direction. The **tricuspid valve**, located between the right atrium and right ventricle, allows blood to flow from the right atrium into the right ventricle and not the opposite direction. The **pulmonary semilunar valve,** positioned between the right ventricle and pulmonary artery, directs the blood from the right ventricle into the pulmonary arteries as it travels to the lungs. The **bicuspid (or mitral) valve,** located between the left atrium and ventricle, allows blood to flow only from the left atrium into the left ventricle. The **aortic semilunar valve,** situated in the orifice of the aorta, permits the blood to be pumped from the left ventricle into the aorta but not the reverse. With each contraction and relaxation of the heart, the blood flows

---

pericardium
is a double-layered membrane that encloses the heart.

epicardium
is the protective outer layer of the heart.

myocardium
is the cardiac muscle.

endocardium
is the thin, innermost layer of the heart.

septum
is the wall that separates the heart's chambers.

tricuspid valve
of the heart allows blood to flow from the right atrium into the right ventricle.

pulmonary semilunar valve
of the heart directs blood from the right ventricle into the pulmonary arteries.

bicuspid or mitral valve
of the heart allows blood to flow from the left atrium into the left ventricle.

aortic semilunar valve
of the heart permits the blood to be pumped from the left ventricle into the aorta.

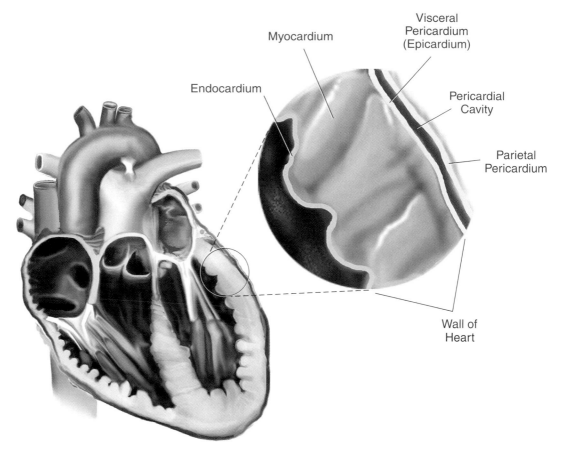

Figure 5.45

Wall of the heart, including pericardium.

arteries
are thick-walled muscular and elastic vessels that transport oxygenated blood from the heart.

arterioles
small blood vessels between the arteries and the capillaries.

capillaries
are the smallest blood vessels and connect arterioles with the venules.

venules
are microscopic vessels that continue from the capillaries and merge to form veins.

in, travels from the atriums to the ventricles, and is then driven out to be distributed all over the body (Figure 5.46).

The impulses that generate the rhythmical heartbeat originate within the heart muscle. A system of specialized cardiac tissue initiates rhythmic impulses that transmit throughout the cardiac muscle and stimulate it to contract. This occurs without stimulation by outside nerve fibers or other agents. Even though the rhythmic heart contractions are initiated within the heart muscle, there is a complicated neurological heart monitoring system that regulates the heart rate. Impulses from the *vagus* (**VAY**-gus) *nerve* and the *sympathetic nervous system*, help regulate the force of contraction and the heart rate. In a normal adult, the heart beats about 60 to 80 times a minute.

The Blood Vessels

The **arteries, arterioles, capillaries, venules,** and **veins** transport blood from the heart to the various tissues of the body and back again to the heart. The construction of all blood vessels, except the capillaries, is similar. The innermost layer is made up of endothelium; the middle layer is smooth muscle; and the outer layer is tough, protective connective tissue. The arteries and arterioles have thicker walls than veins and venules. The farther from the heart, the finer and more delicate the vessels become. The capillary walls are made up of only a single layer of simple

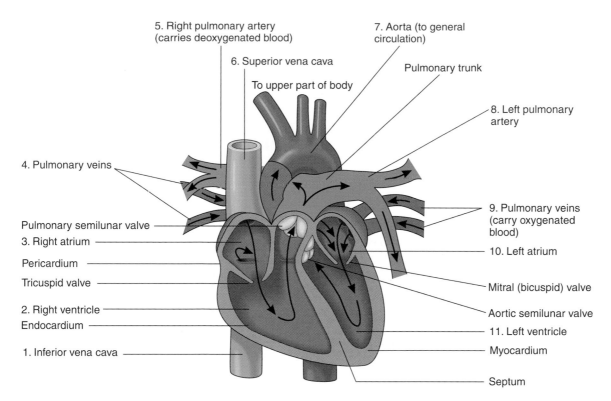

5. Right pulmonary artery
(carries deoxygenated blood)

6. Superior vena cava

To upper part of body

7. Aorta (to general
circulation)

Pulmonary trunk

8. Left pulmonary
artery

4. Pulmonary veins

Pulmonary semilunar valve

3. Right atrium

Pericardium

Tricuspid valve

2. Right ventricle

Endocardium

1. Inferior vena cava

9. Pulmonary veins
(carry oxygenated
blood)

10. Left atrium

Mitral (bicuspid) valve

Aortic semilunar valve

11. Left ventricle

Myocardium

Septum

Figure 5.46
Anatomy of the heart.

squamous epithelium to allow the passage of nutrients and wastes from and into the bloodstream. There are as many as 60,000 miles of continuous blood vessels that make up the circulatory system of an adult human.

Arteries and Arterioles

Arteries are thick-walled muscular and elastic vessels that transport oxygenated blood (except for the pulmonary artery) under relatively high pressure from the heart. The main artery of the body is the **aorta** (ay-OR-tuh), which arches up from the left ventricle of the heart, extending over and down along the vertebral column. Arteries branch into smaller and smaller branches until eventually they become microscopic arterioles that control the rate of flow of blood into the capillaries. Arteries vary in size from the aorta, which is about an inch in diameter, to the microscopic capillaries, whose walls are just a single cell in thickness and are only large enough to pass one blood cell at a time.

The smooth muscle tissue in the walls of the arteries and arterioles is richly supplied with nerves from the sympathetic portion of the autonomic nervous system. Impulses from these *vasomotor nerves* cause the smooth muscles of the arterial walls to contract, reducing the diameter of the vessel. This action is called **vasoconstriction**. When the nerve impulses are inhibited, the muscles relax and the diameter of the vessel enlarges or undergoes **vasodilatation**. Changes in the diameter of the vessels affect the blood pressure and flow. The nerve response and control of the small arteries and arterioles regulate the flow of blood to the tissues in direct proportion to the tissue's specific needs.

veins
are thinner-walled blood vessels that carry deoxygenated blood and waste-laden blood from capillaries back to the heart.

aorta
is the main artery of the body.

vasoconstriction
is the contraction of the arterial walls.

vasodilation
is the relaxation and enlargement of the arterial walls.

Capillaries

Capillaries are the smallest microscopic, thin-walled blood vessels whose networks connect the small arterioles with the venules. The walls of the capillaries are extremely thin and permeable. The most important function of the capillaries is the two-way transport of substances between the flowing blood and the tissue fluids surrounding the cells. Substances move through the capillary walls either by the process of diffusion, filtration, or osmosis. Of these, diffusion is the most prevalent.

In the process of **diffusion,** substances move from an area of higher concentration to an area of lower concentration. Blood entering the capillaries has a higher concentration of nutrients and oxygen than the fluid surrounding the cells, so the oxygen and nutrients diffuse into the tissue spaces. By the same account, the concentrations of metabolic waste products and carbon dioxide are more highly concentrated in the tissue fluid and therefore tend to diffuse into the bloodstream.

The pressure of the blood, especially at the junction of the arteriole and the capillary, tends to push fluids and substances through the capillary wall and into the tissue spaces through a process called **filtration.** Because of a high concentration of proteins and other substances retained in the plasma, there is an osmotic pressure created that tends to draw water into the capillaries from the tissue spaces at almost the same rate as the blood pressure forces fluid out. Through these processes, substances can move back and forth between the bloodstream and tissues to support the needs of the cells and at the same time maintain the volume of the blood at a normal level.

---

diffusion
is a process in which substances move from an area of higher concentration to an area of lower concentration.

filtration
is a process in which blood pressure pushes fluids and substances through the capillary wall and into the tissue spaces.

Blood flow toward the heart

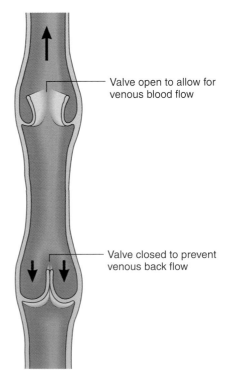

Valve open to allow for venous blood flow

Valve closed to prevent venous back flow

Figure 5.47
Valves in the veins.

Veins and Venules

Venules (**VEN**-yools) are the microscopic vessels that continue from the capillaries and merge to form veins. Veins are thinner-walled blood vessels that carry deoxygenated and waste-laden blood from the various capillaries back to the heart. Many veins, especially those in the arms and legs, have a system of valves that prevent blood from flowing backward in the vein and act as a *venous pump* to move the blood toward the heart. These valves are flaplike structures that protrude from the inside walls of the vein in such a way that blood moving toward the heart pushes past the valve, but if the blood attempts to move in the reverse direction, pressure against the valve forces it closed and blood cannot pass. The venous pump is a phenomenon that results when muscles contract and exert external pressure on the veins, which tends to collapse them. As the vein is repeatedly collapsed, the blood is forced along through the system of valves toward the heart. Massage strokes are very effective at encouraging the blood to move through the veins and therefore should always be directed to follow the venous blood flow toward the heart (Figure 5.47).

The Circulation of the Blood

The blood is in constant circulation from the moment it leaves until it returns to the heart. There are two systems involved in circulation: pulmonary and systemic.

Pulmonary Circulation

Pulmonary circulation is the blood circulation from the heart to the lungs and back again to the heart. During pulmonary circulation, the deoxygenated blood is pumped from the right ventricle of the heart, through the pulmonary arteries, to the capillaries of the lungs, where carbon dioxide is replaced by oxygen. The exchange is continuous. Freshly oxygenated blood returns to the left atrium of the heart through the pulmonary veins.

General or Systemic Circulation

General or **systemic circulation** is the blood circulation from the heart throughout the body and back again to the heart.
The course that blood travels is as follows:

1. The right atrium or auricle receives oxygen-poor blood from the large superior and inferior vena cava.

2. From the right atrium, the venous blood passes through the tricuspid valve into the right ventricle.

3. From the right ventricle, the venous blood is pumped through the pulmonary semilunar valve and is carried through the pulmonary arteries to the lungs to be oxygenated.

4. The freshly oxygenated blood is collected from the capillaries into the pulmonary veins and returned to the heart.

5. The left atrium receives the oxygenated blood from the pulmonary veins.

6. From the left atrium or auricle, the oxygenated blood passes through the bicuspid or mitral valve into the left ventricle.

7. From the left ventricle, the blood is pumped through the aortic semilunar valve and into the aorta.

8. From the aorta, the blood is distributed to the major arteries throughout the body except for the lungs. The blood moves into ever-smaller branches of the arterial system until it flows into the arterioles.

9. From the arterioles, the blood moves into the thin-walled capillaries where the oxygen, nutrients, and fluids move into the tissue spaces and the metabolic wastes and carbon dioxide are reabsorbed into the bloodstream.

10. The blood is then collected from the capillary beds into the venules and then into larger and larger veins until the blood finally flows into the inferior or superior vena cava.

11. This cycle is repeated as the venous blood is brought back again to the right atrium or auricle of the heart (Figure 5.48).

pulmonary circulation
is the blood circulation from the heart to the lungs and back again to the heart.

general or systemic circulation
is the blood circulation from the left side of the heart throughout the body and back again to the heart.

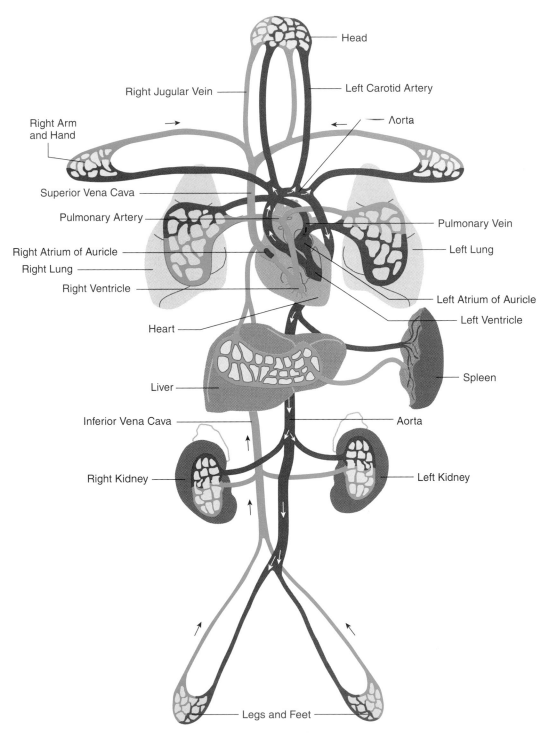

Head

Right Jugular Vein —————— ———— Left Carotid Artery

Right Arm
and Hand ————— →   ← ———— Λorta

Superior Vena Cava —————

Pulmonary Artery ————— ———————— Pulmonary Vein

Right Atrium of Auricle ————— ———— Left Lung

Right Lung —————

Right Ventricle ————— ———— Left Atrium of Auricle

Heart ————— ———— Left Ventricle

———— Spleen

Liver —————

Inferior Vena Cava ————— ———— Aorta

Right Kidney ————— ———— Left Kidney

Legs and Feet

Figure 5.48
Circulation of the blood.

Disorders of the Blood Vessels

Atherosclerosis

Atherosclerosis is characterized by an accumulation of fatty deposits on the inner walls of the arteries. The development of the deposits, called plaque, seems to relate to the level of cholesterol in the blood. The deposits may interfere with blood flow or create a surface where blood clots may form. The walls of affected arteries tend to thicken, become fibrous, and lose their elasticity in a condition called *arteriosclerosis* (ar-TEER-ee-o-skler-O-sis).

Having a family history of atherosclerosis, high blood pressure, a high cholesterol level, a sedentary lifestyle, and smoking increase the chances of developing atherosclerosis. There are really no outward symptoms of atherosclerosis until it has progressed to the point that a related condition appears. Occlusion of a coronary artery is common and results in *angina pectoris* or a heart attack (myocardial infarction, see p. 208). If atherosclerosis causes a thrombus (blood clot) to form or if the clot breaks free to become an embolus, the embolus may become lodged in an artery, and the tissues supplied by that artery will stop functioning. If that happens in the brain, a stroke will result; in the heart, a heart attack will occur; and in the lungs, a pulmonary embolism may result. Advanced atherosclerosis may also affect the aorta, renal arteries, the carotid arteries, or the peripheral arteries of the legs by restricting blood flow to the structures they supply.

Circulatory massage is contraindicated for persons with advanced or diagnosed atherosclerosis. If a prospective client is under a doctor's care or is taking any kind of medication for circulatory conditions, get medical clearance from the physician before proceeding with massage

Phlebitis and Thrombophlebitis

Phlebitis is an inflammation of a vein which might result from injury, surgery, or infection. Symptoms include pain and inflammation along the course of the vein and swelling. Thrombophlebitis signifies the presence of a blood clot (thrombus) in an inflamed vein. It is difficult to determine whether the clot is the cause or the result of the inflammation. Thrombophlebitis usually occurs in the lower extremities and may affect the superficial or deep veins.

A major concern with thrombophlebitis is that a portion of the blood clot may break free to become an embolus that travels through the veins back to the heart, and then to the lungs to cause a pulmonary embolism, which could be life threatening.

Symptoms for thrombophlebitis vary. In fact, the first symptoms may be those of a pulmonary embolism, shortness of breath, pain in the lungs, and coughing. Thrombophlebitis in a superficial vein may be accompanied by signs of inflammation. The vein will be tender to the touch and feel like a hard cord. Deep vein thrombophlebitis is often accompanied by a deep ache in the area of the clot and edema distal to the location of the clot because the venous blood flow is inhibited, causing fluid to remain in the tissues. Thrombophlebitis is a serious condition that requires immediate medical attention. Massage is systemically contraindicated.

Aneurysm

An aneurysm is a local distention or ballooning of an artery due to a weakening wall. It most commonly occurs in the abdominal or thoracic cavity and occasionally in the cranium. It is generally asymptomatic but may cause a feeling of pressure, pain, or edema, depending on the location. The most serious consideration with an aneurysm is that it may rupture, causing internal bleeding and possibly death. Massage is contraindicated.

CVA

A cerebrovascular accident (CVA) or stroke is caused by a disturbance in cerebral circulation. This may be due to an embolism, atherosclerosis, hemorrhage, or a ruptured aneurysm. Symptoms vary according to the area of the brain affected and may include unilateral weakness, paralysis, numbness, dizziness, confusion, blurred or double vision. The aftereffects of a stroke depend on the severity and what portion of the brain was involved. About 25 percent of strokes are fatal; 25 percent have no lasting effects; and 50 percent result in some physical impairment. Disability from a CVA may include partial to full paralysis to one side of the body, possible memory loss, vision loss, loss of the ability to speak, and/or personality changes that may range from mild to extreme. The onset of a CVA requires immediate medical attention. Massage in the acute stage is contraindicated but may be very beneficial during rehabilitation under a physician's supervision.

Myocardial Infarction

Commonly known as a heart attack, a myocardial infarction is the result of a reduced blood flow in the coronary arteries supplying the heart muscle due to atherosclerosis, narrowed vessels, or an embolus. The reduced blood flow causes a lack of oxygen and nutrients that damages or kills the portion of the heart muscle supplied by the occluded artery. The seriousness of the heart attack is determined by the location and the extent of the damaged heart tissue. Symptoms include pressure or aching around the heart and often radiating into the left arm, back, or jaw. Immediate hospitalization is required; fewer than 30 percent of those inflicted survive. Massage is contraindicated during the acute stage but may be incorporated during rehabilitation under a doctor's supervision.

Varicose Veins

Varicose veins are characterized by protruding, bulbous, distended superficial veins particularly in the lower legs. Extensive back pressure in the veins due to prolonged standing or blockage causes the veins to enlarge and stretch to the point that the valves become incompetent. The weight of the blood further distends the veins, and more valves become dysfunctional, perpetuating the condition. Increased pressure in the veins also increases pressure in the capillaries and often results in edema. Severe varicose veins are contraindicated for all but the lightest massage. Darkened veins that are not elevated or painful and the small, isolated spider veins are safe for moderate or light massage.

Hematoma

A **hematoma** is the result of bleeding under the epidermis and sometimes deep within the tissues of the body. A superficial hematoma, commonly referred to as a bruise, is recognized by its black-and-blue or purplish color and localized pain. The color fades to a greenish yellow as macrophages move into the site to clean up the debris. Deep hematomas or bleeding deep between the muscle sheaths may or may not show discoloration but will be painful to the touch. Massage is contraindicated during the acute stages of a hematoma; however, it may be applied gently around the periphery to sooth the area and promote circulation in the subacute stages.

> **hematoma**
> is a mass of blood trapped in some tissue or cavity of the body and is the result of internal bleeding.

Edema

Edema is a condition of excess fluid in the interstitial spaces. Edema is characterized by swelling of the tissues due to the excess fluid. The cause of edema is an imbalance in fluid pressures within the capillaries. The pressure imbalance may be caused by obstructions in the veins or lymph vessels, high capillary pressure or porosity, or kidney malfunction that results in fluid retention. Edema may be associated with a weakened heart, congested liver, chemical imbalance, or a local injury or infection. Edema is a local contraindication for classic massage techniques. Some types of edema respond well to specialized lymph massage techniques. (See Chapter 18, p. 715, Lymph Massage.)

The Blood

Blood is the nutritive fluid circulating throughout the blood-vascular system. It is salty and sticky, has an alkaline reaction, and maintains a normal temperature of 98.6°F (37°C). The amount of blood varies according to a person's size as well as some other factors. An average-sized male (about 160 pounds) will have approximately 11 pints of blood or about one sixteenth to one twentieth of the body's weight. The skin may hold as much as one half of all the blood in the body.

Chief Functions of Blood

1. The blood carries water, oxygen, food, and secretions to all areas of the body.

2. It carries away carbon dioxide and waste products to be eliminated through the excretory channels.

3. It helps to equalize the body temperature, thus protecting the body from extreme heat and cold.

4. It aids in protecting the body from harmful bacteria and infections through the action of the white blood cells.

5. It coagulates (clots), thereby closing injured blood vessels and preventing the loss of blood through hemorrhage.

Composition of Blood

The blood is a liquid connective tissue consisting of a fluid component (blood plasma) and a solid component that consists of red corpuscles, white corpuscles, and blood platelets. Plasma constitutes from 50 to 60 percent of the blood volume.

Blood Cells

Red corpuscles (red blood cells) or *erythrocytes* (e-**RITH**-row-sites) are double concave disk-shaped cells colored with a substance called **hemoglobin** (hee-mow-**GLOW**-bin). The function of the red corpuscles is to carry oxygen from the lungs to the body cells and transport carbon dioxide from the cells to the lungs. The red blood cells are confined to the blood vessels and do not circulate outside the blood-vascular system. The red blood cells are formed in the red bone marrow. They are far more numerous than the white blood cells and account for as much as 98 percent of the blood cells.

The blood itself is bright red in the arteries (except in the pulmonary artery) and dark red in the veins (except in the pulmonary vein). This change in color is due to the color change of hemoglobin as the result of a gain or loss of oxygen as the blood passes through the lungs and other tissues of the body.

White corpuscles (white blood cells), also called *leukocytes,* differ from red blood cells in many respects. They are larger in size, colorless, and can change their shape and other properties according to their location and function. White corpuscles are produced in the spleen, lymph nodes, and the red marrow of the bones. Leukocytes can squeeze between the cells that comprise the capillary walls and move through the intercellular spaces with an amoeba-like motion. The most important function of these cells is to protect the body against disease by combating different infectious and toxic agents that may invade the body. Most leukocytes actually engulf and digest harmful bacteria and other foreign elements in a process called **phagocytosis** (fag-o-sigh-**TOE**-sis). Our bodies also manufacture specialized leukocytes that produce antibodies that protect us from specific disease organisms and are an important part of our **immune system.**

Blood platelets or *thrombocytes* are colorless, irregular bodies, much smaller than the red corpuscles. They are formed in the red bone marrow. These bodies play an important role in the clotting of the blood over a wound (Figure 5.49).

---

red corpuscles
or erythrocytes, carry oxygen from the lungs to the body cells and transport carbon dioxide from the cells to the lungs.

hemoglobin
an iron-protein compound in red blood cells capable of carrying oxygen from the lungs to the cells and carbon dioxide from the cells.

white corpuscles
or leukocytes, protect the body against disease by combating infections and toxins that invade the body.

phagocytosis
is a process in which leukocytes engulf and digest harmful bacteria.

immune system
helps keep people safe from foreign invaders and diseases.

blood platelets
or thrombocytes, are colorless, irregular bodies, much smaller than red corpuscles.

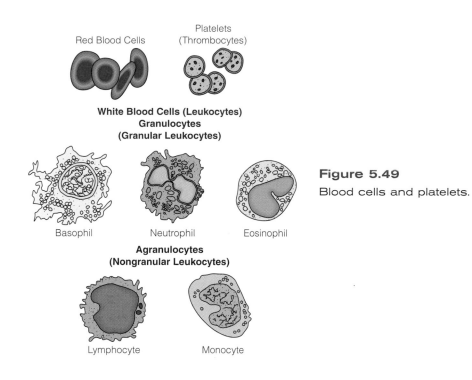

Figure 5.49

Blood cells and platelets.

Blood Coagulation or Clotting

When a blood vessel is damaged, several things happen to prevent severe blood loss. The blood platelets adhere to the ragged edges of the injured vessel, especially to the collagen fibers surrounding the blood vessel. They immediately begin to change shape as protrusions form from their cell membrane and they stick together to create a platelet plug. Platelets also release *serotonin* (seer-o-**TOE**-nin), which is a vasoconstrictor that causes a vascular spasm that temporarily closes the blood vessel.

The tissue damage causes an enzyme to be released that acts on one of the components in the plasma (fibrogen) to activate and form threads of *fibrin*. The fibrin tends to stick to the damaged blood vessels, forming a meshwork that entraps other platelets and blood cells in a *blood clot*.

Plasma

Plasma is the fluid component of the blood, strawlike in color, in which the red corpuscles, white corpuscles, and blood platelets are suspended. About 90 percent of plasma is water. The remaining plasma is made up of about 7 percent proteins and 1.5 percent other substances. It functions to regulate fluid balance and pH and to transport nutrients and gases. Plasma is derived from the food and water taken into the body (Figure 5.50).

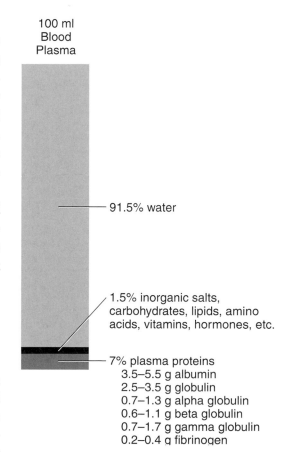

100 ml
Blood
Plasma

— 91.5% water

— 1.5% inorganic salts, carbohydrates, lipids, amino acids, vitamins, hormones, etc.

— 7% plasma proteins
3.5–5.5 g albumin
2.5–3.5 g globulin
0.7–1.3 g alpha globulin
0.6–1.1 g beta globulin
0.7–1.7 g gamma globulin
0.2–0.4 g fibrinogen

Figure 5.50

Composition of plasma. Plasma, which is primarily water, contains about 7% protein and 1.5% other substances.

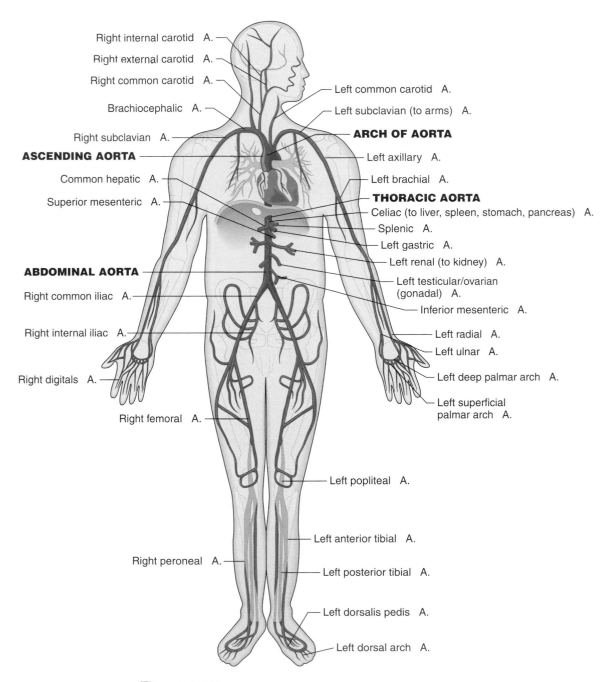

Figure 5.51a

Circulatory system.

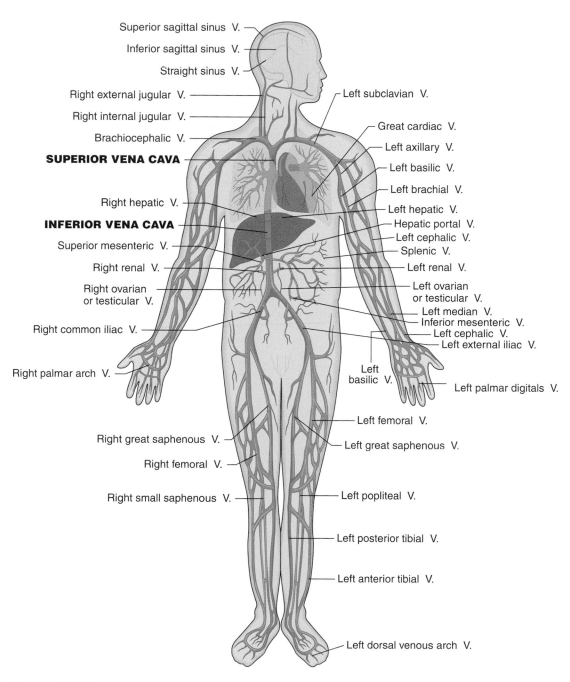

Figure 5.51b
Circulatory system.

Diseases of the Blood

Hemophilia

Hemophilia is characterized by extremely slow clotting of blood and excessive bleeding from even very slight cuts. This disease is hereditary, but men are the chief sufferers. Women may, however, transmit this blood condition to their sons.

Anemia

Anemia refers to a number of conditions in which there is a rapid loss or inadequate production of red blood cells. In this condition, the oxygen-carrying capacity is reduced, resulting in a lack of body strength and paleness of the complexion.

Anemia is more a symptom of a condition than an actual disease. Some forms of anemia are related to nutritional deficiencies that inhibit red blood cell production. *Nutritional anemia* may be due to dietary deficiencies of iron, folic acid, or B_{12}, all of which are essential for the production of hemoglobin. Severe lack of protein or copper may also contribute. If the deficiency were due to inadequate amounts of the nutrient in the diet, replenishing the missing nutrient would reverse the anemia. In *pernicious anemia,* perhaps the most serious nutritional anemia, the stomach does not produce enough intrinsic factor needed to assimilate B_{12}. B_{12} supplementation, usually in the form of monthly injections, is required.

Nutritional anemia is not a contraindication for massage; however, no amount of massage will improve the condition until the proper nutrients are restored to promote red blood cell production.

Hemorrhagic anemia is the result of excessive blood loss either from large wounds or internal bleeding such as bleeding ulcers or excessively heavy menstruation.

Aplastic anemia occurs when the bone marrow slows or stops the production of blood cells. Infection, exposure to certain types of radiation or poison, cancer, or autoimmune disease may inhibit the bone marrow's ability to produce red and white blood cells and platelets. In some cases, if detected early enough, a bone marrow transplant may successfully reverse aplastic anemia.

Hemolytic anemia refers to a number of conditions where the red blood cells die prematurely. One form, *sickle cell anemia,* is an inherited condition where the hemoglobin molecule changes to a rodlike shape after delivering its oxygen to the cells (Figure 5.52). Eventually this causes the red blood cell to change from a smooth, round, doughnut shape to a curved, sharp, sickle shape that is prone to getting stuck in small capillaries and causes clots to form. The process deprives tissues or organs of oxygen-carrying blood and produces periodic episodes of pain. Complications include infections, strokes, ulcerated sores on the legs, blindness, and organ damage that may cause death. Sickle cell anemia is inherited, and there is no cure, although proper medical care may alleviate symptoms and reduce the frequency and number of episodes.

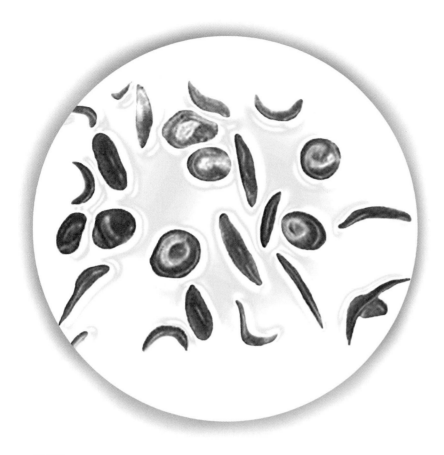

Figure 5-52

Sickle cell anemia is an inherited disorder in which abnormal hemoglobin causes red blood cells to assume a sickle shape.

General massage is systemically contraindicated for hemorrhagic, hemolytic, and aplastic anemia.

Secondary anemia is a complication of or accompanies other serious conditions such as hepatitis, leukemia, kidney disease, bleeding ulcers, or other acute infectious diseases. The anemia usually dissipates as the associated condition heals. Massage is contraindicated as long as the primary condition and the associated anemia persist.

Leukemia

Leukemia is a form of cancer in which there is an uncontrolled production of white blood cells. These cells do not fully mature, and they remain virtually nonfunctional. As a result, the person's resistance to disease is reduced. There are two major types of leukemia: Myeloid leukemia begins in the bone marrow, and lymphoid leukemia begins in the white-cell-producing portions of the lymphoid tissue. The leukemic cells soon metastasize into other areas of the body, producing leukemic cells and demanding excessive amounts of metabolic elements, resulting in severe tissue degeneration. Common effects are severe anemia, spontaneous bleeding, a tendency toward infections, and eventually death.

Arteries of the Head, Face, and Neck

The common carotid arteries are the main sources of blood supply to the head, face, and neck. They are located on either side of the neck, and each artery divides into an internal and external branch. The internal branch of the common carotid artery supplies the cranial cavity, whereas the external branch supplies the superficial parts of the head, face, and neck. The arteries, like the muscles and nerves, are named in accordance with the parts of the body that they serve (Figure 5.53).

Table 5.6 presents the names and functions of the important arteries of the body.

Table 5.7 presents the names and functions of the important veins of the body.

Table 5.6
Important Arteries of the Body

NAME	FUNCTION
Head and Neck	
Facial Artery	Supplies blood to face and pharynx
Temporal Artery	Supplies blood to forehead, masseter muscle, and ear
Common Carotid Arteries:	
Internal branch	Supplies blood to cranial cavity
External branch	Supplies blood to surface of head, face, and neck
Branches of External Carotid Artery	
Ophthalmic artery	Supplies blood to the eyes
Supraorbital artery	Supplies blood to the eye socket, forehead, and side of the nose
Frontal artery	Supplies blood to forehead
Parietal artery	Supplies blood to the crown and the sides of head
Posterior auricular artery	Supplies blood to the scalp and back of ear
Submental artery	Supplies blood to chin and lower lip
Superior labial	Supplies blood to upper lip and center of nose
Trunk	
Aorta	Forms main trunk of arterial system and subdivides to form large and small branches
Subclavian artery	Supplies blood to neck, chest, and upper part of back
Coronary artery	Supplies blood to heart muscles
Common iliac artery	Supplies blood to abdominal wall
External iliac artery	Supplies blood to lower limb
Internal iliac artery	Supplies blood to pelvic organs and inner thigh
Upper Extremities	
(The following arteries are for one side of the body)	
Axillary artery	Supplies blood to shoulder, chest, and arm
Brachial artery	Supplies blood to the arm and forearm
Radial artery	Supplies blood to forearm, wrist, and thumb side of hand
Ulnar artery	Supplies blood to forearm, wrist, and small finger side of hand
Lower Extremities	
(The following arteries are for one side of the body)	
Femoral artery	Supplies blood to lower part of abdominal wall, pelvic organs, and upper thigh
Popliteal artery	Supplies blood to knee and leg
Anterior tibial artery	Supplies blood to leg
Posterior tibial artery	Supplies blood to leg, heel, and foot
Dorsalis pedis artery	Supplies blood to foot

Figure 5.53

Arteries of the head, face, and neck.

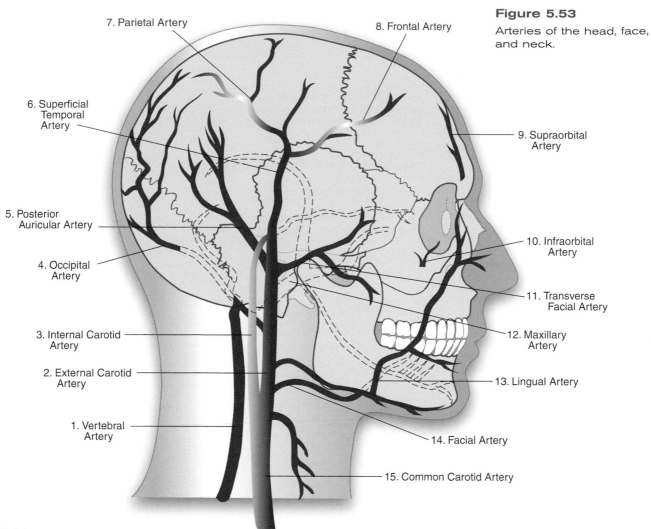

7. Parietal Artery

8. Frontal Artery

6. Superficial Temporal Artery

9. Supraorbital Artery

5. Posterior Auricular Artery

4. Occipital Artery

10. Infraorbital Artery

11. Transverse Facial Artery

3. Internal Carotid Artery

2. External Carotid Artery

12. Maxillary Artery

13. Lingual Artery

1. Vertebral Artery

14. Facial Artery

15. Common Carotid Artery

Table 5.7

Important Veins of the Body

NAME	FUNCTION
Head and Neck (Figure 5.54, next page)	
Facial vein	Receives blood from face and empties into internal jugular vein
Internal jugular vein	Receives blood from cranial cavity and from surface of face and neck
External jugular vein	Receives blood from deep parts of face and from the surface of cranium
Temporal veins	Receives blood from the temporomaxillary region of the head
Maxillary anterior vein	Receives blood from the anterior portion of the face
Ophthalmic vein	Receives blood from the eyes
Supraorbital vein	Receives blood from the forehead and eyebrows
Frontal vein	Receives blood from the anterior portion of the scalp
Superior and inferior labial veins	Receives blood from the upper and lower lips
Trunk	
Innominate veins	Receives blood from internal jugular and subclavian veins
Coronary veins	Receives blood from heart muscles
Common iliac vein	Receives blood from external and internal iliac veins and empties into inferior vena cava
Inferior vena cava	Receives blood from abdomen, pelvis, and lower limbs
Superior vena cava	Receives blood from head, neck, thorax, and upper limbs

continues

Table 5.7

Important Veins of the Body (continued)

NAME	FUNCTION
Upper Extremities	
(The following veins are for one side of the body.)	
Cephalic vein	Receives blood from radial side (front) of arm
Basilic vein	Receives blood from ulnar side (outside) of arm
Axillary vein	Returns blood from arm to heart
Lower Extremities	
(The following veins are for one side of the body.)	
Great saphenous veins	Receives blood from the inner side of front leg
Small saphenous vein	Receives blood from back of leg
Popliteal vein	Receives blood from anterior and posterior tibial veins
Femoral vein	Receives blood from feet, legs, and thigh

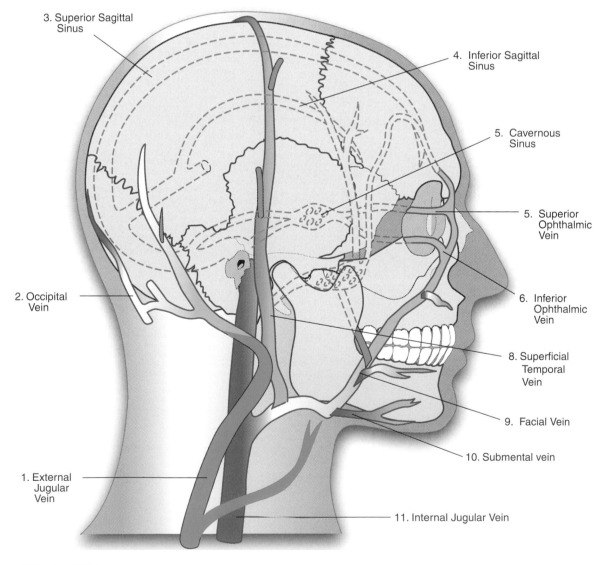

Figure 5.54

Veins of the head, face, and neck.

THE LYMPH-VASCULAR SYSTEM

The lymphatic system acts as an aid to, and is interlinked with, the blood-vascular system. Lymph is derived from the blood and is gradually shifted back into the bloodstream. The lymph-vascular system includes the lymph, lymphatics, lymph ducts, lymph nodes, and lacteals. Also considered a part of the lymph system are the tonsils, the spleen, and the thymus gland.

Function of the Lymph System

The lymphatics collect excess tissue fluid, invading microorganisms, damaged cells, and protein molecules that are too large or too toxic to return directly to the blood system through the capillary walls. These materials are transported from the interstitial spaces through the lymph vessels, are filtered through the lymph nodes, and eventually rejoin the blood near the junction of the subclavian and jugular veins. The lymphoid tissue contains vast numbers of lymphocytes, white blood cells that are an important element of the body's immune system (Figure 5.55a and b).

Lymph and Tissue Fluid

Lymph is a straw-colored fluid that is derived from and is very similar to the tissue fluid or interstitial fluid of the body part from which it flows. By bathing all cells, tissue fluid acts as a medium of exchange, trading to the cells its nutritive materials and

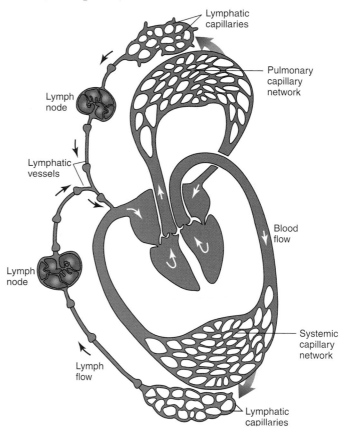

Figure 5.55a

Interaction of blood and lymph system.

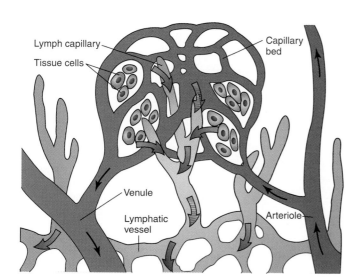

Figure 5.55b

Lymph capillaries begin as closed-end tubules in the tissue spaces near blood capillaries.

receiving in return the waste products of metabolism. Most of the fluid that filters through the capillary walls to surround the cells is eventually reabsorbed into the capillaries. However, about 10 percent of the fluid enters the lymph capillaries and returns to the blood through the lymph system.

Lymph-Collecting Vessels

Lymph capillaries are located throughout the body with the exception of the epidermis of the skin, the central nervous system, the bones, and the endomyseum of most muscles. **Lacteals** (**LAK**-tee-als) are lymphatic capillaries located in the villi of the small intestine. The walls of the lymph capillaries are constructed of endothelial cells that overlap at the edges yet are not securely attached. The endothelial cells have fine filaments that anchor the lymph capillaries in the tissue and help the capillaries to open in response to fluid pressure or the gentle stretching and relaxation of the tissues. This arrangement creates flaplike valves that allow fluid from the tissue spaces to enter the lymph capillaries (Figure 5.56).

Lymph Pathways

After being collected in the lymph capillaries, lymph flows into **lymphatics,** which merge into larger and larger lymphatics. The pathways of the lymphatics are closely associated with the veins of the body. The lymphatics continue to merge until the lymph flows into one of two large lymph ducts and finally back into the blood.

Lymph from the legs, abdomen, left arm, left side of the head, neck, and chest flows into the **thoracic duct** *(left lymphatic duct).* Lymph from the thoracic duct re-enters the bloodstream through the left subclavian vein

---

lacteals

are lymphatic capillaries located in the villi of the small intestine.

---

lymphatics

small, intermediate lymph vessels.

---

thoracic duct

is the largest lymph vessel that collects lymph from both legs and the left side of the rest of the body.

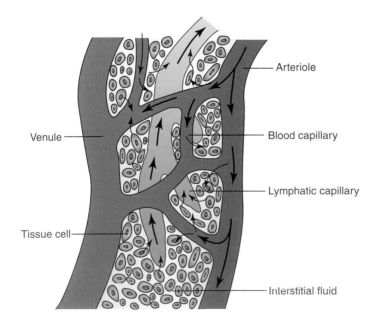

Figure 5.56a

Relationship of lymph capillaries, tissue cells, and blood capillaries.

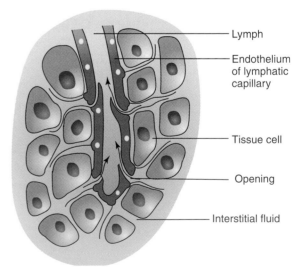

Figure 5.56b

Lymph capillary in tissue cells showing valves and filaments.

and from there flows into the superior vena cava and into the right atrium of the heart. Lymph from the right side of the head, neck, chest, and the right arm flows into the right lymphatic duct. Lymph from the right lymphatic duct re-enters the bloodstream at the right subclavian vein.

Unlike the blood-vascular system where the blood flows through a relatively closed circuit of arteries, capillaries, and veins, lymph moves through a closed-end system from the body tissues to the heart (Figure 5.57a and b).

The Movement of Lymph

Lymph is collected from the interstitial spaces into the lymph capillaries. It travels through the lymphatics and lymph nodes, into the right or left lymphatic duct, and finally back into the bloodstream. Unlike the blood-vascular system where the heart pumps the blood, the lymph system has no internal pump. The structure and arrangement of lymphatics resemble those of the veins except that the lymphatic capillaries are

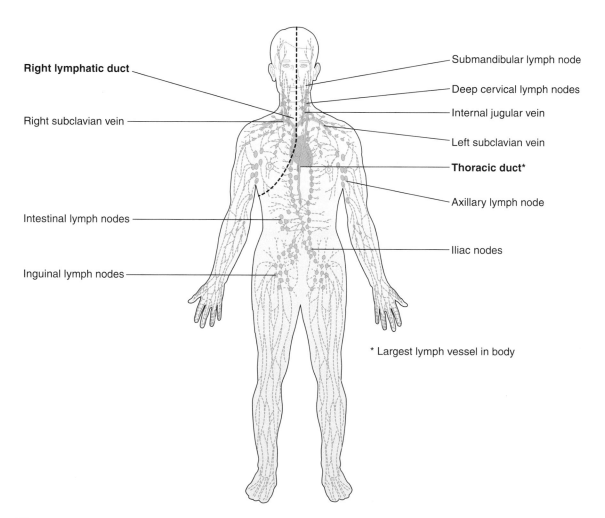

Figure 5.57a

The lymphatic system and lymphatic ducts. (*From* Human Anatomy and Physiology *by Joan G. Creager. Copyright 1983 by Wadsworth, Inc. Reprinted by permission of Wadsworth Publishing Company, Belmont, CA 94002.*)

continues

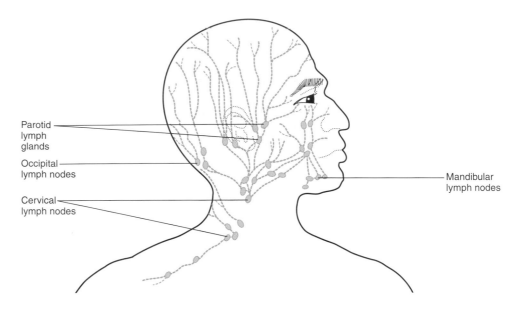

Parotid
lymph
glands

Occipital
lymph nodes

Cervical
lymph nodes

Mandibular
lymph nodes

Figure 5.57b

The lymphatic system and lymphatic ducts found in the head.

closed, whereas the veins are a continuation from the arteries and capillary beds. Also resembling the veins, the lymph vessels contain a system of valves that allow fluid movement in only one direction. The walls of the larger lymphatics are similar to veins. The inner surface is a thin layer of endothelial cells; the middle layer is made up of smooth muscle tissue surrounded by tough connective tissue. The action of the smooth muscle combined with external forces on this extensive system of valves creates a *lymphatic pump*.

Beginning in the smallest lymph capillaries, the endothelial cells that form the capillary walls overlap in such a way that they form microscopic valves that allow the movement of fluids into the capillary, but the slightest back pressure closes the openings so that once inside, the fluid does not escape. Within the lymphatics, flaplike valves protrude from the inside of the vessel walls that prevent backflow.

When a segment of a lymph vessel is compressed, the pressure on the fluid in that segment forces the previous valve to close and the next one to open as the fluid moves through the valve and progresses toward the heart. The external pressure that activates the lymphatic pump is supplied primarily from the contraction of the skeletal muscles. Other factors that may contribute are movement of body parts, breathing, contractions of smooth muscles in the larger lymph vessels, arterial pulsation, and compression of tissues from outside the body (such as massage).

Lymph Nodes

Lymph nodes are made of *lymphoid tissue* and are located along the course of the lymphatics. They are oval or rounded masses from the size of a pinhead to an inch in length and resemble the shape of a bean.

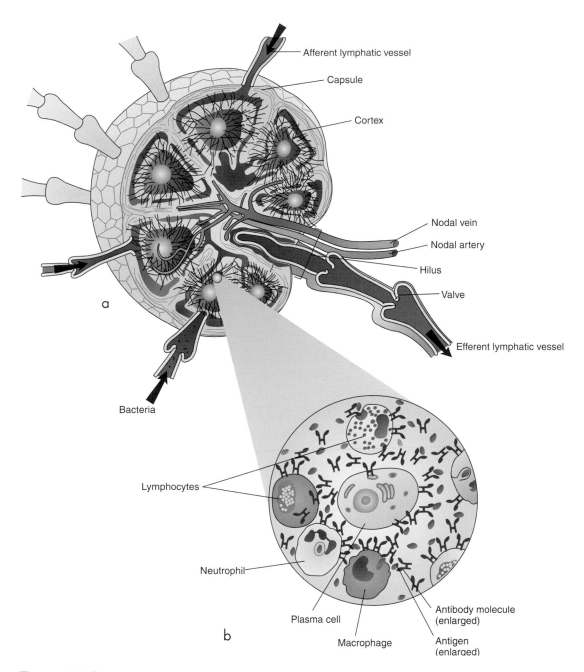

Figure 5.58
(a) Cross section of lymph node; (b) white blood cells destroying bacteria.

Lymph nodes contain a large concentration of lymphocytes and serve to filter and neutralize harmful bacteria and toxic substances collected in the lymph, thereby preventing the spread of infection to other parts of the body (Figure 5.58).

Lymph nodes are found in the following regions of the body:

1. Back of the head, draining the scalp

2. Around the neck muscles, draining the back of the tongue, pharynx, nasal cavities, and the roof of the mouth

3. Under the floor of the jaw, draining the floor of the mouth

4. Upper extremities, in the bend of the elbow, under the armpit, and under the pectoral muscle

5. Abdomen and pelvis, along the blood vessels in these regions

6. Lower extremities, in back of the knee and the groin

Regional lymph nodes are named according to their location in the body:

Node	Location
Submandibular	Beneath the mandible
Occipital	Base of the skull
Axillary	Armpit
Inguinal	Groin
Supratrochlear	Elbow
Popliteal	Behind the knee
Mammary	Breast
Femoral	Thigh
Tibial	Leg
Cervical	Neck

Healthy tissue depends on good lymph circulation. Correct massage can increase lymphatic circulation and clear the lymph spaces as well as drain sluggish lymph nodes. The purpose of lymph drainage is to cleanse and regenerate the tissues and organs of the body. Massage stimulates the movement of lymph and the formation of lymphocytes that produce antibodies, increasing the body's resistance to infection. (See Lymph Massage, Chapter 18, p. 715.)

IMMUNE SYSTEM

The immune system is a remarkable system that helps keep people safe from a variety of "foreign" invaders and diseases. It consists of a complex array of organs, cells, and molecules distributed throughout the body. Keeping infection-causing organisms such as bacteria and viruses, as well as parasites and fungi, out of the body and destroying any that get in is the mission of the immune system.

Specialized white blood cells (lymphocytes) play a major role in the immune response. White blood cells originate in bone marrow. Some migrate to the thymus, where they develop into specialized types of immune cells (T-cells). From the bone marrow and thymus, white blood cells are transported through the blood and lymph and gather in lymph nodes and other immune organs, including the spleen, tonsils, adenoids, appendix, and small intestine, where they may encounter antigens. (An **antigen** is anything that can trigger an immune response.)

Lymphatic vessels and blood vessels transport white blood cells throughout the body to sites of infection. Lymphatic vessels also transport lymph-carrying microorganisms and dead cells from distant infections into lymph nodes, where they can be digested and eliminated.

antigen

is anything that can trigger an immune response.

Lymphocytes, called B-cells and T-cells, are the main types of immune cells and bear the major responsibility for immune response. They recognize and coordinate an attack against specific microorganisms.

The B-cell is responsible for the production of antibodies (proteins that can bind to specific molecular shapes), and the T-cell (two types) is responsible for helping the B-cell to make antibodies and for killing damaged or "different" cells (all foreign cells except bacteria) within the body. The two main types of T-cells are the "helper" T-cell and the cytotoxic T-cell (CDT cell).

The immune system is amazingly complex. It can recognize millions of different enemies and produce secretions and cells to match up with and wipe out each one of them. Whenever any foreign substance or agent enters the body, the immune system is activated. Both B- and T-cell members respond to the threat, which eventually results in the elimination of the foreign substance or agent from the body.

The marvel of your immune system is its ability to distinguish between what's "you" and belongs from what's "foreign" and does not belong. Every substance—from a dust mite to the flu virus to one of your own cells—carries its own "chemical ID card," marked by a unique molecular pattern on its surface. All your body's cells have the same molecular pattern. White blood cells learn to recognize and ignore cells identified by your body's own pattern and react strongly against antigens. They become the "soldiers" in your "immune army."

In abnormal situations, the immune system can mistake self for nonself and attack itself. The result is called **autoimmune disease.** Some forms of arthritis and diabetes are autoimmune diseases. In other cases, the immune system responds inappropriately to a seemingly harmless substance such as ragweed pollen or cat hair. The result is allergy, and this kind of antigen is called an **allergen.**

> **autoimmune disease**
>
> occurs when the immune system mistakes self for nonself and attacks itself.

> **allergen**
>
> an antigen that can cause an allergic response in some people.

B-Cell System

B-cells work chiefly by producing antibodies. When a B-cell intercepts an antigen, it produces a specific antibody that fits to and disables the invading body. Each B-cell is designed to make a specific antibody, and each antibody is designed to battle a specific microorganism. B-cells also develop into plasma cells that manufacture millions of identical antibody molecules and pour them into the bloodstream. An antibody matches an antigen much as a key matches a lock. Whenever antibody and antigen interlock, the antibody marks the antigen for destruction by other scavenging cells of the immune system. Other B-cells transform into rapidly multiplying memory cells that circulate throughout the body, preparing it for the next encounter with this antigen.

T-Cell system

T-cells coordinate immune defenses and kill organisms in cells on contact. T-cells are active against bacterial infection, fungi, cancerous cells, transplanted tissue, wounded cells harboring pathogens, and so on. T-cells produce lymphokines, which draw macrophages, neutrophils, and eosinophils toward sensitized T-cells, and activate macrophages, which then inhibit viral reproduction.

T-cells originate in the thymus and also become localized in lymphoid organs. A variety of T-cells have been identified:

- Killer T-cells attack antigens directly.

- Helper T-cells enable the other T-cells and most B-cells to perform their functions. They activate B-cells, causing the appropriate ones to transform into plasma cells and flood the bloodstream with antibodies. T-cells are destroyed by the HIV virus in AIDS, resulting in a depressed immune response that allows infection by a variety of microorganisms and the growth of certain tumors.

- Suppressor T-cells monitor and adjust the level of antibodies and counteract the action of helper T-cells.

Other White Blood Cells

phagocytosis
is a process in which leukocytes engulf and digest harmful bacteria.

phagocytes
blood cells that are able to engulf and digest cellular debris and foreign bodies in the tissues.

Other important types of white blood cells associated with the immune system, including macrophages and granulocytes, remove neutralized antibody-antigen complexes and organisms by **phagocytosis**, a process of engulfing and digestion. **Phagocytes**, the name for these large white blood cells, comes from the Greek word meaning "eaters." Their main function is to gobble up foreign bodies—a speck of dust or pollen to a virus. The macrophage is one type of phagocyte that migrates out of the bloodstream into the tissue spaces. As scavengers, macrophages rid your body of worn-out cells and other debris. They also play a vital role in initiating the immune response. Other white blood cells—neutrophils, eosinophils, and basophils—are also "cell eaters." In addition, they release powerful chemicals that destroy microorganisms. Mast cells are responsible for the recruitment of other inflammatory cells, mainly through releasing their contents of inflammatory mediators, such as histamine, protein-breaking enzymes, leukotrienes, and heparin. They are most important in allergic disorders.

How the System Works

The immune system responds to external factors such as bacteria, viruses, toxins, and foreign proteins, and internal ones, including potential tumors and damaged normal tissue. In addition, many diseases, such as some forms of diabetes and arthritis, may result from altered immune processes that target healthy normal tissue. The term "antigen" is short for "antibody-generating." An antigen can be any type of molecule that is encoded in such a way that the body does not recognize it as one of its own and therefore provokes an immune response. The immune system responds by producing antibody proteins that selectively bind to and usually inactivate the antigen.

When an antibody binds to an antigen, a complementary set of chemical reactions is initiated. The sequence of events involved in this kind of immune response can be summarized in this series of steps:

- Invading microorganisms initially encounter whatever macrophages, neutrophils, or B- and T-cells might be present in the immediate vicinity.

- Pathogenic destruction by local phagocytes produces chemical messengers.

- Inflammation is initiated.

- Chemical signals are sent to the bone marrow, where the production of white blood cells and phagocytes increases.

- More macrophages, neutrophils, and lymphocytes are drawn to the site of invasion.

- Any antibodies present at the site of infection lock onto their antigen.

- T-cells are brought into action, directly killing some pathogens and making others more susceptible to attack by phagocytes.

- Debris from this interaction produces strong attracting signals for more phagocytes and lymphocytes.

- The killer T-cells attack antigens directly, and T-cells begin to produce lymphokines.

Immunity, Natural and Acquired

Immunity refers to all the physiological mechanisms used by the body as protection against foreign substances. These foreign substances include such common infectious organisms as bacteria, viruses, and parasites such as fungi, worms, and single-cell protozoa, as well as drugs, foods, chemicals, and various inhalants (e.g., pollens).

Innate immunity is present from before birth, consisting of many nonspecific factors and blood-based immunity from the mother.

Acquired immunity, a more specialized form of immunity, is the result of an encounter with a new substance, which triggers events that induce an immune response specific against that particular substance. This involves B lymphocytes, T lymphocytes, and macrophages. When people are exposed to a new antigen, it usually takes several days to a week for the immune system to develop an immunity, which corresponds to the time needed for the B-lymphocytes to be mobilized and activated for antibody production to counteract the antigen invasion. Whenever T-cells and B-cells are activated, some of the cells become *memory cells*. The next time an individual encounters the same antigen, the immune system is set to stop the infection before it starts.

When you are vaccinated, **vaccines** containing microorganisms that are either dead, weakened, or altered forms of a live infectious organism stimulate an immune response usually without causing the accompanying illness. The resulting memory cells provide immunity for years or even a lifetime.

innate immunity
is present from before birth.

acquired immunity
results from an encounter with a new substance, which triggers events that induce an immune response specific to that particular substance.

vaccine
contains microorganisms that are either dead, weakened, or altered forms of a live infectious organism that stimulates an immune response without causing an illness.

Protective Functions of the Immune System

Fever

Fever is an abnormally high body temperature that is an immune system response to a viral or bacterial infection, or sometimes it is a response to major tissue damage. Normal body temperature is 98.6°F (37°C), although it may fluctuate a degree in either direction. A body temperature above 99.8°F is considered a fever. Fevers of 104°F or above are serious and require medical care. Sustained fevers of 107°F or higher may cause permanent brain damage or death. If a fever is accompanied by any of the following signs, a doctor should be consulted immediately:

- Significant stiff neck and pain when you bend your head forward
- A severe headache
- Persistent vomiting
- Difficulty breathing
- Severe swelling of your throat
- Unusual skin rash
- Unusual eye sensitivity to bright light
- Mental confusion
- Extreme listlessness or irritability
- Abdominal pain or pain when urinating

A fever is an indication that the body is working to get rid of a pathogen. Although uncomfortable, unless it is dangerously high or lasts more than 48 hours, it is advantageous to allow the fever to eradicate the invader. For instance, viruses that cause colds and other respiratory infections thrive in cooler temperatures. By creating a fever, your body is helping to eliminate the virus. Common complications of prolonged fever are dehydration and acidosis (bloodstream that is too acidic), so it is important to drink plenty of water and get plenty of rest.

When an infectious virus or bacteria enters the body, it is attacked by certain white blood cells. In response, the white blood cells produce a substance called interleukin-1 that travels to the brain, where a series of chemical reactions cause—among other things—the hypothalamus to reset the body's thermostat. The muscles and glands of the body respond, metabolism increases, superficial blood vessels constrict, shivering and the "chills" begin, and the body's core temperature begins to rise. The increased body temperature helps to fight the invading pathogens by increasing the production of T-cells, which stimulates B-cells to produce antibodies. The heart rate increases to increase the distribution of white blood cells. The antiviral agent interferon becomes more active.

A fever will usually resolve itself as the pathogen is controlled. As the fever breaks, the body often responds by sweating to cool the body down. This is a sign that health is being restored.

Massage is contraindicated during a fever.

Inflammation

Inflammation is an immune system response to a local infection or injury that acts to isolate and resolve the damage and protect the body from invasion. Inflammation is a reaction to tissue damage. The damage may be from trauma, a burn, laceration, toxic chemical, or an infectious agent. When a cell is damaged, it releases certain proteins, such as histamines and cytokines that set off a chain reaction:

● Immediately, vasoconstriction occurs to prevent excessive bleeding.

● This is soon followed by a period of vasodilatation where the capillaries dilate and become more permeable, allowing white blood cells, antibodies, clotting factors, and other important substances to flood the area. This accounts for the inflammatory heat and swelling.

● Platelets and fibrin begin to form clots to close off broken blood vessels. This not only stops blood loss, it prevents pathogens and other harmful substances from entering the bloodstream.

● Neutrophils and macrophages neutralize and phagocytize pathogens.

● Fibroblasts migrate to the area and begin producing collagen fibers to start mending the torn and damaged tissues. Collagen produces scar tissue that continues to form after the initial, acute inflammation subsides.

The first four steps represent the acute inflammation stage. The classic signs of acute inflammation are pain, heat, redness, swelling, and sometimes loss of function and itching. The acute inflammatory stage for an injury such as a wound or sprain/strain is usually 24 to 72 hours. The subacute stage of scar tissue formation and repair may take days, weeks, months, or even years, depending on the nature and extent of the injury.

Massage during the acute stage of inflammation, when swelling, pain, and heat are present, is contraindicated. Massage during the subacute stages, when scar tissue is forming and the tissues are rebuilding, may be invaluable to ensure that strong, pliable, and flexible tissue develops.

Dysfunctions of the Immune System

When the immune system is weakened or overwhelmed, a variety of conditions can occur:

● Allergy—This response is an overreaction by the immune system to an otherwise harmless substance such as pollen or pet dander. Contact with an allergy-causing substance, or allergen, triggers production of a specific kind of antibody that causes immune cells in the mucous lining of your eyes and airways to release inflammatory substances, including histamine. Release of histamine leads to the familiar symptoms of allergy and asthma—redness and swelling of the eyes, sneezing, coughing, difficult breathing, nasal congestion, and hives. A more severe allergic reaction is anaphylactic shock, which may occur in previously sensitized individuals as a result of a bee sting, a food reaction, or an injected or ingested drug. In this case, the bronchioles constrict, breathing becomes difficult, and cardiac failure may result unless emergency treatment is given with an injection of epinephrine to dilate the airways and stimulate the heartbeat.

- Autoimmune diseases—In these conditions, the body makes antibodies and T-cells directed against its own cells. Insulin-dependent diabetes, for example, may be partly caused by an attack on the pancreas by a person's own antibodies. Self-destructive antibodies are also associated with chronic muscle weakness (myasthenia gravis), rheumatoid arthritis, and multiple sclerosis. No one knows what causes the immune system's recognition process to break down this way. Scientists believe multiple factors—heredity, viruses, certain drugs, or even sunlight—may play a role.

- Cancers of the immune system—When immune cells reproduce uncontrollably, the result is a cancer of the immune system such as leukemia, multiple myeloma, or lymphoma.

- Immune-deficiency diseases—These conditions occur when one or more parts of the immune system are deficient or missing. These defects can be inherited or acquired from a viral infection such as AIDS. They also can be caused by the toxic effects of radiation or some drugs.

HIV/AIDS

HIV disease occurs when the human immunodeficiency virus (HIV) enters a person's body. HIV specifically infects CD4+ lymphocytes, the very cells necessary to activate both B-cell and cytotoxic T-cell immune responses. Without helper T-cells, the body cannot make antibodies properly, nor can infected cells containing HIV (an intracellular pathogen) be properly eliminated. Consequently, the virus can multiply, kill the helper T-cell in which it lives, infect adjacent helper T-cells, and repeat the cycle, until eventually there is a substantial loss of helper T-cells and the body's ability to fight infection weakens.

A person with HIV infection may remain healthy for many years. During this time, enough of the immune system remains intact to provide immune surveillance and prevent most infections. Eventually, when a significant number of CD4+ lymphocytes have been destroyed and when production of new CD4+ cells cannot match the rate of destruction, failure of the immune system leads to the appearance of clinical AIDS. The term "AIDS" applies to the most advanced stages of HIV infection.

According to the Centers for Disease Control (CDC), a diagnosis of AIDS is made when the count of CD4+ T-cells falls below 200 per cubic millimeter of blood. (Healthy adults usually have CD4+ T-cell counts of 1,000 or more.) In addition, the definition of AIDS includes 26 clinical conditions that can affect people with advanced HIV disease. Most AIDS-defining conditions are opportunistic infections that rarely cause harm in healthy individuals. In people with AIDS, however, these infections are often severe and sometimes fatal because the immune system is so ravaged by HIV that the body cannot fight off certain bacteria, viruses, and other microbes. HIV infection always evolves to clinical AIDS over time, though the speed at which this evolution occurs may vary.

The first cases of AIDS were noticed in 1980. HIV was first identified in 1984 by French and American scientists, but the human immunodeficiency virus did not get its name until 1986.

HIV is spread most commonly by sexual contact with an infected partner or through contact with infected blood. Women can transmit HIV to their fetuses during pregnancy or birth. HIV also can be spread to babies through the breast milk of infected mothers. Although researchers have detected HIV in the saliva of infected individuals, no evidence exists that the virus is spread by contact with saliva, such as by kissing. Scientists also have found no evidence that HIV is spread through sweat, tears, urine, or feces. HIV is not spread through casual contact such as the sharing of food utensils, towels, bedding, swimming pools, telephones, or toilet seats. HIV is not spread by biting insects such as mosquitoes or bedbugs.

In the health care setting, workers have been infected with HIV after being stuck with needles containing HIV-infected blood or, less frequently, after infected blood contacts the worker's open cut or splashes into a mucous membrane (e.g., the eyes or inside the nose). This risk can be reduced if health care workers follow universal precautions, treating all blood, semen, or vaginal secretions, no matter from whom the fluid comes, as if they contained HIV. Health care workers must wash their hands between patients; wear gloves, masks, gowns, and eyewear when doing certain procedures; and disinfect or sterilize appropriate equipment.

Massage is not contraindicated for people with HIV unless they are severely ill with one of the many opportunistic diseases. Precautions must be taken because the client has a weakened immune system and risks picking up infections from the therapist. The therapist must avoid any open lesions or wounds and be cautious of any bodily fluids. Massage should not be performed if the therapist has cuts or abrasions on her own hands unless wearing gloves for protection. When working with people in advanced stages, work under the direction of the physician. With strict hygiene precautions, touch and massage are a valuable therapy for people inflicted with HIV and AIDS.

REVIEW

Important Veins of the Body

Matching Test I

Insert the letter of the proper term in front of each definition.

_____ 1. receives blood from eyes   a. femoral vein

_____ 2. receives blood from heart   b. ophthalmic vein

_____ 3. receives blood from face   c. coronary veins

_____ 4. receives blood from outer arm   d. facial vein

_____ 5. receives blood from legs   e. basilic vein

True or False Test I

Carefully read each statement and decide whether it is true or false; draw a circle around the letter T or F.

1. T F Both the internal and external jugular veins return blood from the head, face, and neck to the heart.

2. T F The inferior vena cava receives blood from the abdomen and upper limbs.

3. T F The popliteal vein is located in the lower extremities.

4. T F The innominate veins are found in the upper extremities.

5. T F The superior vena cava receives blood from the head, neck, thorax, and upper limbs.

Important Arteries of the Body

Matching Test II

Insert the letter of the proper term in front of each definition.

_____ 1. supplies blood to heart   a. ophthalmic artery

_____ 2. supplies blood to eyes   b. subclavian artery

_____ 3. supplies blood to face   c. frontal artery

_____ 4. supplies blood to forehead   d. coronary artery

_____ 5. supplies blood to chest   e. facial artery

True or False Test II

Carefully read each statement and decide whether it is true or false; draw a circle around the letter T or F.

1. T F The posterior auricular artery supplies blood to the scalp.

2. T F The aorta does not form large and small branches.

3. T F The axillary artery supplies blood to the shoulder, chest, and arm.

4. T F The external branch of the common carotid artery supplies blood to the cranial cavity.

5. T F The external iliac artery supplies blood to the upper limbs.

SECTION QUESTIONS FOR DISCUSSION AND REVIEW

1. Name the important parts comprising the circulatory system.
2. What are the two divisions of the circulatory system?
3. What is the function of the heart?
4. Name the protective covering of the heart and describe its function.
5. Name the chambers of the heart in the order that blood would pass through them.
6. Which nerves regulate the heartbeat?
7. What is the function of the arteries?
8. What is an arteriole?
9. Which nerves control the movements of the arterial walls?
10. What is the function of the capillaries?
11. What is the function of the veins?
12. What is a venule?
13. What is the purpose of the venous pump?
14. Name the main artery of the body.
15. Name two circulatory systems of the blood-vascular system.
16. What vein carries freshly oxygenated blood?
17. Which constituents are found in the blood?
18. What is the primary function of the red blood cells?
19. What is the primary function of the white blood cells?
20. Which substances are carried by the blood to the body cells?
21. Which substances does the blood carry away from the body cells?
22. In what ways does the blood protect the body?
23. What is the normal temperature of the blood?
24. Name the parts of the lymph system.
25. What is the major function of the lymph-vascular system?
26. What is the major function of the lymph glands or nodes?
27. Which regions of the body contain lymph nodes?
28. From what is lymph derived?
29. Into which blood vessels does the lymph return?
30. What is meant by lymph drainage?
31. What are lacteals?
32. Of what value is massage to the health of the lymphatic system?
33. What determines names of lymphatics?
34. What is the lymphatic pump and how does it work?
35. Trace the flow of lymph from just before it enters the lymph system until it leaves.

neuron
is the structural unit of the nervous system.

nerve cell
is the same as a neuron.

nerve fibers
projections from the body of the nerve cell that carry nervous impulses.

5 | THE NERVOUS SYSTEM

The nervous system controls and coordinates the functions of other systems of the body so that they work harmoniously and efficiently. The nervous system is composed of the brain, spinal cord, and peripheral nerves. The primary function of the nervous system is to collect a multitude of sensory information; process, interpret, and integrate that information; and initiate appropriate responses throughout the body.

The functions of the nervous system are

1. To rule the body by controlling all visible and invisible activities
2. To control human thought and conduct
3. To govern all internal and external movements of the body
4. To give the power to see, hear, move, talk, feel, think, and remember

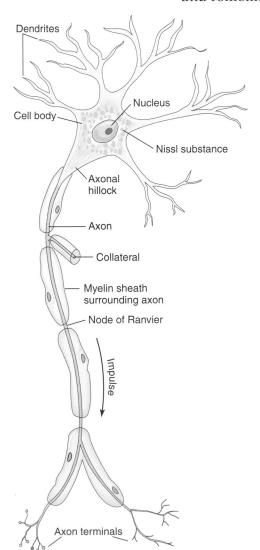

Figure 5.59

Common neuron.

Neurons and Nerves

A **neuron** is the structural unit of the nervous system. A neuron is the **nerve cell** (cell body) including its outgrowth of long and short projections of cytoplasm, called **nerve fibers**. There are two types of nerve fibers. A neuron has numerous multi-branched **dendrites** that connect with other neurons to receive information and a single **axon** that conducts impulses away from the cell body. The axons of most nerves are covered by a myelin sheath that is made of fatty Schwann cells. The myelin insulates the nerve and aids in the conduction of the nerve impulse. The nerve cell stores energy and nutrients that are used by the cell processes to convey nerve impulses throughout the body. Neurons have the ability to react to certain stimuli (irritability) and to transmit an impulse generated by that stimulus over a distance or to another neuron (conductability). Impulses are passed from one neuron to another at a junction called a **synapse** (**SIN**-aps). When an impulse reaches the end of an axon, a chemical **neurotransmitter** is released at the synapse that acts on the membrane of the receptive neuron to pass the impulse along. Almost all the nerve cell bodies are contained in the brain and spinal cord, while their fibers extend outward to make up the nerves (Figure 5.59).

Functionally, there are three types of neurons:

Sensory neurons (afferent neurons) originate in the periphery of the body and carry impulses or messages from sense organs to the brain where sensations of touch, cold, heat, sight, hearing, taste, or pain are interpreted and experienced.

Motor neurons (efferent neurons) carry nerve impulses from the brain to the effectors (the muscles or glands that they control).

Interneurons (internuncial neurons) are located in the brain and spinal cord and carry impulses from one neuron to another. They function to transmit and direct impulses from one place in the spinal cord or brain to another.

A nerve fiber is the extension from a neuron. A **nerve** is a bundle of nerve fibers held together by connective tissue that extends from the central nervous system to the tissue that the neurons innervate. Nerves have their origin in the brain and spinal cord and distribute branches to all parts of the body.

Sensory nerves, or **afferent nerves,** carry sensory impulses from a variety of sensory receptors toward the brain or spinal cord. *Motor nerves,* termed *efferent nerves,* carry impulses from the brain or spinal cord to the muscles or glands. Most nerves contain both sensory and motor fibers and are called *mixed nerves.*

Anatomically, the nervous system is divided into two main divisions: the central nervous system and the peripheral nervous system.

Central Nervous System

The **central nervous system** (CNS) is the main control center for the human organism. It is responsible for our thoughts and emotions, for receiving and interpreting incoming sensory information, and for disseminating appropriate motor responses to maintain safety and homeostasis. The CNS consists of the *brain* and *spinal cord*. The CNS is surrounded by bone and is covered by a special connective tissue membrane called the **meninges** (me-NIN-jeez). More specifically, the brain is housed in the cranium, and the spinal cord is housed in the vertebral canal of the spine. The meninges has three layers. The outer layer, the **dura mater** (DOO-ruh MAY-ter), is a protective fibrous connective tissue sheath covering the brain and spinal cord. The **pia mater,** the innermost layer, is attached to the surface of the brain and spinal cord and is richly supplied with blood vessels to nourish the underlying tissues. Between the dura and pia mater is a thin netlike membrane called the **arachnoid mater,** sometimes referred to as the arachnoid space. The arachnoid mater provides a space for the blood vessels and the circulation of cerebrospinal fluid (Figure 5.60).

Cerebrospinal fluid is a clear fluid derived from the blood and secreted into the inner cavities or ventricles of the brain. The fluid circulates through the ventricles and then down through the central canal of the spinal cord and into the arachnoid space. The brain and spinal cord are surrounded by cerebrospinal fluid and indeed seem to be suspended by the fluid. Cerebrospinal fluid carries some nutrients to the nerve tissue and carries wastes away, but its main function is to protect the CNS by acting as a shock absorber for the delicate tissue.

---

dendrites
connect with other neurons to receive information.

axon
conducts impulses away from the cell body.

synapse
the junction where nerve signals jump from one nerve to another.

neurotransmitter
is a chemical that sends a nerve signal across a synapse.

sensory neuron
carries impulses from sense organs to the brain.

motor neuron
carries nerve impulses from the brain to the effectors.

interneuron
carries impulses from one neuron to another.

nerves
are bundles of fibers held together by connective tissue that originate in the brain and spinal cord and distribute branches all over the body.

afferent nerves
carry impulses toward the spinal cord and brain.

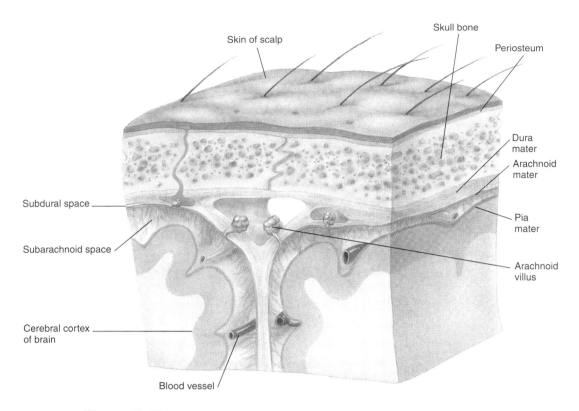

Figure 5.60

Meninges of the central nervous system.

central nervous system
consists of the brain and spinal cord.

meningitis
is an acute inflammation of the pia mater and arachnoid mater around the brain and spinal cord.

dura mater
is the outer layer of the meninges.

pia mater
is the innermost layer of the meninges.

arachnoid mater
is the middle space of the meninges.

The Brain

The *brain,* the principal nerve center, is the body's largest and most complex nerve tissue, containing in excess of 10 billion neurons and innumerable nerve fibers (Figure 5.61). It is located in and protected by the cranium. It controls sensations, muscles, glandular activity, and the power to think and feel (emotions). The brain includes the following:

1. The *cerebrum,* the largest portion making up the front and top of the brain, presides over such mental activities as speech, sensation, communication, memory, reasoning, will, and emotions. The cerebrum is divided by a central fissure into right and left cerebral hemispheres that are connected by bundles of nerve fibers called the *corpus callosum* that provide communication between the right and left hemispheres. It is interesting to note that sensory and motor functions from the right side of the body are processed on the left side of the brain and the sensory and motor activities from the left side of the body are processed and controlled by the right side of the brain.

2. The *cerebellum,* the smaller part of the brain, located below the cerebrum and at the back of the cranium, helps maintain body balance, coordinates voluntary muscles, and makes muscular movement smooth and graceful.

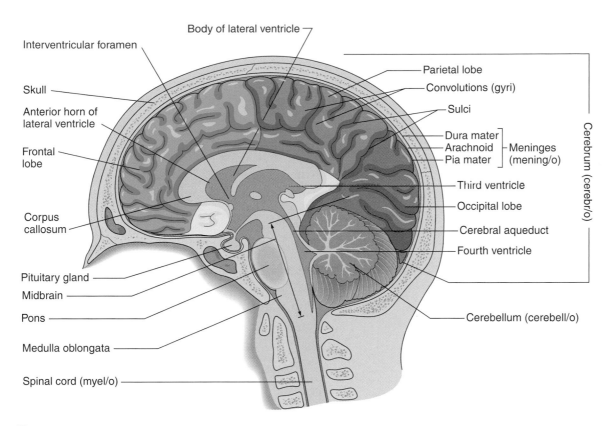

Figure 5.61
Cross section of the brain.

3. The *diencephalon,* which includes the hypothalamus, thalamus, pineal and pituitary glands, is located in the center of the brain. The thalamus is a relay center for sensory information coming into the brain. The hypothalamus governs the pituitary gland, thereby having a regulatory effect on the autonomic system and the endocrine glands. The pituitary gland, considered to be the master gland because its hormones control other endocrine glands, is located at the base of the brain in the sella turcica of the sphenoid bone.

4. The *brain stem* has three parts: the midbrain, the pons, and the medulla oblongata. These contain intricate masses of nerve fibers that relay and transmit impulses from one portion of the brain to another.

The midbrain contains the main nerve pathways connecting the cerebrum and the lower nervous system as well as certain visual and auditory reflexes that coordinate head and eye movements with things seen and heard.

The pons, located between the midbrain and the medulla oblongata, relays nerve impulses between the cerebrum and the medulla and from the cerebrum to the cerebellum.

cerebrospinal fluid
flows through and around the brain and spinal cord to nourish and protect them.

peripheral nervous system

consists of all the nerves that connect the CNS to the rest of the body.

The medulla oblongata is an enlarged continuation of the spinal cord that extends from the foramen magnum to the pons and connects the brain with the spinal cord. Control centers within the medulla oblongata regulate movements of the heart and control vasoconstriction of the arteries and the rate and depth of respiration.

Spinal Cord

The spinal cord extends downward from the brain and is housed in and protected by the vertebral column. It extends down from the medulla oblongata to the level of the first lumbar vertebrae. The spinal cord consists of 31 segments, each segment being the site of attachment of a pair of spinal nerves. The spinal cord functions as a conduction pathway for nerve impulses traveling to and from the brain as well as a reflex center between incoming and outgoing peripheral nerve fibers (Figure 5.62).

The Peripheral Nervous System

The **peripheral nervous system** consists of all the nerves that connect the central nervous system to the rest of the body. It includes the spinal nerves, the cranial nerves, and all their branches. Peripheral nerves send sensory impulses to the brain and spinal cord and transmit motor impulses from the brain to the muscles, glands, and visceral organs. The peripheral nervous system is divided into the **autonomic nervous system** and the *somatic nervous system*. Basically, the somatic system involves those nerves connecting the CNS, the voluntary muscles, and skin; the autonomic nervous system connects the CNS to the visceral organs such as the heart, blood vessels, glands, and intestines.

Cranial Nerves

There are 12 pairs of **cranial nerves** that connect directly to some part of the brain surface and pass through openings called foramina on the sides and base of the cranium. They are classified as *motor* or *sensory* nerves and *mixed* nerves, which contain both motor and sensory fibers.

The cranial nerves are named numerically according to the order in which they arise from

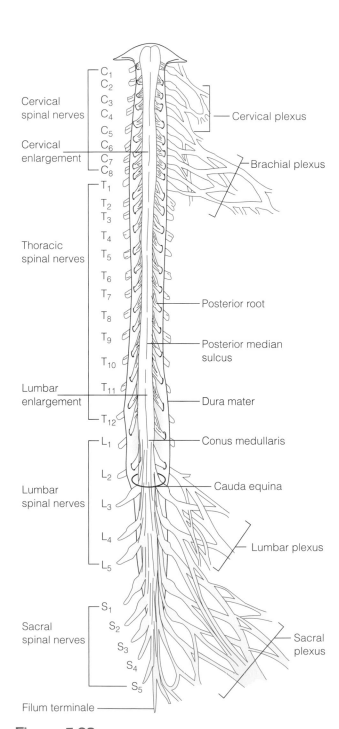

Figure 5.62

Spinal cord and spinal nerves.

Table 5.8

Classification of Cranial Nerves

CRANIAL NERVE	TYPE OF NERVE	LOCATION	FUNCTION
i. Olfactory nerve	Sensory nerve	Nose	Sense of smell
ii. Optic nerve	Sensory nerve	Retina of eye	Sense of sight
iii. Oculomotor nerve	Motor nerve	Muscles of eye	Controls eye movements
iv. Trochlear nerve	Motor nerve	Obliquus superioris muscle of eye	Rotates eyeball downward and outward
v. Trigeminal or trifacial nerve	Motor and sensory nerve	Face, teeth, and tongue	Controls sensations of the face and movements of the jaw and tongue
vi. Abducent nerve	Motor nerve	Recti muscles of eye	Rotates eyeball outward
vii. Facial nerve	Motor and sensory nerve	Face and neck	Controls facial muscles of expression and some muscles of the neck and ear
viii. Acoustic or auditory nerve	Sensory nerve	Ear	Sense of hearing
ix. Glossopharyngeal nerve	Motor and sensory nerve	Tongue and pharynx	Sense of taste
x. Vagus or pneumogastric nerve	Motor and sensory nerve	Pharynx, larynx, heart, lungs, and digestive organs	Controls sensations and muscular movements relating to talking, heart action, breathing, and digestion
xi. Spinal accessory nerve	Motor nerve	Shoulder	Controls movement of neck muscles
xii. Hypoglossal nerve	Motor nerve	Tongue and neck	Controls movement of the tongue

the brain, and by names that describe their type, function, or location (Figure 5.63 and Table 5.8).

Spinal Nerves

Thirty-one pairs of spinal nerves emerge from the spinal cord and are numbered according to the level of the vertebra where they exit the spine. All spinal nerves are mixed nerves that contain both sensory and motor nerve fibers to provide two-way communication between the CNS and the body. Each spinal nerve has an anterior and a posterior root. The anterior root contains motor neurons, and the posterior root contains sensory neurons.

Spinal nerves number

- 8 pairs of cervical nerves
- 12 pairs of thoracic nerves
- 5 pairs of lumbar nerves
- 5 pairs of sacral nerves
- 1 pair of coccygeal nerves

autonomic nervous system

regulates the action of glands, smooth muscles, and the heart.

cranial nerves

twelve pairs of nerves that emerge from the brain through openings in the base of the cranium.

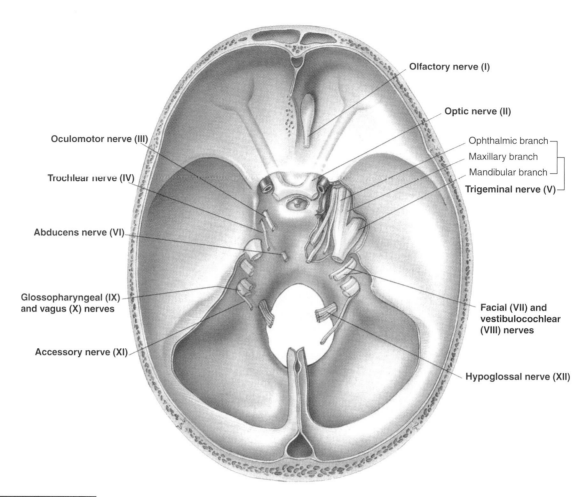

Figure 5.63
Cranial nerves.

cervical plexus
consists of the four upper cervical nerves that supply the skin and control the movement of the head, neck, and shoulders.

brachial plexus
is composed of four lower cervical nerves and the first pair of thoracic nerves that control arm movements.

lumbar plexus
is formed from the first four lumbar nerves.

The four upper cervical nerves form the **cervical plexus,** which supply the skin and control the movement of the head, neck, and shoulders.

The four lower cervical nerves and the first pair of thoracic nerves form the **brachial plexus,** which controls the movement of the arms by way of the musculocutaneous, radial, median, and ulnar nerves. The next 11 pairs of thoracic nerves supply the muscles, skin, and organs in the thorax.

The first four lumbar nerves form the **lumbar plexus,** whose nerves supply the skin, the abdominal organs, hip, thigh, knee, and leg. The femoral and obturator nerves reach the upper parts of the leg.

Portions of the forth and fifth lumbar nerves, the first, second, third, and fourth sacral nerves form the **sacral plexus.** The spinal nerves that form the sacral plexus divide and merge to form several collateral nerves and one main branch, the **sciatic** (sigh-AT-ic) **nerve.** The sciatic nerve is the largest and longest nerve in the body. The sciatic nerve consists of two nerves in the same nerve sheath: the common peroneal nerve and the tibial nerve. The sciatic nerve serves the hamstrings and the lower leg and foot.

Another portion of the fourth sacral nerves, the fifth sacral nerve and the coccygeal nerve, forms the **coccygeal plexus** (kok-SIJ-ee-al **PLEK**-sus). The coccygeal nerves supply the skin and muscles around the coccyx (Figure 5.64 to Figure 5.66).

> **sacral plexus**
> is formed from the fourth and fifth lumbar nerves, and the first four sacral nerves.

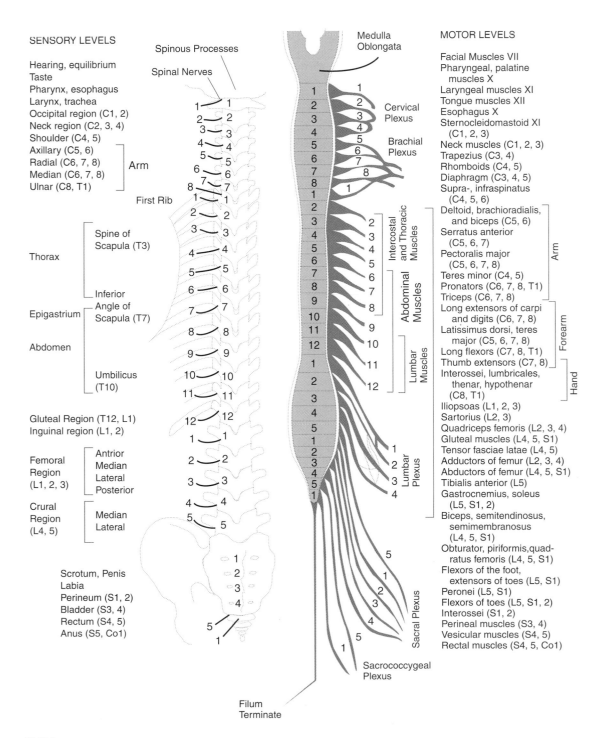

SENSORY LEVELS

Hearing, equilibrium
Taste
Pharynx, esophagus
Larynx, trachea
Occipital region (C1, 2)
Neck region (C2, 3, 4)
Shoulder (C4, 5)
Axillary (C5, 6)
Radial (C6, 7, 8)
Median (C6, 7, 8)   Arm
Ulnar (C8, T1)

Thorax — Spine of Scapula (T3)
         — Inferior
Epigastrium — Angle of Scapula (T7)
Abdomen
            Umbilicus (T10)

Gluteal Region (T12, L1)
Inguinal region (L1, 2)

Femoral Region (L1, 2, 3)   Antrior Median Lateral Posterior

Crural Region (L4, 5)   Median Lateral

Scrotum, Penis
Labia
Perineum (S1, 2)
Bladder (S3, 4)
Rectum (S4, 5)
Anus (S5, Co1)

Spinous Processes
Spinal Nerves
First Rib
Filum Terminate

Medulla Oblongata
Cervical Plexus
Brachial Plexus
Intercostal and Thoracic Muscles
Abdominal Muscles
Lumbar Muscles
Lumbar Plexus
Sacral Plexus
Sacrococcygeal Plexus

MOTOR LEVELS

Facial Muscles VII
Pharyngeal, palatine muscles X
Laryngeal muscles XI
Tongue muscles XII
Esophagus X
Sternocleidomastoid XI (C1, 2, 3)
Neck muscles (C1, 2, 3)
Trapezius (C3, 4)
Rhomboids (C4, 5)
Diaphragm (C3, 4, 5)
Supra-, infraspinatus (C4, 5, 6)
Deltoid, brachioradialis, and biceps (C5, 6)
Serratus anterior (C5, 6, 7)
Pectoralis major (C5, 6, 7, 8)
Teres minor (C4, 5)
Pronators (C6, 7, 8, T1)   Arm
Triceps (C6, 7, 8)
Long extensors of carpi and digits (C6, 7, 8)   Forearm
Latissimus dorsi, teres major (C5, 6, 7, 8)
Long flexors (C7, 8, T1)
Thumb extensors (C7, 8)
Interossei, lumbricales, thenar, hypothenar (C8, T1)   Hand
Iliopsoas (L1, 2, 3)
Sartorius (L2, 3)
Quadriceps femoris (L2, 3, 4)
Gluteal muscles (L4, 5, S1)
Tensor fasciae latae (L4, 5)
Adductors of femur (L2, 3, 4)
Abductors of femur (L4, 5, S1)
Tibialis anterior (L5)
Gastrocnemius, soleus (L5, S1, 2)
Biceps, semitendinosus, semimembranosus (L4, 5, S1)
Obturator, piriformis, quadratus femoris (L4, 5, S1)
Flexors of the foot, extensors of toes (L5, S1)
Peronei (L5, S1)
Flexors of toes (L5, S1, 2)
Interossei (S1, 2)
Perineal muscles (S3, 4)
Vesicular muscles (S4, 5)
Rectal muscles (S4, 5, Co1)

Figure 5.64

Spinal nerves showing plexuses, motor and sensory functions.

sciatic nerve
is the largest and longest nerve in the body.

coccygeal plexus
is formed from a portion of the fourth sacral nerves, the fifth sacral nerve, and the coccygeal nerve.

Tables 5.9 to 5.15 present the names, functions, and distribution of the nerves of the neck, chest, head and face, abdomen, back, arms and hands, legs and feet, respectively.

Sensory Receptors

Sensory input from a neuron is initiated from a variety of sensory receptors. They can be categorized as mechanoreceptors, thermoreceptors, photoreceptors, chemoreceptors, and nociceptors.

Mechanoreceptors respond to mechanical stimulation or tissue distortion such as touch, pressure, vibration, and stretch. Examples of mechanoreceptors include the ruffini end organs, Pacini corpuscles, and Merkel disks in the skin and the proprioceptors located in the muscles, fascia, and joints. The latter include the muscle spindle cells and the Golgi tendon organs.

Thermoreceptors are located in the skin and in the mouth. Two types of thermoreceptors detect heat or cold.

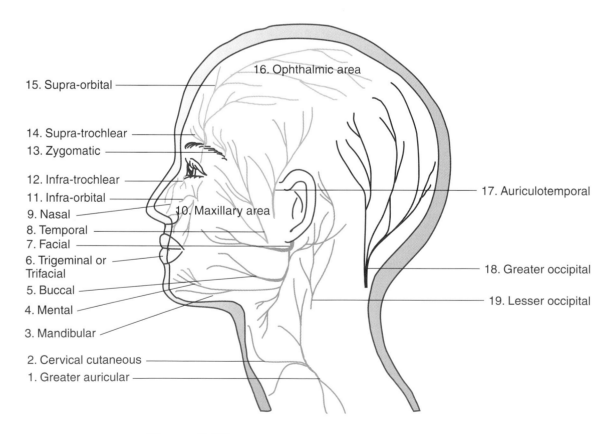

Figure 5.65

Nerves of head, face, and neck.

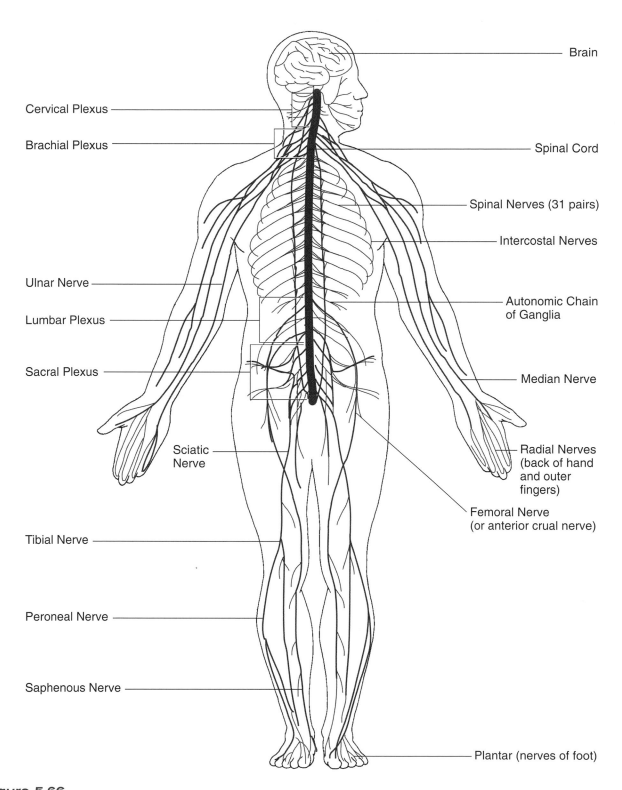

Brain

Cervical Plexus

Brachial Plexus

Spinal Cord

Spinal Nerves (31 pairs)

Intercostal Nerves

Ulnar Nerve

Lumbar Plexus

Autonomic Chain
of Ganglia

Sacral Plexus

Median Nerve

Sciatic
Nerve

Radial Nerves
(back of hand
and outer
fingers)

Femoral Nerve
(or anterior crual nerve)

Tibial Nerve

Peroneal Nerve

Saphenous Nerve

Plantar (nerves of foot)

Figure 5.66

The nervous system.

Table 5.9
Nerves of the Neck

NAME	FUNCTION	DISTRIBUTION
Auricular, great	Sensation	Skin of neck
Colli, superficial	Sensation	Skin of neck and throat
Dental, inferior	Sensation-Motion	Mylohyoid muscle
Digastric	Motion	Stylohyoid and posterior portion of digastric muscle
Hypoglossal	Motion	Geniohyoid and omohyoid muscles
Mylohyoid	Motion	Mylohyoid and anterior part of digastric muscle
Spinal accessory	Motion	Neck muscles
Stylohyoid	Motion	Stylohyoid and posterior part of digastric muscle
Suboccipital	Motion	Muscles of back and neck
Cervical, superficial	Sensation	Skin of front of neck
Occipital, greater	Sensation-Motion	Muscles of back of neck
Pneumogastric	Sensation-Motion	Larynx or voice box

Table 5.10
Nerves of the Chest

NAME	FUNCTION	DISTRIBUTION
Pneumogastric	Sensation-Motion	Heart and lungs
Phrenic	Motion	Diaphragm
Suprasternal	Sensation	Skin over top of breastbone
Thoracic, external anterior	Motion	Pectoralis major
Thoracic, internal anterior	Motion	Pectoralis major and minor
Thoracic, external posterior	Motion	Serratus anterior
Thoracic, spinal	Sensation-Motion	Muscles and skin of chest
Cervical (8)	Sensation-Motion	Trunk and upper extremities
Dorsal (12)	Sensation-Motion	Muscles and skin of chest and trunk

Two types of *photoreceptors* located in the retina of the eyes, rods, and cones are sensitive to light and detect color. They give us the ability to see color and form.

Chemoreceptors located in the mouth and nose are sensitive to certain chemical stimuli and give us the sense of taste and smell. Chemoreceptors in certain arteries are sensitive to CO_2 and pH changes in the blood and affect respiration and other involuntary functions to maintain homeostasis.

Table 5.11

Nerves of the Head and Face

NAME	FUNCTION	DISTRIBUTION
Auriculotemporal	Sensation	Side of scalp
Auditory	Sensory nerve of hearing	Ear
Abducent	Motion	Obliquus externus muscle of eye
Trochlear	Motion	Obliquus superior muscle of eye
Auricular, anterior	Sensation	Skin of external ear
Auricular, great	Sensation	Side of neck and ear
Auricular, posterior	Motion	Epicranius and auricularis posterior muscle
Buccal	Motion	Buccinator and orbicularis oris muscles
Dental, inferior	Sensation-Motion	Teeth of lower jaw and skin of chin
Facial	Sensation-Motion	Muscles of expression
Frontal	Sensation	Skin of forehead
Glossopharyngeal	Sensation-Motion	Muscles and mucous membranes of pharynx and back of tongue
Infraorbital	Sensation	Skin of cheek and lower eyelid
Infratrochlear	Sensation	Skin of lower eyelid and side of nose
Mandibular	Sensation-Motion	Teeth and skin of lower jaw and cheeks
Masseteric	Motion	Masseter muscle
Maxillary	Sensation	Nasal pharynx, teeth of upper jaw and skin of cheek
Mental	Sensation	Skin and mucous membrane of nose
Occipital, greater	Sensation-Motor	Skin over back part of head
Occipital, lesser	Sensation	Skin behind ear and on back of scalp
Oculomotor	Motion	Levator palpebrae superioris, recti muscles and obliquus inferior muscle of eye
Olfactory	Sensory nerve of smell	Nose
Ophthalmic	Sensation	Tear glands, eye membrane, skin of forehead and nose
Optic nerve	Sensory nerve of sight	Retina of eye
Orbital	Sensation	Skin of temple
Supraorbital	Sensation	Skin of forehead
Pterygoid, external	Motion	External pterygoid muscle
Pterygoid, internal	Motion	Internal pterygoid muscle
Trigeminal or trifacial	Sensation-Motion	Skin of face, tongue, teeth and muscles of mastication
Supratrochlear	Sensation	Skin of upper eyelid and root of nose
Pneumogastric	Sensation-Motion	Pharynx
Temporal	Motion	Temporal muscle

Nociceptors detect pain and are located in nearly every tissue in the body except the brain. They respond to extreme stimuli (pressure, sound, heat, and cold) and tissue damage. Nociceptors serve as a protective function by informing us when something is wrong, it hurts. Usually pain is felt where the nociceptors are affected; however, at times pain may be referred—such as with trigger points or with visceral pain.

Table 5.12

Nerves of the Abdomen

NAME	FUNCTION	DISTRIBUTION
Hypogastric	Sensation-Motion	Muscles and skin of abdominal wall
Ilio-hypogastric	Sensation-Motion	Muscles and skin of lower abdomen
Ilio-inguinal	Sensation-Motion	Obliquus internus abdominis muscle and skin of groin
Intercostal	Sensation-Motion	Muscles and skin of upper abdomen
Lumar (5)	Sensation-Motion	Front of lower abdomen
Pneumogastric	Sensation-Motion	Stomach

Table 5.13

Nerves of the Back

NAME	FUNCTION	DISTRIBUTION
Coccygeal	Sensation-Motion	Coccygeus muscle and skin over coccyx of spine
Gluteal, inferior	Motion	Gluteus maximus muscle
Gluteal, superior	Motion	Gluteus medius muscle
Intercostal	Sensation-Motion	Muscles and skin of back
Subscapular	Motion	Latissimus dorsi muscle
Suprascapular	Motion	Supraspinatus and infraspinatus muscles
Spinal accessory	Motion	Trapezius muscle
Supra-acromial	Sensation	Skin over shoulder
Iliac	Sensation	Skin of gluteal region
Sacral (5)	Sensation-Motion	Multifidus muscles of spine and gluteal region

Table 5.14

Nerves of the Arms and Hands

NAME	FUNCTION	DISTRIBUTION
Cervical (8)	Sensation-Motion	Upper extremities
Circumflex	Sensation-Motion	Deltoid, teres minor, shoulder joint, and overlying skin
Cutaneous, internal	Sensation	Skin of inner part of forearm
Interosseous, anterior	Motion	Deep flexor and pronator muscles of forearm
Interosseous, posterior	Sensation-Motion	Muscles and skin of back of forearm and wrist
Median	Sensation-Motion	Pronator and flexor muscles of forearm, external lumbricales, and skin of fingers
Musculocutaneous	Sensation-Motion	Flexors of upper arm and skin of external part of forearm
Musculospiral	Sensation-Motion	Extensor muscles of entire arm and hand, and skin of back of forearm
Radial	Sensation	Back of hand and outer fingers
Subscapular	Motion	Teres major and subscapularis muscles
Ulnar	Sensation-Motion	Flexor carpi ulnaris and flexor digitorum profundus muscles, elbow and wrist joints, and skin of fingers

Table 5.15

Nerves of the Legs and Feet

NAME	FUNCTION	DISTRIBUTION
Crural	Sensation	Skin of upper thigh
Musculocutaneous of leg	Sensation-Motion	Peroneal muscles and skin of external part of lower leg and foot
Obturator	Sensation-Motion	Adductor muscles of thigh, hip and knee joints, and skin of inner portion of thigh
Pectineal	Motion	Pectineus muscle
Popliteal, external Peroneal, common	Sensation-Motion	Extensor muscles of lower leg and foot and overlying skin
Popliteal, internal	Sensation-Motion	Flexor muscles of lower leg and foot and overlying skin
Sacral	Sensation-Motion	Muscles and skin of lower extremities
Saphenous, external	Sensation	Skin of foot and toe
Saphenous, internal	Sensation	Skin of inner part of knee, leg, ankle, and dorsum of foot
Sciatic, great	Sensation-Motion	Flexor muscles of thigh, leg, foot, and skin of calf and sole
Sciatic, small	Sensation	Skin of back of thigh
Tibial, anterior	Sensation-Motion	Extensor muscles of foot and toes and skin of dorsum of foot
Tibial, posterior	Sensation-Motion	Flexor muscles of foot and toes, and skin of sole
Cutaneous, dorsal	Sensation	Top of foot
Plantar	Sensation-Motion	Sole of foot, deep muscles of foot and toes

The Autonomic Nervous System

Autonomic means self-governing. The **autonomic nervous system** regulates action of glands, smooth muscles, and the heart. It controls the circulation of blood, the activity of the digestive tract, respiration, and body temperature. These activities are not under conscious control and are considered involuntary. The autonomic nervous system consists of motor neurons that originate in the central nervous system. The autonomic nervous system is further subdivided into the *sympathetic* and *parasympathetic* nervous systems. Neurons from both systems supply the same visceral organs (except the adrenals) and are said to be complementary. The sympathetic system excites and the parasympathetic system inhibits in such a way as to maintain internal homeostasis in an ever-changing external environment.

The nerves of the **sympathetic nervous system** originate in the thoracolumbar (thoracic and lumbar portions of the spine) between T-1 and L-2 and enter a double chain of small *ganglia* (**GANG**-glee-uh) (masses of neurons) that extend along the spinal column from the base of the brain to the coccyx. Within these ganglia, neurons synapse with

> **autonomic nervous system**
>
> regulates the action of glands, smooth muscles, and the heart.

> **sympathetic nervous system**
>
> supplies the glands, involuntary muscles of internal organs, and walls of blood vessels with nerves and prepares the body for energy-expending circumstances.

other neurons before continuing to their target organs. These ganglia are connected with each other and with the central nervous system by nerve fibers. The sympathetic nervous system supplies the glands, involuntary muscles of internal organs, and walls of blood vessels with nerves.

The activity of the sympathetic system is primarily to prepare the organism for energy-expending, stressful, or emergency situations. Stimulation of the sympathetic nerves can bring about rapid responses, such as increased respiration, dilated pupils, and increased heart rate and cardiac output. Blood vessels dilate, and the liver increases conversion of glycogen to glucose for more energy. There is increased mental activity and production of the adrenal hormones epinephrine and norepinephrine. All these activities prepare us to meet emergencies.

The **parasympathetic nervous system** counteracts the action of the sympathetic system. The general function of the parasympathetic division is to conserve energy and reverse the action of the sympathetic division. The effects of parasympathetic activity are reduced heart rate, respiration, and blood pressure and increased digestion and elimination. The parasympathetic nervous system is most active when the individual is calm and in a state of relaxation.

Parasympathetic nerve fibers that serve the organs and glands of the thorax and abdomen are part of the vagus nerve. Pelvic portions of the parasympathetic system arise from the second, third, and fourth sacral spinal nerves. Parasympathetic nerve fibers associated with parts of the head are included in the III, VII, and IX cranial nerves (Figure 5.67a and b).

> **para-sympathetic nervous system**
>
> functions to conserve energy and reverse |the action of the sympathetic division.

Reflexes and Reflex Arcs

A **neurological pathway** is the route that a nerve impulse travels through the nervous system. The usual nerve path consists of a stimulus that initiates an impulse along a sensory nerve fiber to the spinal cord to communicate with an indeterminable number of interneurons (depending on how complicated or intricate the response is) and finally a response impulse along motor nerves to the associated effectors, producing the resultant action.

> **neurological pathway**
>
> is the route that a nerve impulse travels through the nervous system.

The simplest form of nervous activity that includes a sensory and motor nerve and few if any interneurons is called a **reflex.** The nerve pathway of a reflex is called a **reflex arc.** A simple reflex, such as a knee jerk, involves just two neurons (sensory and motor) that pass into and out of the spinal cord without influencing any other nerve centers. Another type of reflex called the withdrawal reflex (flexor reflex) occurs when a person touches something sharp or hot and immediately pulls away, thereby preventing excessive injury. Reflexes are automatic, unconscious, involuntary responses to a stimulus and are responsible for many of the body's activities, such as sneezing, coughing, and swallowing, as well as many involuntary activities such as heart rate, breathing rate, and blood pressure. More complex reflexes affect parts of the body distant from the point of stimulation (Figure 5.68).

> **reflex**
>
> is the simplest form of nervous activity, which includes a sensory and motor nerve.

> **reflex arc**
>
> is the nerve pathway of a reflex.

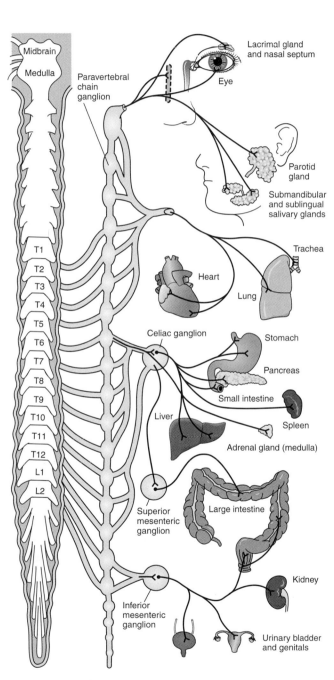

Figure 5.67 (a)

Nerves of the sympathetic division of the autonomic nervous system communicate through a chain of ganglia located along each side of the spine.

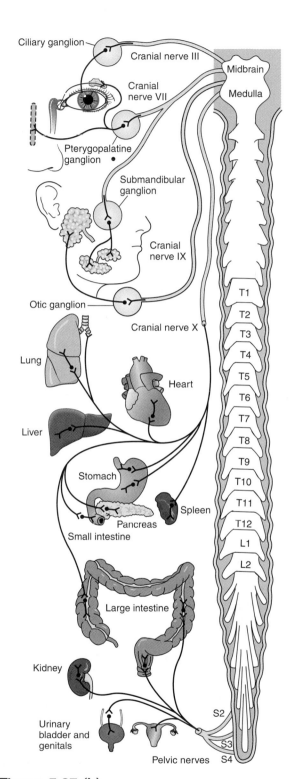

Figure 5.67 (b)

Nerves of the parasympathetic division of the autonomic nervous system.

Figure 5.68

Simple reflex arc; knee-jerk reflex.

The areas of the body that are particularly sensitive to reflex influences are

1. The skin of the back between the shoulders
2. The side of the chest between the fourth and sixth ribs
3. The skin at the upper and inner portion of the thigh
4. The skin overlying the gluteal muscles
5. The sole of the foot

Proprioception

Peripheral nerves are classified as either motor nerves or sensory nerves. Sensory nerves can be further classified as exteroceptors and proprioceptors according to their location and the sensations they record. **Exteroceptors** are located throughout the body and record conscious sensations such as heat, cold, pain, and pressure. **Proprioceptors** respond to the unconscious inner sense of position and movement of the body known as *kinesthesia* (kin-es-**THEE**-zee-uh). They sense where the body is and how it moves.

Proprioception is a system of sensory and motor nerve activity that provides information to the central nervous system about the position and rate of movement of different body parts. Proprioception also provides information as to the state of contraction and position of the muscles and in so doing helps to prevent injury to the joints and muscles from excessive stretches or contractions and makes possible the coordination of smooth and accurate motion.

Proprioceptors are specialized nerve endings located in the muscle, tendons, joints, or fascia. Two major categories of proprioceptors are

exteroceptors

record conscious sensations such as heat, cold, pain, and pressure throughout the body.

proprioceptors

sense where the body is and how it moves.

the **muscle spindle cells** and the **Golgi tendon organs**. Their sensory input goes no farther than the brain stem, so their activity is all unconscious.

Spindle cells are located largely in the belly of the muscle. They are made up of specialized contractile tissue called intrafusal muscle fibers. Coiled around the center of the intrafusal muscle fibers are the annulospiral or primary receptors. A secondary sensory nerve receptor, often referred to as a flower-type receptor, is located adjacent to the annulospiral receptor. These sensory nerve ends of proprioceptive neurons relay information directly to the spinal cord. These receptors continuously sense movement in the spindles and in the muscle fibers surrounding them, alerting the CNS as to the length and stretch of the muscle as well as how far and fast the muscle is moving.

The *Golgi tendon organs* (GTOs) are multibranched sensory nerve endings located in the muscle-tendon junction where muscle fibers attach to tendon tissue. The GTOs measure the amount of tension produced in muscle cells as a result of the muscle's stretching and contracting. They also monitor the amount of force pulling on the bone to which the tendon attaches.

The proprioceptive receptors located in and around the joints sense angulation and pressure. Other pressure-sensitive nerve endings are situated throughout all planes of connective tissue, and together these supply sensory information to the central nervous system to give a concise body image of soft tissue and of joint position and movement (Figure 5.69).

How Proprioceptors Work

Proprioceptors sense tissue distortion. Each time the tissue is compressed, decompressed, twisted, or distorted in a specific way or there is a pressure on or movement in the body, these nerves record that change with the central nervous system. These messages feed the integrative areas of the brain with richer and more detailed information about every body part. The information is continually assembled into an overall body image that is the brain's way of knowing what the body is doing.

Neurological Disorders

Diseases of the nervous system have many causes. They may result from birth defects, trauma, or degenerative disease. They may be caused by infection, blood clots, tumors, or hemorrhage. Some diseases manifest as abnormal muscular activity, while others affect functional and mental activities. Only physiologically based diseases will be discussed here.

Multiple Sclerosis

Multiple sclerosis (MS) is a degenerative nerve disease that affects the body's ability to control the muscles. MS usually occurs in young adults between the ages of 20 and 50 and is the result of the breakdown of the myelin sheath, which inhibits nerve conduction. Symptoms vary from minor to debilitating depending on the area of the brain or spinal cord

muscle spindle cells
sensory organs in muscle that detect the rate of stretch in muscles.

Golgi tendon organs
are multibranched sensory nerve endings located in tendons.

multiple sclerosis
occurs in young adults and results from the breakdown of the myelin sheath.

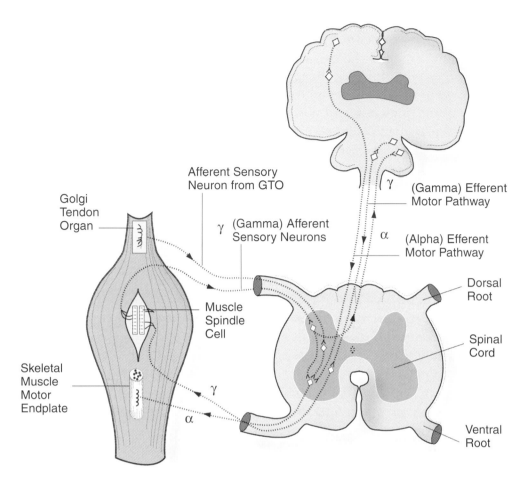

Figure 5.69

Proprioceptors' role in coordination of muscle movement.

affected and the extent of damage to the myelin sheath or nerves. Symptoms may include muscle weakness, spasticity, loss of coordination or balance, and loss of bladder control. Speaking becomes difficult, vision is affected, and there may be memory loss and difficulty concentrating. The progress of the disease varies with periods of remission and exacerbation. A person may have an episode, totally recover, and never have another attack; or a person may have an attack, recover, then later have another attack, followed by another and another, progressively becoming more and more debilitated. There is no cure, but medication to alleviate symptoms, physical therapy, and psychological counseling are useful in counteracting the effects of the disease. Massage is systemically contraindicated during the acute stages when the extra stimulation would tend to exacerbate the condition. During the subacute phase and when in remission, gentle massage is beneficial to counter stress, spasticity, and depression.

Parkinson's Disease

Parkinson's disease occurs as the result of the degeneration of an area of the cerebrum that produces the neurotransmitter dopamine. Without dopamine, another nearby area of the cerebrum loses the abil-

| **Parkinson's disease** |
| occurs as a result of the degeneration of certain nerve tissues which regulate body movements. |

ity to balance the activity of the prime movers and their antagonists, resulting in the lack of coordination and difficulty in moving experienced by those afflicted with the disease. It generally develops late in life and is characterized by tremors and shaking, especially in the hands. Muscles stiffen as movement slows and becomes more deliberate as many of the postural reflexes are lost. A gradual and progressive rigidity of the muscles, especially the flexors, cause a stooped posture and a labored, shuffling gait. Changes in the vocal cords affect speech until it becomes little more than a whisper. Because of the progressive nature of the disease, it is usually accompanied by anxiety and depression. Massage is useful to maintain flexibility, relax muscles, and relieve anxiety and depression. The massage therapist must work under the supervision of the client's physician when working with people with Parkinson's disease.

Amyotrophic Lateral Sclerosis

Amyotrophic lateral sclerosis (ALS), also known as *Lou Gehrig's disease,* is a progressive, eventually fatal, neurological condition that causes the motor neurons of the brain and spinal cord to degenerate and die causing weakness, spasticity, and atrophy of the voluntary muscles. It usually attacks people between the ages of 40 and 60, though there have been cases reported in people older and younger. It affects nearly twice as many men as women. Early symptoms may be weakness or twitching of a leg, arm, or hand or slurred speech depending on which nerves are involved. As the disease progresses, more muscles throughout the body become involved affecting the ability to move, speak, swallow, and even breathe. There is no known cure for ALS. Fifty percent of those diagnosed die within 3 to 5 years, and 90 percent succumb within 10 years, usually from complications of paralysis or the loss of respiratory function. ALS only attacks the motor neurons and does not affect the intelligence, memory, personality, or the ability to taste, smell, and hear or the sense of touch. In the earlier stages of the disease, massage may be helpful to relieve spasticity and stress. Because ALS is not contagious, does not spread through the blood and lymph, or affect the sensory nerves, massage is not contraindicated and may provide a great amount of comfort and relief. As the disease progresses, massage should be given under the physician's supervision and in coordination with the health care team.

Spinal Cord Injury

A *spinal cord injury* (SCI) is caused by trauma or disease to the vertebral column or to the spinal cord itself. Most injuries are caused by trauma to the vertebral column that results in pinching, bruising, or tearing of the spinal cord. The injury affects the ability of the nerve fibers in the cord to transmit impulses to and from the brain and results in loss of sensation and movement of the parts of the body controlled by the spinal nerves that exit the spinal cord below the site of the injury. Each spinal cord injury is different according to the level of the injury and the extent of damage to the spinal cord. Injury of the cervical spine (C-1 through T-1) results in *tetraplegia* or **quadriplegia,** affecting the neck, shoulders,

> **quadriplegia**
>
> is paralysis of the arms and legs caused by a stroke or spinal cord injury.

paraplegia
paralysis of the lower extremeties; does not affect the arms or hands.

skin brushing
a light, brisk brushing using a dry vegetable bristle bath brush.

cerebrovascular accident
or stroke, is caused by a blood clot or ruptured blood vessel in or around the brain that subsequently destroys nerve tissue.

hemiplegia
is unilateral paralysis caused by a stroke.

epilepsy
is a neurological condition in which there is an abnormal electrical activity in the CNS without apparent tissue abnormalities.

arms, hands, and legs. If the injury is between T-2 and S-5, and only the mid-lower chest, stomach, legs, and feet are affected, the condition is called **paraplegia.** The higher the level of injury, the more sensory and motor deprivation occurs. An SCI is a *complete injury* when there is no motor or sensory function below the injury level and *incomplete* when not all the spinal nerve fibers are affected and there is still some sensory and motor function below the injury site.

Massage can be very beneficial for people with spinal cord injury, but it requires some special consideration. Massage applied above the injury level, where there is normal sensation and mobility, is similar to massage on an able-bodied individual and is helpful in addressing compensation patterns that accompany living in a wheelchair. Below the injury level, there is no sensation or it is impaired and muscle tissue is atrophied, spastic, or brittle. The feet and ankles may have edema because of lack of movement. Massage directed toward the muscles is generally contraindicated. However, light massage or **skin brushing** may help reduce edema and improve the quality of the skin. If done regularly, gentle range of motion will help maintain flexibility, prevent contractures, and reduce spasms. Because of mobility impairments, special care must be taken when transferring a client with an SCI to and from the massage table. Clear communication will help determine what assistance is needed and how to provide it.

Stroke (CVA)

Stroke or **cerebrovascular accident** (CVA) is the result of a blood clot or ruptured blood vessel in or around the brain and the subsequent destruction of nerve tissue. It is the third leading cause of death in the United States, behind cancer and heart disease, and is the leading cause of adult onset disability. The effect of the stroke depends on the location and extent of damaged tissue. There may be loss of vision in one or both eyes, loss of the ability to speak or understand language, loss of memory, or personality changes. Often, a stroke causes paralysis on one side of the body, opposite the side of the brain in which the damage occurred. The extent of the paralysis is relative to the extent of the neurological damage. The condition of unilateral paralysis caused by a stroke is called **hemiplegia.** Massage can be a beneficial part of stroke rehabilitation when given under medical supervision and with consideration of related cardiovascular precautions. Because hemiplegia may involve sensory deprivation and muscle paralysis, deep massage directed toward the muscles is contraindicated.

Epilepsy

Epilepsy is a neurological condition in which there is abnormal electrical activity in the CNS without apparent tissue abnormalities. Epilepsy is characterized by seizures, some of which are so mild that they are barely noticeable, whereas others may be so extreme that the person loses consciousness and is thrown into uncontrollable convulsions. People with epilepsy generally can live normal, productive lives with the use of appropriate medication. Massage is inappropriate during a seizure; however, massage is indicated for a person with a history of seizure disorder.

Viral or Bacterial Infections

Many diseases that affect the nervous system are the result of an invading virus or bacteria. Causes of such infections may vary from contaminated wounds and bites from animals or insects to infections elsewhere in the body. Viral infections include poliomyelitis, encephalitis, and shingles.

Polio

Poliomyelitis (po-lee-o-my-e-**LIE**-tis), or *polio,* is a crippling or even deadly disease that affects the motor neurons of the medulla oblongata and spinal cord, resulting in paralysis of the related muscle tissues. Symptoms of polio include fever, gastrointestinal discomfort, stiff neck, and headache. If detected early, its devastating effects can be minimized. The development of the Salk and Sabin vaccines has nearly eradicated this terrible disease. Post-polio syndrome occurs in polio victims years or even decades after the initial infection and causes degenerative muscle weakness and fatigue. Massage is beneficial in both polio and post-polio syndrome as part of a physician-directed treatment.

Encephalitis

Encephalitis (en-sef-a-**LIE**-tis) refers to several related viral diseases that cause an inflammation of the brain or the meninges. The infection is sometimes spread due to a carrier such as an animal or bird by way of a mosquito bite or may arise as a secondary infection from measles, mumps, or chickenpox. Symptoms may include headache, fever, disoriented behavior, and often seizures. Serious cases may result in nerve or brain damage and may cause paralysis, emotional disturbances, or even death.

Meningitis

Meningitis (men-in-**JIGH**-tis) is an acute inflammation of the pia and arachnoid mater around the brain and spinal cord. This is often a secondary infection due to bacteria traveling from the middle ear, upper respiratory tract, lungs, or sinuses or due to polio or mumps viruses. Symptoms include severe headache, stiff neck, high fever, chills, delirium, and often convulsions or even coma. Antibiotic treatment is usually effective. If untreated, permanent brain damage usually results with possible blindness, deafness, retardation, or paralysis.

Diagnosis of encephalitis and meningitis is made with a spinal tap or lumbar puncture, in which a hollow needle is inserted into the spinal canal in the lumbar area to determine the constituents and pressure of the cerebrospinal fluid. Massage is systemically contraindicated during the active stage of encephalitis or meningitis. However, for a client with a history of either that has no current symptoms, massage is quite appropriate.

Shingles

Shingles is an acute inflammation of a nerve trunk and the dendrites at the end of the sensory neurons by the herpes zoster virus. The symptoms include a band of pain around the torso and a rash with water blisters that erupt in a confined area on one side of the body. Seldom does the rash cross the midline of the body. Shingles may develop from an exposure to herpes or chickenpox viruses, a reaction to a medication, or trauma. Massage is contraindicated due to the risk of infection and because it would be very painful. Immediate medical attention is recommended.

Neuritis

Neuritis literally means inflammation of a nerve. Neuritis is not a disease but a symptom of some other condition such as a herniated disk, herpes zoster, or diabetes mellitus. Neuritis affects the nerves of the peripheral nervous system. Because most peripheral nerves are both sensory and motor, neuritis may cause weakness or paralysis and may be painful. The pain associated with neuritis is called *neuralgia*. Generalized neuritis affecting a number of nerves (polyneuritis) may be due to nutritional deficiency, alcoholism, chemical poisoning, allergies, and viral or bacterial infections. Usually the symptoms of neuritis subside when the cause is resolved. Rest, a diet rich in B vitamins, and therapy such as massage are helpful. The appropriateness of massage depends on the cause of the neuritis and is decided on a case-by-case basis. Local massage is contraindicated in the area of the inflamed nerve.

Sometimes neuritis will affect a specific nerve (mononeuritis). Pain or partial paralysis along the course of the affected nerve could be the result of disease, pressure on, or injury to the nerve. A common form of neuritis is the result of injury or pressure on the sciatic nerve called *sciatica*. The sciatic nerve is exposed to many sites of possible irritation as it exits the spine and courses through the pelvis and down the leg. Depending on the severity, sciatica results in burning pain or paresthesia (pins and needles) through one buttock and down the back of the leg and into the foot that may be accompanied by muscle weakness or paralysis. Skilled massage is very effective to relieve sciatica if it is caused by soft tissue conditions of the muscles or ligaments. However, massage is contraindicated if the sciatica is caused by a herniated disk, spondylosis (bone spurs on the vertebra), or other conditions within the spine. It is important to have a diagnosis and clearance from a physician before proceeding.

A *pinched nerve* can refer to any of a wide variety of conditions where pressure on a nerve is responsible for pain, numbness, or a reduction of function in the tissues supplied by the nerve. The pinched nerve could be a result of *nerve compression* or *nerve entrapment.*

Nerve compression or impingement is due to bone or cartilage pressing against the nerve such as a herniated vertebral disk pressing against a spinal nerve. Symptoms may include sharp pain at the site of the lesion, radiating pain along the course of the nerve, tingling, numbness, or weakening of the affected muscle.

Nerve entrapment is caused by soft tissue such as muscle, fascia, tendon, or ligament putting pressure against a nerve. The nerve may be trapped within constricted soft tissue as a result of overuse or injury. Or constricted soft tissue may be pressing the nerve against bone as in thoracic outlet syndrome. Symptoms of nerve entrapment vary according to nerve involvement and severity from mild to intense local or radiating pain, numbness, burning, or weakness in the affected muscles. Massage is indicated to relieve the constricted soft tissues responsible for the entrapment.

Thoracic Outlet Syndrome

Thoracic outlet syndrome (TOS) is caused by a compression or entrapment of the brachial nerve plexus and/or blood vessels going to or from the arm that results in pain, paresthesia, numbness, and/or weakness in the shoulder, neck, and arm. The brachial plexus originates as the spinal nerves C-5 to T-1. The nerves travel through the spinal foramen, between the anterior and medial scalene muscles, between the clavicle and first rib, under the pectoralis muscle near its attachment to the coracoid process, and on down the arm. The axillary artery and the subclavian vein lay parallel to the nerve between the clavicle and first rib, under the pectoralis muscle and through the axilla. Compression along the course of the nerve or blood vessels will cause symptoms in the arm or along the course of the nerve. Occasionally, the cervical nerve will be impinged by a spinal misalignment, bulging disk, or bone spur on the vertebra. Hypertonicity of the scalene muscles may compress the brachial nerves while tension in the pectoralis minor muscle may compress the nerves and blood vessels against the first rib causing TOS symptoms down the arm. TOS due to muscular involvement can be effectively relieved with massage. However, if the TOS is from bone spurs, herniated disk, or pressure from a cervical rib, massage will offer little or no relief.

Carpal Tunnel Syndrome

Carpal tunnel syndrome (CTS) is the result of compression of the median nerve as it passes through the anatomical tunnel of the wrist that causes pain and weakness in the thumb and/or first three fingers. There are different conditions that cause CTS. A common cause is the same activity of the hand and wrist repeated hour after hour, day after day (repetitive stress injury) such as meat cutting, typing, or cashiering that results in hypertrophy of the tendons passing through the carpal area or fibrosis of the connective tissues. This causes pressure on or irritation to the median nerve. Fluid retention and edema may also cause pressure on the nerves in the wrist causing CTS. A number of other conditions may mimic CTS such as herniated disks, thoracic outlet syndrome, or shoulder and wrist injuries. It is important to have a definitive diagnosis before providing massage on a client with CTS symptoms. Edematous CTS responds well to gentle massage to drain the excess fluids from the arm. CTS due to fibrotic buildup or hypertrophy may or may not respond to massage. Always work conservatively. If massage around the wrist exacerbates the symptoms, stop immediately! If the client experiences relief and improvement, proceed slowly and cautiously.

REVIEW

Nerves of the Head and Face

Matching Test I

Insert the letter of the proper term in front of each definition.

_____	1. sense of hearing	a. facial nerve
_____	2. sense of smell	b. trifacial nerve
_____	3. sense of sight	c. auditory nerve
_____	4. supplies skin of face	d. olfactory nerve
_____	5. supplies muscles of expression	e. optic nerve

True or False Test I

Carefully read each statement and indicate whether it is true or false; draw a circle around the letter T or F.

1. T F The great auricular nerve supplies the epicranius muscle.

2. T F The frontal and supraorbital nerves supply the skin of the forehead.

3. T F The abducent nerve supplies the obliquus superior muscle of the eye.

4. T F The trigeminal nerve supplies the muscles of mastication.

5. T F The auriculotemporal nerve supplies the side of the scalp.

Nerves of the Neck and Chest

Matching Test II

Insert the letter of the proper term in front of each definition.

_____	1. supplies neck muscles	a. greater occipital nerve
_____	2. supplies front of neck	b. phrenic nerve
_____	3. supplies back of neck	c. pneumogastric nerve
_____	4. supplies heart and lungs	d. superficial cervical nerve
_____	5. supplies diaphragm	e. spinal accessory nerve

True or False Test II

Carefully read each statement and decide whether it is true or false; draw a circle around the letter T or F.

1. T F The cervical nerves supply the trunk and the lower extremities.

2. T F The suboccipital nerve supplies the back of the neck.

3. T F The dorsal and spinal thoracic nerves supply the muscles and skin of the chest.

4. T F The pneumogastric nerve supplies the heart and lungs but not the larynx.

5. T F Branches of the thoracic nerve supply the pectoralis major, pectoralis minor, and serratus anterior muscles.

Nerves of the Abdomen and Back

Matching Test III

Insert the letter of the proper term in front of each definition.

_____	1.	supplies lower abdomen
_____	2.	supplies upper abdomen
_____	3.	supplies shoulders
_____	4.	supplies stomach
_____	5.	supplies trapezius muscle

a. supra-acromial nerve
b. iliohypogastric nerve
c. pneumogastric nerve
d. spinal accessory nerve
e. intercostal nerve

True or False Test III

Carefully read each statement and decide whether it is true or false; draw a circle around the letter T or F.

1. T F The sacral, coccygeal, and suprascapular nerves supply various muscles of the spine.
2. T F The subscapular and suprascapular nerves supply the same muscles of the back.
3. T F The lumbar nerves supply the upper part of the abdomen.
4. T F Superior gluteal nerve supplies the gluteus medius muscle.
5. T F Subscapular nerve supplies latissimus dorsi muscle of the back.

Nerves of the Arms and Hands

Matching Test IV

Insert the letter of the proper term in front of each definition.

_____	1.	supplies elbow joint
_____	2.	supplies shoulder joint
_____	3.	supplies skin of back of arm
_____	4.	supplies deltoid muscle
_____	5.	supplies muscles of forearm

a. median nerve
b. ulnar nerve
c. circumflex nerve
d. radial nerve
e. subscapular nerve

True or False Test IV

Carefully read each statement and decide whether it is true or false; draw a circle around the letter T or F.

1. T F The subscapular nerve supplies the teres minor muscle.
2. T F The cervical nerves supply the upper extremities.
3. T F The musculospiral nerve supplies the extensor muscles of the entire arm and hand.
4. T F The musculocutaneous nerve supplies the pronator muscles of the upper arm.
5. T F The ulnar nerve supplies the skin of the fingers.

Nerves of the Legs and Feet

Matching Test V

Insert the letter of the proper term in front of each definition.

_____	**1.** supplies soles of foot	a. small sciatic nerve
_____	**2.** supplies upper thigh	b. obturator nerve
_____	**3.** supplies inner portion of thigh	c. crural nerve
_____		d. external saphenous nerve
	4. supplies back of thigh	
_____	**5.** supplies foot and toe	e. plantar nerve

True or False Test V

Carefully read each statement and decide whether it is true or false; draw a circle around the letter T or F.

1. T   F   The obturator nerve supplies the hip and knee joints.

2. T   F   The internal popliteal nerve supplies the extensor muscles of the lower leg and foot.

3. T   F   The sacral nerve supplies the muscles and skin of the lower extremities.

4. T   F   The anterior tibial nerve supplies the flexor muscles of the foot and toes.

5. T   F   The dorsal cutaneous nerve supplies the top of the foot.

SECTION QUESTIONS FOR DISCUSSION AND REVIEW

1. What is the primary function of the nervous system?

2. Name the main parts of the nervous system.

3. Name and describe the general structure of a nerve cell.

4. What abilities do neurons have that enable them to transmit nerve impulses?

5. What is a synapse?

6. Describe three types of neurons.

7. Describe the structure of a nerve.

8. What is an efferent nerve?

9. What is an afferent nerve?

10. What is a mixed nerve?

11. What are the two divisions of the nervous system?

12. What is the CNS and where is it located?

13. Define meninges and name its layers.

14. What is cerebrospinal fluid and what is its function?

15. What are the main parts of the brain?

16. Where is the peripheral system located?

17. What are the divisions of the peripheral nervous system?

18. How many pairs of cranial nerves branch out from the brain?

19. Identify the cranial nerves by name and number.

20. How many pairs of spinal nerves branch out from the spinal cord?

21. Describe how the spinal nerves are numbered.

22. What is a nerve plexus?

23. Name the important spinal nerve plexuses and the body areas they supply.

24. What is the function of the autonomic nervous system?

25. Name and contrast the two divisions of the autonomic nervous system.

26. Which organs are supplied by the sympathetic nervous system?

27. What is a reflex action?

28. What is proprioception?

29. Name two categories of proprioceptors, including where they are located and the information they record.

6 THE ENDOCRINE SYSTEM

The endocrine system comprises a group of specialized glands that affect the growth, development, sexual activity, and health of the entire body, depending on the quality and quantity of their secretions.

The major function of the endocrine system is to assist the nervous system in regulating body processes.

Glands of the Body

Glands are specialized organs that vary in size and function. The circulatory and nervous systems closely interact with the glands. The glands act as chemical factories, with the ability to remove certain constituents from the blood to produce specialized secretions. There are two main classifications of glands. **Exocrine** (**EK**-sow-krin) or *duct glands* possess tubes or **ducts** leading from the gland to a particular part of the body. Various skin and intestinal glands belong to this group. The other group, known as *ductless* or **endocrine glands,** depend on the blood and lymph to carry their secretions to various affected tissues.

The chemical substances manufactured by the endocrine glands are known as hormones. Hormones, sometimes referred to as the body's chemical messengers, are specialized so that they act on specific tissues (target organs) or influence certain processes in the body. Some hormones stimulate other endocrine or exocrine glands. Some have a profound effect on physical or sexual development. Others regulate

> **exocrine**
> or duct glands possess tubes or ducts leading from the gland to a particular part of the body.

> **endocrine**
> or ductless glands depend on the blood and lymph to carry their secretions to various affected tissues.

metabolism or body chemistry. (See Table 5.16 on glands and their associated hormones.) The endocrine glands operate cooperatively with one another and the nervous system to maintain a state of homeostasis within the organism. Some of the endocrine glands exert a regulatory influence over the other glands. The effect of their hormones may either stimulate or restrain the activity of another gland. Under- or overfunctioning of any ductless gland will upset the delicate balance of the entire chain of endocrine glands.

Among the important endocrine glands are the pituitary gland, thyroid gland, parathyroid glands, adrenal glands, sex glands (gonads), and pancreas. Other organs that have hormone-producing tissue include the pineal gland, the hypothalamus, the kidneys, the placenta, and intestinal mucosa.

Most diseases or dysfunctions of the endocrine system are the result of overactivity or underactivity of one or more glands. Overactive or **hyperactive glands** oversecrete hormones due to lack of regulation or glandular tumors. Underactive or hypoactive glands secrete insufficient amounts of their hormones. Hypoactive glands may be diseased, underdeveloped, injured by trauma, surgery, or radiation, or they may not be receiving proper stimulation and regulation. Individual glands will be discussed as to their primary function and some effects of hyper- or hypoactivity (Figure 5.70).

hyperactive glands
oversecrete hormones due to lack of regulation or glandular tumors.

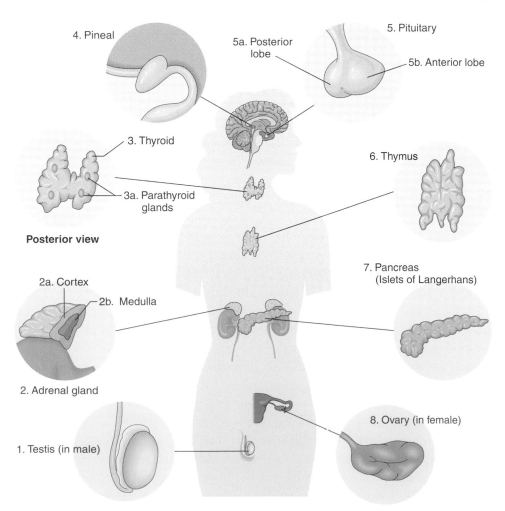

Figure 5.70
The endocrine system.

Table 5.16

Endocrine Glands and Their Hormones

GLAND	HORMONE	PRINCIPAL FUNCTIONS
Anterior pituitary	ACTH (adrenocorticotropin)	Stimulates adrenal cortex to produce cortical hormones; aids in protecting body in stress situations (injury, pain)
	TSH (thyroid-stimulating hormone)	Stimulates the thyroid to produce thyroxin
	FSH (follicle-stimulating hormone)	Stimulates growth and hormone activity of ovarian follicles; stimulates growth of testes; promotes development of sperm
	GH (human growth hormone)	Promotes growth of all body tissues
	LH (Luteinizing hormone)	Causes development of corpus luteum at site of ruptured ovarian follicle in female; stimulates secretion of testosterone in male
	Lactogenic hormone	Stimulates secretion of milk by mammary glands
Posterior pituitary	ADH (antidiuretic hormone; vasopressin)	Promotes reabsorption of water in kidney tubules; stimulates smooth muscle tissue of blood vessels
	Oxytocin	Causes contraction of muscle of pregnant uterus; causes ejection of milk from mammary glands
Adrenal cortex	Cortisol (95% of glucocorticoids)	Aids in metabolism of carbohydrates, proteins, and fats; active during stress
	Aldosterone (95% of mineralocorticoids)	Aids in regulating electrolytes
	Sex hormones	May influence secondary sexual characteristics in male
Adrenal medulla	Epinephrine and norepinephrine	Increases blood pressure and heart rate; activates cells influenced by the sympathetic nervous system plus many not affected by sympathetics
Pancreatic islets	Insulin	Aids transport of glucose into cells; required for cellular metabolism of foods, especially glucose; decreases blood sugar levels
	Glucagon	Stimulates the liver to release glucose, thereby increasing blood sugar levels
Parathyroids	Parathormone	Regulates exchange of calcium between blood and bones; increases calcium level in blood
Thyroid gland	Thyroid hormone (thyroxine and triiodothyronine)	Increases metabolic rate, influencing both physical and mental activities; required for normal growth
	Calcitonin	Decreases calcium level in blood
Ovarian follicle	Estrogens (e.g., estradiol)	Stimulates growth of primary sexual organs (uterus, tubes, etc.) and development of secondary sexual organs such as breasts, plus changes in pelvis to avoid broader shape
Corpus luteum (in ovaries)	Progesterone	Stimulates development of secretory parts of mammary glands; prepares uterine lining for implantation of fertilized ovum; aids in maintaining pregnancy
Testes	Testosterone	Stimulates growth and development of sexual organs (testes, penis, others) plus development of secondary sexual characteristics such as hair growth on body and face and deepening of voice; stimulates maturation of sperm cells

The Pituitary Gland

The pituitary gland is a small gland about the size of a cherry that produces a number of hormones that regulate many body processes. The pituitary gland is located in a depression just behind the point where the optic nerves cross on the floor of the cranium called the sella turcica of the sphenoid bone. The **pituitary gland** is often called the *master gland* because many of the hormones it secretes stimulate or regulate other endocrine glands. The pituitary gland is regulated by impulses and secretions from the hypothalamus. It has an anterior and posterior lobe, each of which secretes different hormones.

The anterior lobe of the pituitary produces and secretes the following:

- *Somatotropic* or *growth hormone.* This hormone stimulates the growth of bones, muscles, and organs. A deficiency of this hormone will inhibit mental and physical growth.

- *Thyroid-stimulating hormone (TSH).* This hormone regulates the thyroid gland.

- *Adrenocorticotropic hormone (ACTH)* stimulates the adrenal cortex.

- *Gonadotropic hormones* regulate the development and function of the reproductive systems in women and men.

- *Prolactin* stimulates the production of milk in a woman's breast.

The posterior lobe of the pituitary stores and secretes the following:

- *Antidiuretic hormone* stimulates the kidneys to reabsorb more water, thereby reducing urine output.

- *Oxytocin* causes the uterus to contract (during and after childbirth) and causes the letdown of breast milk.

Hyperpituitarism (high-per-pi-**TOO**-i-tar-izm) is most notably observed as the production of excessive amounts of growth hormone. If the hypersecretion occurs before puberty, the activity in the growth plates of the bones is accelerated and produces a giant, a condition known as *giantism.* If the hyperpituitarism occurs after puberty when a person has reached full height, the effects are different. The bones of the hands, feet, face, and spine enlarge in a condition called *acromegaly* (ak-row-**MEG**-a-lee). There is excessive growth in some soft tissues as the lips and nose enlarge and the lower jaw protrudes. Hyperactivity of the pituitary is usually due to a tumor.

Hypopituitarism can result from inadequate stimulation from the hypothalamus or from destruction of the pituitary gland. Because the secretions of the pituitary gland act to stimulate other endocrine glands, deficient pituitary secretions inhibit the actions of the target glands.

The Thyroid Gland

The thyroid gland, situated on either side of the trachea, produces three hormones. **Thyroxin** and **triiodothyronine** (trigh-ioh-do-**THIGH**-ro-neen) both act to stimulate the metabolic rate of the body. Thyroid hormones regulate the cellular consumption of oxygen and therefore the production of heat and energy in body tissues. The proper manufacture of these hormones requires adequate iodine in the blood. Proper diet assures adequate iodine, which helps to prevent goiter (enlarged thyroid).

Secretions from the pituitary gland control the rate of production of thyroxin. When the level of thyroxin in the blood is low, the pituitary releases *thyroid-stimulating hormone (TSH),* which stimulates the thyroid to produce more thyroxin to be secreted directly into the bloodstream. When there is an adequate level of thyroxin in the blood, the pituitary stops releasing TSH into the blood and thyroxin production is inhibited.

The thyroid also produces **calcitonin** (kal-si-**TOE**-nin), a hormone that is antagonistic to the parathyroid hormone and helps control the calcium level of the blood.

Hyperthyroidism is the excessive functional activity of the thyroid gland. Often the thyroid gland enlarges to create a *goiter.* Symptoms of hyperthyroidism include heart palpitations, rapid pulse, profuse sweating, insomnia, nervousness, and excitability. Graves' disease, a form of hyperthyroidism, is characterized by strained, tense facial expression and bulging eyes.

Hyperthyroidism is generally treated by destroying some or all of the thyroid gland with radioactive iodine therapy or by surgically removing part or all of the thyroid gland.

Hypothyroidism is a condition of deficient thyroid activity. Symptoms are the opposite of hyperthyroidism with slow heart rate; sluggish mental and physical activity; bloated, edemic appearance; and muscle weakness. **Cretinism** (**KREE**-tin-izm) is congenital hypothyroidism due to an error in fetal development in which the thyroid fails to develop or is underactive. Thyroxin is essential to physical and mental health and development. Lack of it in young children results in a dwarfed stature and mental retardation. Hypothyroidism is easily treated with oral thyroxin supplementation.

Parathyroid Glands

Two pairs of parathyroid glands, situated on each lobe and behind the thyroid, produce **parathormone,** which regulates the blood level of calcium. When the blood calcium is low, the parathyroid secretes parathormone, which stimulates the activity of the osteoclasts in the bones. Thus calcium from the bones is absorbed into the blood. When blood calcium levels are high, calcitonin has an opposite effect as calcium is deposited in the bones. In this way parathormone and calcitonin have an antagonistic yet cooperative action in maintaining proper calcium levels in the blood.

Hyperparathyroidism causes loss of calcium from the bones and excessive excretion of calcium and phosphorus from the kidneys. The bones become brittle and prone to fracture, and there is a tendency toward kidney stones and disease.

Hypoparathyroidism results in low blood calcium. The low blood calcium makes the nervous activity hypersensitive. The main characteristic of hypoparathyroidism is **tetany,** a sustained muscle contraction that usually affects the hands and feet.

calcitonin
is a hormone that controls the level of calcium in the blood.

cretinism
is caused by a lack of thyroxin during fetal development and results in a dwarfed stature and mental retardation.

parathormone
regulates the blood level of calcium.

tetany
a sustained muscle contraction that usually affects the hands and feet.

The Thymus

The thymus is located behind the sternum and above the heart. It has endocrine and lymphatic functions and in most people is active until puberty, at which time it begins to diminish. The thymus produces a number of related hormones that are essential in developing and maintaining our immune system. The main purpose of the thymus is to stimulate lymphoid tissue to produce lymphocytes.

The Pancreas

The pancreas is located behind the stomach and has both endocrine and exocrine functions. It produces digestive enzymes that are excreted into the small intestine through the pancreatic duct. This is the exocrine function. Scattered throughout the pancreas are small groups of specialized cells called *islets* (**islets of Langerhans**) that produce the hormones *insulin* and *glucagon,* which are secreted directly into the bloodstream.

> **Islets of Langerhans**
> found in the pancreas, produce insulin and glucagon.

Insulin regulates the movement of glucose across the cell membrane so that when there is an increased level of glucose in the blood (such as after meals) secretion of insulin into the blood causes a rapid intake of glucose by most tissues in the body, especially the muscles, liver, and adipose tissue. Insulin also plays an important role in protein and fat transport and metabolism.

Diabetes mellitus is a condition caused by decreased output of insulin by the pancreatic islets. When insulin is deficient, blood glucose is elevated, and glucose is not transported across the cell membrane, so there is not enough glucose in the cells for proper cell metabolism. Because the glucose is not used by the cells, blood glucose remains high and glucose is discharged by the kidneys into the urine. Glucose in the urine is the major sign of diabetes. Without being able to use glucose for metabolism, the body resorts to the abnormal breakdown of proteins and fats. Long-term fat and protein breakdown lead to serious complications of diabetes. Fat metabolism causes an increase in the lipids in the blood and a decrease in pH. The decrease in pH could cause the person to go into a coma. Increased blood lipids cause artherosclerosis. Circulation is generally poor. Occluded arteries in the heart can cause heart failure. Poor circulation to the retina of the eyes results in blindness. Vascular disorders in the legs result in poor healing and often gangrene, which sometimes leads to amputation.

> **diabetes mellitus**
> is caused by decreased output of insulin by the pancreas.

Treatment of diabetes is in the form of controlled diet, exercise, and a controlled program of insulin injections.

Glucagon, also produced by specialized cells in the islets of Langerhans, has an effect antagonistic or the opposite of insulin. When the glucose level in the blood is low, glucagon acts to convert glycogen stored in the liver into glucose, thereby increasing the glucose level in the blood.

The Adrenal Glands

The *adrenal glands* are situated on top of each kidney. The adrenal glands each have two distinct parts, the *medulla* and the *adrenal cortex,* that produce different hormones.

The two principal hormones produced by the medulla are *epineph-rine* (ep-i-**NEF**-rin) (also called adrenaline) and *norepinephrine*. Stimulation of the adrenal medulla comes from the sympathetic nervous system, and the actions of adrenaline and norepinephrine cause a similar effect throughout the body as direct stimulation to the organs by the sympathetic nervous system. Known as the "fight or flight" hormones, they cause the bronchioles to dilate, the heart rate to increase, the blood pressure to elevate, and glycogen to convert to glucose, flooding the bloodstream and preparing the muscles to do an extraordinary amount of work to respond to any emergency situation.

The adrenal cortex produces a group of hormones called *cortico-steroids* (kor-ti-ko-**STEER**-oyds). Over 30 steroids have been identified. One group, called *mineralocorticoids,* affects the extracellular electrolytes—especially sodium and potassium. The most important of these is *aldos-terone* (al-**DOS**-ter-own), which regulates the sodium/potassium balance in the extracellular fluid and in the blood. In the absence of mineralo-corticoid secretions, potassium levels would increase, sodium levels would fall, and the volume of blood would decrease. Without the administration of aldosterone or mineralocorticoid therapy, the patient would go into shock and die in a matter of days.

Another group, the *glucocorticoids,* affects carbohydrate, protein, and fat metabolism. Our bodies produce increased levels of these hormones in response to stress. The most important steroid of this group is *cortisol* (**KOR**-ti-sol), also known as *hydrocortisone*. These hormones have the ability to repress or resolve conditions of inflammation and enhance the rate of healing of damaged tissue.

The production of hormones by the adrenal cortex is stimulated by the adrenocorticotropic hormone (ACTH) from the pituitary gland.

Hyperadrenalism is the excessive release of adrenal hormones into the bloodstream. The effects and symptoms of hyperadrenalism depend on which hormones are secreted in excess. **Cushing's syndrome** results from excess glucocorticoid production and is characterized by obesity (especially in the trunk), muscle weakness, elevated blood sugar, hypertension, and arteriosclerosis.

Hypoadrenalism, also called Addison's disease, is due to the failure of the adrenal cortex to produce aldosterone and cortisol. The disease is characterized by weight loss, muscle fatigue or atrophy, low blood pressure, and darkened skin pigmentation.

The Sex Glands

The sex glands (gonads) are both duct and ductless glands. The male and female sex glands manufacture the reproductive cells and sex hormones that are required for fertility and reproduction. In the male, the **testes** produce **testosterone,** a potent androgen that is primarily responsible for the development of the reproductive structures. Another function involves the development of secondary sexual characteristics such as the voice, body hair, and body structure.

Cushing's syndrome

results from excess glucocorticoid production and is characterized by obesity, muscle weakness, elevated blood sugar, and hypertension.

testes

are two small, egg-shaped glands that produce the spermatozoa.

testosterone

is a male hormone responsible for development of secondary sexual characteristics.

---

estrogen

is a female hormone responsible for development of secondary sexual characteristics.

---

progesterone

a female hormone that prepares the uterine lining for implantation, aids maintaining pregnancy, and stimulates development of mammary glands for nursing.

---

ovaries

are glandular organs in the pelvis that produce the ovum and female sex hormones.

Estrogen and **progesterone** are the two essential hormones produced in the **ovaries** of the female reproductive system. In the female, estrogen nearly parallels the actions of testosterone regarding the development of secondary sexual characteristics. Estrogen also regulates the development of the reproductive organs, the mammary glands, and menstruation.

SECTION QUESTIONS FOR DISCUSSION AND REVIEW

1. What is the composition of the endocrine system?

2. What is the major function of the endocrine system?

3. What is an important difference between a duct and ductless gland?

4. Why are the glands dependent on an adequate nerve and blood supply?

5. Are sebaceous (oil) glands classified as duct or ductless glands?

6. What is the function of a ductless or endocrine gland?

7. Which glands function as both duct and ductless glands?

8. Which glands produce hormones?

9. Why are hormones important to the body?

10. Name the endocrine glands.

11. What is the nature of most endocrine dysfunctions?

12. Why is the pituitary gland called the master gland?

13. What are the two hormone-producing parts of the adrenal glands?

14. What is the endocrine function of the sex glands?

REVIEW

Matching Test I

Match the hormone in the left list with the gland that produces it by writing the appropriate letter in the space provided.

_____	1. gonadotropic hormone	a. pituitary gland
_____	2. adrenaline	b. thyroid gland
_____	3. insulin	c. parathyroid
_____	4. antidiuretic hormone	d. thymus gland
_____	5. thyroxin	e. adrenal cortex
_____	6. testosterone	f. adrenal medulla
_____	7. ACTH	g. pancreas
_____	8. cortisol	h. ovaries
_____	9. progesterone	i. testes
_____	10. aldosterone	
_____	11. somatropic hormone	
_____	12. glucagon	
_____	13. epinephrine	
_____	14. parathormone	
_____	15. TSH	

Matching Test II

Match the hormone with the best description of its function by writing the appropriate letter in the space provided.

_____	**1.** gonadotropic hormone	a.	stimulates the thyroid
_____	**2.** TSH	b.	affects growth
_____	**3.** glucagon	c.	regulates blood calcium
_____	**4.** thyroxin	d.	stimulates metabolic rate
_____	**5.** epinephrine	e.	promotes carbohydrate metabolism
_____	**6.** ACTH	f.	stimulates adrenal cortex
_____	**7.** somatropic hormone	g.	fight or flight response
_____	**8.** cortisol	h.	converts glycogen to glucose
_____	**9.** insulin	i.	resolves inflammation
_____	**10.** parathormone	j.	affects sex organs

7 | THE RESPIRATORY SYSTEM

To carry on the vital functions of the organism, the cells of the body require a continual supply of oxygen and the removal of carbon dioxide. Without a constant supply of oxygen, a human being would die within a matter of minutes. The vital exchange of oxygen and carbon dioxide is accomplished by the respiratory system.

The respiratory system includes the nose, nasal cavity, pharynx, larynx, trachea, bronchial tubes, and the lungs. The lungs are composed of spongy tissue, blood vessels, connective tissue, and microscopic air sacs called *alveoli* (al-**VEE**-o-ligh). A network of very fine capillaries bring the blood in close contact with the thin walls of alveoli (Figure 5.71).

Respiration

Respiration is the exchange of carbon dioxide and oxygen that takes place at three levels in the body:

1. External respiration is the exchange between the external environment and the blood and takes place in the lungs.

2. Internal respiration is the gaseous exchange between the blood and the cells of the body.

3. Cellular respiration or oxidation occurs within the cell.

Respiration begins as air is inhaled through the nose and passes through the nasal cavity where it is warmed, moistened, and filtered. It passes through the pharynx and larynx and into the trachea. The trachea divides into two bronchi, which subdivide into smaller and smaller branches of the *bronchial tree*. The air moves through the *bronchioles* until it reaches the ends of the air passages that terminate in clusters of air sacs called *alveoli*. The thin porous walls of the alveoli are surrounded by

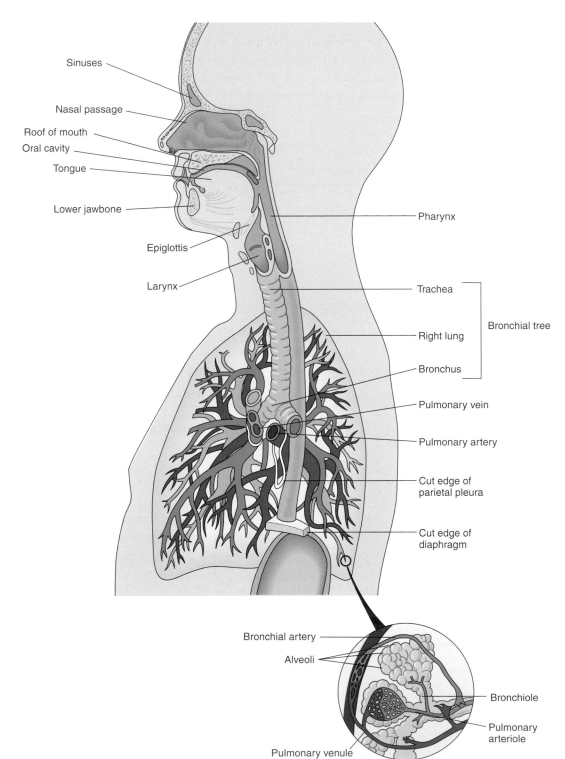

Figure 5.71
Respiratory organs
and structures.

capillaries of the pulmonary circulatory system. The blood entering the
lungs through the pulmonary arteries has a high concentration of carbon
dioxide that has been picked up from the cells of the body and a low concentration of oxygen. The concentration of oxygen in the alveoli is
greater than in the blood. Likewise, concentrations of carbon dioxide in

the blood are higher than in the alveoli. Therefore, through the process of diffusion, carbon dioxide moves from the blood to the lungs and is exhaled while oxygen moves from the lungs into the bloodstream and is carried by the red blood cells back to the heart and then circulated throughout the body.

Oxygenated blood moves into the capillaries of the systemic circulation. Differences in concentration of the gases between the blood and tissue fluid cause oxygen to diffuse into the tissue fluid while carbon dioxide diffuses out of the fluid and into the blood. A similar diffusion process takes place between the tissue fluid and the cells.

Once in the cells, the oxygen is used in cellular respiration to produce energy. Some of that energy is used by the cell to function. The rest is in the form of heat. The waste products of cellular respiration include carbon dioxide and water, which migrate back into the bloodstream to be eliminated. The carbon dioxide is carried by the red blood cells and the plasma to the lungs, where it diffuses out of the blood into the alveoli to be expelled from the lungs with the next exhalation.

Breathing

External respiration, also called *ventilation* or *breathing,* involves the act of inhaling and exhaling air, resulting in an exchange of gases between the blood and alveoli. With each inhalation, the intercostal muscles contract, raising the ribs and expanding the thoracic cavity. At the same time the diaphragm contracts and is pulled down, causing the lungs to draw in air. Exhalation occurs as the intercostals and the diaphragm relax, returning to their neutral positions and pushing the air out of the lungs. Forced exhalation involves the contraction of the internal intercostal muscles, which collapse the rib cage, and the contraction of the abdominal muscles, which force the abdominal viscera against the diaphragm, further reducing the area of the thoracic cavity. The maximum intake of oxygen and expulsion of carbon dioxide is accomplished during deep breathing, which involves exaggerated movements of both the ribs and diaphragm.

Depending on the individual's lung capacity, the natural rate of breathing for an adult is between 10 and 20 times a minute. The rate of breathing is increased by the demand for oxygen by such things as increased muscular activity.

A healthy respiratory system is maintained by avoiding air pollution, toxic chemicals, and smoking. Deep breathing, regular exercise, and a healthy diet all help to keep the respiratory system functioning normally. Should the massage practitioner notice that a client has trouble breathing normally, it is wise to suggest that the client see a physician. There is a great deal more to the respiratory system than has been covered in this brief overview. Study Figure 5.71 to be sure that you understand the location of the major parts of the respiratory system.

Disorders of the Respiratory System

Common Cold

Also known as an upper respiratory tract infection (URTI), the common cold is a viral infection caused by over 200 different viruses, which is usually spread through physical contact. A cold has a variety of symptoms that include nasal discharge and congestion, mild fever, sore throat, dry coughing, and headache. Massage is contraindicated in the acute stage of the common cold because the respiratory system is already overtaxed and massage will only tend to stir up more toxins and exacerbate the symptoms. When the viral infection has progressed to the postacute stage, massage can help the body recover more quickly. It is important to gain the patient's permission to do so, as massage at this stage may cause the patient to feel as though the virus is relapsing. The effect, however, is that the massage accelerates the healing process and turns three days of recovery into one day of feeling sick again.

Influenza

Influenza, or the flu, is a viral infection that is similar to the common cold. It can also be spread through physical contact, but unlike a cold, it can be spread via airborne viruses as well. Flu symptoms include high fever and achiness, both of which should last no more than three days. After the fever subsides, symptoms such as coughing, sneezing, congestion, and general malaise may follow for up to two weeks. A common complication of influenza is that with the body in a weakened condition, the possibility of secondary bacterial infections such as bronchitis or pneumonia increases. This is a particular concern for people with pre-existing lung conditions, the elderly, or the very young. Massage is contraindicated for all stages of the flu except the very end of the subacute stage when it may help to flush out residual toxins and help the body recover more efficiently. Even at this stage, massage may cause the patient to feel as though the virus is relapsing, so it is important to inform the client and gain permission before proceeding.

Pneumonia

Pneumonia, or pneumonitis, is a word that describes any type of inflammation of the lungs. There are many different viruses and types of bacteria that cause pneumonia. Symptoms vary widely from coughing, chills, high fever, and achiness to chest pains, cyanosis, thickened yellow/green phlegm, and blood-streaked phlegm. There is a different medical treatment for each type of pneumonia, but massage treatment is the same for any type of pneumonitis. Massage should only be applied to pneumonia patients when the infection has reached the subacute stage and, even then, only under medical supervision. Percussive massage, especially, has proven to assist in loosening phlegm from alveoli into the bronchial tubes. Massage is contraindicated in any other stage of infection.

Sinusitis

Sinusitis refers to the swelling or inflammation of the paranasal sinus cavities. This condition may occur as a reaction to allergies, nasal obstructions, or infection. Symptoms include localized tenderness, pressure headaches, runny nose, congestion, or facial and tooth pain. As long as no viral or bacterial infection is present, massage can be beneficial to a patient suffering from sinusitis. However, in any case wherein infectious acute sinusitis is possible, massage is contraindicated.

Tuberculosis

Tuberculosis is a highly infectious airborne disease that can begin in the lungs and spread through other parts of the body. Tuberculosis, or TB as it is commonly called, is caused by an infection of the microbacterium tuberculosis bacteria. It begins as a bacterial infection that can incubate in the body without detection by sealing itself away in fleshy pockets called *tubercles*. Tubercles are most likely to form in the lungs. However, the bacteria may be transported through the bloodstream with tubercles forming in other parts of the body such as the bones and kidneys. Once the infected body's immune system weakens, the bacterial infection turns into a disease that is highly contagious. The World Health Organization thought the disease was wiped out by the 1970s, but in the late 1980s, it made a frighteningly successful comeback with a new mutation that is surprisingly drug-resistant. AIDS patients, cancer patients undergoing chemotherapy, and anyone who has a severely weakened immune system is at more risk of contracting the disease from the bacteria, whereas a person with a strong immune system may have the infection for many years before contracting the disease.

The bacterial infection rarely has any symptoms. The disease, however, has a wide variety of symptoms, including night sweats, fatigue, and a cough that will start dry and begin to be productive of bloody or pus-filled phlegm. Massage is contraindicated for tuberculosis in either form because it may assist in spreading tubercles throughout the body, thereby having a devasting effect on the patient. Therapists also have their own health to consider; they would not be beneficial to any of their patients if they contracted the disease.

SECTION QUESTIONS FOR DISCUSSION AND REVIEW

1. What are the major organs of the respiratory system?

2. What is the function of the respiratory system?

3. What is the physical appearance of the lungs?

4. What are the three levels of respiration and where do they take place?

5. What is an alveoli and what is its function?

6. What is breathing?

7. What is the natural rate of breathing for an adult?

8. What is the diaphragm, and what function does it perform?

8 THE DIGESTIVE SYSTEM

digestion

is the process of converting food into substances capable of being used by the cells for nourishment.

absorption

is the process in which the digested nutrients are transferred from the intestines to the blood or lymph vessels.

alimentary canal

consists of the mouth, pharynx, esophagus, stomach, and small and large intestines.

accessory digestive organs

consist of the teeth, tongue, salivary glands, pancreas, liver, and gallbladder.

oral cavity

or mouth, prepares food for entrance into the stomach.

saliva

contains enzymes that begin to digest carbohydrates.

The human body is a living organism made up of millions of cells that perform a multitude of different tasks. Each cell must receive a continuous supply of nutrients to provide fuel for energy and nutritional elements for growth and regeneration. These nutrients come from the food we eat. Food that enters the mouth must undergo many changes before it can be used by the cells for nourishment. This process is carried on by the digestive system. The main functions of the digestive system are **digestion** and **absorption.** Digestion is the process of converting food into substances capable of being used by the cells for nourishment. Absorption is the process in which the digested nutrients are transferred from the intestines to the blood or lymph vessels so that they can be transported to the cells.

The digestive system is composed of the **alimentary canal** and **accessory digestive organs.** The alimentary canal, also known as the gastrointestinal or digestive tract, consists of the mouth (oral cavity), pharynx (throat), esophagus, stomach, small intestine, and large intestine. The accessory organs include the teeth, tongue, salivary glands, pancreas, liver, and gallbladder.

The alimentary canal is a muscular tube that is about five times as long as a person is tall and goes from the lips to the anus. The tube forms a continuous barrier so that material in the digestive tube can be acted on by the digestive juices although it is not yet part of the body or its cellular makeup.

The process of digestion changes the food into a nutritious fluid capable of being absorbed by the blood. Digestion is accomplished through physical and chemical means. The physical means involve the teeth, tongue, and involuntary muscles of the pharynx, esophagus, stomach, and small intestine. The teeth tear and grind the food into small pieces while the tongue mixes and moves the food. After the food is swallowed, the involuntary muscles mix the food with digestive juices and propel it through the alimentary canal. Food is acted on chemically by enzymes and a variety of digestive juices to break it down from complex food substances into simple nutritional molecules that can be absorbed into the bloodstream and through the cell membranes.

The Path of Digestion

The mouth, called the **oral cavity,** prepares the food for entrance into the stomach. In the mouth, the food is masticated (chewed) by the teeth and mixed by the tongue with secretions from the *salivary glands.* **Saliva** contains enzymes that begin to digest carbohydrates. The action of the teeth, tongue, and saliva prepares the food into a soft ball called a *bolus* that slides into the throat and is swallowed by voluntary and reflex actions of the muscles of the pharynx.

Structure of the Alimentary Canal

From the throat to the anus, the walls of the alimentary canal are similar in structure except for specialized modifications that perform particular functions. The wall of the alimentary canal consists of four distinct layers (Figure 5.72):

1. The *mucosa* (myoo-**KO**-suh) or mucous membrane is made up of epithelial cells, connective tissue, and a variety of digestive glands. This layer protects the underlying tissues and functions to carry on secretion and absorption.

2. The *submucosa* consists of connective tissue, nerves, and blood and lymph vessels that serve to nourish the surrounding tissues and carry away the absorbed material.

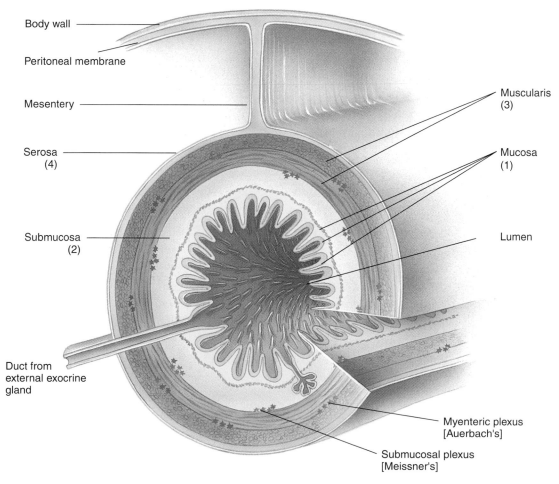

Figure 5.72

Structure of the walls of the alimentary tract.

3. The *muscular layer* has two layers of smooth muscle. The muscle fibers of the inner layer encircle the tube so that when they contract, the diameter of the tube decreases. The outer layer of muscle fibers is arranged longitudinally so that when they contract, the tube shortens.

4. The *serous layer* is the outer covering of the tube. On the stomach and intestines, this layer is continuous with the peritoneum that lines the abdominal cavity.

When food passes from the throat into the esophagus, the smooth muscles of the alimentary canal are stimulated and begin to produce a rhythmic, wavelike motion that propels and churns the food throughout the length of the canal. The wavelike muscular action is called **peristalsis** (per-i-**STAL**-sis).

> **peristalsis**
>
> is the wavelike muscular action of the alimentary canal.

The Stomach

After food travels down the esophagus, it passes through the *cardiac sphincter* and enters the stomach, where it is churned with gastric juices secreted from glands in the wall of the stomach that contain *hydrochloric acid* and protein-digesting enzymes. The mixture of digestive juices, mucus, and food material is called *chyme*. From the stomach, the chyme passes through the *pyloric sphincter* and into the duodenum of the small intestine. Sphincters are muscular valves that allow the passage of food substances in only one direction. The pyloric sphincter also plays an important role in determining how long food is held in the stomach.

The Small Intestine

The *small intestine* is the longest part of the alimentary canal. It consists of three parts: the *duodenum* (doo-o-**DEE**-num), *jejunum* (je-**JOO**-num), and *ileum* (**IL**-ee-um). Thousands of glands in the intestinal walls produce *intestinal digestive juices*. In addition to the intestinal juices, secretions of bile from the liver and *pancreatic fluids* from the pancreas are poured into the duodenum. Bile from the liver and gallbladder is carried through the *common bile duct* and is essential for the breakdown of fats. Pancreatic fluid enters the duodenum by way of the *pancreatic duct* and contains enzymes that act to digest proteins, carbohydrates, and fats (see Table 5.17).

The small intestine is lined with small, fingerlike projections covering the intestinal walls called *villi* (**VIL**-eye) that greatly increase the surface area available for absorption. Each microscopic villus contains a network of blood capillaries and lymph capillaries (lacteals). The end products of digestion pass through the intestinal wall and are absorbed into the blood vessels and the lacteals. Nutrients absorbed into the bloodstream are carried to the liver. Nutrients absorbed by the lymph flow through the cisterna chyli and the thoracic duct before entering the systemic circulation.

Table 5.17

Glands, Digestive Juices, and Enzymes

GLANDS AND JUICE	LOCATION	ENZYMES	CHANGES IN FOOD
Saliva (3) Salivary gland	Mouth	Salivary Amylase (ptyalin)	Begins digestion of starch into simple sugars
Gastric juice Stomach	Stomach wall	Pepsin	Begins digestion of protein into amino acids
Pancreatic juice Pancreas	Small intestine	Amylase Trypsin Lipase	Starches, proteins, fats
Juice from small intestine	Small intestine	Lactase Maltase Sucrase	Breaks down complex carbohydrates to simple sugars
Bile from liver	Small intestine	No enzymes	Breaks down fats into fatty acids

The Large Intestine

After the digestive processes have been completed in the small intestine, the waste (unusable) materials (water and solids) move through the *iliocecal valve* into a small, pouchlike part of the large intestine called the *cecum* (**SEE**-kum). The large intestine (colon) continues upward along the right side of the abdomen to form the *ascending colon.* Then it travels across the abdominal cavity and forms the *transverse colon.* It continues downward on the left side of the abdomen to become the *descending colon.* As the colon reaches the left iliac region, it forms an S-shaped bend known as the *sigmoid colon* that empties into the rectum. The rectum is a temporary storage area for waste. The distal part of the large intestine is the *anal canal,* which ends with the anus, from which fecal matter is expelled.

The functions of the colon include storing, forming, and excreting waste products of digestion and regulating the body's water balance. The colon aids in regulating the body's water balance by absorbing large amounts of water from the undigested material back into the body. Through a process of water absorption and bacterial action, the liquid state of the undigested and indigestible material in the colon is transformed into the semisolid feces, which is eliminated from the rectum. The bacterial action in the colon also synthesizes some B-complex vitamins and vitamin K, which is reabsorbed into the bloodstream (Figure 5.73).

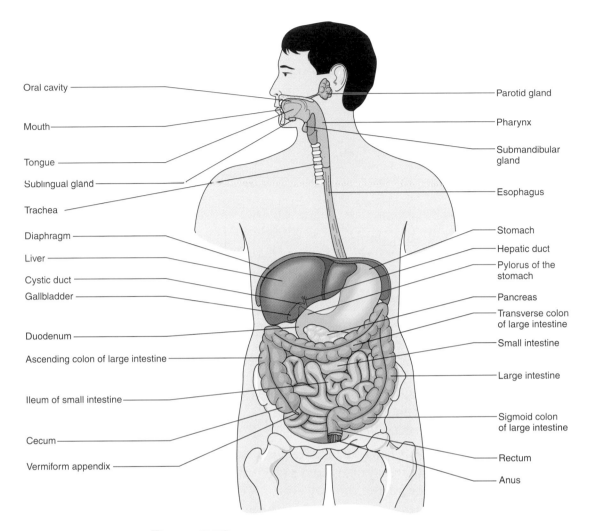

Oral cavity

Mouth

Tongue

Sublingual gland

Trachea

Diaphragm

Liver

Cystic duct

Gallbladder

Duodenum

Ascending colon of large intestine

Ileum of small intestine

Cecum

Vermiform appendix

Parotid gland

Pharynx

Submandibular gland

Esophagus

Stomach

Hepatic duct

Pylorus of the stomach

Pancreas

Transverse colon of large intestine

Small intestine

Large intestine

Sigmoid colon of large intestine

Rectum

Anus

Figure 5.73
The digestive system.

SECTION QUESTIONS FOR DISCUSSION AND REVIEW

1. Which structures compose the digestive system?

2. What is the function of digestion?

3. What is absorption?

4. What are the physical processes of digestion?

5. What chemical agents in the digestive juices aid digestion?

6. What digestive changes occur in the mouth?

7. Describe the general structure of the alimentary canal.

8. What is peristalsis or peristaltic action?

9. What digestive changes occur in the stomach?

10. Name the three parts of the small intestine.

11. Which glands supply digestive secretions to the small intestine?

12. What digestive changes occur in the small intestine?

13. Which structures absorb the end products of digestion?

14. From which organ is the undigested food eliminated from the body?

9 THE EXCRETORY SYSTEM

The Excretory Organs

The food we eat, water we drink, and air we breathe all play an important role in supplying the elements for the body's metabolic activity. As the cells metabolize these elements to produce their specialized substances and energy, waste products are formed that must be carried away and excreted from the body. If retained, these **metabolic wastes** would have a tendency to poison the body.

> **metabolic wastes**
>
> are products formed from cell metabolism.

The function of the excretory system (including the urinary system) is to eliminate or excrete metabolic wastes and undigested food from the body. The organs of the excretory system are the kidneys, liver, skin, large intestine, and lungs.

1. The kidneys excrete uric acid, urea, electrolytes, water, and other wastes through the process of urination.

2. The liver produces urea, which is returned to the blood to be excreted by the kidneys. The liver also discharges bile through the gallbladder and into the intestines.

3. The skin eliminates water and heat through the process of perspiration.

4. The large intestine discharges food wastes through the process of defecation.

5. The lungs exhale carbon dioxide and water vapor through external respiration.

Urinary System

The *urinary system* includes two kidneys, two ureters, the bladder, and a urethra. The **kidneys** are bean-shaped organs located at the back of the abdominal cavity, between the tenth thoracic and third lumbar vertebrae, and kept in place by fibrous connective and fatty tissues. The kidneys are an efficient blood filtration system. The **nephron** (NEF-ron) is the functional unit of the kidney (Figure 5.74). There are 2 to 3 million nephrons in the kidneys. Each day, the nephrons filter 40 to 50 gallons of plasma from the blood. Ninety-nine percent of this fluid is reabsorbed into the bloodstream. The kidneys excrete the remaining water and waste products through the *ureters*. As the kidneys filter the blood, they remove a certain amount of water and nitrogenous waste products of metabolism (such as urea, uric acid, as well as ammonia and some drugs). The ureters

> **kidneys**
>
> are bean-shaped glands that filter the blood.

> **nephron**
>
> is the functional unit of the kidney.

bladder

is an organ where
the urine is stored.

are tubes that carry urine from the kidneys to the **bladder,** where the urine is stored. The bladder is a hollow organ constructed of walls of elastic fibers and involuntary muscles that acts as a reservoir for the urine until it is excreted from the body. When the bladder accumulates about a pint of urine, sensors indicate that it is time to urinate. Voiding or emptying the bladder is accomplished by a voluntary relaxation of a sphincter muscle at the mouth of the urethra and the involuntary contraction of the muscles of the bladder. As the bladder contracts, urine is forced through the *urethra* and out of the body (Figure 5.75a).

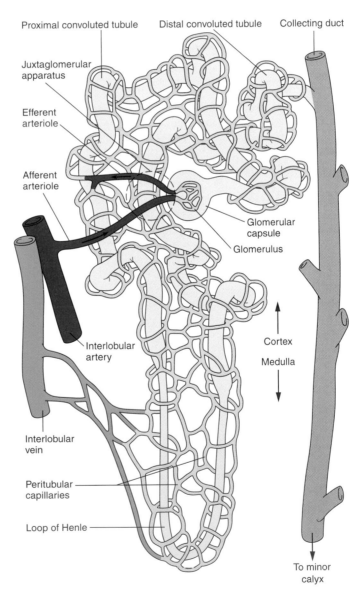

Figure 5.74

Anatomy of the nephron, the functional unit of the kidney.

A *urinalysis* is a chemical examination of the urine that is often part of the routine examination given by most physicians. The presence of white blood cells, blood, glucose, or other chemicals in the urine may be an indication of metabolic imbalance, infection, or numerous other conditions. Normal, healthy urine is a clear yellowish fluid. A change in the color of the urine, such as a reddish or brownish color, may indicate infection or other problems.

The kidneys also function to maintain the body's water balance and acid-base balance. Another function of the kidneys is the production of the hormone *renin,* which acts to regulate blood pressure. When the blood pressure is low, the kidneys are stimulated to release more renin into the bloodstream, which causes blood vessels to contract, thereby raising the blood pressure (Figure 5.75b).

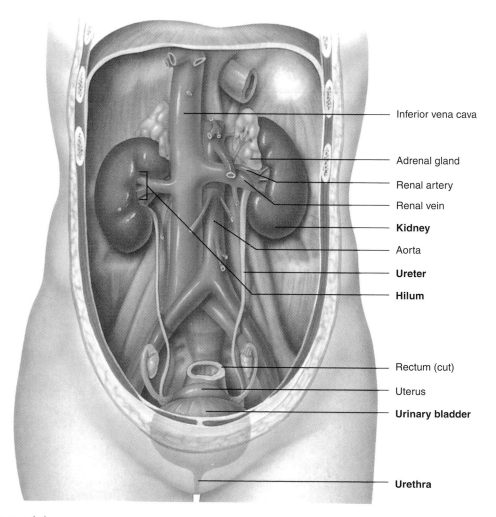

- Inferior vena cava
- Adrenal gland
- Renal artery
- Renal vein
- **Kidney**
- Aorta
- **Ureter**
- **Hilum**
- Rectum (cut)
- Uterus
- **Urinary bladder**
- **Urethra**

Figure 5.75 (a)

Organs of the urinary system.

continues

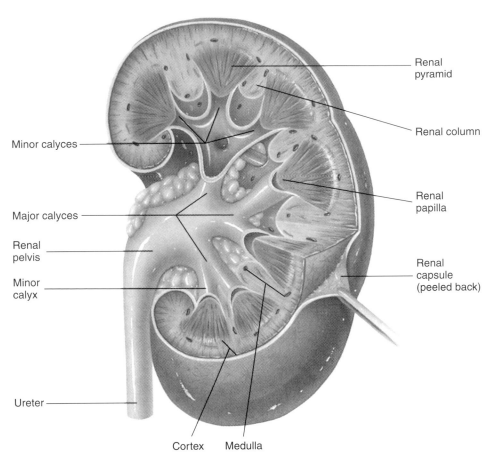

Renal
pyramid

Renal column

Minor calyces

Renal
papilla

Major calyces

Renal
pelvis

Renal
capsule
(peeled back)

Minor
calyx

Ureter

Cortex   Medulla

Figure 5.75 (b)
Internal anatomy of the kidney.

The Liver

The *liver* is the largest organ in the body and is situated on the upper right side of the abdomen, immediately below and in contact with the diaphragm. The liver performs many of the body's chemical functions. The liver neutralizes or detoxifies toxic substances that may have been absorbed from the intestines such as alcohol, food additives, and drugs. The liver functions in a great number of other metabolic processes that include converting glucose to glycogen, changing lactic acid to glucose, producing glucose from noncarbohydrates, changing carbohydrates and protein to fats for storage, producing cholesterol lipoproteins, and breaking down and reforming damaged red blood cells. The liver stores vitamins A, B, and B_{12} and glycogen. The main excretory function of the liver is the formation of urea, which is returned to the bloodstream to be excreted by the kidneys. The liver also produces and excretes bile through the intestines. **Bile** is a bitter, alkaline, yellowish-brown fluid secreted from the liver into the duodenum and contains water, bile salts, mucin, cholesterol, lecithin, and fat pigments. Bile aids in the emulsification, digestion, and absorption of fats and the regulation of alkalinity of the intestines (Figure 5.76).

bile

is a bitter, alkaline, yellowish-brown fluid secreted by the liver that aids in fat digestion.

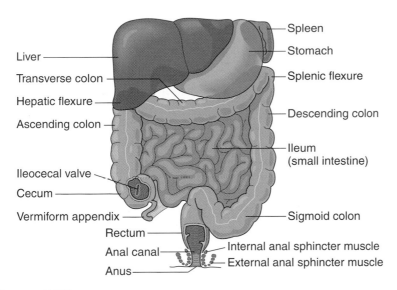

Figure 5.76
The liver.

SECTION QUESTIONS FOR DISCUSSION AND REVIEW

1. Name the five important organs of the excretory system.

2. What happens if waste products are retained within the body instead of being eliminated?

3. What is the function of the excretory system?

4. Name the parts of the urinary system.

5. What is the functional unit of the kidney?

6. Why do most physicians include urinalysis as a part of a routine physical checkup?

7. What colors of urine indicate a problem that needs checking by a physician?

8. Which organ of the body secretes bile?

9. What is the excretory function of the liver?

10 | THE HUMAN REPRODUCTIVE SYSTEM

The reproductive system is the generative apparatus necessary for organisms to reproduce organisms of the same kind and ensure the continuation of their species.

Lower forms of life such as one-celled organisms do not need a partner to reproduce. They do so by nonsexual means, which is called *asexual reproduction.*

In humans (and most multicellular organisms), reproduction is sexual and requires a male and female, each having specialized sex cells. *Gamete* is the term used to describe a reproductive cell that can unite with another gamete to form the cell (zygote) that develops into a new individual. In the male, these cells are *spermatozoa* (sper-ma-to-**ZOE**-uh) and in females, *ovum*. A *zygote* is the fertilized ovum, the cell formed by the union of a spermatozoon with an ovum. A *gonad* is a sex gland that produces the reproductive cell. In the female, the gonad is the *ovary*. In the male, it is the *testes* (Figure 5.77).

It is not within the scope of this book to describe in detail the entire process of human reproduction. The following is a brief summary.

The Male Reproductive System

The functions of the male reproductive system are the production of sperm, the production of the male hormones, and the performance of the sex act. The reproductive system in males includes two testes, two vas deferens, two seminal vesicles, a prostate gland, the bulbourethral glands (Cowper's glands), and the penis.

The male gonads are located outside the body in a pouch situated at the base of and beneath the penis called the *scrotum*. The *testes* are two

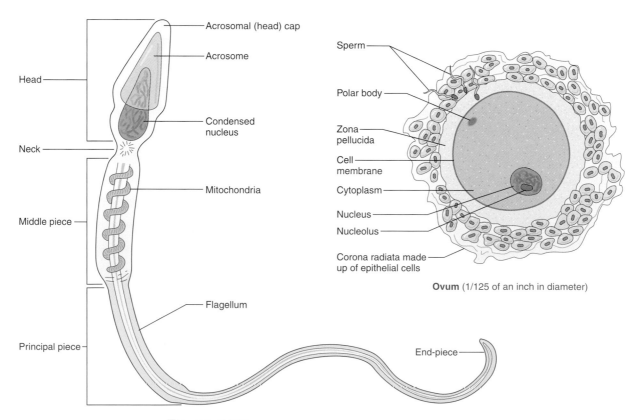

Figure 5.77
Human sperm and ovum.

small, egg-shaped glands made up of minute convoluted tubules, lined with specialized cells that produce the spermatozoa. Other specialized cells in the testes form the male hormone **testosterone.**

Testosterone is essential to the development of the male sexual characteristics, including body hair, masculine voice, sex organs, and sperm production. *Spermatozoa* are tiny detached cells, egg shaped and equipped with a tail that enables them to be motile or to swim. Of the millions of spermatozoa released during ejaculation, only one will fertilize the reproductive cell (egg) produced by the female. The others die within a short time.

The male reproductive system includes a duct system, tubes that transport the spermatozoa from the testes to the outside of the body.

The *epididymis* (ep-i-**DID**-i-mis), located in the scrotum, receives sperm from the testes and stores the sperm until it becomes fully mature. This tube extends upward to become the left or right *vas deferens (ductus deferens)* and continues through a small canal behind the abdominal wall and behind the urinary bladder. The sperm collects in the vas deferens until it is expelled from the body. The vas deferens join with the ducts of the seminal vesicles to form the *ejaculatory ducts*. These two ducts enter the prostate gland, where they empty into the urethra.

The Accessory Glands

The glands of the male reproductive system produce secretions that combine with the sperm to form *semen,* which is excreted from the body during ejaculation.

Seminal vesicles are two convoluted, glandular tubes located on each side of the prostate that produce a nutritious fluid that is excreted into the ejaculatory ducts at the time of emission. The secretions of the seminal vesicles contain simple sugars, mucus, prostaglandin, and other substances to help nourish, protect, and aid the sperm as it travels into the female reproductive system. The *seminal fluid* forms the majority of the semen when ejaculated.

The *prostate gland* lies below the urinary bladder and surrounds the first part of the urethra. The prostate secretes an alkaline fluid that enhances the sperm's motility (ability to swim). The fluid also neutralizes the acidic vaginal secretions, thereby protecting the sperm and increasing its chances of reaching and fertilizing the ovum. Ducts from the prostate enter the ejaculatory ducts. The prostate gland is supplied with muscular tissue that reflexively contracts during ejaculation.

The *Cowper's (bulbourethral) glands* are two pea-sized glands located beneath the prostate gland. They are mucus-producing glands that serve to lubricate the urethra.

The *urethra* serves to convey urine from the bladder and to carry reproductive cells and secretions out of the body.

The *penis* is the male organ of copulation consisting of erectile tissue that may become engorged and erect in order to deposit the sperm-containing semen deep within the female's vagina (Figure 5.78).

testosterone
is a male hormone responsible for development of secondary sexual characteristics.

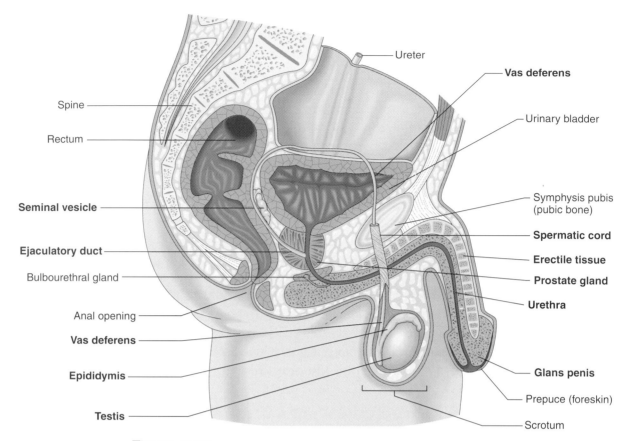

Figure 5.78

The male reproductive system.

The Female Reproductive System

The functions of the female reproductive system are to produce the ovum and female hormones, to receive the sperm during the sex act, and to carry the growing fetus during pregnancy.

The reproductive system in females includes two ovaries, two fallopian tubes (oviducts), a uterus, a vagina, and the vulva or external genitalia.

The *vulva* forms the external part of the female reproductive system. It includes the outer lips called the *labia majora* and the inner, smaller lips called the *labia minora*. On a virgin, within the vulva, a fold of connective tissue, the hymen, partially covers the external orifice of the vagina. The clitoris is a small sensitive body of erectile tissue located at the anterior junction of the labia.

The mons pubis is a pad of fatty tissue over the pubic symphysis.

The Female Internal Organs

The **vagina** is a muscular tube or canal leading from the vulva opening to the cervix and is the lower part of the birth canal. The vagina is the organ that receives the penis and the ejaculated semen during sexual in-

---

vagina

is a muscular tube leading from the vulva to the cervix and is the lower part of the birth canal.

tercourse. Near the vestibule of the vagina are mucus-producing glands called *Bartholen's glands.*

The **uterus** is a pear-shaped, muscular organ consisting of an upper portion, the body, and the cervix or neck. The uterine cavity is small and narrow except during pregnancy, when it expands to accommodate the fetus and a large amount of fluid.

The *oviducts,* also called *fallopian tubes,* are the egg-carrying tubes of the female reproductive system. They extend from the uterus to the ovaries. The **ovaries** (female gonads) are a pair of glandular organs located within the pelvic area. The ovaries perform two functions. They produce the ovum and the female sex hormones, *estrogen* and *progesterone.* The *ovum* is the egg cell capable of being fertilized by a spermatozoon and developing into a new life (Figure 5.79).

During each *menstrual cycle* (the regularly recurring series of changes that take place in the ovaries, uterus, and related structures in the female), a follicle develops in the ovary and produces estrogen (female hormone) as an ovum (egg) matures. Usually only one follicle matures each cycle (approximately every 28 days). **Ovulation** is the discharge of a mature ovum from the follicle of the ovary. A hormone from the pituitary gland, called *luteinizing hormone,* transforms the follicle into the *corpus luteum.* This is a yellowish endocrine body formed in the ruptured follicle of the ovary that produces estrogen and progesterone.

---

uterus

is a pear-shaped, muscular organ that expands during pregnancy to accommodate the fetus.

---

ovaries

are glandular organs in the pelvis that produce the ovum and female sex hormones.

---

ovulation

is the discharge of a mature ovum from the follicle of the ovary.

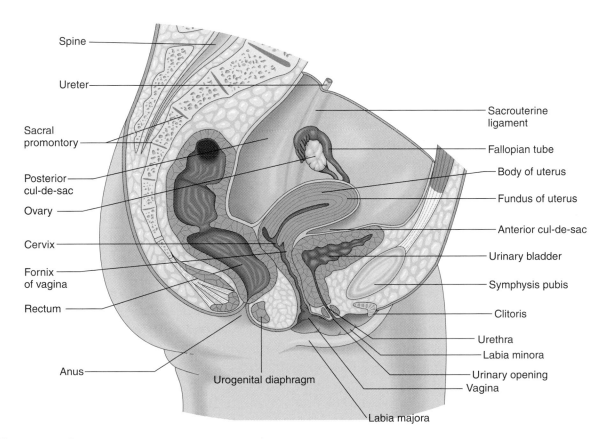

Spine
Ureter
Sacral promontory
Posterior cul-de-sac
Ovary
Cervix
Fornix of vagina
Rectum
Anus
Urogenital diaphragm

Sacrouterine ligament
Fallopian tube
Body of uterus
Fundus of uterus
Anterior cul-de-sac
Urinary bladder
Symphysis pubis
Clitoris
Urethra
Labia minora
Urinary opening
Vagina
Labia majora

Figure 5.79

The female reproductive system.

menstruation
is the cyclic, physiologic uterine bleeding that occurs at about four-week intervals during the reproductive period of the female.

menopause
is the physiological cessation of the menstrual cycle.

pregnancy
or gestation, is the physiological condition that occurs from the time an ovum is fertilized until childbirth.

gestation
same as pregnancy.

fetus
is the developing child from the third month of pregnancy until birth.

These hormones promote the lining of the uterus to thicken in preparation to receive the egg if it should be fertilized. Estrogen also controls the development of secondary female sexual characteristics (breast development, female body contours, etc.).

The ovum is carried into the fimbriated ends of the oviducts by the action of cilia, which produce a current in the peritoneal fluid. The ovum travels down the oviduct toward the uterus. If the ovum (egg) is fertilized by a sperm cell, pregnancy results. If the ovum is not fertilized, the built-up lining of the uterus sloughs off and is expelled along with the menstrual blood and secretions.

Menstruation is the cyclic, physiologic uterine bleeding that normally occurs at about four-week intervals (except during pregnancy) during the reproductive period of the human female. Menstruation begins at puberty and continues until **menopause,** which occurs at about ages 45 to 55. Menopause is the physiological cessation of the menstrual cycle and therefore the end of the child-bearing years.

Pregnancy

Pregnancy, or **gestation** (jes-**TAY**-shun), is the physiological condition that occurs from the time an ovum is fertilized until childbirth. During pregnancy, the fertilized egg develops in the mother's uterus or womb from a single cell, through many stages to a full-term infant. The duration of pregnancy in women is approximately 280 days or 40 weeks.

Embryonic life begins at conception, with the fertilization of the ovum by the sperm, which usually takes place within the first three days after ovulation and the first few hours after copulation. Of the millions of sperm deposited within the vagina, only several hundred reach the ovum. Of those that reach the ovum, only one will penetrate the covering to fertilize the egg. After fertilization, the developing zygote travels down the fallopian tubes and becomes embedded in the uterine wall. The developing form first receives nourishment from the uterine fluids, and then the wall of the uterus until a placenta develops. From about the 12th week, the developing fetus, enclosed in a protective fluid-filled amniotic sac with its own circulatory system, receives nourishment and disposes of its wastes by way of the placenta. The mother's blood and the blood of the fetus never interchange. From the beginning of the third month of pregnancy until birth, the developing child is called a **fetus.** During pregnancy, the mother's metabolism changes due to the demands made on her body systems. Her lungs must provide more oxygen, and her heart must pump more blood. The kidneys must excrete nitrogenous wastes from the fetus and the mother's body.

During pregnancy, the mother needs proper nutrition to provide for the growth of the fetus as well as to maintain the health of all organs as the body prepares for labor and birth.

Following the birth of the child, the mother should maintain her health and that of her child by attention to nutritional needs and by specific exercises to tone and strengthen her muscles.

SECTION QUESTIONS FOR DISCUSSION AND REVIEW

1. What is the reproductive system?

2. What is the difference between asexual and sexual reproduction?

3. What is a gonad?

4. What is a zygote?

5. What are the parts of the male reproductive system?

6. What are the functions of the male reproductive system?

7. What are the parts of the female reproductive system?

8. What are the functions of the female reproductive system?

9. What is the difference between an embryo and a fetus?

10. What is ovulation?

11. What is the approximate duration of pregnancy in women?

PART III

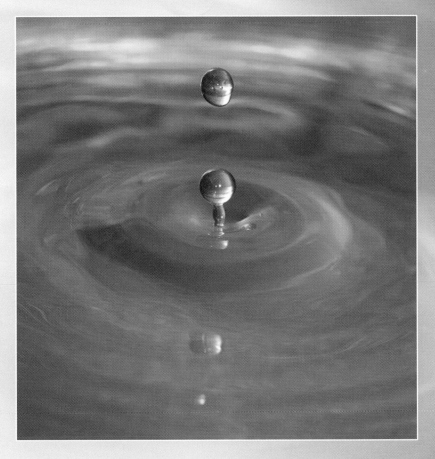

Massage Practice

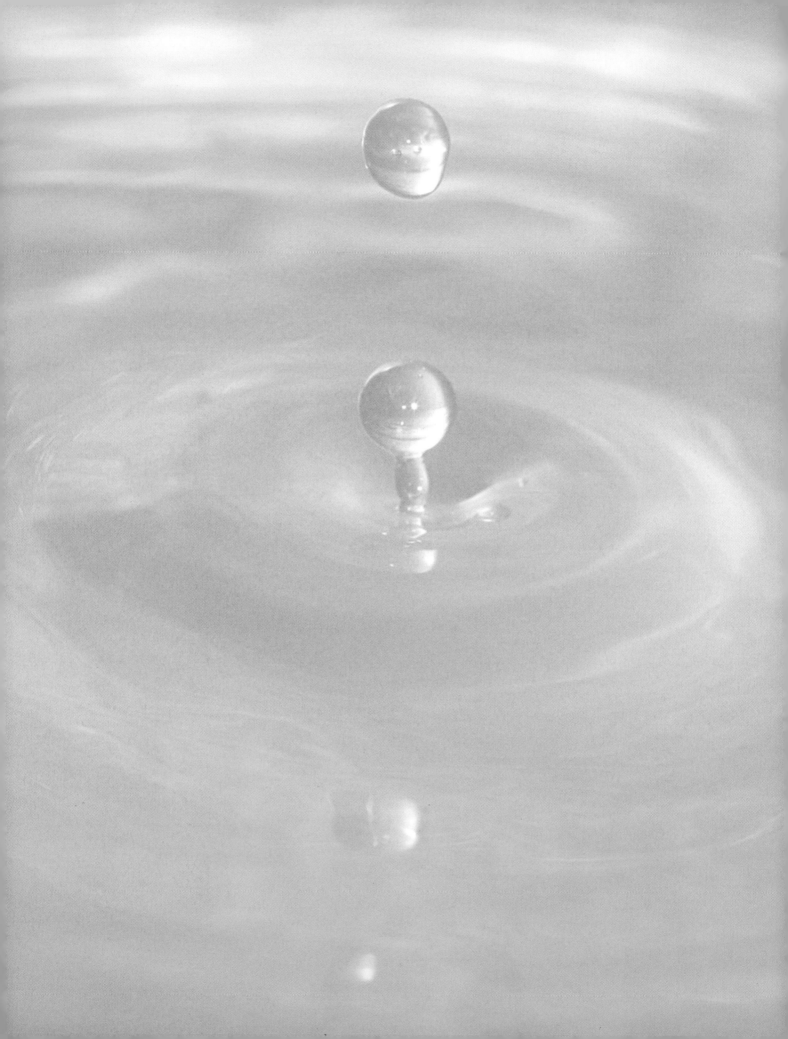

Effects, Benefits, Indications, and Contraindications of Massage

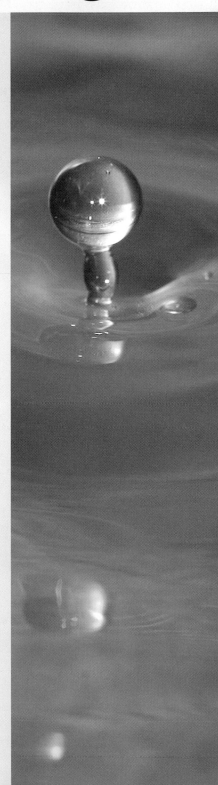

LEARNING OBJECTIVES

After you have mastered this chapter, you will be able to:

1. Explain the physiological effects and benefits of massage.

2. Explain the psychological effects and benefits of massage.

3. Describe the effects of massage on the circulatory, muscular, and nervous systems of the body.

4. Describe the effects of massage on the skin.

5. Explain the main contraindications for massage.

INTRODUCTION

There is much historical evidence to indicate that massage was one of the earliest remedial practices for relief of pain and for the restoration of healthy body functions. Massage is a natural and instinctive method by which minor aches and pains can be soothed away while bringing relief from nervous tension and fatigue.

The term *massage* is applied to different practices, but in the following chapters, the techniques of traditional Western, or what is commonly termed Swedish massage, will be considered. The effects of massage differ from one client to another depending on the needs of the individual and the goals and intentions with which the massage is administered. This is why massage on two different people may render different results. In addition to physical effects from massage therapy, the client may experience mental and emotional reactions. Many healthy people believe that frequent massage helps them to remain physically, mentally, and emotionally fit. They enjoy the relaxed, refreshed, and invigorated feeling they get from a therapeutic massage.

Although massage is not a magic cure-all, it is safe and beneficial for everyone from infants to the elderly, except when there are certain contraindications. A **contraindication** is any physical, emotional, or mental condition that may cause a particular massage treatment to be unsafe or detrimental to the client's well-being. When there is doubt on the part of the practitioner whether to give massage or to recommend a particular stretch, the client should be referred to her primary health care provider and obtain the physician's recommendations in writing. If the

> **Contraindication**
>
> any physical, mental, or emotional condition a client may have that may cause a particular intervention or treatment to be detrimental or unsafe.

client does not have a primary physician, the practitioner may recommend an appropriate health care professional he knows to be familiar with and supportive of the practice of massage therapy.

EFFECTS AND BENEFITS OF MASSAGE

Massage has direct psychological and physiological benefits. Physically, massage increases metabolism, hastens healing, relaxes and refreshes the muscles, and improves the functions of the lymphatic system. Massage helps to prevent and relieve muscle cramps and spasms and improves circulation of blood and lymph, thereby improving the delivery of oxygen and nutrients to the cells as it enhances the removal of metabolic wastes. Because blood carries nutrients to the skin, massage is beneficial in keeping the skin functioning in a normal, healthy manner. Massage therapy is effective in pain management in conditions such as arthritis, neuritis, neuralgia, labor and delivery, whiplash, muscular lesions, sciatica, headache, muscle spasms, and many other conditions.

Psychologically, massage relieves fatigue, reduces tension and anxiety, calms the nervous system, and promotes a sense of relaxation and renewed energy.

There are indications that massage is beneficial in numerous conditions; however, in cases of injury or disease, the client's physician must be consulted before massage treatments are given. Massage has been credited with being of great benefit in helping patients recover from various illnesses or injuries. In some cases, modalities that use heat, light, cold, water, and electricity may be recommended by the client's physician. A physician may recommend massage for both its physical and psychological benefits.

Physiological Effects of Massage

Skillfully applied massage is an effective means of influencing the structures and functions of the body. The specific effects of any massage will vary according to the intent with which it is given, the selection of techniques used, and the condition of the client. Depending on the type and manner of manipulation, a sense of mild relaxation, stimulation, or refreshment may follow massage. Under no circumstances should massage be applied so vigorously that it causes the client to feel exhausted or results in bruised or injured tissues.

There are two physical effects of massage, mechanical and reflex, which may occur separately or together. Mechanical effects are direct physical effects of the massage techniques on the tissues they contact. Reflex effects of massage are indirect responses to touch that affect body functions and tissues through the nervous or energy systems of the body. Gentle stimulation of the sensory nerve endings in the skin, as in superficial stroking, results in reflex effects, either locally or in distant parts of the body. When pressure is applied to the muscles, blood, and lymph vessels, or to any internal structure, both reflex and direct mechanical effects are experienced. Pressure on reflex points, active trigger points, and other pressure points reflexively affects functions or areas of the body away from the actual point of contact.

The immediate effects of massage are noticeable on the skin. Friction and stroking movements heighten blood circulation to the skin and increase activity of the sweat (sudoriferous) and oil (sebaceous) glands. Accompanying the increased flow of blood, there is a slight reddening and warming of the skin. Nutrition to the skin is improved. Massage treatments over a period of time impart a healthy radiance to the skin. The skin tends to become softer, more supple, and of finer texture.

The physiological effects of massage are not limited to the skin. The body as a whole benefits by the stimulation of muscular, glandular, and vascular activities. Most organs of the body are favorably influenced by clinical massage treatments.

Effects of Massage on the Muscular System

Massage encourages the nutrition and development of the muscular system by stimulating its circulation, nerve supply, and cell activity. Regular and systematic massage causes the muscles to become firmer and more flexible. Massage is also an effective means of relaxing tense muscles and releasing muscle spasms.

The supply of blood to the muscles is proportionate to their activity. It is estimated that blood passes three times more rapidly through muscles being massaged than muscles at rest. Petrissage or kneading and compression movements create a pumping action that forces the venous blood and lymph onward and brings a fresh supply of blood to the muscles. Massage aids in the removal of metabolic waste products and helps nourish tissues.

Massage prevents and relieves stiffness and soreness of muscles. Muscles fatigued by work or exercise will be more quickly restored by massage than by passive rest of the same duration.

Muscle tissue that has suffered injury heals more quickly with less connective tissue buildup and scarring when therapeutic massage is applied regularly. Massage can release fascial restrictions and reduce the thickening of connective tissues (hyperplasia), allowing more flexibility; easier, pain-free movement; and improved posture. Friction massage, when properly applied, prevents and reduces the development of adhesions and excessive scarring following trauma.

Massage can have positive effects on the range of motion of limbs that have a limited range due to tissue injury, inflammation, muscle tension, or strain. The client may have experienced discomfort or pain resulting in limited use of a limb or may have stopped using the limb. The limb will need to be taken through the range of motion passively and carefully and the range increased gradually.

Passive movement is the method by which joints are moved through their range of motion with no resistance or assistance by muscular activity on the part of the client. Passive massage movements benefit circulation of the blood and lymph, nourish the skin, relax and lengthen the muscles, soothe the nerves, and lubricate the joints.

Active joint movement in massage refers to exercises in which the voluntary muscles are contracted by the client and either resisted or assisted by the therapist. Active joint movements have beneficial effects similar to exercise. They help to firm and strengthen muscles, improve circulation, and aid the function of related internal organs.

Effects of Massage on the Nervous System

nervous system

controls and coordinates all the body systems and includes the nerves, spinal cord, and brain.

central nervous system

consists of the brain and spinal cord.

peripheral nervous system

consists of all the nerves that connect the CNS to the rest of the body.

sympathetic nervous system

supplies the glands, involuntary muscles of internal organs, and walls of blood vessels with nerves.

parasympathetic nervous system

functions to conserve energy and reverse the action of the sympathetic division.

The **nervous system** consists of the **central nervous system** (brain and spinal cord) and the **peripheral nervous system**. The peripheral nervous system includes the autonomic nervous system, the cranial nerves, and the spinal nerves. The cranial and spinal nerves are made up of somatic (motor) nerves and sensory nerves. The autonomic nervous system is composed of the **sympathetic nervous system** and the **parasympathetic nervous system**.

The sensory nerves and their associated nerve receptors provide input to the central nervous system about what is happening in the body and the surrounding environment. These are the nerves that are influenced by massage. Information from sensory input is processed in the central nervous system, then appropriate responses are sent out via various neurotransmitters, the somatic nerves, and the autonomic nervous system in order to maintain homeostasis.

The effects of massage on the nervous system depend on the direct and reflex reaction of the nerves stimulated. The nervous system can be stimulated or soothed depending on the type of massage movement applied.

Stimulation of the peripheral nerve receptors could have reflex reactions affecting the autonomic nervous system, neurotransmitters in the brain, pain perception, or the underlying joints and muscles of the areas being massaged.

1. **Stimulating massage techniques:**

   a. Friction (light rubbing, rolling, and wringing movements) stimulates nerves.

   b. Percussion (light tapping and slapping movements) increases nervous irritability. Strong percussion for a short period of time excites nerve centers directly. Prolonged percussion tends to anesthetize the local nerves.

   c. Vibration (shaking and trembling movements) stimulates peripheral nerves and all nerve centers with which a nerve trunk is connected.
      D. Knuckle stroking -

2. **Sedative effect of massage techniques:**

   a. Gentle stroking produces calming and sedative results.

   b. Light friction and petrissage (kneading movements) produce marked sedative effects.

c. Holding pressure (ischemic compression) on a sensitive trigger point desensitizes the point and helps release the pathophysiologic reflex cycle that maintains hypertension in the associated muscle.

Effects of Massage on the Autonomic Nervous System

The effects of massage on the autonomic nervous system are mostly reflexive. The autonomic nervous system is divided into the sympathetic nervous system and the parasympathetic nervous system. The sympathetic nervous system is responsible for preparing the body to expend energy in response to emergency situations, commonly referred to as "fight-or-flight" preparation. Activation of the sympathetic nervous system is related to stress, real or perceived. Sympathetic stimulation initiates an accelerated heart rate, blood is diverted to the muscles, elimination and digestion are inhibited, adrenal secretions of **epinephrine/adrenaline** and **norepinephrine** are increased, sweat glands are activated, and the body is more alert and attentive.

epinephrine
"fight" or "flight" hormone that prepares the body to respond to emergencies.

The parasympathetic system is responsible for counteracting the effects of the sympathetic system and establishing the normalizing and restorative functions of a non-alarm state. Stimulation of the parasympathetic system causes a reduced heart rate, increased digestion and elimination, and increased circulation to the internal organs in a relaxation/restorative response. The sympathetic and parasympathetic nervous systems work together to maintain **homeostasis.**

norepinephrine
"fight" or "flight" hormone that prepares the body to respond to emergencies.

Initially, massage seems to alert the sympathetic nervous system. Short, invigorating massage, such as pre-event sports massage or 15-minute chair massage, tends to stimulate the body, leaving it more alert and energized. Longer, relaxing massage, however, seems to affect the autonomic nervous system by sedating the sympathetic nervous system and stimulating the parasympathetic nervous system. As a result, blood levels of epinephrine and norepinephrine are reduced, heart rate and blood pressure are reduced, and the relaxation response is increased.

homeostasis
is the internal balance of the body.

Effects of Massage on Neurotransmitters

Various studies by Tiffany Fields and her associates at the Touch Research Institute in Miami, Florida, have provided compelling evidence that massage promotes relaxation and relieves stress. One study at the institute showed that individuals who received 15-minute massages twice a week exhibited a decreased beta wave and an increased delta wave when given an EEG. These same individuals performed better on math tests, completing the tests in significantly less time and with significantly fewer mistakes. Job-related stress, anxiety, and blood levels of cortisol (the stress hormone) were also reduced (Field, Ironson, Scafidi, et al., 1996). Massage therapy reduces anxiety and enhances EEG pattern of alertness and math computations (*International Journal of Neuroscience, 86,* 197–205, 1996).

Research has shown that massage influences the levels of a number of neurochemicals or elements related to, or that regulate, various physiologic functions. As mentioned previously, massage modulates the blood levels of the stress-related adrenal hormones epinephrine and norepinephrine. Massage has also been found to increase the levels of serotonin, dopamine, endorphins, and enkephalins, neurochemicals related to elevated moods and pain control.

Epinephrine/adrenaline and norepinephrine/noradrenaline are produced in the adrenal medulla and are excreted into the bloodstream in response to stimulation of the sympathetic nervous system. These hormones are also neurotransmitters that stimulate alertness and attentiveness in response to fear or in preparation for the fight-or-flight response. Epinephrine functions in the body; norepinephrine is active in the brain.

Mental and emotional stresses are directly related to increased levels of adrenaline/epinephrine. Low levels of epinephrine and norepinephrine cause drowsiness, low energy, fatigue, and sluggishness.

Short invigorating massage tends to stimulate the production of epinephrine and norepinephrine; while a full, relaxing, one-hour rhythmic massage will decrease the levels of epinephrine and norepinephrine and encourage relaxation.

Dopamine is a neurotransmitter that affects brain functions that control fine movement, emotional response, and the ability to experience pleasure and pain. Elevated levels of dopamine lead to feelings of pleasure and excitement, improvement of mood, alertness, and sex drive. A decline of dopamine in the brain is linked to cognitive and movement problems. Parkinson's disease is caused by the body's inability to produce dopamine.

Serotonin is a neurotransmitter that is synthesized in the brain and found in the brain, bloodstream, and intestinal walls. Serotonin has a broad range of influences, including mood, behavior, appetite, blood pressure, temperature regulation, memory, and learning ability. Serotonin seems to modify behavior in a way that counterbalances the effects of norepinephrine. Where norepinephrine is released in response to stimulants, stress, and anxiety, serotonin promotes a sense of calm and well-being. It seems to regulate moods in a quieting, comforting manner. It suppresses outbursts and irritability while reducing cravings for food or sex. A low level of serotonin is implicated in depression, eating disorders, personality disorders, sleep disturbances, and schizophrenia.

Massage increases levels of available serotonin and dopamine. Increased levels of serotonin and dopamine indicate decreased stress and depression and an elevated mood.

Massage increases the secretions of endorphins and enkephalins in the CNS. These elements are mood elevators and natural painkillers. Endorphins interact with pain receptors in the brain in a very similar manner as morphine and codeine. Besides reducing the sensation of pain, enkephalins and endorphins are related to feelings of euphoria, appetite control, and enhancement of the immune system.

Effect of Massage on Pain

Massage is effective in reducing pain due to a number of neurological processes and conditions. The positive effects of relaxing massage in-

---

dopamine
is a neurotransmitter that controls fine movement, emotional response, and the ability to experience pleasure and pain.

serotonin
is a neurotransmitter that helps regulate nerve impulses and influences mood, behavior, appetite, blood pressure, temperature regulation, memory, and learning ability.

terrupts the transmission of pain sensations of affected nociceptors from entering the central nervous system by stimulating other cutaneous receptors due to what is known as the **gate control theory**. According to the gate control theory, painful impulses are transmitted along small- and large-diameter nerve fibers from nociceptors to the spinal cord and on to the brain. Stimulation of thermo- or mechanoreceptors by rubbing, massaging, icing, or other means is transmitted along the larger fibers and suppresses the pain sensations at the gate where the fibers enter the spinal column. Evidence of this theory can be witnessed in the instinctive practice of briskly rubbing a part of the body that has been bumped or struck by an object in order to relieve the intensity of the pain.

As mentioned before, massage also reduces the sensation of pain by increasing the concentration of endorphins and enkephalins and other pain-reducing neurochemicals in the central nervous system and bloodstream.

Massage can relieve referred myofascial pain and reduce ischemia-related pain by releasing hypersensitive trigger points and restoring circulation to hypertonic muscle tissue.

Certain massage techniques affect the proprioceptive mechanisms of the muscles' spindle receptors and the Golgi tendon organs. Techniques such as compression, positioning, stretching, and pressure alter the feedback circuits and allow new pain-free possibilities for muscle length and function.

gate control theory
the positive effects of relaxing massage interrupts the transmission of pain sensations of affected nociceptors from entering the central nervous system by stimulating other cutaneous receptors.

Effects of Massage on the Circulatory System

Clinical massage affects the quality and quantity of blood coursing through the circulatory system. With the increased flow of blood to the massaged area, better cellular nutrition and elimination are favored. The work of the heart is lessened due to the improvement in surface circulation. Blood pressure and heart rate are temporarily reduced at the same time the systolic stroke volume is increased and capillary beds dilate and become more permeable. Under the influence of massage, the blood-making process is improved, resulting in an increase in the number of red and white blood cells (Figure 6.1). In 1992, studies at Touch Research Institute showed an increase in the presence and activity of T4 killer cells in the bloodstreams of people with HIV after receiving massage, indicating that massage might strengthen the immune system.

An important principle to remember in Swedish massage is to always massage toward the heart. Massage movements should be directed upward along the limbs and lower parts of the body and downward from the head, thereby facilitating the flow of venous blood and lymph back toward the heart and other eliminatory organs.

Massage may influence the blood and lymph vessels either by direct mechanical action on the vessel walls or by reflex action through the vasomotor nerves. Pressure against the vessels not only tones their muscular walls but also propels the movement of the blood. The vasomotor nerves, by controlling the relaxing and constricting of the blood vessels, determine the amount of blood that will reach the area being massaged.

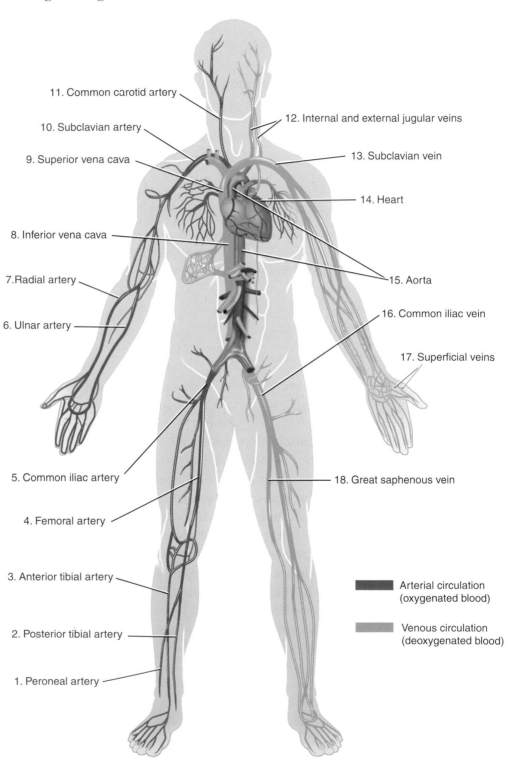

11. Common carotid artery

10. Subclavian artery

9. Superior vena cava

8. Inferior vena cava

7. Radial artery

6. Ulnar artery

5. Common iliac artery

4. Femoral artery

3. Anterior tibial artery

2. Posterior tibial artery

1. Peroneal artery

12. Internal and external jugular veins

13. Subclavian vein

14. Heart

15. Aorta

16. Common iliac vein

17. Superficial veins

18. Great saphenous vein

Arterial circulation
(oxygenated blood)

Venous circulation
(deoxygenated blood)

Figure 6.1
Circulatory system.

Massage movements affect blood and lymph channels in the following ways:

1. Light stroking produces an almost instantaneous, though temporary, dilation of the capillaries, whereas deep stroking brings about a more lasting dilation and flushing of the massaged area.

2. Light percussion causes a contraction of the blood vessels, which tend to relax as the movement is continued.

3. Friction hastens the flow of blood through the superficial veins, increases the permeability of the capillary beds, and produces an increased flow of interstitial fluid. This creates a healthier environment for the cells.

4. Petrissage or kneading stimulates the flow of blood through the deeper arteries and veins.

5. Properly applied, light massage enhances lymph flow and reduces lymphedema.

6. Compression produces a hyperemia (high-per-**EE**-mee-eh) or an increase in the amount of blood stored in the muscle tissue.

Psychological Effects of Massage

The psychological effects of massage should not be underestimated. If the client feels healthier, invigorated, and more energetic, the massage has been worth the effort. In treatment centers for addictions, massage has proven to be an effective therapeutic tool to rebuild a more positive self-image and sense of self-worth. Victims of sexual abuse and rape indicate having an improved self-image and a reduction of an aversion to touch after receiving therapeutic massage. Massage has also been shown to reduce depression and anxiety in adolescents who have experienced sexual or verbal abuse (Fields 1993). People have regular massages as much for psychological as for physical benefit.

Many people suffer from stress and find that massage promotes relaxation and mental alertness as it soothes away minor aches and pains. For some clients, regular massage keeps them feeling more youthful and encourages them to pay more attention to proper nutrition, exercise, and good health practices.

Massage helps clients to become more aware of where they are holding tension, and where they have tight muscles or painful areas. The practitioner may discover areas the client may not have been aware of previously. By getting in touch with, or becoming aware of these conditions, the client can begin to focus on relaxing them both during the massage and on a daily basis. Becoming aware of these trouble spots and responding to them is considered part of preventive maintenance.

CONDITIONS GENERALLY RELIEVED BY MASSAGE

Almost all healthy people occasionally have some physical condition that can be improved by massage. When relief is obtained, there is also a renewed sense of well-being. No matter how well a client may be, a good massage will leave that person feeling even better.

The following conditions are most frequently relieved by regular massage treatment:

1. Stress and tensions are relieved. With the relief of tension and stress, the client feels better able to cope with day-to-day situations.

2. Mental and physical fatigue is relieved, leading to renewed energy and ambition.

3. Pain in the shoulders, neck, and back (when caused by strained muscles or irritated nerves) is relieved.

4. Muscles and joints become more supple. Soreness and stiffness are relieved.

5. Muscle soreness from overexertion can be reduced or prevented.

6. Circulation is improved, thus improving delivery of nutrients to and removal of wastes from the tissues.

7. Digestion, assimilation, and elimination are often improved.

8. Facial massage helps tone the skin, helps prevent blemished skin, and softens fine lines.

9. Headache and eyestrain are often relieved.

10. Deep relaxation is induced and insomnia is often relieved.

11. Muscular spasms are relieved.

12. Obesity (overweight) and flabby muscles can be improved when combined with proper exercise, diet programs, and massage.

13. Pain in joints, sprains, and poor circulation are relieved.

14. Increased circulation of nourishing blood to the skin and other parts of the body encourages healing.

15. Mental strain is reduced, resulting in better productivity.

16. Mildly high blood pressure is temporarily reduced.

17. Renewed sense of confidence and control is experienced.

18. Constrictions and adhesions can be reduced or prevented as traumatized muscle tissue heals.

19. Joint mobility can be increased.

CONTRAINDICATIONS FOR MASSAGE

Although there are many benefits from therapeutic body massage, there are also contraindications of which the professional practitioner must be aware.

Contraindication means that the expected treatment or process is inadvisable. In massage, it means that conditions may exist in which it would not be beneficial to apply massage to a part or all of the body. Contraindications may be absolute, regional, or conditional. A contraindication is absolute when massage is absolutely not appropriate, such as in cases of severe, uncontrolled hypertension; shock; acute pneumonia; or toxemia during pregnancy. Regional or partial contraindications prohibit administering massage to only a local part of the body, such as local contagious conditions, open wounds, or acute neuritis or arthritis, but massaging other areas is fine. Conditional contraindications require the practitioner to adjust the massage when there are health concerns where certain massage techniques may cause discomfort or have adverse effects, though other therapeutic applications are very beneficial. The practitioner must know not only when massage is advised but, more importantly, when it should be avoided, or when certain strokes or movements should not be used.

When you define massage as a form of touch that is applied in a therapeutic manner, then it is true that massage of some form is beneficial to nearly everyone. However, there are situations where particular manipulations may not only be uncomfortable for the client but also could be dangerous.

Many conditions are both indicated and contraindicated for massage. Many conditions respond favorably to massage, whereas others can be aggravated or worsened by specific massage techniques. Certain movements could do more harm than good. Such techniques are contraindicated. It is the responsibility of the practitioner to understand fully the indications and contraindications for massage.

During the first interview or consultation with a client, it is important to obtain information about the state of the client's health and determine any reasons why massage treatments might be inadvisable. A client intake form that includes a medical history is helpful. Careful questioning about the client's conditions is essential in determining whether contraindications exist. When these conditions exist, the client is usually already under the care of a doctor. Most contraindications are conditional. When a client is under the care of a physician, the client should inform the doctor that she is receiving massages and request a written recommendation that includes both precautions and indications for massage. In this way, the practitioner becomes part of a health care team and massage becomes an integral part of the client's health program. In many cases, the physician may not be aware of massage procedures and their benefits. With the client's permission, the practitioner may confer with the physician regarding the client's condition, the effects and benefits of massage, and any precautions or recommendations the doctor may have. It is important for the practitioner to follow any recommendations the physician may have.

Often during the interview or during the course of a massage, conditions that the client may not be aware of become apparent that are contraindicated and should be referred to the attention of a physician. When in doubt, caution is the best policy. The client can be asked (tactfully) to supply a physician's report and/or recommendations before beginning or continuing treatments, or the practitioner could, after receiving the client's consent, ask the client's physician first whether there are questionable circumstances.

Because massage requires a great deal of physical energy on the part of the practitioner, mechanical and electrical apparatus have been devised as aids to manual massage. The hand vibrator is an example. The same contraindications for manual massage also apply when any kind of helpful apparatus is used.

The major contraindications include the following:

- *Abnormal body temperature:* 98.6° F (Fahrenheit), or 37° C (Celsius), is considered normal body temperature, but it may vary depending on the time of day or other factors. The normal body temperature can vary from 96.4° to 99.1° F (35.8° to 37.3° C). Some doctors and therapists say that massage is not recommended when temperature exceeds 99.4° F. If the client feels abnormally warm or feverish, her temperature should be taken to ascertain the advisability of massage treatment. Massage is contraindicated when the client has a fever. Generally a fever indicates that the body is trying to isolate and eliminate an invading pathogen. The body is stepping up its own action in order to confine, narrow down, and eliminate the problem. Therefore, massage would tend to work against the defense mechanisms of the body.

- *Acute infectious disease:* Typhoid, diphtheria, severe colds, influenza, and the like would preclude massage. Giving a massage to an individual who is coming down with an acute viral infection (cold or flu) will intensify the illness and also expose the therapist to the virus. Massage is systemically contraindicated and the client should contact her physician.

- *Inflammation:* When there is acute inflammation in a particular area of the body, massage is not advisable because it could further irritate the area or intensify the inflammation. This is particularly true for spreading or penetrating types of massage manipulations. Inflamed joints do not indicate massage of the joint itself; however, there are some pressure point applications that are useful. Therapeutic touch, which is simply placing your hands on or near the inflamed area, may be helpful.

Although working directly on an area may be contraindicated, working on a reflex or related area or working in an area proximal to the affected area can be useful because it tends to stimulate circulation and the natural healing properties of the body. A reflex point is an area that is distant to the affected area yet, when stimulated, has an effect on that area.

There are numerous types of inflammations. A word with the suffix *-itis* pertains to inflammation. For example, arthritis is an inflammation of the joints, neuritis is an inflammation of a nerve or nerves, dermatitis is inflammation of the skin, and so on. Caution must be used when a client has any kind of inflammation that could be aggravated by massage.

Inflammation due to tissue damage: When tissue is damaged, the body's natural response is inflammation. Inflammation is characterized by swelling, redness, heat, and pain.

If the tissue damage is of a traumatic nature and severe enough, blood vessels may be damaged, resulting in a hematoma (hee-muh-**TOE**-muh). The area may become swollen and discolored. The bluish color is from blood escaping from the damaged blood vessels. Any reddening is a sign of inflammation. Inflammation is the body's natural defense mechanism to protect and speed healing to the tissues.

Inflammation from bacterial infestation: If there is pus or a pus pocket formed, massage is definitely contraindicated. Pus is a combination of dead white blood cells and bacteria. If it is disturbed, there is a chance of spreading the infection. If the pus gets into the bloodstream, there is a chance of a serious systemic infection.

Osteoporosis: This condition leads to deterioration of bone. In advanced stages, bones become brittle, sometimes to the point that they are easily broken. Osteoporosis is prevalent in the elderly and in certain kinds of diseases. The symptoms of osteoporosis may include frailty and stooped shoulders. In women, osteoporosis can be due to reduced estrogen levels. It is best to obtain the advice of the client's physician before giving massage when osteoporosis is indicated (Figure 6.2).

Varicose veins: Varicose veins is a condition in which the valves in the veins break down because of back pressure in the circulatory system. The veins bulge and rupture, usually in the legs. The development of varicose veins is often the result of gravity or obstructed venous flow, as the result of crossing the legs or other sitting postures that inhibit circulation to or from the legs. Varicose veins are often hereditary or can be the result of standing for long hours. In women, the pressure on the large veins in the pelvic area during pregnancy often contributes to this condition.

Blood is pumped through the veins by means of pressure originating in the heart and is helped along by contractions of muscle surrounding the veins. Veins are basically tubes consisting of a layer of endothelial lining and smooth muscle and are

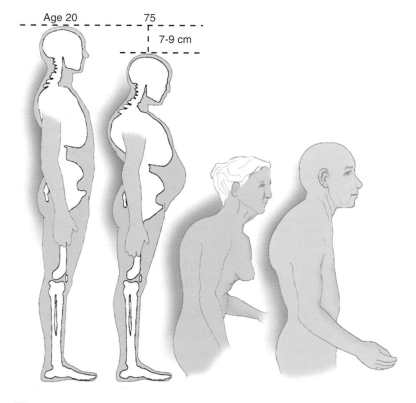

Figure 6.2

Symptoms of osteoporosis often include stooped shoulders.

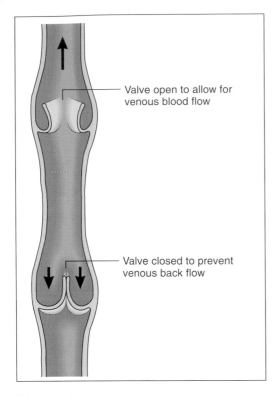

Figure 6.3
A vein valve.

Valve open to allow for venous blood flow

Valve closed to prevent venous back flow

---

phlebitis

is an inflammation of
a vein accompanied
by pain and swelling.

---

thrombophlebitis

is the inflammation
of veins due
to blood clots.

---

embolus

if a piece of a clot
loosens and floats in
the blood.

---

covered with connective tissue. Many veins, especially those in the arms and legs, have a system of valves that prevent blood from flowing backward in the vein and act as a *venous pump* to move the blood toward the heart. These valves are flaplike structures that protrude from the inside walls of the vein in such a way that blood moving toward the heart pushes past the valve, but if the blood attempts to move in the reverse direction, pressure against the valve forces it closed and blood cannot pass. The venous pump is a phenomenon that results when muscles contract and exert external pressure on the veins, which tends to collapse them. As the vein is repeatedly collapsed, the blood is forced along through the system of valves toward the heart (Figure 6.3).

Extensive back pressure in the veins due to prolonged standing or blockage causes the veins to enlarge and stretch to the point that the valves become incompetent. The weight of the blood further distends the veins and more valves become dysfunctional, perpetuating the condition. When veins become abnormally dilated due to excessive back pressure, they rupture and are called *varicose*. Blood then accumulates in enlarged portions of the vein. If the flow of blood becomes obstructed, clotting may occur. When this condition is accompanied by inflammation, it is painful and potentially dangerous. Increased pressure in the veins also increases pressure in the capillaries and often results in edema.

The practitioner will recognize varicose veins as bluish, protruding, thick, bulbous, distended superficial veins usually found in the lower legs. Also to be considered with caution are the small reddish groupings of broken blood vessels that often surround a small, protruding vein. Any deep massage on these areas may set a blood clot loose in the general circulation and cause a serious problem (Figure 6.4).

It is easy to see why massage would be contraindicated in cases of varicosities. However, massage proximal to the affected area might be very helpful, especially superficial (barely touching) techniques.

Phlebitis: Inflammation of a vein accompanied by pain and swelling is called **phlebitis** (fle-BY-tis). Phlebitis may be the result of surgery, or may be secondary to an infection or injury, or may have no apparent precursor. In many cases of phlebitis, a blood clot forms along the wall of the inflamed vein, causing the dangerous condition known as **thrombophlebitis,** or deep vein thrombosis (DVT). If a piece of this clot loosens and floats in the blood, it is called an **embolus** (EM-bo-lus). If this embolus reaches the lungs, it can cause death by pulmonary embolism. If the embolus reaches the brain or the nourishing vessels of the heart, it can bring about stroke or myocardial infarction (heart attack).

Postsurgical: Always obtain the physician's permission before applying massage following surgery. The possibility of thrombosis is increased for a period of time following surgery. Massage over a fresh incision is contraindicated; however, after the initial healing has taken place, specialized connective tissue massage may help reduce excessive scar formation and adhesions. If an incision has already healed, creating excessive scar tissue and adhesions to the neighboring fascia, muscles, or skin, specialized scar tissue massage may be applied to break down the adhesions and reduce the associated pain and discomfort.

Aneurosa: An aneurosa (an-yoo-**RO**-suh) or **aneurysm** (**AN**-yoo-rizm) is a localized dilation of a blood vessel or, more commonly, an artery. It can be caused by a congenital defect, arteriosclerosis, hypertension, or trauma and is generally located in the aorta, thorax, and abdomen and sometimes in the cranium. Although this condition can appear, it is rarely encountered in the massage field, and if suspected, should be referred to medical attention.

Hematoma: A **hematoma** is a mass of blood trapped in some tissue or cavity of the body and is the result of internal bleeding. **Contusions** (kun-**TOO**-zhuns) or bruises are common types of hematomas that are generally not too serious. Contusions usually occur as a result of a blow that is severe enough to break a blood vessel. The escaping blood leaves the familiar black-and-blue spot. The blood quickly clots, and in a matter of time, the body naturally reabsorbs the cellular debris. The bruise changes color to greens and yellows and eventually disappears.

When the hematoma is in the acute phase, massage is contraindicated because of the risk of reinjuring the tissue. After the bruise has changed colors, light massage will enhance circulation to the area and actually assist the healing.

A cranial hematoma is a serious condition that is usually the result of a blow to the head. A broken blood vessel inside the cranium forms a tumorlike mass that puts pressure on the brain. Depending on the location and severity of the hematoma, symptoms range from headache, confusion, and drowsiness to paralysis, loss of consciousness, and death. The only treatment for cranial hematoma is surgery to remove the pressure.

Edema: Edema (e-**DEE**-muh) is a circulatory abnormality that generally appears as puffiness or swelling in the extremities but is sometimes more widespread. Edema is an excess accumulation of fluid in tissue spaces; it has numerous causes. In some instances, massage is indicated, and in others, it is not. If edema is the result of back pressure in the veins due to immobility, massage and mild exercise may prove helpful.

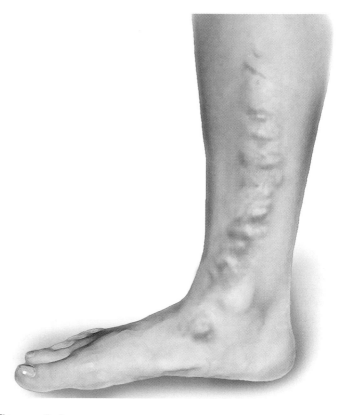

Figure 6.4

Varicose veins appear as bluish, protruding, thick, bulbous, distended superficial veins usually found in the lower legs.

aneurysm
is a local distention or ballooning of an artery due to a weakening wall.

hematoma
is a mass of blood trapped in some tissue or cavity of the body and is the result of internal bleeding.

contusion
or bruise is a common type of hematoma that is generally not too serious.

edema
is a condition of excess fluid in the interstitial spaces.

If, on the other hand, edema is the result of protein imbalance due to breakdown in the kidneys or liver, or is the result of increased permeability (allowing passage especially of fluids) of the capillaries due to inflammation, massage is contraindicated.

When edema is suspected, it can be easily detected by pressing a finger into the area. When the finger is removed and an indentation remains, edema is present. This indentation will take several seconds to return to the level of adjoining skin. This is called *pitting edema*. Local circulatory massage is contraindicated for all cases of pitting edema.

Edema can result from an imbalance of factors that regulate the interchange of fluids between the capillaries and tissue spaces. Other causes can be related to heart or kidney disease, poison in the system (affecting histamine levels that cause increased capillary permeability), or an obstruction of lymph channels. If edema is related to pregnancy and is caused by toxemia (poisons in the blood), massage is definitely contraindicated.

Obviously such conditions should be brought to the attention of a physician. It is essential that the reason for edema is known before massage is performed on the edematous tissue.

Lymphedema: **Lymphedema** is swelling, usually in an extremity, when fluid accumulates in the interstitial spaces because it is not able to pass into and through the lymph channels. Primary lymphedema is a congenital or genetic condition where a portion of the lymphatic system does not develop completely. Secondary lymphedema is the result of trauma, surgery, radiation, infection, or some other event that damages lymph tissue or otherwise interferes with the lymph transport system. Lymphedema is a localized condition. Generalized or deep massage on the limb with lymphedema is contraindicated; however, massage on the rest of the body is okay. Light massage on the affected limb should be done last and be directed from distal to proximal. The most appropriate form of massage to be done on the affected area is manual lymph drainage massage as taught by the Vodder School or other similar methods.

High blood pressure: **High blood pressure** refers to an elevated pressure of the blood against the walls of the arteries. If the client has a history of high blood pressure, her physician should be consulted before treatment. The client may be taking medication to bring the condition under control. Unless it is severe, massage may be of assistance in relieving some of the hypertension that accompanies high blood pressure. Any massage that involves high blood pressure should be soothing and sedating. Low blood pressure is not a consideration in massage.

Cancer: **Cancer** is a conditional contraindication for massage. Many types of cancer spread or metastasize through the blood or lymph channels. Because massage enhances circulation, the application of massage must be modified when working with people with cancer. Massage has proven to have many benefits for people with cancer, including relaxation, pain relief, relief of side effects from cancer treatments, and support of the immune system. It is essential to consult with the client's physician and to be a part of the health support team prior to any treatment. (Refer to page 317, "Massaging People with Cancer.")

---

lymphedema

is an accumulation of interstitial fluid, or swelling, in the soft tissues due to inflammation, blockage, or removal of the lymph channels.

---

high blood pressure

refers to an elevated pressure of the blood against the artery walls.

---

cancer

is the uncontrolled growth and spread of abnormal cells in the body.

Fatigue: In cases of chronic fatigue, the excretory system is already overburdened, and there is little to nourish those overworked and exhausted tissues. When a client is suffering from chronic fatigue, massage should be extremely light and superficial to induce rest and relaxation. Over a period of time, massage helps to restore the client's energy.

Intoxication: Intoxication is a contraindication because massage can spread toxins and overstress the liver.

Psychosis: Psychosis is another condition wherein it is advisable to work directly under the supervision of the patient's doctor.

Medication and drugs: There are times when a client will be taking specific medications or drugs and massage may or may not be recommended. If there is any question concerning the client's condition and possible harmful side effects a massage might cause, the client's physician should be consulted.

Skin problems: The following skin conditions are contraindications. Usually only the affected areas are of concern. For example, a minor laceration on the hand would not prevent massage of other healthy parts of the body. However, as has already been stated, when a condition is of a contagious nature, massage is not given.

Acne	Impetigo	Skin cancer
Boils	Inflammation	Skin tags
Broken vessels	Lacerations	Sores
Bruises	Lumps	Stings and bites
Burns and blisters	Rashes	Tumor
Carbuncles	Scaly spots	Warts
Hypersensitive skin	Scratches	Wounds

Hernia: Hernia is a protrusion of an organ or part of an organ, such as the intestine protruding through an opening in the abdominal wall surrounding it. This is also referred to as a rupture, and massage is not recommended over or near the afflicted area.

Frail elderly people: Frail elderly people may have fragile bones and very sensitive skin. However, gentle massage may be beneficial.

Scoliosis: When a client has scoliosis (sko-lee-**O**-sis), or crooked spine, massage must be recommended by the client's physician. Caution must be exercised (Figure 6.5).

Specific conditions or diseases: It should be obvious to the practitioner that a client who is suffering from *severe asthma* (a chronic respiratory disorder), *diabetes* (deficient insulin secretion), or any type or *heart* or *lung disease* should be under the supervision of a physician. Massage would not be given without the physician's knowledge and advice. This is why it is important to take time during the first consultation (interview) to determine the client's state of health.

When making decisions whether to perform massage on a person who has a medical condition, be conservative. When in doubt, don't! Remember the first and foremost rule: **"Do no harm!"**

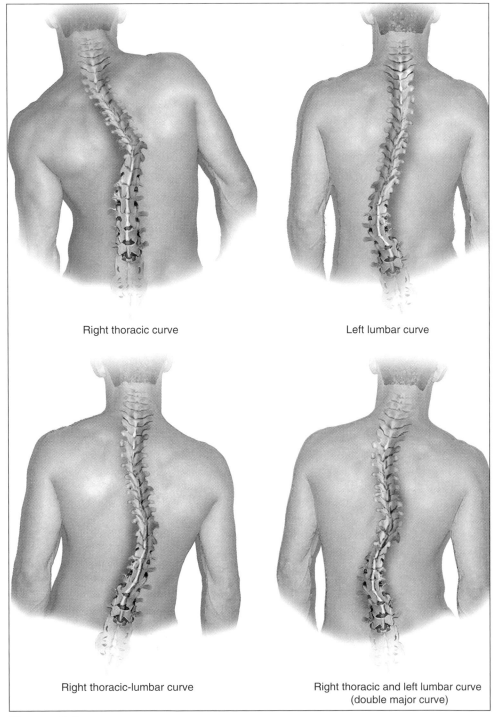

Right thoracic curve

Left lumbar curve

Right thoracic-lumbar curve

Right thoracic and left lumbar curve
(double major curve)

Figure 6.5
Scoliosis is an abnormal lateral curve of the spine.

MASSAGE DURING PREGNANCY

During a normal, healthy pregnancy, massage may be very beneficial in promoting relaxation, soothing nerves, and relieving strained back and leg muscles. Massage also tends to instill a feeling of well-being to both the mother and the unborn child. However, certain situations and conditions exist of which the practitioner must be aware. Toxemia or

pre-eclampsia is a complication of pregnancy that is an absolute contraindication for massage. It is characterized by high blood pressure, edema of the lower extremities, nausea, and diarrhea. A woman with this condition should be under the care of a qualified physician.

Massage should always be soothing and relaxing. No heavy percussion or deep tissue massage should ever be done. Likewise, abdominal kneading or other deep abdominal massage should be avoided. Care should be taken to position the mother in such a way as to assure the comfort of both the mother and the unborn child.

When the client is supine (face up), pillows are used under the knees, head, and upper back. In this position, the weight of the fetus may press on the aorta in such a way as to constrict the flow of blood to the lower body and the fetus. A half-sitting, or semireclining position is preferred (Figure 6.6).

When the client is on her side, pillows are placed under her head and between her knees and legs (Figure 6.7).

> **pre-eclampsia**
> is a condition of pregnancy related to increased blood pressure in the mother that affects the placenta; can also affect the mother's kidney, liver, and brain.

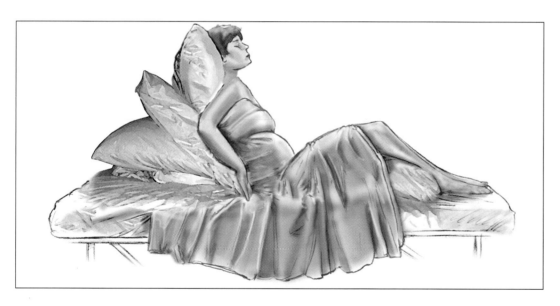

Figure 6.6

In the supine position, the pregnant client should be supported in a semireclining position to prevent pressure from the fetus on the major abdominal blood vessels.

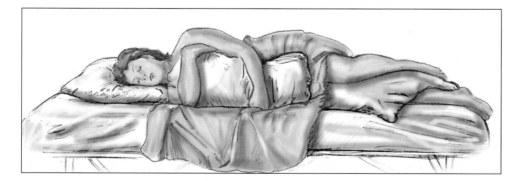

Figure 6.7

When the client is on her side, pillows are placed under her head and upper knee or between her legs.

During the second and third trimesters, lying prone (face down) places pressure on the abdominal area. This position is not only very uncomfortable, but it may be dangerous to the unborn child. A prone position is not advisable unless proper and adequate support is provided. Special bolsters and massage tables are available that provide full and safe support so that even a full-term, soon-to-be mother can lie face down and receive a soothing massage to her back. If there is any question as to the state of health of either the mother or the unborn child, the client's doctor must be consulted before massage is given.

MASSAGE FOR THE CRITICALLY ILL

Massage is becoming a common part of preferred treatment with the critically ill. Many times, conditions are present that are normally contraindicated for massage. However, by making adjustments to the intent and delivery of the massage session, there is literally no contraindication for touch therapy. Depending on an individual's condition, there are precautions and concerns as to how a massage will proceed.

Purpose

The intent of massage for the critically ill is gentle and genuine caring touch therapy to bring comfort, pleasure, and relaxation to an individual at a difficult time of life.

Benefits

- Helps control discomfort and pain
- Improves mobility
- Helps reduce disorientation and confusion by bringing the person back to a more positive body awareness
- Reduces isolation and fear
- Helps to ease the emotional and physical discomforts of the individual
- Allows the individual to develop a more positive attitude about her situation or condition

Considerations and Precautions

It is important for the practitioner to be conscious and aware of the individual's needs. Conditions dictate how much is done and what precautions are used. When in doubt about how or whether to proceed because of a person's condition, be sure to ask. Ask the client first. Generally, clients are very aware of any precautions concerning their condition. It is also important to communicate with the physician or the caregiver in charge.

A critically ill person's physical and emotional condition is constantly changing. Continually assess the client visually, verbally, and tactually and adjust the massage accordingly. The practitioner must be open to the needs of the individual at the moment.

Techniques

Many of the common massage techniques are designed for the relatively healthy person. When working with the critically ill, it is essential to be aware of each individual's needs and tolerances. Many massage techniques are made to stimulate circulation and stir up wastes and toxins. These may not be appropriate when massaging an individual with a critical illness. With the critically ill, the body may be having a hard time eliminating and not tolerate any more wastes being pushed into the system.

Techniques should soothe and add comfort. Touch, slow and gentle stroking, and energy work are the most common choices for massaging the critically ill. Depending on the tolerance of the client, the length of a session may be abbreviated. Rather than a full massage that lasts an hour or more, the situation might call for the back and shoulders or just the feet to be massaged for 15 minutes. This is a time to underdo rather than overdo. It is a time to be supportive and calming. The touch session may only involve holding the client's hand and being there for the person.

Any and all contact that is made is an integral part of the session. Your mere presence is as important as the manipulations you use. Your actions, voice, breathing, and movements should all reflect the caring, nurturing, and compassion of the session. In the words of Irene Smith of Service Through Touch:

> We give massage primarily for relaxation and pleasure. The patient may be under a high level of stress due to fear, pain, and anxiety on the physical, emotional and spiritual levels. Slow, gentle, loving touch is used in order to offer the patient a time of peace and quiet. Peace and quiet and gentleness are three very valuable healing qualities.

PRECAUTIONS FOR WORKING WITH HIV-INFECTED INDIVIDUALS

The **human immunodeficiency virus (HIV)** is the causative agent for **acquired immune deficiency syndrome (AIDS)**. The only way to determine whether an individual is HIV positive is through a simple blood test. Not everyone who is HIV positive develops AIDS. Being HIV positive is no longer a death sentence. Through medication, the progression of the disease can be slowed or stopped.

human immunodeficiency virus (HIV)
is a virus that can multiply and destroy a portion of the immune system.

acquired immune deficiency syndrome (AIDS)
is a condition caused by HIV infection whereby a portion of the immune system is destroyed, making it easy for the infected person to get life-threatening diseases.

Stages of HIV Infection

There is a continuum of stages of HIV infection. After being infected with the virus, there may be absolutely no symptoms for a long period of time. This period may be a matter of months or several years. When the immune system begins to weaken, mild symptoms appear. As the immune system continues to weaken, symptoms become more severe. Symptoms continue to become more severe as the body loses its ability to fight off infections. When an HIV-infected person has a T-cell count of 200 or less and/or is diagnosed with an **opportunistic infection**, that person has AIDS.

Opportunistic infections are caused by organisms that are commonly found in the environment and that many of us already have in our body. Normally our immune system protects us against these bacteria, parasites, fungi, and viruses. With the immune system weakened by HIV, the uncontrolled organisms become deadly. Common opportunistic infections associated with AIDS include:

> **opportunistic infection**
>
> is caused by organisms commonly found in the environment and our bodies that become deadly when the body's immune system is weakened.

- *Pneumocystis carinii pneumonia (PCP).* PCP is caused by a protozoan commonly found in our lungs. When the immune system is weakened, as in AIDS, the organism multiplies and causes the disease. PCP is the most common opportunistic disease of persons with AIDS. Unless you have an immune deficiency, there is no concern about catching PCP.

- *Cryptococcal meningitis.* Cryptococcal meningitis is caused by the fungus *Cryptococcus neoformans.* This fungus is found in the environment and grows in pigeon droppings. Dust containing the fungus is inhaled, and it spreads to the meninges of the central nervous system, creating the symptoms of the disease.

- *Toxoplasmosis.* Toxoplasmosis comes from a protozoan that is usually acquired through eating raw or undercooked meat. If the immune system is weak, the infection may spread to the heart, lungs, or brain. In AIDS patients, the infection often affects the brain, resulting in lesions and neurological complications.

- *Candida.* The fungus *Candida albicans* is normally found in the intestines, mouth, and vagina. When a person's resistance is reduced due to illness, immunosuppressive drugs, or broad spectrum antibiotics, Candida infections can occur. In people with AIDS, Candida infection may appear in the mouth, where it is called *thrush,* or it may appear as a rash on the skin. Do not touch a Candida rash because it may be very sensitive and can spread from one part of the body to another.

- *Herpes.* There are three forms of the herpes virus, all of which are very contagious:

    Herpes simplex I causes fever blisters and cold sores on the face and mouth.

Herpes simplex II causes painful sores around the genitals and anus and is sexually transmitted.

Herpes varicella-zoster is also called *shingles* and causes painful blisters that tend to follow specific nerve pathways.

- *Kaposi's Sarcoma (KS).* KS is a form of cancer of the cells that line certain blood vessels. KS produces lesions that may appear on the skin. The lesions may be bluish to reddish purple and may be smooth or raised. They may be closed, in which case massaging over them is acceptable; or they may be open, in which case the same precautions as with blood products must be observed.

- *Other rashes.* The person with AIDS may have any number of rashes caused by fungi or reactions to medications. Most rashes are contraindicated to massage. Simply avoid the area where there is a rash and proceed to another area of the body.

Transmission of HIV

The virus that causes AIDS is transmitted from person to person only through the exchange of body fluid that contains the virus. The transmission of HIV requires three simultaneous conditions.

1. The virus requires a proper environment to survive. The virus is found in blood, semen, vaginal fluids, and mother's milk in high enough concentrations to be virulent. HIV has also been found in sweat, tears, and rarely in saliva.

2. The substance containing the virus must have a sufficiently large concentration of the virus in order to cause an HIV infection. There is no known case of HIV infection caused by contact with sweat, tears, or saliva.

3. The virus must have a port of entry; that is, there must be a way for the virus to enter the body. Some ways this may occur are: engaging in unprotected sexual activity, sharing needles used for injecting drugs or applying tattoos, receiving transfusions with infected blood, transmitting in utero to an unborn child, or through nursing an infant when you are infected.

Precautions Against Infection

Understanding the stages of HIV infection and the factors necessary for transmission of HIV will help to guide the practitioner when determining what precautions to take.

Always be aware of standard infection precautions when working with any client. These precautions are designed to prevent blood or any other body secretions from entering the practitioner's body through any opening such as open sores or cuts.

The primary infection precaution is thorough hand washing. Thorough hand washing is accomplished by scrubbing the hands vigorously with a germicidal soap before and after each massage session. When deemed necessary, the hands may be washed during the session. The hands are washed before the session to protect the client who may be susceptible to infection. Thorough hand washing after the session protects the therapist and anyone the therapist comes in contact with after the session.

The Use of Gloves

The use of gloves is a secondary infection precaution and never replaces the need for thorough hand washing. Either vinyl or latex gloves may be used. When massaging with oil, latex gloves may break down or tear. Double gloving may be used when added protection is a concern. In situations where the client is susceptible to infection, sterile latex gloves may be used.

A practitioner should use gloves

- when handling blood, feces, or any other body fluids or secretions or linens soiled with them.

- when the practitioner has an open sore, cut, or broken cuticles on the hands.

- whenever you as a practitioner do not feel comfortable without them. (Always explain to your client why you are wearing gloves and get her agreement before proceeding.)

- when the client requests that you wear gloves.

Caring for Equipment

Tables and other surfaces that have been contaminated with blood can be cleaned and sanitized with a 10 percent solution of chlorine bleach. This can be made by mixing one part chlorine bleach with nine parts water. Alcohol can be used to disinfect surfaces contaminated by other body fluids and secretions.

Linens can be disinfected by washing them in hot water with detergent and a cup of bleach and drying them in a hot dryer.

Following these general infection precautions does minimize the risk to you and your clientele. However, it does not eliminate the fact that some risk is involved. If any questions or concerns arise as a result of working with a person who has an HIV infection or any other infectious disease, contact your local infection control center. There is an infection control center located at your local hospital or medical center.

(For more information about massage for HIV-infected persons or massage for the critically ill, contact www.everflowing.org, Service Through Touch, 41 Carl St., #C, San Francisco, CA 94117.)

MASSAGING PEOPLE WITH CANCER

Until recently, massage has been considered to be a contraindication when working with persons with cancer because of the effects it has on blood and lymph circulation and the fear that massage may actually spread the cancer. Pioneers such as Debra Curties, Gayle MacDonald, and others have examined the development of cancer and the mechanics of how it spreads and have concluded that when certain precautions are taken and guidelines followed, the risks of massaging persons with cancer are minimal when weighed against the many benefits provided by skilled touch. Two books recommended for anyone considering working with people with cancer are *Medicine Hands: Massage Therapy for People with Cancer* by Gayle MacDonald and *Massage Therapy and Cancer* by Debra Curties.

Certain types of massage or massage techniques are contraindicated for people with cancer or for those undergoing cancer treatment; however, many techniques provide support and relief to people with this devastating disease. With a clearer understanding of the disease, careful consideration, and some specific guidelines, massage may now be offered to a population that will find great benefit in their increased comfort and enhanced quality of life. In fact, massage is used in many cancer centers and hospitals as an integrated therapy for cancer patients.

People who receive a diagnosis of cancer suddenly face a life-threatening and life-changing situation that will require hard choices and the likelihood of invasive medical procedures. They are suddenly facing a fight against a disease that will deeply affect their mental, emotional, and physical well-being. Adverse physical effects of cancer may stem from the disease itself or from the rather aggressive treatment required to fight it. Common cancer therapies tend to be invasive, painful, stressful, sometimes even disfiguring. Emotional side effects of cancer or its treatment may include mood swings, depression, a sense of hopelessness, confusion, or decreased cognitive skills. Massage provides both physical and emotional support to people dealing with cancer.

Benefits of massage for persons with cancer include pain relief or control and relief from depression. Massage has been effective in reducing nausea, eliminating insomnia, promoting relaxation, reducing anxiety, increasing body awareness, and helping restore a positive body image. Massage induces relief from muscle tension, spasms, and fatigue. Further effects of massage include improved lymph movement, reduced edema and swelling, better digestion and elimination, better flexibility, improved outlook on life, and enhanced self-esteem. Massage restores range of motion and promotes health, and it feels good. It imparts an improved quality of life and a boost to the healing process. The intention of providing massage to people with cancer is to relax, restore, and nurture. Massage provides comfort and support even though it is not necessarily intended to "fix" anything (see Box 6.1).

Massage that reduces stress levels has been found to reduce the levels of cortisol and glucocorticoids in the blood and therefore may inhibit

BOX 6.1 BENEFITS OF MASSAGE TO PERSONS WITH CANCER

Provides some pain relief or control

Reduces nausea

Improves digestion and elimination

Relieves stress

Promotes relaxation

Helps insomnia

Reduces anxiety

Provides some relief from depression

Provides some relief from muscle tension and spasm

Helps improve flexibility

Helps restore range of motion

Improves lymph movement, reduces edema

Increases body awareness

Restores positive body image

Enhances self-esteem

Improves outlook on life

Improves quality of life

Boosts the healing process

Promotes health

Feels good at a time when lots of things feel bad

the spread of the disease. Higher levels of these stress-related hormones have been linked to increased tumor proliferation.

Cancer Metastasis

metastasis
is the spread of cancer from one site to another location in the body.

There is limited knowledge as to why cancer strikes; however, there is more and clearer understanding of how it spreads. **Metastasis** is the manner in which cancer spreads. Metastasis, or proliferation of cancer cells, is a complex process that is still under investigation in the fight against this disease. Even though modern medical practices are very successful at eliminating primary tumors associated with cancer, the fact that the cancer metastasizes to other locations is usually the cause of death. Usually by the time a palpable tumor is detected and diagnosed, metastasis has already started. It is estimated that in 30 to 50 percent of people with cancer, metastasis has begun before they receive their initial treatment.

Cancer spreads in four ways:

- direct invasion of nearby structures
- within body cavities
- via the bloodstream
- via the lymph system

Three stages of metastasis are of concern to the massage therapist (Figure 6.8):

- cells breaking off of the primary tumor
- circulation through the blood and lymph vessels
- implantation of cancerous cells at secondary sites

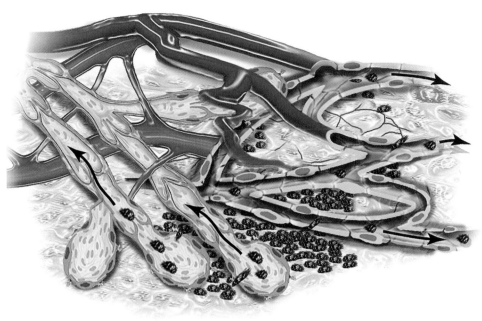

A. Cancer cells shedding

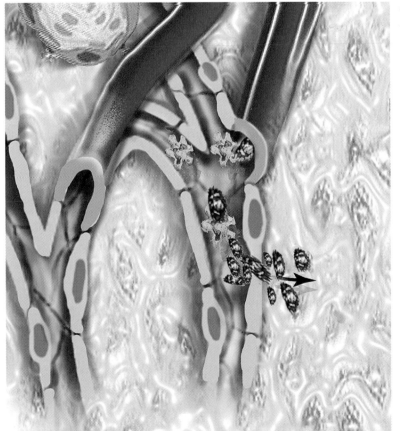

 Cancer cells

 Phagocyte

B. Cancer cells implanting

Figure 6.8
Cancer cells shed from the primary tumor, enter the bloodstream, and implant in a secondary site.

Cancers that metastasize through the bloodstream seem to be the most lethal. The means by which this happens is very complicated. Simply stated, cancerous cells from a tumor slough off and pass through the walls of the blood vessels feeding the tumor. Mechanical processes such as direct pressure or intense movement in the close proximity of a tumor may enhance shedding of cells from a primary tumor. Therefore massage, stretching, or joint movements on or near the site of the tumor are contraindicated especially if the tumor is in superficial tissues. When cancer cells enter the circulatory system, they enter into a very hostile environment in which far less than 1 percent of them survive. Factors that cause their destruction include the fact that cancer cells are not able to absorb nutrients while moving through the bloodstream, the immune system is designed to seek and destroy abnormal cells, and cancer cells are not built to withstand the turbulent forces of movement in the circulatory system. So the longer cancer cells remain in circulation, the less likely they are to survive. Fewer than 1 percent of metastatic cells from a tumor survive in the bloodstream, and less than 1 percent of those cancer cells are able to initiate the metastatic process (Groenwald and Frogge, 1995; Curties, 1994). Cells may clump together to increase their chance at survival. Eventually the cells move into and lodge in a capillary bed, where they adhere to the wall of the blood vessel. With the right conditions, they grow or penetrate the capillary wall, invading the interstitial space and begin growth as a secondary tumor.

Cancerous cells may also enter the bloodstream via the lymph system. Cells shed from the primary tumor and into the interstitial spaces where they are absorbed into lymph capillaries. They travel into lymph vessels and to regional nodes where they are either destroyed by the immune system or proliferate in the node. Malignant cells can enter the bloodstream through the nodal capillaries or pass on through infected lymph nodes to the thoracic or right lymphatic ducts and then into the bloodstream via the vena cava.

If the effects of massage increase the volume and speed of blood and lymph circulation and increase immune function, the agitated hostile environment would be more likely to suppress metastatic cell survival in the bloodstream than support it. The long-held assumption that massage spreads the cancer through the blood and lymph system is largely unfounded and without merit. As of the most current revision of this text, there has been no definitive study done examining whether or not massage affects the spread of cancer.

Implantation at a secondary site happens when viable malignant cells reach the capillary bed of a preferred host tissue. The cancerous cells adhere to the capillary walls, are able to penetrate the capillary wall, move into the new site, and establish themselves as a secondary site. Most cancers seek out and prefer certain host tissues or organs as secondary sites. These patterns of metastasis are clearly documented and must be considered when determining where and how to administer massage techniques. Secondary sites are often in deep, major organs where distal circulatory massage is of minor consequence.

The question is, does massage increase the chances of malignant cells implanting in a secondary site? There is no available data one way or another, so it is prudent to take a precautionary approach. Depending on the site of the primary tumor, massage should be avoided in the area or areas of probable secondary sites, especially if those sites are in superficial tissues. There is no conclusive research regarding the risks of massage during the stages of metastasis; however, by observing certain precautions, the risks of spreading the cancer can be minimized.

It has been shown that people with cancer who receive massage experience many benefits. In studies at Touch Research Facility at the University of Miami, massage has been shown to increase certain immune factors in the bloodstream. Avoiding gentle comfort-giving touch will not stop metastatic cells from breaking away from a primary tumor, moving through the bloodstream, and stopping in host tissues to form secondary tumors, but it will deny a population under myriad stressful conditions the many benefits of skilled touch.

Each situation is different, considering the type of cancer, the stage of the disease, the level of treatment or state of remission, the state of the immune system, the stamina and attitude of the individual, or many other factors. The decision to do massage must be made on an individual basis.

Classifications of Cancer

There are many types of cancer as well as different stages of the disease process. Cancer is defined by type, grade, site, and stage.

The *type* of cancer is determined by the kind of tissue in which the cancer cells begin to develop:

- carcinoma—originates in the epithelial tissue that lines organs and vessels
- myeloma—originates in bone marrow
- sarcoma—originates in the supportive and connective tissues such as muscles, cartilage, and bone
- lymphoma—originates in lymphatic tissue
- leukemia—originates in tissues that form blood cells

Grading involves the examination of tumor cells microscopically that have been harvested through biopsy. The degree of abnormality of the cells determines the grade of the cancer. Grade levels are from 0 to 4, where 0 indicates normal cells and grade 4 indicates highly abnormal, undifferentiated, cancerous cells.

Site refers to the location of the primary tumor and is often reflected in the name describing the cancer. Cancer tumors are usually named after the part of the body where the cancer first began. Its name does not change even if the cancer spreads to another part of the body. For example, if breast cancer spreads (metastasizes) to the lung, it is still named and treated as breast cancer.

Stages of cancer refers to a system of quantifying the status of the primary tumor, the regional lymph node involvement, and the areas of metastasis that uses numerical values to express the extent of involvement of the disease. The treating physician, usually an oncologist, is the best source to obtain information as to the location, type, and extent or probable sites of metastasis of the cancer.

Stage defines the growth of most cancers:

- *Stage I:* Cancer is still small and contained in the original tumor.
- *Stage II:* Cancer has grown and/or spread to nearby lymph nodes.
- *Stage III:* Cancerous cells have spread to regional lymph nodes and/or other tissues in the area.
- *Stage IV:* Cancer is well developed and has spread to other tissues or organs in the body.
- *Recurrent:* Cancer has returned after being treated. It may come back at the original site or another part of the body.

Another classification scheme of staging considers the cancer distribution in terms of primary tumor (T), regional lymph node involvement (N), and extent of metastasis (M). The T component indicates the size and invasiveness of the primary tumor. The N component indicates the absence or extent of invasion of cancer cells in the regional lymph nodes. The M component indicates whether the cancer has spread to other parts of the body.

- Tumor (T)

  T0   No evidence of tumor

  T1–4   Increasing tumor size and involvement
- Node (N)

  NX   Lymph node involvement cannot be assessed

  N0   No evidence of lymph node involvement

  N1–4   Increasing degrees of lymph node involvement
- Metastases (M)

  M0   No evidence of distant metastases

  M1   Evidence of distant metastases

Progression of the Disease

Cancer develops progressively from an alteration in certain cells to uncontrolled growth that invades tissues and organs. Clinically, a person with cancer goes through a succession of experiences as she learns of the disease, makes decisions for treatment, progresses through treatment, and deals with the outcome. Persons with cancer will exhibit different conditions and have varying needs at each level. The phases of progression are:

1. onset
2. diagnosis/pretreatment
3. treatment—surgery, radiation, chemotherapy, alternative, and complementary

4. remission/survivorship

5. advanced terminal/terminal

Choices for massage therapy must be made on a case-by-case basis. A thorough intake procedure, safe practice, and informed client consent become essential.

Intake Procedure for Persons with Cancer

During the intake consultation, a medical history is taken to gather information about the client, the type of cancer, stage of the cancer, the course of treatment (type and timing), the side effects, the names of the treating physicians, as well as the level of health, stamina, and emotional state of the client. Become as informed as possible. Learn about the kind of cancer, where it is located, primary secondary sites (areas where the particular cancer tends to metastasize to), type of treatment, side effects of the treatment, treatment schedule, symptoms of the cancer, and the treatment. Questions that cannot be answered by the client may be referred to the client's doctor. The Internet is also a rich source of information about different types of cancer and treatment (see Box 6.2).

Adjust the Massage to the Client's Health Status

An individual's level of health may vary greatly depending on where the client is in the progression of the disease or treatment. Attitude, stamina, and health status influence the choice of massage treatment.

Adjust the Massage to the Cancer Site

Many cancers have a specific location where there is a tumor, whereas some, such as leukemia or lymphoma, have no specific location. By knowing the location of the cancer, the therapist can avoid circulatory

---

BOX 6.2 IMPORTANT CONSIDERATIONS WHEN CONSIDERING MASSAGE FOR PERSONS WITH CANCER

The type and location of cancer

The stage of progression of the cancer

Possible secondary sites of metastasis

The treatment type and stage

The condition of the immune system

The stamina of the person

The attitude of the person

The belief and desire of the person regarding massage

The purpose of the massage

Therapist's intention and quality of touch

massage or pressure to the local area of the cancer or its possible sites of metastasis. Massage that puts pressure on the site of a tumor is contraindicated due to the concern of dislodging tumor cells. If there is a secondary site where the cancer is suspected to have spread, local and regional massage is contraindicated in that area as well.

Adjust the Massage to the Cancer Treatment

Cancer treatments are often quite invasive and have numerous side effects, many of which must be taken into consideration by the massage therapist. Side effects from cancer intervention may last for days, weeks, or even years after treatments are completed. Massage, when applied with knowledge and understanding, may provide relief for some of the unpleasant treatment side effects. These same treatments and their accompanying side effects are the reason for many massage modifications and contraindications.

Types of Cancer Treatment

After a person receives a diagnosis of cancer, a course of treatment is prescribed. The treatment depends on the type and stage of the cancer and may include one or a combination of the following:

- Surgery
- Chemotherapy
- Radiation
- Bone marrow transplant
- Treatment with other drugs such as steroids, narcotics, and antidepressants
- Complementary and alternative therapies

Surgery

Surgery is often the first intervention in cancer treatment. Generally, the primary tumor and often the local or regional lymph nodes are surgically removed. Recent surgery increases the chance of a blood clot or thrombus forming in a blood vessel such as in a vein in the leg or in the area of the surgery. This is a serious consideration for the massage therapist because circulatory massage could dislodge the clot and it would become a floating embolus in the bloodstream. The embolus would circulate back to the heart and then into the pulmonary arteries where it would eventually lodge in one of the smaller arteries and become a pulmonary embolism, which is a life-threatening condition.

Because of the concern of thrombosis, massage on or around the incisions from surgery is contraindicated. Also massage to the lower limbs is contraindicated for postsurgical patients. Always consult the client's physician to determine when it is safe to massage the lower extremities or the incision after surgery, asking the physician specifically when the danger of thrombosis is past.

The site of the incision is a local contraindication unless the therapist has specific training in working with scar tissue and adhesions and has the physician's approval. Reasons for being a contraindication include: it is the site of a recent tumor; the tissue is actively healing, and there may be clotting; and it may still be inflamed or irritated.

Another postoperative concern is infection, either at the incision site or systemically. The postsurgical client is often in the hospital under close supervision so that any sign of infection is quickly treated. Any areas of infection or inflammation are contraindicated for massage, and the client should be immediately referred to the doctor. A common side effect or symptom of cancer surgery or other treatment is fever. When fever is present, massage is contraindicated.

Surgery often involves the removal of regional lymph nodes that sometimes will cause lymphedema in the limb distal to the missing nodes. Excess fluid fills the interstitial spaces of the limb distal to the affected lymph nodes due to interference in the normal lymph channels. General massage or massage techniques that apply pressure to the affected areas are contraindicated in that they may exacerbate the condition. Only light manual lymph drainage techniques may be employed, and only after consulting with the treating physician.

During the client intake, the therapist should be very thorough in determining the kind of surgery, when it was done, the location and extent, if lymph nodes were removed, and how well the client recovered. When the therapist has formulated a treatment plan, she should check with the treating physician and get an informed consent from the client before proceeding with massage therapy.

Chemotherapy

Chemotherapy uses chemicals usually administered intravenously or orally to kill, sterilize, or weaken the cancer cells so that other chemical or radiation treatments will hopefully eradicate the cancer. Some types of chemotherapy can target specific cancer cells or specific properties of those cells; however, many types of therapies cannot differentiate, so many fast-growing normal cells are affected. Dosages are controlled to obtain the maximum effect on the cancer without overwhelming the normal tissues.

Many side effects of chemotherapy stem from the destruction of the fast-growing cells of the respiratory organs, digestive tract, and bone marrow and include nausea, diarrhea, vomiting, mouth sores, constipation, skin rashes, weight loss, fever, hair loss, reduced white and red blood cell count, reduced platelet count, pain, fatigue, and nervous symptoms such as vertigo and peripheral neuropathy. Each of these side effects has implications for the massage therapist.

Effects from chemotherapy may range from mild to severe with the most difficult time within the first 24 to 72 hours following treatment. General massage during this time may be too taxing, whereas short gentle touch sessions may help reduce muscle tension, anxiety, and nausea.

Clients receiving chemotherapy may have an IV catheter located semipermanently on their body. Care must be taken not to disturb the catheter either with positioning or massage.

When white blood cell counts are low, the immune system is compromised and the client is more vulnerable to infection. Therapists should avoid contact if they or anyone in their close surroundings (family or colleagues) is ill.

If the treatment has reduced the client's platelet count, the client may be prone to bruising or bleeding because platelets control clotting. The therapist may need to adjust the massage to prevent bruising or damaging delicate tissues.

Reduced red blood cell counts cause anemia, which results in fatigue, intolerance to cold, occasional dizziness, and shortness of breath. The therapist should consider keeping the session brief and light to avert fatigue and keep extra blankets handy to avoid chilling the client. Be careful when helping the client up from the table in case of dizziness.

Hair loss or alopecia may or may not be accompanied by irritation on the scalp. This condition must be approached delicately because of the client's body image. It is important to ask the client about any scalp condition and any desire for touch. The client may choose to keep a wig or head covering on during the massage, or the client may want a thorough head massage. Care must be taken to not get lotion or oil on the head covering or hairpiece. Any scalp irritation is a contraindication for massage.

Digestive abnormalities are common with chemotherapy. Nausea and diarrhea contraindicate general circulation massage, especially joint movements and rocking that can cause more queasiness. Light comforting touch or massage to specific areas of discomfort may be very helpful. The location of the nearest restroom should be pointed out to the client just in case the need arises to get there in a hurry.

Chemotherapy may cause skin rashes, dryness, or lesions. It may also cause areas to become supersensitive. These conditions contraindicate local massage. If you massage someone with open, weeping lesions, local and regional massage are contraindicated, and the therapist should wear gloves to prevent contact with fluids that may be present on the sheets, hands, or other parts of the body. It is best to be safe.

Weight loss (cachexia) is common due to chemotherapy and the ravaging effects of later stages of the disease. The loss of adipose and muscle tissue, especially if the patient is confined to bed, increases the possibility of pressure sores. Massage may help prevent pressure sores from forming but is contraindicated on or close to decubitus sores/ulcers. Muscle loss may result in stiff or hypermobile joints. If range of motion (ROM) is used, it must be done carefully and gently. Fatigue and a loss of stamina often accompany weight loss. The massage must be adjusted to support, not tire, the client.

Some forms of chemotherapy may affect the central or peripheral nervous system, causing pain, burning, or tingling sensations. If your client has these symptoms, talk with the client's doctor to determine the cause and what you may do. Peripheral neuropathy, a common side effect, causes numbness, burning, tingling, or pain in the feet and hands. Gentle massage sometimes relieves symptoms; however, deep pressure or any methods that exacerbate the symptoms are contraindicated.

If a person is receiving chemotherapy, the preferred time to receive massage may be before the chemotherapy treatment. Massage given before the invasive treatment may help relieve stress and lower anxiety levels, which may result in less severe reactions to the treatment. Massage may be resumed after the chemotherapy when the side effects have subsided to the point that the individual can easily tolerate touch. Family members may be shown slow stroke back massage and neck and shoulder relaxation massage to assist their loved ones through this difficult time.

Persons with cancer, especially those in treatment, experience increased stress that may result in increased muscle tension accompanied with fatigue and pain. Massage works wonders, when applied within the client's safe practice limits, to alleviate muscle tension and associated symptoms.

Radiation

Radiation therapies usually beam radiation directly at a tumor site in order to either destroy the cancer cells and reduce the tumor size or more often destroy cancer cells' capability to reproduce. The problem is that the cancer cells cannot be singled out and normal tissue cells in the irradiated area are also damaged. In some cases, a larger area or the whole body may be irradiated. In these instances, only the patient is exposed to the radiation, and there is no concern of radiation exposure to the therapist or others. For some types of cancer treatment, an implant or radioactive iodine is used. In these instances, the patient is isolated until the danger of exposure to others is reduced to safe levels.

To help control or aim the radiation, spots are inked or tattooed on the patient's body. These spots are not to be tampered with as long as the patient is undergoing treatment.

Massage for Persons Receiving Radiation

There are no clear massage protocols while an individual is undergoing radiation. Each case must be considered under its own merits. The therapist should consult the treating physician regarding the advisability of working in the area being treated. After a radiation session, the client may experience fatigue and/or nausea, which preclude massage until those symptoms pass. The area being irradiated requires special consideration. The irradiated tissue is very fragile and may continue to degrade for a period of time after the actual treatment, much as a sunburn gets worse even after exposure has ceased. The patient is usually under doctor's orders regarding care of or using lubricants on the affected area. The massage therapist should regard these instructions carefully. Abide by all restrictions regarding touch or lubricants. Avoid working on the area for three to five days or until the burning effects completely subside. If there are any lesions, wait until they are completely healed. Remember, the damaged tissue is not only on the surface. There may be similar conditions at the exit site of the radiation. Local and regional massage is contraindicated to radiation sites. Affected areas of the skin may remain sensitive to heat and pressure long after treatment.

A locally radiated area does not preclude massage on other parts of the body, although the massage may need to be modified to accommodate for other side effects such as nausea or fatigue. In the case of fatigue, modify the massage session in consideration of the stamina of the client by using light, nonintrusive techniques in an abbreviated session. If the client is experiencing nausea, avoid joint movements, rocking, or passive movement techniques that might aggravate the nausea. If the radiation has destroyed any lymph nodes, lymphedema may be a concern. Follow the same guidelines discussed in the previous section on surgery.

Massage seems to be more effective before chemotherapy and radiation treatments because it seems to improve the client's outlook and reduces anxiety. As a result, recovery from the treatment is quicker, and many of the side effects such as fatigue and nausea seem less drastic.

Transplants

Bone marrow and stem cell transplant therapies are some of the most drastic treatments done. They involve whole body radiation followed by transplant surgery so that more rigorous chemotherapy can be done. The patient's health is very compromised. The individual's immune system is weakened, and the person may be in isolation. Total body irradiation may result in extensive skin burns. It is a time when the patient is debilitated and weak from repeated interventions in the attempt to fight the cancer.

Massaging Persons with Cancer

To provide safe and effective massage, the therapist must find out as much about the treatment and the client as possible. Most people in cancer treatment are very knowledgeable about their condition. They will know of any restrictions. If the client is in the acute stage of the disease and in treatment, work closely with the medical team and the client when formulating a treatment plan. The treating physician may provide a massage recommendation or prescription and agree to inform the massage therapist of any changing conditions that may influence the choice of massage treatment.

In this difficult time, massage must be gentle, supportive, and compassionate. The massage session is one of the few times the patient experiences soothing, noninvasive, and pleasurable touch.

Adjust the massage session to the cancer, the treatment, and the client's level of health. Most special considerations have to do with site restrictions, positioning, pressure sensitivity, or stamina. If the client fatigues easily or has a low energy level, adjust the massage accordingly. This can be done by shortening the length of the session, lightening the pressure, and slowing the pace of the massage. How much adjustment is made in these areas depends on the client's condition and needs. Listen to your client, and be there for your client. Careful questioning, observation, and intuition are key to determining a course of action. It is better to do too little than too much. It is not a time to fix anything or further deplete a client's energy, but to provide relaxation, comfort, and ease.

When a treatment plan is developed and discussed with the client along with the potential risks and benefits, the client should sign an informed consent form releasing the therapist from any liability regarding the proliferation of the disease. Then massage, within safe parameters, can proceed. The client makes the decision to proceed; nevertheless, it is wise to do less rather than more.

As people progress deeper into the disease and become more ill, the benefits they receive from massage increase. In hospice settings where patients have a prognosis of less than six months to live, massage has been shown to improve the quality of a person's experience by reducing pain, muscle tension, and anxiety and improving circulation, appetite, sleep, and general comfort. Skilled touch communicates a sense of caring, comfort, and acceptance.

This is a time for nurturing touch. When light Swedish techniques may even be too much, modalities such as Reiki, therapeutic touch, or mild polarity may be used. When working with persons with cancer, they are not the only ones to consider. Spouses and close family members are also under increased stress and can benefit from massage. Many times, family members who are part of the client's support group can be taught simple or specific massage techniques so that they can provide caring touch to the persons with cancer on a more routine basis. This not only provides additional comfort to the client, it also empowers family members by giving them something positive they can do to support their loved one.

There are many conditions during the course of cancer that warrant precautions regarding the application of massage; however, at any stage of the disease, some form of skilled touch provides many benefits welcomed by the person with the disease.

Guidelines for Massaging Persons with Cancer

- Before any massage is given to a new client, a complete medical history is taken.
- The physician/oncologist is consulted, and a recommendation for massage is obtained.
- A treatment plan is developed, and the client is fully informed about the effects of massage therapy before giving informed consent.
- When doing massage, use light to moderate pressure, shorter sessions, and positioning for comfort.
- Deep massage is contraindicated in that it overstresses the body.
- Massage or direct pressure in the local area of the tumor as well as the regional area where affected lymph nodes may reside is contraindicated.
- Avoid circulatory massage at probable secondary metastatic sites.
- Avoid massage treatment in the event of infection or fever.

- Adjust massage according to the current state of client's health:
  - Know the stage of the disease and the client's stamina, attitude, and emotional state.
  - Adjust the type of massage, depth, duration, and speed.
  - Consult with client, caregiver, family, and physician.
- Adjust massage according to the treatment regime.

Table 6.1
Endangerment Sites

ENDANGERMENT SITES	LOCATION	STRUCTURES OF CONCERN
Interior to the ear	Notch posterior to the ramus of the mandible	Facial nerve, external carotid artery, styloid process
Anterior triangle of the neck	Bordered by the mandible, sternocleidomastoid muscle, and the trachea	Carotid artery, internal jugular vein, vagus nerve, lymph nodes
Posterior triangle of the neck	Bordered by the sternocleidomastoid muscle, the trapezius muscle, and the clavicle	Brachial plexus, subclavian artery, brachiocephalic vein, external jugular vein, and lymph nodes
Axilla	Armpit	Axillary, median, musculocutaneous and ulnar nerves, axillary artery, axillary nerve, and lymph nerves
Medial Brachium	Upper inner arm between the biceps and triceps	Ulnar, musculocutaneous and median nerves, brachial artery, basilic vein, and lymph nodes
Cubital area of the elbow	Anterior bend of the elbow	Median nerve, radial and ulnar arteries, median cubital vein
Ulnar notch of the elbow	The funny bone	Ulnar nerve
Femoral triangle	Bordered by the sartorius muscle, the adductor longus muscle, and the inguinal ligament	Femoral nerve, femoral artery, femoral vein, great saphenous vein, and lymph nodes
Popliteal fossa	Posterior aspect of the knee	Bordered by the gastrocnemius (inferior) and the hamstrings (superior and to the sides); tibial nerve, common peroneal nerve, popliteal artery, popliteal vein
Abdomen	Upper area of the abdomen under the the ribs	Right side, liver and gallbladder; Left side, spleen; Deep center, aorta
Upper lumbar area	Just inferior to the ribs and lateral to the spine	Kidneys (avoid heavy percussion)

- Consult with medical personnel.

- Consider the client's state of fatigue, nausea, and well-being.

- Be aware of chemotherapy concerns—low blood counts, white cell, red cell, platelet; IV ports.

- Be aware of radiation concerns—skin rashes and burns, hair loss, tissue fragility, infection, fatigue.

- Be aware of surgery concerns—increased chance of blood clots, hemorrhage, thrombosis; avoid massage on site of incision; specialized scar massage may be started in four to six weeks, after approval from doctor.

- Be aware of a client's impaired awareness to pain or sensory loss—may be due to disease-related neurological damage, pharmaceuticals, depression, surgery, or near-death withdrawal. Proceed with caution.

- Adjust your treatments to best serve the client—obtain client feedback from previous sessions along with current needs to adapt the session to best serve the client's needs.

ENDANGERMENT SITES

Certain areas of the body warrant consideration when being massaged because of the underlying anatomical structures. Because of the possibility of injury to the structures by certain massage manipulations, these areas are sites of potential endangerment. In most of these areas, major nerves, blood vessels, or vital organs are relatively exposed and vulnerable to deep manipulations or direct pressure. Table 6.1 presents a list of the endangerment sites, their location, and the anatomical structures of concern.

QUESTIONS FOR DISCUSSION AND REVIEW

1. What are the main physiological benefits of massage?

2. What are the main psychological benefits of massage?

3. What are the two physical ways massage affects the body?

4. Which body systems are said to benefit from regular therapeutic massage?

5. In what way does the muscular system benefit from massage?

6. What massage movements promote circulation in muscles?

7. How does massage relieve sore and stiff muscles?

8. What massage technique prevents the formation of adhesions and fibrosis in muscles?

9. What are the immediate effects of massage on the skin?

10. How does massage affect the nervous system?

11. What massage movements have a stimulating effect on the nervous system?

12. What massage techniques have a sedative effect on the nervous system?

13. What is the effect of massage on the circulatory system?

14. Why are all massage movements directed toward the heart?

15. Which massage movements increase the flow of blood and lymph?

16. In what way does improved circulation of the blood benefit the skin?

17. When should massage be avoided?

18. What is the meaning of contraindication as it relates to massage?

19. Why does the practitioner need to take the client's medical history?

20. Why should the therapist keep a fever thermometer on the premises?

21. What should the practitioner do when a client has a condition that appears to be a contraindication to massage?

22. What are the signs of inflammation?

23. How should massage be applied in the case of local inflammation?

24. How do you recognize varicose veins?

25. What is a hematoma and how is it massaged?

26. How does massage benefit a woman during a normal, healthy pregnancy?

27. How does massage benefit an individual who is critically ill?

28. How is the HIV/AIDS virus transmitted from person to person?

29. Why is massage contraindicated for people with cancer?

30. What are some of the benefits of massage for people with cancer?

31. How can the practitioner reduce the chances of promoting metastasis when massaging people with cancer?

32. What are the stages of cancer?

33. What are the common treatments for cancer?

34. What are some important considerations when determining to massage people with cancer?

35. When a person is receiving chemotherapy or radiation, when is a good time for them to receive massage and why?

36. What modifications can be made to massage for a client who tends to fatigue easily?

37. Why are certain areas of the body sites of potential endangerment?

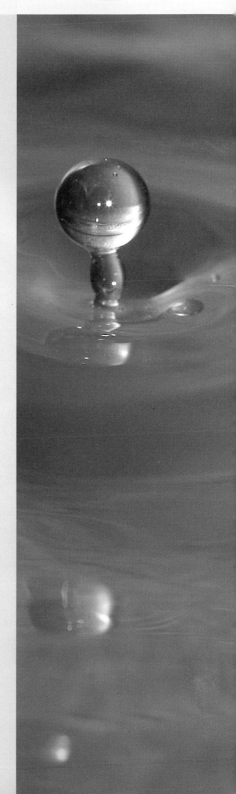

Equipment and Products

LEARNING OBJECTIVES

After you have mastered this chapter, you will be able to:

1. Prepare a checklist of supplies and equipment needed for therapeutic massage.

2. Describe various products and their use.

3. Select a massage table.

4. Check and adjust lighting for the massage room.

5. Check all equipment for safety and readiness.

INTRODUCTION

The practice of therapeutic massage is a part of the health care profession. It is important that a practitioner present herself in a professional and friendly manner at all times. Professionalism is an attitude that is manifested in yourself and your business. Your clients will expect you to project a professional image by your speech, your appearance, your courtesy, and your good manners. Technical competence and the ability to express yourself are also professional ingredients. A massage practitioner should project an image of confidence and yet be relaxed.

Generally, a client coming for a massage anticipates a relaxing, rejuvenating experience. In order to provide such an experience, a number of conditions are desirable, if not necessary. The professional and friendly manner in which the practitioner presents herself will provide a certain confidence to the client. The appearance and atmosphere of the massage facility will affect the client's overall response. Cleanliness, a sense of order, and sanitation are essential factors. Comfortable yet professional furnishings will add to the client's confidence. Privacy and the absence of distractions or interruptions are important considerations. The facilities in which you work should reflect a professional appearance yet at the same time be comfortable and relaxing.

When considering the comfort of the client, adequate heat, ventilation, and indirect lighting are important. Relaxing music is an option that many practitioners employ. An awareness of the factors that enhance the massage experience enables the practitioner to incorporate these factors when planning her facilities.

YOUR PLACE OF BUSINESS

The location of your massage business is an important consideration and will be discussed extensively in Chapter 19. The image of your place of business makes an impression on your massage clients and therefore must be considered when establishing a business.

A national survey of massage practitioners conducted by Knapp and Associates in 1990 indicates that approximately one third of massage therapists operate a private practice out of their home, one third from a private office or clinic, and the remaining third practice in another facility such as a health club, resort, health professional's office or salon, or the like. More recent surveys conducted in 2002 show nearly identical numbers. Regardless of the location of the business, the internal environment of the facility reflects directly on the impression the client will have of the therapist and of the services the therapist offers.

Clients coming into your place of business will be influenced by the environment and the people with whom they come in contact. The decor should be professional yet comfortable, clean yet not sterile, relaxed and free of distractions and safety hazards. In a massage establishment, space should be allotted for the exclusive practice of massage. Although this is necessary for a client's privacy and comfort, it also gives a more professional image. Some practitioners go to their clients' homes in addition to or rather than maintaining a studio and office space. The equipment used, as well as the appearance and actions of the therapist, when doing in-home massage or outcalls to an office, hotel, or other facility directly reflect on the perception of the client. Whether the massage facility is in the practitioner's home, the client's home, or a separate office, standards of cleanliness, safety, and professionalism must be observed.

Sanitation and Safety in Your Workplace

Whether working in a small salon or studio with little space or a large, luxurious spa, the space and equipment must be kept clean and neat. The massage facility and the equipment should be checked regularly to eliminate situations that may cause injury to the therapist or client. Passageways must be kept clear. Surfaces and linens must be sanitized and equipment checked against failure. The main concern is the protection of the client's health and comfort. (See Chapter 8, "Sanitary and Safety Practices," for more on this important topic.)

Equipment and Supplies

Depending on the extent and dimensions of the massage business, the specific equipment and supplies that are necessary or preferred will vary somewhat. However, there are a number of items that are essential to a smooth and efficient massage business operation. The actual practice of giving a massage requires the use of certain equipment and supplies. The manner of conducting consultations, record keeping, and other business operations will somewhat dictate related equipment and materials. Whether or not hydrotherapy and bathing are available in the practice will influence the selection of equipment and related supplies.

The setting of a massage operation will also influence the selection of equipment and supplies. A massage business that is operated out of a home will vary from a massage concession on a cruise ship or the athletic massage offered to a professional sports team. Most massage operations have some consistent needs. For the purpose of this chapter, consider an independent massage practitioner operating out of the home or a small office.

There are generally three areas of operation or activity in a massage business: the massage area, the business area, and the bathroom or hydrotherapy area. The massage area is where the client actually receives the massage treatment. Often in a small operation, the massage area is also where the client disrobes and gets dressed. The massage area must be of an adequate size for the necessary equipment and for the practitioner to move around comfortably to perform the massage.

The business area is where the practitioner keeps records, does consultations, answers the telephone, and carries out other business activities related to the massage practice. All this may take place in the massage room or in an adjacent room, or the activities may be divided so that some things such as client records and consultations happen in close proximity to the massage area and other activities take place elsewhere.

Every massage area must have access to a clean restroom. Massage tends to stimulate kidney activity. It is not possible to relax when one needs to relieve one's bladder or bowels. Ideally there should be a place for the client to shower or bathe before the massage. The restroom also provides a facility for the practitioner to wash his hands before and after each massage.

Ancillary services to the actual massage vary widely. The availability of such services as steam baths, showers, exercise facilities, hot packs, or hot baths will affect the procedures the client follows preceding and following the massage. If the ancillary services are part of the massage operation, the required equipment and related supplies will be dictated by the services offered.

Equipment and supplies should be checked frequently to be sure they are in proper condition and that enough are on hand.

Each booth or room should have the appropriate furnishings and equipment for the treatments to be given. All equipment should be checked regularly for fitness and safety. All supplies must be kept in a clean, sanitized condition. Supplies such as oils, linens, and paper products should be selected and ready before the client enters the booth or room.

Below are general lists of equipment and supplies for the different areas. The lists may not include many optional items, especially in the ancillary areas. Examine the lists and add items you feel would enhance your massage business.

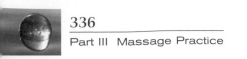

The Massage Area

Massage table

Stool

Supply storage cabinet

   Facial tissues

   Cotton-tipped swabs

   Sterilizing agents

   Alcohol or other sterilizing agents

   Analgesic oil or gel

Bolsters or pillows (face cushion)

Linens (an adequate supply)

   Sheets and towels for draping

   Pillow and bolster covers

Blankets, wraps, and/or robes

Lubricants, oils, creams,
   powders, and liniments

Dressing area (privacy space
   with chair, hangers, and
   wraps)

Indirect lighting

Desk or table and chair
   Record cards and supplies

Clock

Covered waste basket

The Business Operation Area

Desk and chairs

Business telephone and
  answering machine

Appointment book

Filing system

Stationery and stamps

Pencils, pens, stapler, tape, etc.

Bathroom/Bathing Area

Antibacterial soap

Paper hand towels

Clean bath towels for each client

Robes or wraps

Shampoo and bath soap

Disposable water cups

Hydrotherapy Area

Hydrotherapy equipment
  and related supplies

Towels and robes

THE MASSAGE ROOM

Studio Space

A massage room needs to be a minimum of 10 feet wide and 12 feet long. This allows enough space for all necessary equipment as well as enough room to move around the massage table. It also allows space for a desk, chair, and supply table or cabinet. A stool is also a handy item to have in the massage room, because there are times when the practitioner can sit down while working on the client's neck, face, feet, or hands. Sitting for a few minutes can give much needed rest when working long hours (Figure 7.1).

Temperature of the Massage Room

The temperature of the massage room should be comfortable. The room should be warm enough that the client does not chill. If the client becomes chilled, it is very hard for him to relax. About 72° F is warm enough for most clients and at the same time is cool enough to keep the practitioner from getting uncomfortably warm while working. The room should be warmed in advance because it is easy for the client to become chilled, especially after oil or lotion has been applied to the skin. In a room that is cooler, auxiliary blankets, electric mattress pads, or other heating devices must be used to ensure the client's warmth.

The massage room must be well ventilated. Performing a massage requires considerable exertion on the part of the practitioner. For proper relaxation, the client needs a good supply of fresh air. With poor ventilation, the room would become stuffy, and the air may acquire an offensive odor. Proper ventilation ensures an abundant supply of fresh air.

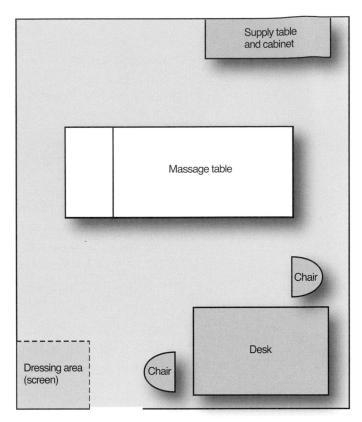

Figure 7.1

The minimum size for a massage room is about 10 by 12 feet. This allows room for a table, desk, chairs, supply cabinet, and room to move around the table to perform the massage.

Lighting

It is difficult for either the practitioner or the client to be comfortable when the lighting in the room is harsh and glaring. In addition, colored lights such as red or blue can make the client feel uncomfortable. Reflective or soft, natural light is preferred. Dimmer switches enable you to change the light easily. Avoid direct overhead lighting or any light that could shine directly into the client's eyes (Figure 7.2).

Use of Music

A stereo and supply of soothing music may provide another dimension to a relaxing massage. Although you may like music playing while you work, you must remember that some people find it distracting and prefer absolute quiet. You may wish to have a selection of soothing music available and ask the client what he prefers. If there is outside noise that may be distracting, music will mask it. Obviously, you should not attempt to match the rhythm of massage movements to the tempo of the music.

The Massage Table

As a massage therapist, one of your most important possessions will be a massage table that fits your needs. Your massage table is your main piece of equipment and, next to your hands, the most important regarding

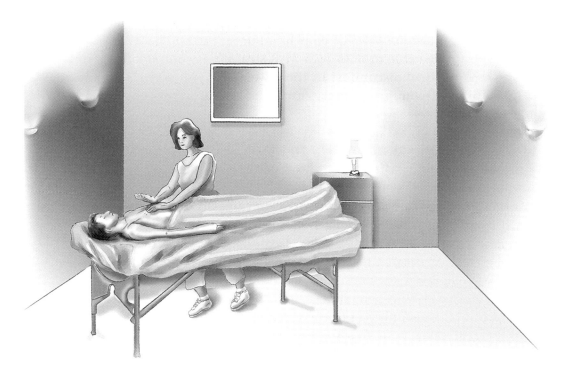

Figure 7.2

Avoid direct overhead lighting in the massage room. Soft natural light from a shaded window or indirect light from wall or table lamps is preferred.

your comfort and that of your clients. One of your concerns should be that the table is stable, firm, and comfortable. If you will be working in an office or studio, a stationary table may be your best choice. If your situation is temporary, or if you prefer the freedom of taking your equipment with you, choose a good portable table. If you travel to do massage, the table must be portable and light enough for you to carry. Regardless of your choice, check the construction carefully. The table should not shake, rock, or squeak. Seldom will new equipment display these problems, but you must consider what will happen after the table has been used for several hundred treatments.

A massage table allows you to move about or to change positions easily and when necessary, without breaking the rhythm of the massage movements.

The optimum height of the massage table is dependent on a number of factors, including the kind or style of massage being done, the height of the practitioner, the size of the client, and the personal preferences of the practitioner. The table must be the right height to give you the leverage needed and to prevent fatigue of your back, neck, arms, and shoulders. The height of the table is determined by your height so that you are not at a disadvantage when reaching and applying pressure. A good indicator for the proper height of a massage table is to stand in an erect yet relaxed manner and measure the distance from the floor to the styloid process on the ulnar (little finger) side of your forearm. This is approximately the optimum height for the table. Another way to test the height of a table is to place the palm of your hand flat on the table. While doing this, you should be able to hold your arm straight at your side. If, after a few sessions you feel discomfort in the lower back, the table is probably too low. If the discomfort is in the upper back, shoulders, or arms, the table is probably too high.

Several stationary and portable models have legs that can be adjusted up or down by removing and replacing wing nuts or thumbscrews. These are advantageous if people of different heights use the same table, or if various techniques used require different table heights. Some stationary tables have a height adjustment button and are operated by hydraulic force or electricity. Though costly, this type of table is very useful when dealing with the elderly or disabled, who might have difficulty getting on a table of normal height, or when several different practitioners use the same table.

The width of a massage table is approximately 28 inches with an additional inch allowed for padding, or approximately 29 inches wide. Tables narrower than 27 inches do not give enough arm support for large clients. Tables wider than 30 inches become awkward when the practitioner is required to reach to the opposite side of the client. The width of the table is somewhat dependent on the height of the practitioner. A taller practitioner will find it somewhat easier to reach across a wider table and easier to carry a wider portable table when it is folded.

A good length for a massage table is about 76 inches. Most tables are about 68 to 72 inches long, which may be too short for tall clients. The padding on the massage table should be firm so that pressure applied by the practitioner to the client is absorbed by the client's body and not pushed into the table. About 1 to 2 inches of high-density foam is the best material to use. Padding should extend beyond the edge of the framework of the table by about half an inch all around to ensure the comfort of the client, who might place a hand or foot over the edge. A good quality vinyl is the best covering for the massage table because it is durable and easy to keep clean. To care for high-quality vinyl, clean it regularly with a mild detergent. Avoid extended contact with massage or body oils, alcohol, or chlorine bleach. These substances cause the vinyl to become brittle and crack. Use a carrying case when transporting portable tables and try to avoid extreme temperatures. If the table gets either extremely hot or cold—because it has been stored in a car, for instance—allow the vinyl to return to room temperature before using.

Tables come in a variety of designs. Often the bed of a massage treatment table will fold up or down in a variety of configurations. This is to accommodate specific therapy situations and may be of no use to the general massage practitioner. An exception is the headpiece that adjusts up or down to alleviate cervical strain. Accommodations for the face may be in the form of a hole in the end of the table or a padded extension to the end of the table. These additions allow the client to lie face down with the cervical spine straight, taking the strain off the neck and upper back.

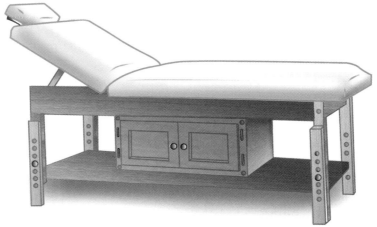

Studio table with adjustable head piece.

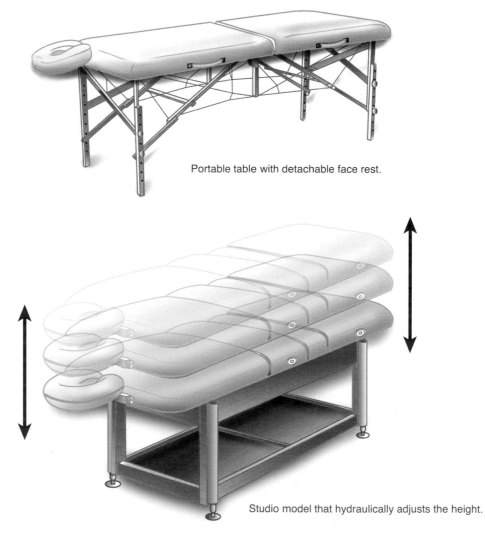

Portable table with detachable face rest.

Studio model that hydraulically adjusts the height.

Figure 7.3

Massage tables come in a variety of styles.

Some massage tables include a number of accessories, like a face cradle. The face cradle is a valuable addition for the comfort of the client. Many tables have face cradles that adjust to a number of positions to ensure comfort (Figure 7.3). Some tables include side extensions to support the arms of larger clients. Another valuable accessory for your portable massage table is a carrying case to protect the table when transporting it from one location to another. Besides protecting the table, the carrying case has extra handles and straps to make lifting and carrying the table easier. Many cases also have a large pocket for carrying linens and supplies.

The table is the massage therapist's main piece of equipment. A professionally designed massage table is recommended. There are several reputable table manufacturers in the United States. Tables from these companies tend to be good tables. Most companies have a range of prices depending on accessories, such as adjustable face rest, special covering, or extra foam cushion. Some companies even sell kits so that the customers can assemble their own table. A few companies have a variety of tables such as portable tables, studio tables, and hydraulic tables. In looking through publications such as the *Massage Magazine* or *Massage Therapy Journal,* the student or practitioner can glean information and phone numbers from numerous table manufacturers.

Regardless of the company or the price of the table you select, there are several factors to keep in mind when choosing a table. They include but are not limited to;

- Adjustable legs
- Face rest (some adjustability is a benefit)
- Vinyl covering (for easy cleaning)
- Easy setup and take-down
- Stability and durability
- Carrying case (for easy carrying and for protection)
- Good warranty

Bolsters and Pillows

To position a client comfortably on the massage table, it is helpful to have a variety of supportive devices such as pillows and bolsters. Bolsters come in a variety of sizes and shapes. They may be round, half-round, rectangular, or specially shaped to support a particular part of the body. Specially manufactured body support systems are available. Six- or 8-inch round bolsters, made of foam and covered with vinyl, that are nearly as long as the table is wide are very common. These are placed under the client's knees when he is face up or under the ankles when he is face down in order to reduce the strain in his lower back. It is important that the vinyl does not come in contact with the client's skin. The bolster can be slipped either under the sheet covering the table or into a pillowcase.

Vinyl-covered bolsters can be cleaned with the same mild detergent used to clean the massage table.

It is also a good idea to keep three or four bed pillows on hand for special positioning situations such as side-lying positions or for extra support under the abdomen or head. Pillowcases on pillows and bolsters must be changed between clients.

Massage Linens

In the practice of massage, linens are used to cover the massage table, the client, the face cradle, bolsters, and pillows. The type of services offered and the style of draping used will determine what linens are needed. Single-sized (twin) fitted or flat sheets can be used as table coverings. Single-sized (twin) flat sheets, bath sheets, beach towels, large- or regular-sized bath towels can be used as drapes for clients. Pillowcases are used for pillows and possibly for bolsters. Washcloths, hand towels, pillowcases, or specially made covers may be used on face cradles.

Clean linens are used for every client. The amount or number of linens needed will depend on the number of clients seen in a day and how often laundry is done. If laundry is done daily, there should be enough linens to last for two days. If laundry is done weekly, there should be enough linens to last one and a half to two weeks.

Popular fabrics for sheets include percale, cotton, cotton blends, and flannel. White, light pastels, and pale floral prints launder and tolerate bleach well. Darker colors tend to fade and show oil stains. When linens become stained, see-through, or threadbare, they should be replaced. Some oil manufacturers sell products that effectively remove oil stains and odors from linens.

Some practitioners prefer to use towels or a combination of towels and sheets for draping. A variety of towel sizes may be used. A bath sheet or large beach towel can be used as a top cover. A large bath towel may be used in combination with a top sheet to hold it in place or as a partial drape. A small bath towel is used as an upper torso (breast) drape. If the service includes bathing facilities, extra towels must be available for drying.

Besides sheets, towels, and pillowcases, the practitioner should keep a couple of light flannel, cotton, or wool blankets on hand for situations to prevent the client from being chilled. The blanket is used over the top of the usual draping to provide extra warmth, security, and comfort. Even though the blankets do not come into direct contact with the client, they should be of a material that is easy to launder occasionally.

Massage Lubricants

Good quality lubricants are some of the practitioner's most important products. The primary purpose for using lubricants is to reduce the friction between the practitioner's hands and the client's skin. The choice of lubricant depends on the style of massage, the needs of the client, and the preference of the practitioner. The practitioner may choose a lotion, cream, or massage oil. Massage oils are the most commonly used lubricant. There is such a wide variety of massage lubricants available from a number of manufacturers and distributors that it may be difficult to choose the powders, oils, creams, or lotions you will want to stock. Quality is important.

Mineral oils are not recommended for massage because they are a petroleum-based product and tend to dry the skin and clog the pores. A combination of vegetable-based oils such as coconut, sweet almond, apricot, olive, peanut, sesame, grape seed, or sunflower oils are mild and easy to work with and provide natural nutrients to the skin. A pleasant combination is coconut and almond oils. Some clients or practitioners may be allergic to nut products and therefore sensitive to oils such as almond. It is important to use fresh oil, because rancid oil has a strong offensive odor. If oil remains on sheets and sets for a while, it will saturate the fibers and develop an offensive odor.

Oils, creams, and lotions have different qualities. Lotions provide a more limited glide that decreases as the area is worked. Most lotions absorb into the skin, become sticky, and provide nutrients to the skin. Lotions are often the choice of deep tissue practitioners because they allow penetration without irritation. Because it does absorb into the skin so readily, lotion may need to be reapplied often.

Massage creams are being offered by more specialty manufacturers as an alternative to massage oil. Massage creams often provide special properties that may stimulate, sooth, warm, cool, or provide special nutrients to the area being massaged. Massage creams are often less oily, may be water based instead of oil based, and have gliding properties similar to oils, but creams are usually considerably more expensive.

As a therapist, experiment with different products until you find the ones that you and your clients prefer. After you have found your preference, it is more economical to buy in larger quantities. If you buy oil in bulk, some should be transferred to smaller bottles. These bottles should be kept filled to the top because it is the air space in the bottle that causes the oil to become rancid. When oil does not have a pleasant smell but is not rancid, a few drops of oil of lemon, clove, cinnamon, musk, or some other essential oil may be added. Usually a few drops of concentrate to a cup of oil will be enough to give a hint of scent. Use scented oils cautiously. Clients may be sensitive to, may be allergic to, or simply do not like certain fragrances. When an oil or cream is being used as a carrier for an essential oil as an aromatherapy treatment, the oils should be mixed specifically for the client at the time of application. Oils and concentrated fragrances can be purchased from supply houses or are usually available at drugstores. Some practitioners like to mix their oils and then place them in unbreakable, easy-to-handle bottles with dispenser tops. This prevents spillage (Figure 7.4). All lubricants must be kept in and dispersed from containers in a manner that prevents contamination.

Some clients may have very oily skin or may not tolerate oil. For these clients, a light powder such as cornstarch may be preferred. Even though powder does not provide the lubrication you get with oil, the same

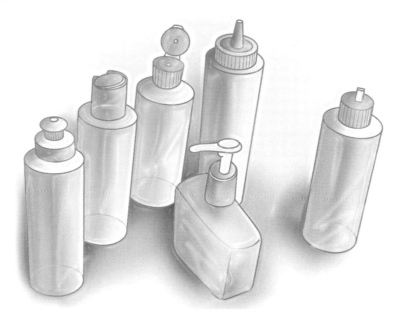

Figure 7.4

Oil bottles with a variety of dispenser tops.

massage movements can be done effectively with powder, and some clients prefer powder. You must avoid inhaling talc when using it for massage.

There are excellent creams and lotions on the market. Always read the label to be sure that you know the product's ingredients and that it is safe to use for massage. It is a good idea to have on hand a dictionary of cosmetic ingredients so that you can look up unfamiliar words. When possible, consult a pharmacist or dermatologist. The federal Food and Drug Administration (FDA) endeavors to control the distribution of products that contain harmful substances. However, what may be harmless to the majority of people may cause an allergic reaction in someone with a sensitivity to a particular substance. During the consultation or before applying a substance to the face or body, it is best to determine whether the client is allergic to any substance. When in doubt, give a patch test before proceeding with the application.

To give a patch test, first wash the area of the inner bend of the elbow with mild soap and warm water. Rinse the area, and then apply a small amount of the product to the skin. Allow 15 to 30 minutes to see whether there is a reaction such as signs of itching, inflammation, and sensitivity, or a stinging sensation. If so, do not use the product. If there are no signs of inflammation or the aforementioned sensations, the product is considered mild enough to use. If the client does begin to have a reaction to a lubricant—for instance, the skin where the lubricant was applied becomes inflamed—immediately remove all lubricant with soap and water. The client can then decide to discontinue the massage or to continue using a different lubricant. Unfortunately, most reactions happen several hours after the application and after the client leaves the facility.

Some people with allergies to fragrances and other cosmetic substances may need to have a patch test given 24 hours before a treatment. In such cases, the client will usually be under the care of a physician, who can give guidance on which products to use and which to avoid. Clients who are sensitive to some products may prefer to supply their own lubricants. There are lubricants on the market that are labeled "hypoallergenic." These products have been tested and found safe for most people even if they do have sensitivities. It is good practice to have some hypoallergenic products on hand to use in situations where clients have known sensitivities to commonly used products.

Most nonprescription products are considered safe for the general public. Most practitioners keep a variety of lubricants on hand to better serve the needs and wishes of their clients. Alcohol is kept available for sanitation purposes. It is also used to remove excess oil from the client's skin following massage, before the client dresses.

QUESTIONS FOR DISCUSSION AND REVIEW

1. What kind of an image should a massage practitioner project to clientele?

2. What are some important considerations when preparing a space to do massage?

3. Approximately how much space is optimal for a massage space?

4. Why should equipment and supplies be inspected periodically?

5. Why is it important to prepare a checklist of supplies and equipment?

6. What kinds of products are usually used for body massage?

7. What is the approximate temperature for the massage room?

8. Why is it important to be able to adjust the height of the massage table?

9. What type of lighting is preferred in the massage room?

10. Why should the client be asked about background music?

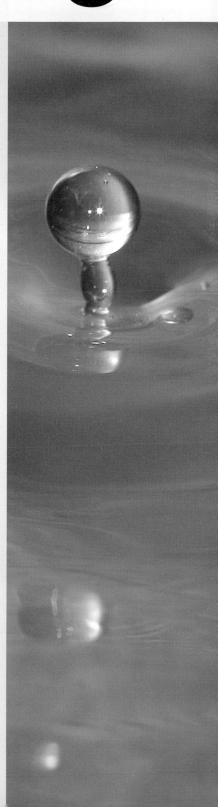

Sanitary and Safety Practices

LEARNING OBJECTIVES

After you have mastered this chapter, you will be able to:

1. Explain the need for laws that enforce the strict practice of sanitation.

2. Sanitize implements and other items used in massage procedures.

3. Explain the difference between pathogenic and nonpathogenic bacteria.

4. Explain the importance of cleanliness of person and of surroundings as protection against the spread of disease.

5. Explain how various disinfectants, antiseptics, and other products are used most effectively.

6. Explain the role of safety in the massage therapy business.

INTRODUCTION

The everyday practice of sanitation and safety is the activity of protecting yourself and your clientele against injury or disease. An awareness of hazardous conditions and the elimination of those situations will prevent an injury before it occurs. Likewise the implementation of sanitary practices to curtail the spread of infectious agents will reduce or eliminate the possibility of you or a client becoming ill as a result of "picking up a bug" at your place of business.

It is the practitioner's responsibility to provide a safe and sanitary facility. The client depends on and expects this service and is not likely to return to a facility that is unsanitary, cluttered, or unsafe.

In recent years, great progress has been made in the control and prevention of disease. In the medical profession, sanitation and sterilization are required procedures that are taken for granted. Every state has laws that make the practice of sanitation mandatory for the protection of public health. In the personal service professions, every precaution must be taken to protect the health of clients as well as the health of practitioners. The nature of the personal service business determines the procedures for the extent of sanitation and sterilization. For example, in the cosmetology profession, a comb or brush used on one client may not be used on another until it has been thoroughly cleansed and sterilized. The esthetician (skin care specialist) must apply products only with sterilized applicators. The massage practitioner may not use the same kinds of implements or have need for the same sanitation procedures; however, appropriate and recommended procedures must be followed diligently.

The massage practitioner need not be a biologist to have some understanding of transmission of disease and to be aware of the importance of impeccable cleanliness at all times. Contagious diseases, skin infections, and other problems can be caused by the transfer of infectious material by unclean hands and nails and by unsanitary equipment and supplies. Therefore, the primary concern is that any item (for example, linens, apparatus) that comes in contact with the client is clean and sanitary. The practitioner's hands must be sanitized by washing with soap (preferably an antibacterial soap) and warm water before touching each client. The premises must also be clean at all times.

PATHS OF DISEASE AND INFECTION

The cause or source of disease may be genetic, metabolic, the result of a deficiency, due to a cancerous condition, or due to an infectious agent. Infectious diseases are caused by minute living organisms called pathogens. Disease-causing pathogens may be transmitted from an infected host to a new host either directly or indirectly in a number of ways. To infect a new host, a pathogen must make contact with (contaminate) and then find entry into (infect) the organism. Pathogens gain entry to the body in a variety of ways that can be called paths of infection or paths of transmission. Certain pathogens must enter the body in a specific manner for the body to become infected. Common paths of infection include ingestion, inhalation, direct contact with mucous membranes, skin contact, and invasion through broken skin. Contaminated food or water can contain organisms or parasites that cause illness, including food poisoning, giardia, hepatitis, typhoid, ringworm, and others. Respiratory infections are often the result of inhaling tiny airborne pathogens by simply being in close proximity to a contagious individual who is coughing, sneezing, or simply talking. The airborne pathogens are inhaled into the respiratory tract and infect the mucous membranes of the upper tract or the more delicate tissues of the lungs. Mucous membranes of the sexual organs are the site of sexually transmitted diseases by either direct contact with infected tissue (herpes, warts) or with bodily fluids (syphilis, gonorrhea, HIV).

Healthy skin is a major defense against the invasion of pathogens. However, contact with certain infectious agents can cause an infection or exacerbate conditions like fungal infections, scabies, poison ivy, or poison oak. When the surface of the skin is broken, the possibility of pathogenic invasion increases drastically. Cuts and wounds must be cleaned, covered, and cared for so that they do not become infected.

The massage practitioner is most concerned with infectious diseases that spread via the transmission of pathogens. Pathogens commonly encountered in the massage practice include bacteria, viruses, and fungi.

Bacteria are minute, unicellular microorganisms exhibiting both plant and animal characteristics. They are also called *germs* or *microbes* and are most numerous in dirt, refuse, unclean water, and diseased tissues. Bacteria exist on the skin, in the air, in body secretions, underneath the free edges of the nails, and elsewhere. There are hundreds of different kinds of bacteria that can only be seen under a microscope. Bacteria are classified as either *nonpathogenic* (harmless) or *pathogenic* (harmful). Nonpathogenic bacteria, the beneficial and harmless type, are the most numerous and perform useful functions, such as aiding the digestive process and other bodily functions. (Figure 8.1).

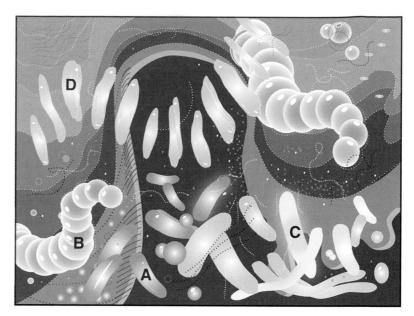

Figure 8.1

A variety of nonpathogenic bacteria thrive in the large intestine: (A) bacteroides, (B) peptostreptococcus, (C) lactobacillus, (D) eubacterium.

Pathogenic bacteria, though not as numerous, are of greater concern to us because they produce disease. Parasites belong to this group because they require living matter for their growth and reproduction. We are primarily concerned with understanding and identifying pathogenic bacteria in order to deal with them more effectively. Figure 8.2 shows the three general forms of bacteria: *cocci* (**KOCK**-sigh), *bacilli* (ba-**SIL**-eye), and *spirilla* (spy-**RIL**-uh). To the right of the name and shape of the bacteria are listed the types of bacteria and the common diseases or conditions with which they are associated (Figure 8.2 to Figure 8.5).

A **virus** is defined as any of a class of submicroscopic pathogenic agents that are capable of transmitting disease. Viruses are parasitic in that they thrive only within the cells of a living host (plant, animal, or human). They invade living cells and control their activity to produce

virus
is class of submicroscopic pathogenic agents that transmit disease.

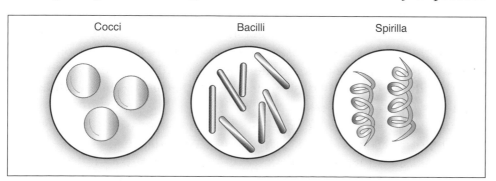

Figure 8.2

Three general forms of bacteria.

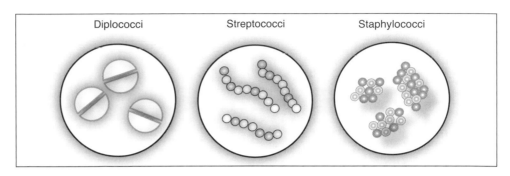

Figure 8.3

Groupings of bacteria.

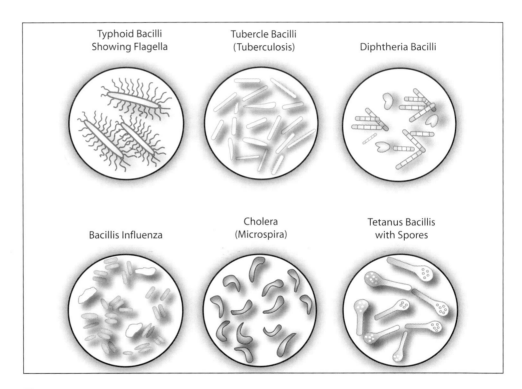

Figure 8.4

Six disease-producing bacteria.

more viruses, often along with toxic substances (Figure 8.6). The cell dies and releases the viruses to invade other cells. A virus may act as an antigen and cause the system to produce antibodies. The virus often has the ability to change its characteristics quickly, which makes viral infections hard to treat by chemical means. Viruses are the cause of many diseases such as the common cold, smallpox, some forms of pneumonia, and childhood diseases like mumps and measles. A virus is also the causative agent for AIDS.

Fungi are parasitic organisms that thrive in a warm, moist environment and are found mostly in humans on the skin and mucous membranes. Molds and yeasts are considered fungi. Fungal infections tend to be tenacious and resist treatment. Common fungal infections include athlete's foot, ringworm, candida, and vaginal yeast infections.

fungus (pl. fungi)

is a diverse group of organisms potentially capable of causing disease that thrive or grow in wet or damp areas.

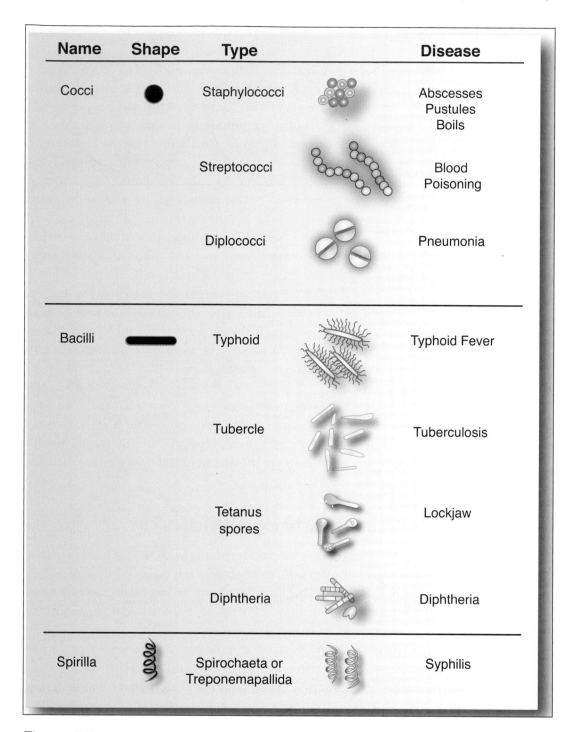

Name	Shape	Type		Disease
Cocci	●	Staphylococci		Abscesses Pustules Boils
		Streptococci		Blood Poisoning
		Diplococci		Pneumonia
Bacilli	▬	Typhoid		Typhoid Fever
		Tubercle		Tuberculosis
		Tetanus spores		Lockjaw
		Diphtheria		Diphtheria
Spirilla	𖤘	Spirochaeta or Treponemapallida		Syphilis

Figure 8.5

Pathogenic (harmful) bacteria and the common diseases or conditions with which they are associated.

Pathogens become a menace to health when they are able to invade the body. Immunity is the body's natural ability to resist infection by harmful bacteria after they have entered the body. Healthy people are able to resist infection better than those with low resistance. Healthy skin is one of the body's most important defenses against invasion of harmful pathogens. Fine hairs in the nostrils, mucous membranes, and tears in

Figure 8.6
Schematic of virus replication.

the eyes also help to defend against pathogens. Inflammation (redness and swelling) is a sign that white blood cells, or leukocytes, are working to destroy harmful microorganisms that have invaded the body. The body also produces antibodies, which inhibit or destroy harmful bacteria. **Antibodies** are a class of proteins produced in the body in response to contact with antigens (toxins, enzymes, etc.) that serve to immunize the body against specific antigens.

The massage practitioner must take special precaution with a client who has a contagious disease or infection and suggest that the client see a physician. The practitioner also has a duty to protect her own health. For example, the practitioner's hands may pick up bacteria from the client's skin. If hands are not cleaned, bacteria can be spread.

The best protection against the spread of disease is to keep yourself and your surroundings clean and sanitary. Maintaining high standards of cleanliness requires constant supervision. Board of health regulations should be observed in maintaining clean massage facilities at all times.

MAINTAINING SANITARY CONDITIONS

The transmission of infectious microorganisms such as bacteria, viruses, and fungi is the cause of many of the diseases that plague humanity. It is not possible or practical to eliminate all these pathogens from our environment; however, by the practice of sanitary procedures, it is possible to greatly reduce the spread of infectious disease.

There are three main levels of removing pathogens from implements and surfaces: sterilization, disinfection, and sanitization.

Sterilization is the most complete process that destroys all living organisms on an object or surface, including bacterial spores. Sterilization is the process used on surgical instruments in hospitals. This is a difficult and time-consuming process that is generally unnecessary in a massage practice. It would be impractical if not impossible to sterilize the surfaces in a massage studio.

Disinfection is the next level of decontaminating pathogens, which is nearly as effective as sterilization except that it does not destroy bacterial spores. Disinfectants are powerful substances that disinfect implements and nonliving surfaces. Professional-strength disinfectants must be used with care and according to the manufacturer's instructions. Disinfectants are not used as hand cleaners because they may damage the skin with prolonged or repeated contact.

antibodies

are a class of proteins produced in the body in response to contact with antigens that immunize the body.

sterilization

is the most complete process that destroys all living organisms, including bacterial spores.

disinfection

is the next level of decontamination, nearly as effective as sterilization, but it does not kill bacterial spores.

Federal law requires that manufacturers provide certain information with disinfectants, including instructions for proper use, a list of active ingredients, safety precautions, a list of the organisms against which the product is effective, and a material safety data sheet (MSDS) with information about potentially hazardous materials contained in the disinfectant. Disinfectants, when used properly, are safe and effective. However, improperly used, they become potentially dangerous. The best way to ensure the proper use of disinfectants is to read and follow the manufacturer's instructions.

Common disinfectants used today are phenols (Lysol®), chlorine bleach, and alcohol.

The third level of decontamination and the one practiced extensively in the massage studio is **sanitation.** Sanitation significantly reduces the number of microorganisms and pathogens found on a surface. Sanitation is generally done with soaps or detergents and water. Hand washing is a good example of an important sanitary practice.

The primary precaution in infection control is thorough hand washing. Thorough hand washing is accomplished by vigorously scrubbing the hands, preferably with an antibacterial soap and warm water. The hands are first moistened. The soap is applied and worked into a good lather. Special care is given to scrub between the fingers, between the finger and thumb, around the nails, and, if appropriate, up the arms. The hands are then rinsed thoroughly and dried with a clean towel.

The practitioner's hands should be washed with an antibacterial soap before and after each session. Washing the hands before the massage protects the client. Thorough hand washing after the massage protects the practitioner and anyone the practitioner may come into contact with later.

There may be situations or conditions in your practice when special hygienic precautions are warranted. As a rule, massage is not done in situations where there is highly contagious or infectious disease present. It is also a rare occasion when the practitioner might be exposed to any body fluids. It is important for the practitioner to recognize these situations and observe Universal Precautions.

Your massage practice may find you working with a client who is in a weak and vulnerable condition or who is in the contagious stage of a disease yet is showing no symptoms. Hygienic practices, especially concerning hand washing and protection, is essential to the health and safety of the client, the practitioner, other clients, and personnel associated in any way with the practice.

It is important to keep the massage studio or work area, dispensary, implements, and equipment in a sanitary condition. Supplies such as towels, blankets, and sheets should be clean and fresh for each client. After each use, linens should be stored in a covered container until they can be laundered in hot water and dried in a hot dryer. If there is concern that the linens have been contaminated, one cup of chlorine bleach can be added to the wash water. Disposable products such as towels and sheets may be used and fresh ones supplied for each client.

sanitation
is the third level of decontamination practiced in the massage studio and is done with soaps or detergents and water.

Although the massage practitioner may not use a wide range of mechanical aids or electrical equipment, anything used on the client's body must be kept sanitized. There are disinfectants, antiseptics, and fumigants that kill or retard the growth of bacteria. Some are commercially prepared, economical to use, and quick acting. General antiseptics are alcohol, hydrogen peroxide, sodium hypochlorite, and boric acid. Disinfectants are stronger than antiseptics.

universal precautions
is a system of infection control that protects persons from exposure to blood and bloody body fluids.

Universal Precautions

Universal Precautions (Box 8.1) is a system of infection control designed to protect persons from exposure to blood and/or bloody body fluids. With Universal Precautions, all blood and body fluids are to be considered potentially infectious for diseases such as HIV, hepatitis A, B, C, and other bloodborne pathogens.

BOX 8.1 WHAT ARE THE COMPONENTS OF UNIVERSAL PRECAUTIONS?

1. Hand washing with soap and water is mandatory before and after contact with every client. Use disposable paper towels. Hands and other skin surfaces should be washed immediately and thoroughly if contaminated with blood or other body fluids.

2. Gloves must be worn if the skin of the practitioner's hands is not intact. Practitioners who have lesions or weeping dermatitis on their hands should refrain from doing massage until the condition heals.

3. Gloves shall be worn when there is potential for direct contact with body fluids, mucous membranes, nonintact skin of clients, handling of items or surfaces soiled with blood or body fluids. Gloves shall be immediately discarded after use.

4. Gloves should be put on prior to beginning a task and removed when the task is complete. Hands must be washed after removal of gloves.

5. Linen soiled with blood or body fluids must be gathered without undue agitation and placed in a leakproof bag for transportation to the laundry or soiled linen container.

6. Laundry: Because the risk of disease transmission from soiled linen is negligible, hygienic and commonsense storage and processing of clean and soiled linen is recommended. Soiled linens should be handled as little as possible. Linens should be washed with detergent in hot water and dried in a hot dryer. For contaminated linens, one cup of chlorine bleach can be added to the wash.

7. Housekeeping: Walls, floors, and other surfaces are not directly associated with transmission of infections; therefore, attempts to disinfect or sterilize are not necessary except for the area of a specific spill. However, cleaning and removal of soil should be done routinely, using products that, according to the manufacturer's instructions, are effective for the sanitation.

Sanitizers

A **wet sanitizer** is any receptacle large enough to hold a disinfectant solution in which the objects to be sanitized can be completely immersed. A cover is provided to prevent contamination of the solution. Wet sanitizers can be obtained in various sizes and shapes (Figure 8.7).

Before immersing objects such as hand brushes in a wet sanitizer, be sure to wash them thoroughly with hot water and soap, and rinse them thoroughly with clear water. This procedure prevents contamination of the solution. In addition, soap and hot water remove most of the bacteria.

After items are removed from the disinfectant solution, they should be rinsed in clean water, wiped dry with a clean towel, and stored in a dry or cabinet sanitizer until needed.

Some implements can be washed with hot water and soap, immersed in alcohol, wiped dry, and then placed in a sterile container until needed.

Moist heat is the method of boiling objects in water at 212° F (100° C) for about 20 minutes. A vessel known as an autoclave is sometimes used in the medical field for sterilization purposes.

Disinfectants

Some disinfectants in general use (Table 8.1) are:

- Chlorine bleach
- Ethyl or grain alcohol
- Cresol (Lysol®)

Common household *chlorine bleach* is effective for disinfecting surfaces, implements, and linens. For surfaces and implements, prepare a 1:10 solution by combining one part bleach with nine parts water. Immerse implements for at least 10 minutes. (*Note:* This bleach solution will discolor dyed material.) For linens, add one cup bleach to hot water during the wash cycle.

> **wet sanitizer**
>
> is any receptacle large enough to hold a disinfectant solution in which the objects to be sanitized can be completely immersed.

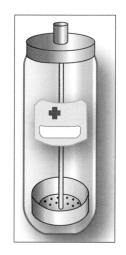

Figure 8.7
Wet sanitizer.

Table 8.1
Approved Chemicals

NAME	FORM	STRENGTH	HOW TO USE
Sodium hypochlorite (household bleach)	Liquid	10% solution	Immerse implements in solution for 10 or more minutes
Alcohol	Liquid	70% solution	Immerse implements or sanitize electrodes and sharp cutting edges for 10 or more minutes
Cresol or Lysol®	Liquid	1% to 5% solution	Use to clean floors, sinks, and restrooms

Ethyl or grain alcohol comes in liquid form. Electrodes and like implements can be sanitized in 70 percent solution. Alcohol can be used as a rinse to sanitize the hands.

Cresol or Lysol® (1 to 5 percent) can be used for cleaning floors, sinks, restrooms, and so on. Commercially prepared solutions are available.

It is important to read directions on all containers when mixing any sanitizing agent.

When in doubt about antiseptics and disinfectants approved for use in your studio or work area, consult your local health department or state board of health.

Proper Practices for Sanitizing Surfaces in a Massage Facility

- Floors
- Massage tables and bolsters
- Restrooms

It is good business practice to keep a massage business facility clean. Clients or patrons expect and appreciate coming into a place that is clean and orderly. For health reasons, it is also important to keep your place of business sanitary. You will have many different individuals passing through your business. They may be carrying with them a great variety of bacteria and other pathogens. To reduce the possibility of these pathogens being passed on to you or the patrons of your business, it is important to exercise good sanitary practices.

Floors

- Carpets: Keep well vacuumed and shampoo when necessary.
- Solid floors: Sweep daily, sanitize with detergent and water, disinfect with Lysol®-type product or a commercial-grade disinfectant.

Other surfaces

- Sanitize all surfaces with cleaning solution (soap and water or commercially prepared solution).

Massage tables and bolsters

- Use spray-type cleaner or soap and water to remove oils.
- Disinfect with disinfectant-type cleaner (10 percent chlorine bleach solution, Lysol®, alcohol, or other comparable cleaner/disinfectant).

Restrooms

- Sanitize all surfaces with detergent and water.
- Disinfect with commercial disinfectant or Lysol®-type product.
- Use 1:10 solution of chlorine bleach to water.

- Spray or wipe the surface with the recommended disinfectant, then wipe dry. Spray again and allow the surface to air dry. Be sure to wear gloves when using a disinfectant to prevent skin irritation. If using a spray bottle, be sure not to inhale the mists.

- Supply restrooms with paper towels, toilet paper, paper cups (in a dispenser), and a liquid antibacterial hand soap.

All products used in the application of massage services must be stored in closed containers that are clearly labeled. Massage oil should be in unbreakable containers with dispenser tops that allow the practitioner to easily dispense the amount of oil or lotion needed without contaminating the remaining contents of the bottle. Using an unbreakable bottle reduces the risk of spillage or breakage should the bottle slip and fall on the floor.

Salves and creams should be removed from containers with spatulas or other implements rather than with the fingers. This reduces the chance of the products being contaminated. Lids should be kept on containers, and the outside of the containers should be kept clean.

SUMMARY OF PRECAUTIONS

1. Keep yourself and your clothing clean.

2. Wash and sanitize your hands with soap and warm water before and after every client. A good hand brush should be used for scrubbing, particularly around the nails, and then the hands should be rinsed and wiped dry. If there is cause for suspicion of bacterial contamination, a mild alcohol solution can be used to rinse the hands.

3. Keep all products, implements, and areas used during massage in a sanitary condition. This includes surfaces where items are placed.

4. Keep lubricants (oils, creams, and lotions) in contamination-proof dispensers and containers. If a jar-type container is used, never remove the product directly with your fingers. Avoid cross-contamination by using a disposable tongue depressor or a spatula that can be sanitized between uses. Be sure that all products are correctly labeled to prevent using the wrong product.

5. Use clean linens for every client. Linens and towels should be laundered in hot water and soap and dried in a hot dryer. Chlorine bleach should be added for its germicidal benefits. Clean linens should be stored in closed cabinets. To prevent a rancid odor, sheets and towels should be laundered the day they are used. Generally, laundry products and fabric softeners will eliminate odor. However, once sheets and towels have become rancid, they should be discarded.

Some oils (peanut, olive, mineral, almond) tend to be hard to remove from fabric. Oil will usually wash out if sheets and towels are laundered immediately. When it is not possible to launder as often as needed, practitioners should use disposable sheets. Commercial products are available from most massage oil manufacturers to remove rancid oil and odors from linens.

6. Wear vinyl gloves or another appropriate covering if you have broken skin or infections on your hands.

7. Do not perform massage if you have a contagious illness that could be passed on by contact or being in close proximity with others.

8. If a client has a contagious condition, take precautions to protect yourself, your client, and others from spreading the infection. If it is an acute condition, such as a respiratory infection, or accompanied by fever, massage is contraindicated, and you may suggest rescheduling the appointment. If it is a regional condition, avoid the area. If it is a general condition that does not preclude massage and the client is under medical care, consult with the physician or medical team to determine the best way to proceed.

9. Keep all areas of the workplace and furnishings clean and sanitary. This includes restrooms, dressing rooms, and work space.

10. The place of business should be well ventilated and kept at a comfortable temperature. Floors, walls, windows, and the like should all reflect your concern for cleanliness and pride in your place of business. Practitioners should know and practice all the rules of sanitation issued by their state board and department of health.

SAFETY PRACTICES AND PROCEDURES FOR MASSAGE THERAPISTS

Massage and massage therapy is a personalized health service that usually involves interaction between client and practitioner and does not involve the use of hazardous equipment or practices. However, there are safety issues that the massage student and practitioner must keep in mind. Safety is an attitude put into practice that is concerned with the prevention of situations and elimination of conditions that may lead to injury of the massage practitioner or client. To ensure the health and safety of everyone concerned, safety considerations must focus on (1) the facility and equipment, (2) the massage practitioner, and (3) the client.

The Facilities

The facilities include the building that houses the massage facility, the facility itself, and the equipment and space within the facility. Safety precautions in the facility include housekeeping, sanitation, fire policy, and heating and ventilation.

Housekeeping/Sanitation

- Keep all halls and walkways clear.

- Keep all carpets vacuumed and cleaned.

- Keep all solid floors cleaned and sanitized.

- Sanitize all restroom and bathing facilities.

- Make sure all floors in wet areas are slip proof.

- Sanitize all equipment surfaces that come in contact with clients (table surfaces, linens, applicators, and vibrators, etc.).

- Disinfect hydrotherapy tubs, steam cabinets, shower stalls, and wet tables between each use.

- Maintain hand-washing facilities (germicidal soap, sanitary or paper towels, clean and sanitary area).

- Linens are commercially laundered or washed in hot water with detergent and dried in a hot dryer. Bleach is available and used when there is any chance of contamination.

- Clean linens are stored in a closed cabinet. Soiled linens are stored in a covered container or stored outside the massage room.

Equipment

- Check all equipment for safety and stability (tables, stools, chairs, etc.).

- Each time a table is set up, check all hinges and locks for stability.

- Maintain all equipment (electrical cords, lubrication, etc.).

- Store equipment and linens properly.

Fire Safety

- Maintain functioning smoke and carbon dioxide detectors.

- Be familiar with the location and use of fire extinguishers.

- Clearly indicate fire exits.

- Be aware of evacuation procedures.

- Establish a policy regarding the use of open flames, candles, incense, and the like.

- Contact your local fire department for a fire safety inspection.

First Aid

- Keep a maintained first aid kit on the premises.

- Make sure that all personnel know the location of the first aid kit.

- As many staff members as possible should learn first aid and cardiopulmonary resuscitation (CPR) techniques.

- Keep emergency information posted in plain view near all telephones, including telephone numbers for the fire and police departments, ambulance, hospital, emergency room, doctors, and taxis.

Heat and Ventilation

The practice of massage generally requires that the massage room be somewhat warmer than normal. This necessitates either turning up the thermostat or using auxiliary heating devices.

- Maintain and service heating and ventilation systems regularly.
- Use only UL-approved auxiliary heating devices.
- Regularly inspect auxiliary heating devices.
- Turn off auxiliary heating devices when not in use.

Practitioner Personal Safety

- When lifting equipment or clients, use proper body mechanics and lifting techniques to prevent muscle strain and injury (Figure 8.8).
- Use proper body mechanics and techniques when practicing massage to prevent muscle strain and overuse syndromes resulting in back, shoulder, or arm injury.
- Use equipment and adjunctive modalities properly and according to manufacturers' instructions and recommendations.
- All practitioners should maintain a current first aid and CPR certification.
- Know the location of the first aid kit.
- Wash hands before and after every treatment.

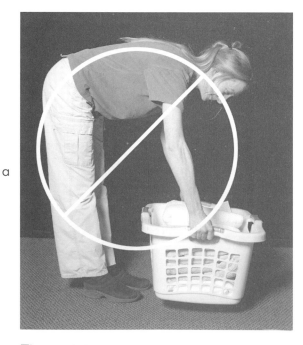 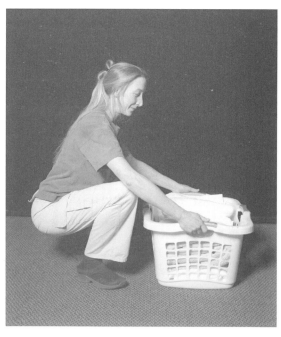

a   b

Figure 8.8

Proper lifting: (a) Lifting with poor body mechanics, using back muscles. (b) Lifting with good body mechanics, using leg muscles with object close to body.

- Know contraindications for massage and perform only procedures that cause no injury and are within your scope of practice.

- When doing an in-house massage, inform an associate of the location, name of the client, the time of the appointment, and the time you plan to complete the appointment. When you have completed the appointment, contact your associate to indicate that you have finished.

Client Safety

- Understand the paths of infection and ensure clients' protection with sanitary practices.
  a. Use clean linens with each client.
  b. Wash hands before and after each client.
  c. Provide sanitary bathing facilities and restrooms.
  d. Avoid open wounds and sores.
  e. Do not practice massage if you are ill and/or contagious.

- Provide safe, clear entryways and passages.
  a. Keep walkways clear and well lighted.
  b. Provide nonskid walkways and floors.

- Assist clients on and off of the massage table.

- Check to make sure that clients are not sensitive or allergic to products used.

- Use proper procedures in dealing with illness and injury. Refer to proper medical authorities when conditions indicate.

- Do no harm!

QUESTIONS FOR DISCUSSION AND REVIEW

1. Why do all states have laws pertaining to sanitation?

2. Why is it particularly important for a massage practitioner to practice rules of sanitation?

3. Why should the practitioner have some knowledge of bacteria?

4. What is the difference between pathogenic and nonpathogenic bacteria?

5. What is the main purpose of the body's production of antibodies?

6. Name three forms of pathogenic (harmful) bacteria.

7. What is the best prevention against the spread of harmful bacteria?

8. What should you do before using any disinfectant or antiseptic product?

9. Why are disinfectants used in the practice of massage?

10. What is the best method for keeping the hands and nails clean?

11. Which strengths of cresol or Lysol® are most suitable for cleaning floors, sinks, or restrooms?

12. What is sterilization?

13. What is safety?

14. What are the four areas of concern for safety in a massage practice?

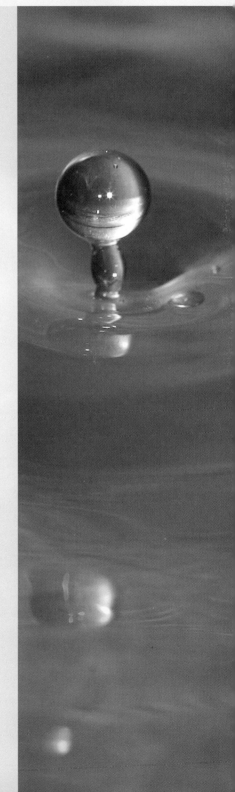

The Consultation

LEARNING OBJECTIVES

After you have mastered this chapter, you will be able to:

1. Explain the importance of the consultation before a massage.
2. Demonstrate how to screen clients while making appointments.
3. Demonstrate how to determine the needs and expectations of the client.
4. Explain why it is important to set policies during the first consultation.
5. Define a treatment plan.
6. Explain what records should be kept and why it is important to keep them updated.

INTRODUCTION

A consultation is a meeting in which views are discussed and valuable information is exchanged. During preliminary consultations between massage practitioners and prospective clients, clients give pertinent information about who they are and why they are seeking the services of the therapist. Practitioners inform clients about the services they provide.

The extent of the consultation depends on the type of massage services offered and the reason the client has come for the session. A relatively healthy client coming for a general, relaxing, wellness massage will require only a brief consultation to determine the client's preferences, needs, and concerns; review pertinent information from the client intake form; explain policies and procedures; and determine that there are no contraindications. However, a client coming with a prescription from a doctor, seeking relief from pain acquired from an auto accident, or seeking reimbursement from insurance, will require a more extensive consultation, assessment, and record keeping. Consultation practices discussed in this chapter are for practitioners in the wellness, personal service sector. Assessment procedures for therapeutic applications will be discussed in Chapter 13.

MAKING THE FIRST APPOINTMENT

The first contact between a practitioner and a prospective client is often the first time the client makes an appointment for a massage. During this first contact, important information can be exchanged to determine whether making the appointment for the massage is appropriate. The prospective client may be looking for services that the therapist does not provide, or it may be determined that massage is contraindicated for the conditions of the would-be client. Screening prospective clients with a couple of questions can save valuable time for both the would-be client and the practitioner as well as eliminate difficult or inappropriate situations. Three questions help screen prospective clients:

- What is your previous experience with massage?
- How did you find out about my services?
- What is your main reason for making this appointment?

Without going into detail, responses to these questions will clarify whether an appointment is desired and appropriate. (We discuss making appointments in Chapter 20).

THE CONSULTATION

The consultation is a time to gather and exchange information. During the consultation, the therapist has the opportunity to

- Greet the client and introduce himself
- Determine the client's needs and expectations
- Explain procedures
- State policies
- Perform a preliminary assessment
- Formulate a treatment plan
- Obtain informed consent from the client

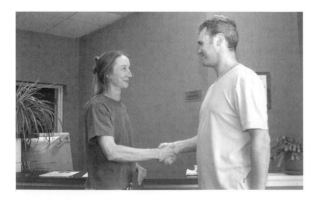

Figure 9.1

The consultation allows the therapist to gather information and helps set the tone of the therapeutic relationship.

The consultation is an interview process that helps determine the course of treatment and sets the tone of the therapeutic relationship between therapist and client. Often, the first consultation is the first time the therapist and client meet. First impressions are lasting impressions. The image the therapist exhibits will influence the client's respect and confidence (Figure 9.1). Be prepared by having everything needed for the interview and massage session organized and ready. Greet the client in a professional and friendly manner. Be courteous and sensitive. Keep the consultation relaxed yet directed toward pertinent information.

An effective consultation depends on clear communication. The practitioner must not only be able to explain policies and procedures so that the client can understand them, but must also listen to and understand clearly the needs and wants of the client. To communicate clearly, it is helpful for the practitioner to be aware of the client's level of intelligence and communicating style, as well as the client's emotional and mental condition. Communicate on a level with the client and in a manner the client comprehends. Some people communicate better by seeing things or by reading or writing information. Others do better talking and listening or by being able to touch and feel things. Be aware of how the client best expresses himself and respond in the same manner. Create an atmosphere of receptivity and develop a rapport with the client by listening carefully and being genuinely interested in his concerns. Personalize the connection by maintaining visual contact, using the client's name and listening attentively during the consultation. Observing and mirroring the client's body language, voice tone, and language can also enhance rapport. Good rapport provides the basis for trust, mutual respect, openness, and harmony that enhances the therapeutic relationship.

Not all communication is by spoken word. Nonverbal communication in the way of posturing, gestures, and facial expressions may accompany verbal communication or may be expressed on its own. Nonverbal communication, sometimes known as body language, often "speaks louder than words" and provides clues to a person's emotional, subconscious, or even physical condition. Be observant of the way a client holds his body, sits, or moves for clues to where he holds tension, pain, or how confident or uncomfortable he might be. Does the client seem to be open and engaged in the consultation or is the client reserved and reluctant to participate? Sometimes verbal and nonverbal communications are not congruent. The words say one thing, and the body or expression says another. For instance, if a client is telling you how good he feels and how well things are going for him at the same time his head and shoulders are down and his voice is weak and shaky, you may want to continue inquiring into the reasons for seeking massage and provide feedback that his body language is sending a different message.

Nonverbal communication is also an important consideration during the massage. Facial expressions such as serene smiles or grimaces and subtle sounds such as moans and groans provide feedback to the practitioner that the selected massage procedures are appreciated or perhaps too aggressive. Fidgeting, muscle contractions, and flinches indicate discomfort and the need to alter the massage in some way. When a nonverbal message is given and received, the practitioner may want to verbalize feedback to the client to clarify the message and ensure that the interpretation is correct.

Also, as a practitioner, be aware of your own nonverbal expression and body language and how they might affect the client. A practitioner who is attentive, is responsive, and maintains eye contact from the same elevation will make a much better impression than a practitioner who sits across a desk, shuffling papers, or who stands above the client or turns his back while busying himself with other tasks during the consultation.

---

nonverbal communication

also known as body language, is how an individual's posturing, gestures, and facial expressions provide information about his mental, emotional, or physical condition.

The practitioner's body language should send the message that the practitioner is open, friendly, confident, and professionally interested in the client during the consultation and throughout the therapeutic relationship. During the consultation, the practitioner will ask questions to determine client concerns and conditions. Ask pertinent questions and listen closely to the responses. Questions that require an explanatory response are preferred to those that can simply be answered with a yes or no. Questions like, "Describe your areas of discomfort and show me where you feel it" provide more information than "Do you have discomfort?" When you do ask a question, listen attentively to the response and allow as much time as necessary for the client to completely answer the question. To make sure that you understood the client's response, summarize what was said and state it back to the client. This will give the client a chance to agree or clarify what was said. This practice vastly reduces the possibility of misinterpreting any information.

The preliminary consultation is the first opportunity for the client and therapist to meet one another and to clarify their intentions and expectations for the massage and to agree on some goals. The first consultation is the time for the client to learn about the therapist and the kind of therapies offered and get some idea about the expected outcome. The practitioner is ethically bound to provide information as to credentials, training, the massage procedures to be used, and the expected results so that the client can make a choice to participate in those services based on a clear understanding of the information provided. It is during this first consultation that the therapist learns about the client's conditions, needs, and expectations and determines whether there are any partial or general contraindications for massage or whether there is any reason to refer the client to another health practitioner. The therapist uses the information gained during the consultation to adapt the massage services to best serve the client's needs. The purpose of the consultation is to exchange information regarding the client's conditions and expectations and the services offered by the therapist and to determine whether they are compatible. During this consultation, enough information is exchanged so that the client can give **informed consent** for the services to be received.

The preliminary consultation is the most extensive; forms are filled out, policies set, an assessment done, and a treatment plan created. However, each session should begin with a short question-and-answer session to determine any changes in conditions or course of treatment.

EXPLAIN PROCEDURES AND STATE POLICIES

During the first consultation, practitioners clearly explain their operational and client interaction policies. When policies concerning such things as missed or late appointments, payment of fees, and sexual boundaries are clearly stated, misconceptions and awkward situations are avoided. Some practitioners include a disclaimer that their services are not a medical treatment. There is no specific manner to present these

informed consent
is a client's written authorization for professional services based on adequate information from the massage therapist about the massage, including expectations, potential benefits, possible undesirable effects, and professional and ethical responsibility.

policies. They may be posted, printed on the intake forms, or verbalized. Regardless of how they are expressed, set only those policies you are willing to uphold.

When the reasons for the client visit are clear and client expectations are stated, practitioners can explain the services they offer and how those services will be of benefit to the client. Practitioners can also explain any procedures they use during the treatment sessions or procedures clients will need to follow during their visits. It is important to keep clients informed about what is being done and why. This is especially important if it is the client's first visit to the place of business and/or first massage. (See Box 9.1.)

During the consultation, the client usually will want to know how the massage treatments will be beneficial. Being able to answer the client's questions adds to the practitioner's credibility as a professional and helps to build client confidence.

BOX 9.1 POLICIES AND PROCEDURES

Procedures and policies should be explained during the initial consultation. It is advisable to have policies and procedures printed in a document the client reads. The therapist may choose to review important policies and procedures to make sure that the client understands them.

Policies and procedures include:

- *type of services offered.* List the modalities or types of therapy offered. Provide an explanation of the benefits, risks, and limitations of the therapy. List any specialty areas, groups, or conditions in which you specialize.

- *qualifications of therapists.* Provide information regarding your schooling, special training, licenses, years of experience, professional affiliations.

- *business policies.* Define your appointment policy, including your work schedule, days and hours you are available for appointments, and how long in advance an appointment can be made or canceled. State your policy for late or missed appointments and the length of sessions. State that information shared during the session and all client files are confidential except when subpoenaed by a court of law. Before client information is shared for medical or insurance purposes, the client will be asked to sign a Release of Medical Information form. State your policies regarding sexual boundaries.

- *fees.* List your fees for different lengths of sessions or different services. Define the kinds of payment accepted: cash, check, credit card, do you bill, accept insurance (under what circumstances). Do you offer discounts for multiple sessions or referrals? Do you offer a sliding scale?

- *session procedures.* Describe a common massage session and what the client can expect. Include the intake and assessment time, undresssing and draping procedures, the sequence of the massage, use of oils or lubricants, policy on talking during massage, the use of music or not, and any special or restricted activity following massage.

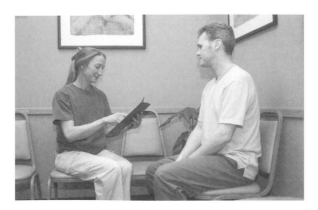

Figure 9.2

Review the client's responses on intake and medical history questionnaires to determine whether further information about the client is needed.

DETERMINING THE CLIENT'S NEEDS AND EXPECTATIONS

To perform services that directly benefit clients, it is necessary to understand their reasons for seeking your services. What are the client's main and secondary concerns? Has the client received massage previously? What type of massage does the client prefer? What are the client's expectations for the session? What does the client expect to get out of the treatment, what are the goals? Are those goals reasonable, what will it take for the client to be satisfied? What conditions might benefit from your services? Are there any conditions that contraindicate massage? Is it necessary to refer the client to another health care provider before providing any massage services?

To get an understanding, you must ask questions and pay close attention to the responses. Two ways to ask questions are written and verbal. Written questions are in the form of intake and medical history questionnaires that the client fills out. When the forms are completed and you review them, a number of verbal questions may be appropriate to clarify the written answers or to gain more specific information about clients and their reason for coming. Important responses should be recorded in the client's file (Figure 9.2).

INTAKE AND MEDICAL HISTORY FORMS

Client intake forms and medical history forms provide vital information that the therapist uses to formulate a treatment strategy. The information requested on intake and medical history forms varies according to the kind of massage services offered or the needs of the therapist. Examples of intake and medical history forms have been included in this chapter to provide ideas (Figure 9.3).

By reviewing the forms, the therapist can reduce the time required to interview the client. After the prospective client has filled out the forms and the therapist has reviewed the information, the client is interviewed in order to elaborate on questions that may need more in-depth consideration. Information gained during the interview is recorded and becomes part of the client's permanent record.

When reviewing consultation forms with the client, it is important to be tactful. If a client questions why you are asking certain questions, explain your reasons. For example, on the form you ask: "What do you do with the majority of your time (hobbies, outside work)?" The client's answers give you clues about what area of the client's body may be carrying stress. The client's answer to the question, "Have you had any surgery?" gives you clues to health problems and contraindications. The question

Massage Clinic
Client Information Form

Name_____ Birth Date _____

Address _____ Telephone _____

_____ Business Phone _____

City/State/Zip _____ Social Security # _____

Occupation _____ Other Activities_____

General Health Condition_____ Blood Pressure _____

List any serious or chronic illness, operations, chronic virus infections, or traumatic accidents you have had. _____

Are you in recovery for addictions or abuse?_____

Are you under a doctor's, chiropractor's, or other health practitioner's care? _____

If so, for what condition(s)? _____

Are you on any medication?_____ If so, what? _____

Do I have permission to contact your doctor/therapist?_____

Names of doctors, chiropractors, or health practitioners:

Name_____ Name _____

Address _____ Address _____

Telephone _____ Telephone _____

Why did you come for our services? (relaxation, pain, therapy, etc.)_____

_____

What results would you like to achieve with our work? _____

Have you had any massage therapy before?_____If so, when and why? _____

_____

How did you find out about our services? _____

Were you referred to this office? _____ By whom? _____

In case of emergency notify: Name_____Phone _____

I have completed this information form to the best of my knowledge. I understand the massage services are designed to be a health aid and are in no way to take the place of a doctor's care when it is indicated. Information exchanged during any massage session is educational in nature and is intended to help me become more familiar and conscious of my own health status and is to be used at my own discretion.

Our time together is precious, and I agree to cancel 24 hours in advance. Unless there is an emergency, if I miss an appointment, I agree to pay the full appointment fee.

Date_____ Signature _____

Figure 9.3

Sample client intake information form.

"Have you received massages before?" allows you to determine what the client's expectation and preference may be. The question "How did you find out about our massage services?" gives you information about the kind of advertising that is most effective.

BODY DIAGRAMS

Body diagrams of the male or female figure are helpful when the client has some painful sore or stiff areas that may require attention. Give the client a few minutes to indicate these areas on the diagram, and then discuss the condition and allow the client to explain his symptoms. After clients have indicated the location of their discomforts on the diagram, ask them to touch or point to the area(s) on their own body. Add notes to the diagram to clarify and record clients' comments about their conditions (Figures 9.4 and 9.5).

The practitioner may direct more questions to assess the situation. Questions specifically relating to the client's condition will help to determine the course the massage sessions will take. Questions may also reveal other conditions that may or may not be related to the primary condition. Thorough assessment will also expose any contraindications for massage.

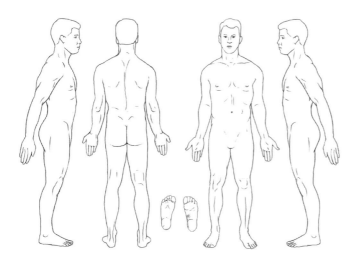

Figure 9.4

Male body diagram. On the diagram, mark as follows: Put an X on any painful area. Rate pain on a scale of 1 to 10. Shade in any stiff or sore areas. Circle areas of other concern and describe the condition.

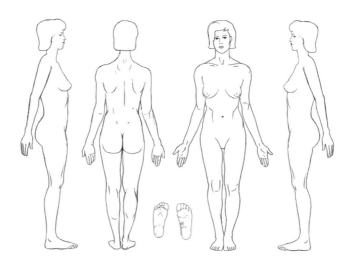

Figure 9.5

Female body diagram. On the diagram, mark as follows: Put an X on any painful area. Rate pain on a scale of 1 to 10. Shade in any stiff or sore areas. Circle areas of other concern and describe the condition.

PRELIMINARY ASSESSMENT

To determine what massage procedures to perform on a prospective client or whether it is advisable to refer the client to another health professional, the therapist must understand as much about the client and his condition as possible. An assessment that includes a client history, observation, and examination will help disclose problems and the physiological basis for the client's complaints.

The extent of the assessment will depend on the type of massage service being offered. A nonspecific relaxing body massage, for instance, would require a brief assessment to determine any special areas of concern and whether there are any contraindications. However, a therapeutic massage session to address some specific concerns or musculoskeletal dysfunction would require a more in-depth assessment.

The history includes information gained from the medical history form, answers to questions, and descriptions that clients offer. Observation includes noticing how clients hold their body and how they move. It includes noticing how they react to questions or manipulative tests. Examination uses various manipulative and verbal tests to help determine more precisely the tissues or conditions involved. (Assessment for therapeutic application is discussed in Chapter 13.)

The assessment process does not end with the consultation but continues throughout the massage. As the massage proceeds, the practitioner monitors the client and the condition of the tissues and modifies or adapts the massage to best serve the needs of the client.

DEVELOP A TREATMENT PLAN

The treatment plan is an outline the practitioner can follow when giving massage treatments. The plan takes into consideration information from the intake and medical history forms, the interview, and preliminary assessment to formulate session goals and choose massage techniques. A general treatment strategy may cover several sessions, but every session should have a treatment plan.

The intake and medical history forms provide past information about the client. If this is not the first session, records from previous sessions provide valuable information. The interview provides additional information concerning the client's reasons for coming and preferences. A further assessment will indicate more about the client's current condition.

By combining and reviewing the information, a strategy or plan of action can begin to evolve. The client's needs, wants, and preferences become more apparent. Indications and contraindications are determined. Referral to other professional or health practitioners might be suggested. A discussion between the client and practitioner can prioritize what the client wants to work on. Options can be discussed.

Goals for the session(s) are proposed, and modalities and techniques are chosen accordingly. When the client is informed of, comfortable with, and understands the proposed plan, the client gives informed consent and the plan is put into action.

INFORMED CONSENT

Informed consent is an educational process that ensures that the client has received and understands the nature and extent of the massage services. It is a way for the clients to be more in control of their health practice. When the client has received adequate information regarding the practitioner's credentials, the services offered, policies and procedures used during the sessions, the client is able to give informed consent. The practitioner will describe the massage techniques to be employed along with projected effects and outcomes, including benefits and possible side effects. As the client receives disclosure of the nature of the services being offered, the client can knowledgeably agree to proceed. The client may agree to proceed with the procedure, suggest modifications, or even refuse the treatment. In the vast majority of situations, the client will consent to proceed with the practitioner's recommended protocol. The client has full right of refusal; that is, the client has the right to modify or

---

Informed Consent

I (name of client) _____ have received, read and understand the policies and procedures of (name of establishment) _____. (Name of therapist) _____ has informed me of her/his qualifications, the kind of massage services to be provided, the benefits, risks and the goals of the session(s) that we have agreed upon. I understand that I retain the right to withdraw my consent at any time during any session.

I (name) _____ understand that the massage services provided by (name of therapist) _____ are intended to promote relaxation and circulation, and relieve stress, muscle tension, spasms and related pain. I understand that the massage therapy is not a substitute for medications or medical treatment and that the massage therapist does not diagnose illness nor prescribe medical treatment or perform spinal manipulations.

I have informed the therapist of my medical and physical condition and of medications I use, and I agree to update the therapist of any changes in my health profile. I release the therapist of any liability if I fail to do so.

If I experience any discomfort or pain during any session, I will immediately inform the therapist so adjustments can be made to the treatment.

Client signature _____ Date _____

Consent to treat a minor

I, the parent or legal guardian of (dependent's name) _____ authorize (therapist's name) _____ to provide massage treatments to my dependent or child.

Parent or Guardian signature _____ Date _____

Figure 9.6

Informed consent form. (Copyright ©2006 by Delmar Cengage Learning. All Rights Reserved. Permission to reproduce for clinical use granted.)

withdraw consent to continue treatment at any time during any session. If this happens, the practitioner must comply regardless of any prior consent the client may have given.

The initial informed consent may take place during the initial consultation and again when the initial treatment or care plan is completed. It is preferred, and actually required in some jurisdictions, that an informed consent form be signed and kept in the client's file (see Figure 9.6 for an example of an informed consent form). Consent to proceed may be given many times throughout the therapeutic relationship. After the initial informed consent is completed, the practitioner should continually inform the client at any appropriate time that a new or unexpected procedure is being employed so that the client is aware and can give consent to proceed.

Informed consent is an ongoing process. After the initial informed consent form is signed and filed, future sessions may continue with assessments and the creation of updated care plans. The care plan will include anticipated outcomes, possible side effects, the number and length of sessions, and the modalities the therapist will use. When the plan is ready, it is discussed with the client for input, and when satisfied, the client can sign it indicating continued informed consent.

CLIENT FILES

The client file is the vehicle that practitioners use to document the work they have done with the client. The information a practitioner keeps in the client files varies as much as the massage routines of different practitioners. Updated client files ensure the practitioner's access to current information regarding the client. Information that is often found in a client file includes intake information (name, address, phone, etc.), medical information and history, treatment plan, informed consent, Medical Information Release forms, recorded session or SOAP notes, financial records, and billing information. Keeping accurate records is a tedious but essential part of a professional operation.

SOAP CHARTING

The most popular method of recording client and session information in many health care professions is SOAP notes. The acronym SOAP stands for Subjective, Objective, Assessment or Application, and Planning. SOAP charts are used to document information from the initial interview and then to update information from each session (see Figures 9.7 and 9.8).

Information recorded under each heading of the SOAP notes includes the following:

- *Subjective:* Initial interview; anything the client tells the therapist— health history, present symptoms, aggravating conditions, what makes it better, what makes it worse, how it started. Information is derived from intake and client history forms and from the client

INITIAL INFORMATION

Name_____ Date_____

S **Subjective**

(Symptoms, frequency, duration, intensity, how it started, aggravating/relieving activities, etc.)

Client's experience, expectations, and goals:

O **Objective**

Observations, tests, and results:

Treatment goals:

A **Assessment & Applications**

Massage treatment given:

Changes due to massage:

P **Planning**

Homework:

Plan for next session:

Long-range plans and goals:

Figure 9.7
SOAP chart used during initial consultation.

```
                    SESSION NOTES

Name                              Date
_____                 _____

S


O


A


P
```

Figure 9.8
SOAP chart used for updating session notes.

interview. Update subjective information at the beginning of each session—present condition, changes noticed since the last session. Any information provided by the client or his physician and the client's expectations or goals for the session are recorded.

- *Objective:* Any information the therapist gathers from history taking, observation, interview, or assessment procedures and tests. The therapist's treatment goals are noted. Information from the subjective and objective assessments is used to design the massage session.

- *Assessment or application:* Records what was done in the session and changes in symptoms or responses by the client to the procedures used in the session. Session goals are reviewed, and subjective and objective changes as a result of the session are recorded. Any progress, either negative or positive, relative to the massage session is documented.

- *Planning:* Records suggestions for future sessions or any recommendations suggested to the client. By taking into account what you did and found during the session, the next session is planned, as well as a more extended treatment plan (frequency and number of sessions) with more long-range goals. (For more detailed information on SOAP charting, refer to *Hands Heal: Documentation for Massage Therapy* by Diane L. Thompson, Lippincott, Williams and Wilkins.)

UPDATING RECORDS

It is necessary to keep records of all services. Records should be accurate and complete and should provide information concerning treatments given, products used, the state of the client's health, and accurate financial information. Any unique information regarding the client, reactions to treatment, or changes in the client's condition should be noted. All data should be recorded with each treatment, including any special information that may be needed as a reference.

Keeping accurate records of the client's condition, tolerance, and reactions permits you to render more effective treatments and to achieve better results.

Your concern for the client's well-being helps to establish mutual confidence. Reviewing updated records before a client comes in for a return visit refreshes your memory about the client's condition, treatments given, and the client's likes and dislikes. This not only allows you to plan the session, but it refamiliarizes you with the client, which impresses the client and increases client confidence in you. On the other hand, a practitioner who relies on memory and forgets important factors about a client from one session to the next may lose the trust that is so necessary in a therapeutic relationship.

The practitioner never discusses or gives out personal information about clients. All records should be kept in a secure place. A practitioner does not divulge information about a client's personal matters without the written consent of the client, and then only when the exchange of such information is for the client's benefit. The practitioner often works closely with a client's physician when dealing with certain physical conditions; therefore, the confidence of both client and physician must be respected.

When the practitioner feels that a client's physician should be consulted before beginning massage treatments, the practitioner should talk this over with and obtain written permission from the client.

Client files, as well as any information about the client, are kept confidential between the client and practitioner except when pertinent information is shared with other health professionals the client is seeing or with the client's insurance company and then only after the client has been informed and has signed a release of information form. A release of information form contains the client's name, the therapist's name, the name of the person(s) the information is being given to, and the time frame in which the information may be released

---

Release of Information

I (client's name) _____ authorize (practitioner's name) _____
to release and/or exchange information and records concerning my health or health
treatments during the time period of _____ to _____ with (other
professional's name) _____. I retain the right to revoke this
permission at any time either verbally or in writing.
This authorization is valid until (date) _____

Client signature _____ Date _____

Figure 9.9

Release of Information. (Copyright © 2006 by Delmar Cengage Learning. All Rights
Reserved. Permission to reproduce for clinical use granted.)

(see Figure 9.9). The completed form is signed, dated, and kept in the
client files. A copy of the release form is included in the shared information. The only other time information from a client is given out is
if it is ordered by a court of law.

QUESTIONS FOR DISCUSSION AND REVIEW

1. Why is the consultation important to the success of the massage
   treatment?

2. What is included in a preliminary client assessment?

3. Why is a preliminary assessment advisable when doing
   therapeutic massage?

4. What is a treatment plan?

5. How is a treatment plan developed?

6. What is informed consent?

7. What information is disclosed by whom to obtain informed
   consent?

8. Why is it important to keep accurate records?

9. What information is included in a client's file?

10. Why is it important to inform the client of pre-massage
    procedures?

11. Why should the massage practitioner anticipate questions
    the client may ask and be able to answer them?

Classification of Massage Movements

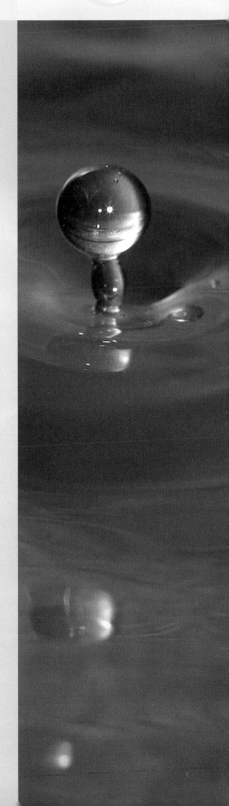

LEARNING OBJECTIVES

After you have mastered this chapter, you will be able to:

1. Describe the six major categories of massage movements.

2. Explain Swedish (classic) massage techniques.

3. Demonstrate mastery of basic massage movements.

4. Demonstrate passive and active joint movements.

5. Explain and demonstrate rhythm and pressure as applied to therapeutic body massage.

INTRODUCTION

Massage movements are to therapeutic massage what words are to language or notes to music. To practice massage, some understanding of the movements is imperative. The more mastery therapists have of the movements, the better they are able to create a work of art each time they choose and combine movements according to each situation. There are any number of massage manipulations and possible combinations of strokes, so a massage can be tailored to the specific needs of each client. Regardless of whether a massage routine is standard or specialized to the specific needs of the client, there is much more to applying strokes than the movement of the hands. The continuous interaction of the client and therapist, the purpose for the session, and the intent with which each manipulation is delivered affect the delivery and outcome of the massage.

CLASSIFICATION OF MASSAGE MOVEMENTS

The following movements are the fundamental manipulations used in Swedish massage and are the foundation of most massage styles practiced today. The massage practitioner must understand the indications for and effects of the manipulations. Most massage treatments combine one or more of these movements, as divided into the six major categories:

1. Touch
   a. Superficial
   b. Deep

2. Gliding or effleurage movements

   a. Aura stroking

   b. Superficial

   c. Deep

3. Kneading movements

   a. Kneading or petrissage

   b. Fulling

   c. Skin rolling

4. Friction

   a. Circular friction

   b. Transverse or cross-fiber friction

   c. Compression

   d. Rolling

   e. Chucking

   f. Wringing

   g. Vibration

      • Manual

      • Mechanical

5. Percussion movements

   a. Hacking

   b. Cupping

   c. Slapping

   d. Tapping

   e. Beating

6. Joint movements

   a. Passive joint movements

   b. Active joint movements

      • Active assistive movements

      • Active resistive movements

The intention with which a massage is given or a technique is applied will greatly influence its effect. Each manipulation is applied in a specific way for a particular purpose. The practice of massage becomes scientific only when the practitioner recognizes the purpose and effects of each movement and adapts the treatment according to the client's condition and the desired results.

Control over the results of a massage treatment is possible only when the practitioner regulates the intensity of the pressure; the speed, length, and direction of the movement; and duration of each type of manipulation.

UNDERSTANDING MASSAGE MOVEMENTS

The practitioner must understand the movement to be applied to a particular part of the body. For example,

- Light movements are applied over thin tissues or over bony parts.

- Heavy movements are indicated for thick tissues or fleshy parts.

- Gentle movements are applied with a slow rhythm and are soothing and relaxing.

- Vigorous movements are applied in a quick rhythm and are stimulating.

While applying the movements, the practitioner must pay close attention to the overall response of the client as well as the response of the tissue or body part to which the manipulation is being applied and adjust the application accordingly.

An important rule in Swedish massage is that most manipulations are directed toward the heart (centripetal). Many massage techniques are intended to enhance venous blood and lymph flow and therefore are directed toward the heart and the eliminative organs. Only strokes light enough that they do not affect fluid flow may be directed away from the heart. When a massage movement is directed away from the heart, it is said to be centrifugal.

The duration of a massage treatment should be regulated. Usually a therapeutic full-body massage takes about one hour, but some practitioners take more or less time. A prolonged massage can be fatiguing to some clients. When a student is learning massage, a full-body massage can take an hour and a half to two hours. This is not unusual because it takes practice for movements to become smooth and efficient. After a while, an hour will be plenty of time to accomplish the desired results. There are times when the practitioner will require more time, so the duration of massages varies. Knowledge and experience are prerequisites to judge the client's special need and adjust the massage session accordingly.

DESCRIPTION OF THE BASIC MASSAGE MOVEMENTS

All hands-on therapies use physical contact as the primary modality. Indeed, it is this caring human contact that makes massage therapy unique.

Touching: Touch, in the context of the classification of massage techniques, refers to the stationary contact of the practitioner's hand and the client's body. Touch is the placing of the practitioner's hand, finger, or body part (such as forearm) on the client without movement in any direction. The pressure exerted may vary from very light to very deep depending on the intention. Skillfully and purposefully applied touch achieves physiological and psychological (soothing) effects.

Gliding is the practice of gliding the hand or forearm over some portion of the client's body with varying amounts of pressure or contact according to desired results.

> **touching**
>
> refers to the stationary contact of the practitioner's hand and the client's body.

Kneading lifts, squeezes, and presses the tissues.

Friction refers to a number of massage strokes designed to manipulate soft tissue in such a way that one layer of tissue is moved over or against another.

Vibration is a continuous trembling or shaking movement delivered by either the practitioner's hand or an electrical apparatus. Vibration may be classified as a type of friction.

Percussion is a rapid striking motion of the practitioner's hands against the surface of the client's body, using varying amounts of force and hand positions.

Joint movement is the passive or active movement of the joints or articulations of the client.

APPLICATION OF MASSAGE STROKES

Touch

Touch is the first technique in developing a therapeutic relationship. Touch may be in the form of a handshake or a pat on the shoulder (Figure 10.1). In the course of a massage, touch constitutes the first and last contact of the practitioner with the client. The practitioner begins the massage with a gentle, noninvasive superficial touch to make first contact and enter the client's personal space. This provides the client the opportunity to become more receptive to the practitioner's touch and presence. The practitioner can use this moment of stationary contact to tune in and connect with the client before proceeding with the session. At the conclusion of the session, when the practitioner has finished the final relaxing strokes, as a completing gesture, a brief stationary contact provides closure for the practitioner and signals the client that the session is finished.

All massage techniques use physical contact, but the quality and sense of touch convey the intent and the power of the movements. Touch is the primary communication tool used by the massage therapist. The sense of touch tells clients what is happening to their bodies and gives practitioners information about the condition and response of the tissues they are working on. The quality of touch continually transmits information from the therapist's hands to the client in direct response to the information communicated by the client and her body.

Light or superficial touch is purposeful contact in which the natural and

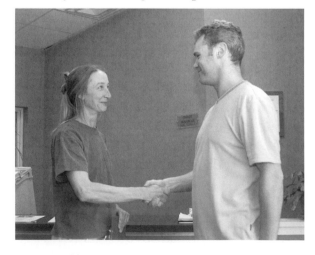

Figure 10.1

A friendly greeting conveys a message of confidence and concern.

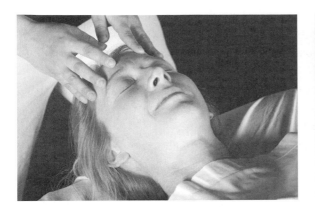

Figure 10.2a
Gentle contact allows the client to unwind.

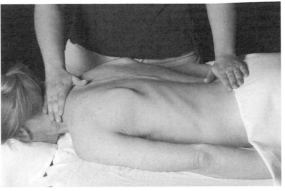

Figure 10.2b
A light touch at the base of the spine, the base of the neck, or the top of the head is a nice way to say hello or good-bye to the client's body.

evenly distributed weight of the practitioner's finger, fingers, or hand is applied on a given area of the client's body. The size of that area may be regulated as necessary by using one or more fingers, the entire hand, or both hands. Some therapeutic techniques employ touch almost exclusively (*jin shin do*, acupressure, polarity, therapeutic touch, *Reiki*). Touch can be remarkably effective in the reduction of pain, lowering of blood pressure, control of nervous irritability, or reassurance for a nervous, tense client. If a person has signs of contraindications for a basic massage, or is in a fragile condition, a complete treatment using light touch exclusively is acceptable. The main objective of light touch is to soothe and to provide a comforting connection that is calming and allows the powerful healing mechanisms of the body to function (Figure 10.2a and b).

Touch Using Deep Pressure

Deep pressure is performed with one finger, thumb, several fingers, or the entire hand. The heel of the hand, knuckles, or elbow can be used according to desired results. The application of deep pressure is used when calming, anesthetizing, or stimulating effects are desired. Deep pressure may be used with other techniques such as cross-fiber friction, compression, or vibration. Deep pressure is useful in soothing muscle spasms and relieving pain at reflex areas, stress points in tendons, and trigger points in muscles. In addition to extensive use in trigger-point therapy, deep pressure is a technique often applied in reflexology, sport massage, acupressure, and *shiatsu* (these methods are discussed in Chapters 16 and 18). When using deep pressure, caution must be used to stay within the pain tolerance of the client. It is essential to use good body mechanics when applying deep pressure to prevent injury to the practitioner. Practitioner body mechanics dictate that undue strain is not exerted to hyperextend any joint. Body mechanics are used in such a way that the "pressure" is delivered through body movement rather than simply hand and upper-body strength (Figure 10.3a to f).

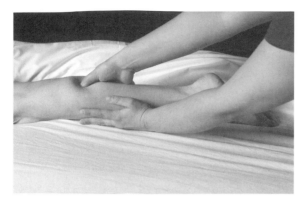

Figure 10.3a

Deep pressure using thumb. Notice the alignment of therapist's thumb and arm to ensure that pressure is directed into client with minimal stress to therapist's joints.

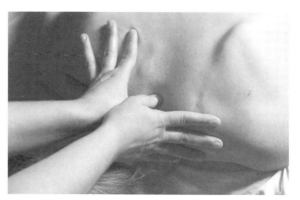

Figure 10.3b

A braced thumb applies deep pressure.

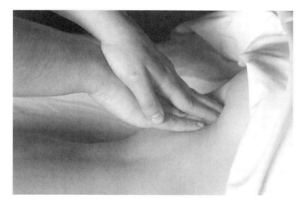

Figure 10.3c

Deep pressure applied with braced fingers.

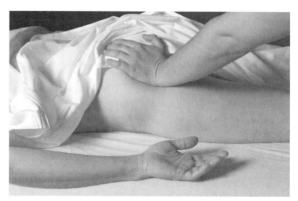

Figure 10.3d

Deep pressure applied with heel of hand.

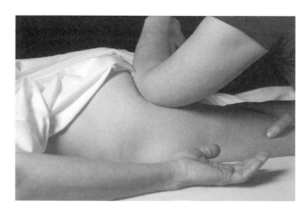

Figure 10.3e

Deep pressure applied with elbow.

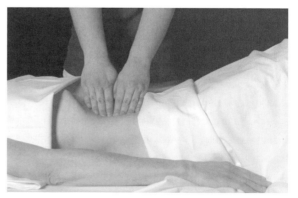

Figure 10.3f

Deep pressure to the abdominal area.

Gliding Movements

Gliding may be done using a varying amount of pressure and length of strokes. Gliding strokes glide over the client's entire body, body part (arm or leg), or a specific area (muscle or reflex).

Ethereal Body or Aura Stroking

This type of stroking is done with long, smooth strokes wherein the practitioner's hands glide the length of the client's entire body or body part, coming very close to but not actually touching the body surface. Generally the movement is in one direction only, with the return stroke being farther from the body. The intention is to affect the energy fields that, according to some philosophies, surround or permeate the body. The direction of the stroking may be along the surface of the body to enhance or impede the natural flow.

The application of this soothing stroke is done only when the surrounding circumstances are very quiet and relaxed and the patient is receptive. It is sometimes used as the final stroke of a massage (Figure 10.4).

Feather stroking

Feather-stroking movements use very light pressure of the fingertips or hands with long flowing strokes.

The application of feather stroking, sometimes called "nerve stroking," is usually done from the center outward and is used as a final stroke to individual areas of the body. Two or three such strokes will have

gliding
is the practice of gliding the hand over some portion of the client's body with varying amounts of pressure.

feather stroking
requires very light pressure of the fingertips or hands with long flowing strokes.

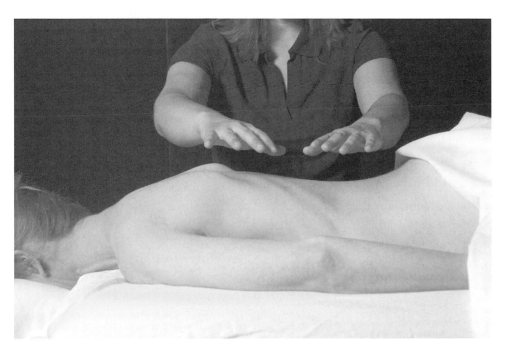

Figure 10.4

Ethereal or aura strokes do not touch the surface of the client's body.

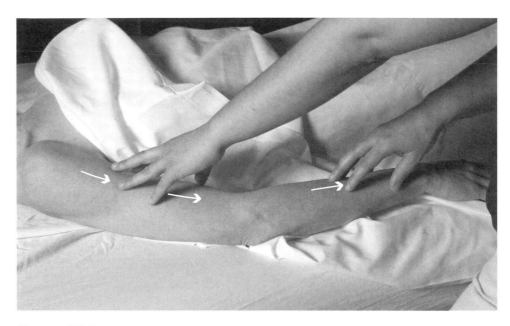

Figure 10.5
Feather strokes (nerve strokes) use the lightest touch of the fingertips.

a slightly stimulating effect on the nerves, whereas many repetitions will have a more sedating response (Figure 10.5).

Gliding or Effleurage

Effleurage is a succession of strokes applied by gliding the hand over a somewhat extended portion of the body. Effleurage is perhaps the most frequently used manipulation in Swedish or Western massage. The term *effleurage* stems from the French verb *effleurer,* meaning to skim or flow. There are two varieties of effleurage: superficial and deep. Superficial gliding strokes employ a very light touch. In gliding strokes, the pressure becomes firmer as the hand glides over the surface of the body. The technique of effleurage or gliding is accomplished either with the fingers, thumbs, the palm of the hand, the knuckles, or the forearm.

> **effleurage**
> is a succession of strokes applied by gliding the hand over an extended portion of the body.

1. Over large surfaces, such as the limbs, back, chest, and abdomen, the gliding movement is performed with the palm of one or both hands.

2. Over small areas, such as the face or hands, the movement is performed with the fingers or thumbs.

3. For very deep gliding strokes, the palms of the hands, the fingertips, the thumbs, the knuckles, or sometimes the forearms are used.

Superficial Gliding

> **superficial gliding**
> is when the practitioner's hand conforms to client's body contours so that light pressure is applied to the body from every part of the hand.

Superficial gliding strokes are generally applied prior to any other movement. The practitioner's hand is flexible yet firm and controlled so that as it glides over the body, it conforms to the body contours in such a way that there is equal pressure applied to the body from every part of the hand. Superficial gliding strokes accustom the client to the practitioner's contact and allow the practitioner to assess the body area being massaged. Light strokes are used to distribute any lubricant that may be used and to prepare the area for other techniques. As the practitioner's hands glide over the tissues, they sense variations that indicate where specific techniques will be applied. Effleurage is interspersed between other techniques to clear the area and soothe the intensity of some deeper manipulations. In Swedish or Western massage, effleurage is generally the first and the last technique used on an area of the body. Slow, gentle, and rhythmic movements produce soothing effects. Rhythmic strokes should be applied in the direction of the venous and lymphatic flow.

Although superficial stroking appears to be simple, its technique is mastered only by long practice. The practitioner's hand should be relaxed in order to mold the surface of the body part being massaged. The pressure and speed of movement should remain constant. Upon completion of the stroke, the practitioner's hand may be elevated and directed to the starting point. In some cases, the hands stay in contact by exerting more pressure centripetally (toward the heart) and then reduce the pressure and lightly stroke (feather stroke) the body to return to the starting point of the stroke. In this way, the practitioner always maintains contact with the client.

Superficial gliding strokes are a valuable application for overcoming a general tired feeling or restlessness. This movement is particularly soothing to nervous or irritated people. Nervous headaches and insomnia (sleeplessness) are often relieved by gentle gliding strokes of the forehead.

Deep Gliding

The term **deep gliding** indicates that the manipulation uses enough pressure to have a mechanical effect. The depth of the gliding movement depends on three factors: the pressure exerted, the part of the hand or arm used, and the intention with which the manipulation is applied. Deep gliding may be applied with the thumb, braced fingers, knuckles, forearm, or elbow, depending on the area of the body or tissues involved. Deep gliding strokes do not involve the use of excessive force. The pressure should never be so forceful as to cause bruising or injury to the tissues. Deep gliding strokes are especially valuable when applied to the muscles. It is most effective when the part under treatment is in a state of relaxation. Then the slightest pressure of the surface will be transmitted to the deeper structures. Deep gliding strokes have a stretching and broadening effect on muscle tissue and fascia. It also enhances the venous blood and lymph flow. If the practitioner uses too much force, the client's body will respond with a protective reflex that will cause muscles to contract, thereby negating the desired effects of the treatment. Deep gliding strokes generally follow the direction of the muscle fibers. On the extremities, the movements are always directed from the end of a limb toward the center of the body. Generally, the movement is toward the heart or in the direction of venous and lymph flow, with the return stroke

> **deep gliding**
>
> indicates that the manipulation uses enough pressure to have a mechanical effect.

being much lighter and away from the center of the body. The exception to this rule is deep, short strokes applied to the muscle attachments and tendons. When directed from the tendon toward the muscle belly, these strokes tend to stretch the tendon and cause a reflexive relaxation of the muscle. Indications for the use of deep gliding strokes may include increasing fluid movement, stretching underlying tissues, separating and broadening tissues, increasing relaxation, and palpating deeper tissues (Figure 10.6a to g and Figure 10.7a to h).

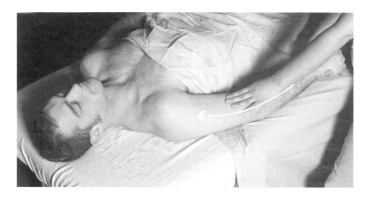

Figure 10.6a
Effleurage or gliding strokes are applied in the direction of venous blood and lymph flow.

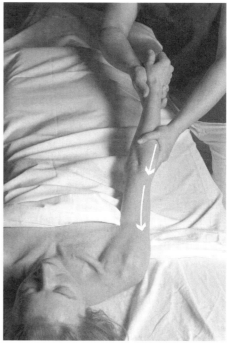

Figure 10.6b
A V-stroke can be used for superficial or deep gliding strokes.

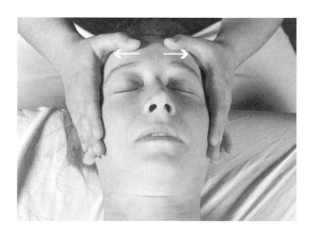

Figure 10.6c
Digital effleurage to the forehead.

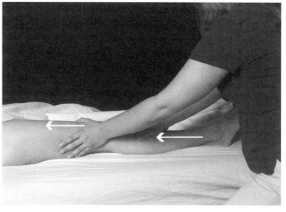

Figure 10.6d
Direction of effleurage on the lower leg. The stroke may continue all the way up the leg to the hip.

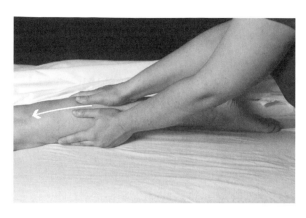

Figure 10.6e

Stroking the entire length of the leg with two hands.

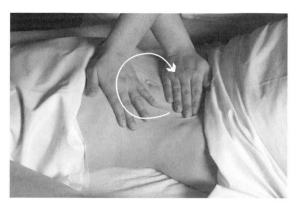

Figure 10.6f

Stroking the abdomen in a circular movement.

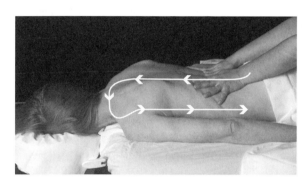

Figure 10.6g

Stroking the entire back.

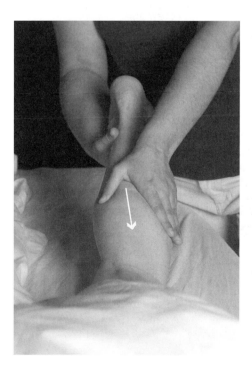

Figure 10.7b

Circular effleurage should be applied following the path of the colon.

Figure 10.7a

V-stroke applied to the posterior leg is used for superficial or deep gliding.

continues

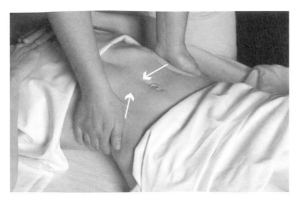

Figure 10.7c

Inward deep gliding strokes of muscles over the stomach area and the abdominal region.

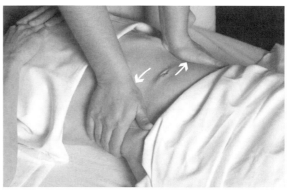

Figure 10.7d

Outward deep gliding strokes to the muscles of the stomach area and the abdominal region.

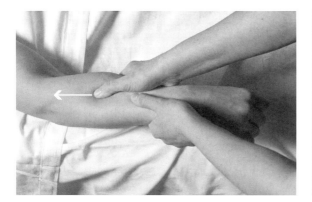

Figure 10.7e

Deep gliding or "stripping" using the thumb on the forearm.

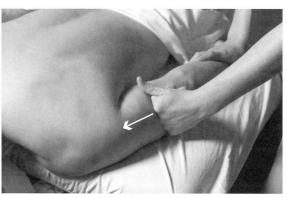

Figure 10.7f

Deep gliding using a loose fist or knuckles on the triceps.

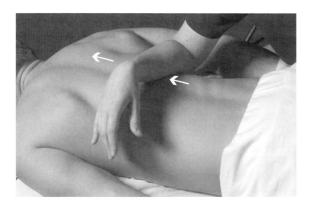

Figure 10.7g

Deep gliding using the forearm and elbow on the back.

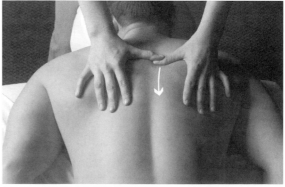

Figure 10.7h

Deep gliding "stripping" using braced thumbs on the back.

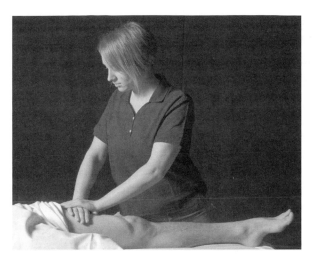

Figure 10.8
When using deep techniques, the practitioner must use good body mechanics to direct the manipulation into the client and at the same time protect herself from injury.

When using deep gliding strokes, the practitioner must use good body mechanics to prevent strain and overuse syndrome injuries. Hand and arm positions should direct the force of the manipulation into the client. The practitioner's shoulders remain down and relaxed, and hyperextension of the wrists, fingers, or thumbs must be avoided (Figure 10.8).

Kneading Movements or Petrissage

In Swedish massage, kneading or petrissage is used on all fleshy areas of the body. The term *petrissage* comes from the French verb *petrir,* which means to knead or mash. Like deep gliding, kneading enhances the fluid movement in the deeper tissues and can help break up superficial adhesions. Skillfully applied, kneading helps reduce adhesions and stretch muscle tissue and fascia. In this movement, the skin and muscular tissues are raised from their ordinary position and then squeezed, rolled, or kneaded with a firm pressure, usually in a circular direction.

On large areas of the body, both hands work alternately as a unit. The tissue is lifted with the palm of the fingers of one hand into the palm of the other hand. Then the process is reversed so that the fingers of the other hand lift the tissue into the palm and base of the opposite hand. The hands alternate in a rhythmical, circular pattern over the entire body part being massaged. Over smaller structures, such as the arms, the flesh is grasped between the fingers and heel of the hand or the thumb. In both cases, the maximum amount of flesh is drawn up into the palm and gently and firmly pressed and squeezed as if milking the tissues. On an area such as the arm, one hand may be used to apply the manipulation while the other hand stabilizes the arm, or both hands may alternate grasping the tissue on each side of the arm. Over smaller structures, such as the hands or fingers, the flesh is held between the thumb and fingers.

Fulling is a kneading technique in which the practitioner attempts to grasp the tissue and gently lift and spread it out, as if to make more space between the layers of tissue or muscle fibers. Often done with both hands simultaneously, the fleshy body part is gathered up between two hands, then raised and separated by the thenar eminence and thumbs as it is gently stretched across the fibers of the tissue.

Skin rolling is a variation of kneading in which only the skin and subcutaneous tissue are picked up between the thumbs and fingers and rolled. As the fingers alternately and continuously pick up and pull the skin away from the deeper tissues, the thumb glides along in the direction of the movement, stretching the underlying fascia. Skin rolling warms, stretches, and begins to separate adhesions between fascial sheaths. When beginning to learn this technique, it is best to use both hands. Use NO lubricant for the technique. Gather up a roll of skin between the thumb and fingers. Continue to gather in more skin with the fingers as you slowly progress along the surface of the body. The thumb supports the roll of skin and slowly slides along as more skin is picked up by the fingers (Figure 10.9a to e, Figure 10.10, and Figure 10.11).

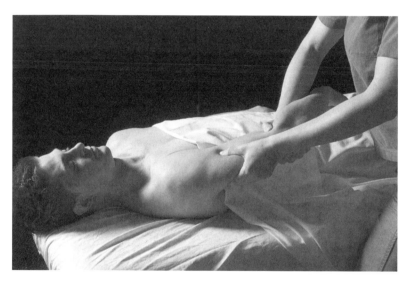

Figure 10.9a
Kneading the triceps and biceps.

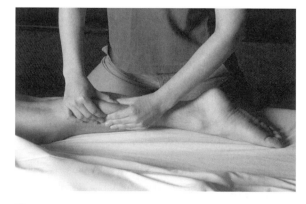

Figure 10.9b
Kneading the calf muscles.

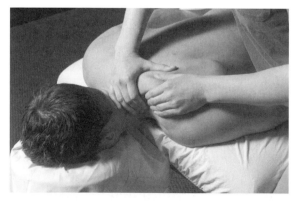

Figure 10.9c
Petrissage of the trapezius muscles.

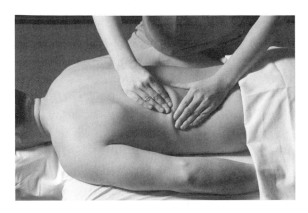

Figure 10.9d

Petrissage is applied to the entire side that is opposite the practitioner. This takes several passes.

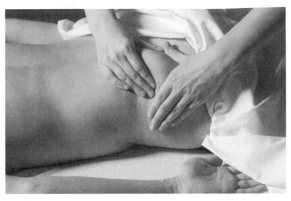

Figure 10.9e

Kneading over the gluteals.

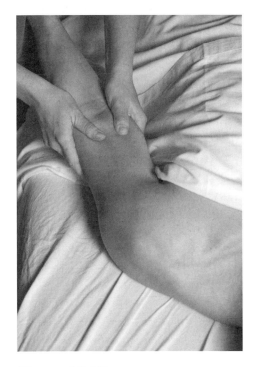

Figure 10.10

For fulling movement, grasp the flesh between the fingers and palms of the hand.

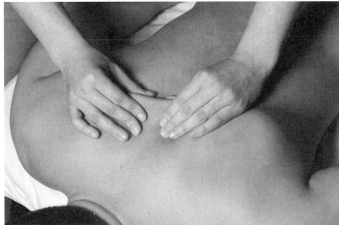

Figure 10.11

Skin rolling lifts the superficial tissues away from the muscles and other deeper tissues.

Friction

Friction movements involve moving more superficial layers of flesh against the deeper tissues. Whereas kneading is done by lifting and pulling the flesh away from the skeletal structures and squeezing in such a way as to milk out the body fluids, friction presses one layer of tissue against another layer in order to flatten, broaden, or stretch the tissue. Friction is done in such a way that it also increases heat. As heat increases, the metabolic rate increases. Friction also increases the rate at which exchanges take place between the cells and the interstitial fluids (fluids situated between the cells and vessels in the tissues of an organ or body part). The added heat and energy also affect the connective tissue surrounding the muscles, making them more pliable so that they function more efficiently.

Friction helps to separate the tissues and to break down adhesions and fibrosis, especially in muscle tissue and fascia. It softens the amorphous (massed) ground substance between layers of fascia. Friction also aids in absorption of the fluid around the joints. Friction has a marked influence on the circulation and glandular activity of the skin. With friction strokes, the area usually becomes red. This indicates an increased flow of blood to the area and that more blood is being rushed to the surface of the skin.

Friction strokes involve moving a more superficial layer of tissue against deeper layers of tissue. This requires pressure on the skin while it is being moved over its underlying structures. The skin and the hand move as a unit against the deeper tissues. Over muscular parts or fleshy layers, friction is applied with the palms of the hands, the flat of the fingers, or the thumbs. Over small surfaces, friction is applied with the fleshy parts of the fingertips or thumbs.

Friction movements may be circular or directional. In **circular friction,** the fingers or the palm of the hand contact the skin to move it in a circular pattern over the deeper tissues. Circular friction is intended to produce heat and stretch and soften the fascia. Circular friction is a general stroke used to warm the area in preparation for more specific or deeper work. The palm or pads of the fingers make contact with the skin and move the skin and more superficial tissues over the deeper layers in a small circular pattern. The fingers or hand DO NOT slide over the skin in a circular manner, although the hand may move along to cover an extended area with circular friction. The intent is to move one layer of tissue over a deeper layer, resulting in a gentle stretching and warming of the area.

Circular friction is also valuable for palpating an area when assessing the condition of the underlying tissues. When working deeply on an area, circular friction and superficial gliding strokes are useful to soothe and calm the client before, after, and interspersed with deep techniques.

Directional friction may be either cross-fiber or longitudinal friction. **Cross-fiber friction,** as the name implies, is applied in a transverse direction across the muscle, tendon, or ligament fibers. Cross-fiber friction is usually applied with the tips of the fingers or the thumb directly to the specific site of a lesion. The intention of cross-fiber friction is to broaden, separate, and align the fibrous tissue. The stroke is broad enough to cover the tissue and deep enough to reach the tissue. When massaging a fibrous band, the cross-fiber friction stroke is not so broad that it snaps across the fiber. The fingers do not move over the skin but move the skin and superficial tissues across the target tissue. Another method of applying cross-fiber friction in some situations is to apply

---

circular friction

is movement in which the fingers or palm of the hand move the superficial tissues in a circular pattern over the deeper tissues.

---

cross-fiber friction

is applied in a transverse direction across the muscle, tendon, or ligament.

compression to an affected area and move the limb in such a way that the underlying bone provides the frictioning movement. This technique is especially applicable to points near the elbow by compressing the points and rotating the forearm (see Figure 10.12f).

Cross-fiber or transverse friction is a preferred technique for rehabilitation of fibrous tissue injuries. When the injury is healing, transverse friction, when properly applied, promotes the formation of elastic fibrous tissue. At the same time, it reduces the formation of fibrosis and scar tissue, so the healed injury retains its original strength and pliability. Applied to old injury sites, cross-fiber friction breaks down some of the adhesions and fibrosis, increasing pliability and reducing the chance of reinjury to the area.

In longitudinal friction, the practitioner's hand moves in the same direction as the tissue fibers. This tends to stretch the tissue and align the collagen fibrils within the fascia (Figure 10.12a to f).

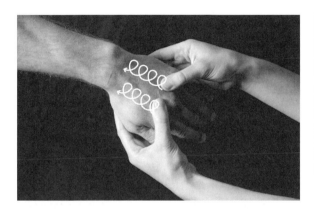

Figure 10.12a
Circular friction of the muscles of the hand.

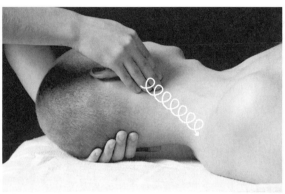

Figure 10.12b
Circular friction of the back of the neck.

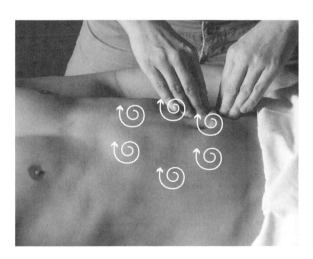

Figure 10.12c
Circular friction over the area of the intestines.

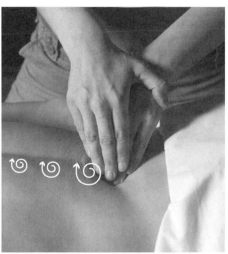

Figure 10.12d
Friction applied to the muscles along the spine.

continues

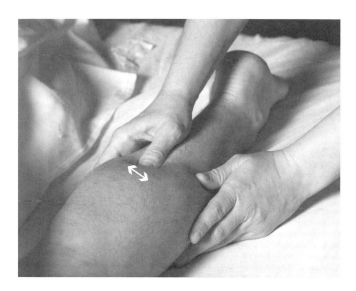

Figure 10.12e
Cross-fiber friction may be applied to the musculotendinous junction of the posterior leg.

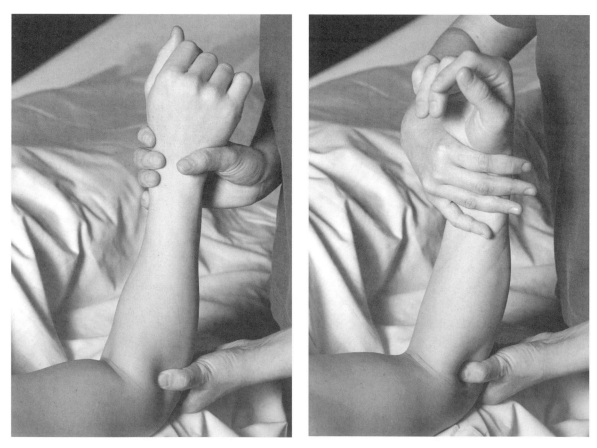

Figure 10.12f
Cross-fiber friction may be applied by compressing a point and moving the underlying bone.

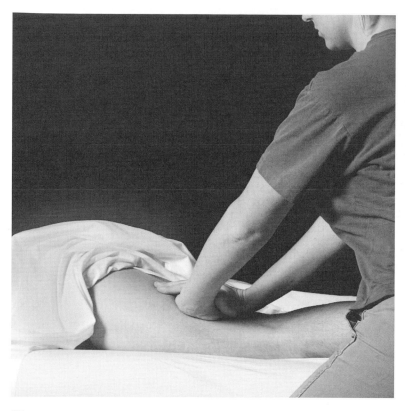

Figure 10.13

Two-handed compression applied to the hamstrings.

> **compression**
>
> is rhythmic pressing movements directed into muscle tissue by either the hand or fingers.

Another form of friction sometimes classified by itself is **compression**. As the name implies, compression is rhythmic pressing movements directed into muscle tissue by either the hand or fingers. *Palmar compression* is done with the whole hand (palm side) or the heel of the hand over the large muscular areas of the body. Palmar compression is a rhythmical pumping action directed into the muscle perpendicular to the underlying bone. Compression can be done over clothing and without the use of lubricant. Compression movements cause increased circulation and a lasting hyperemia in the tissue. Compression is a popular movement used in pre-event sports massage. The intention is to bring more blood and fluid into the tissues, preparing them to exert maximum energy sooner and for a longer period of time (Figure 10.13).

Other manipulations that are considered friction include rolling, wringing, chucking, shaking, and vibration. Chucking, rolling, wringing, and shaking are variations of friction employed principally to massage the arms and legs (see Figure 10.14a to i).

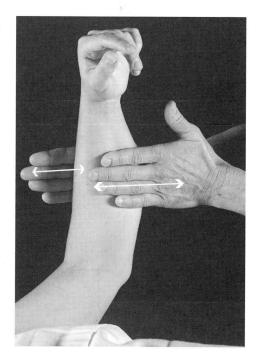

Figure 10.14a

Rolling the arm.

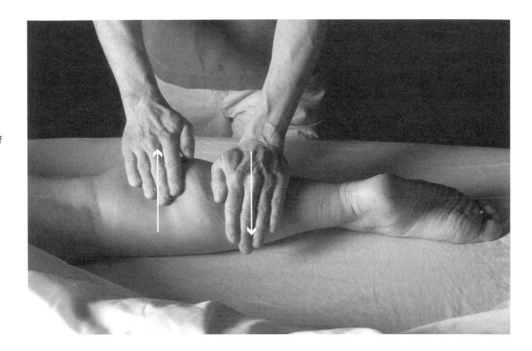

Figure 10.14b
Wringing the muscles of the leg.

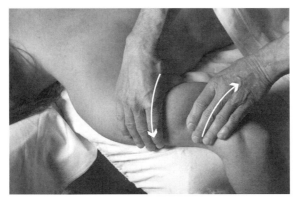

Figure 10.14c
Wringing the muscles of the arm.

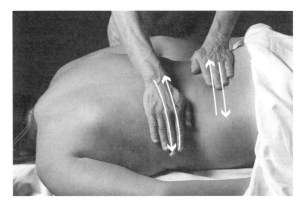

Figure 10.14d
Wringing the muscles of the lower back in a backward and forward movement.

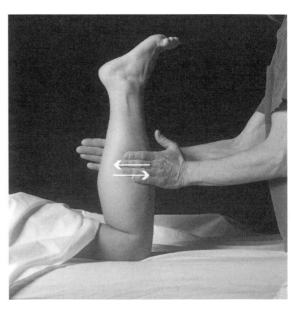

Figure 10.14e
Rolling the muscles of the leg.

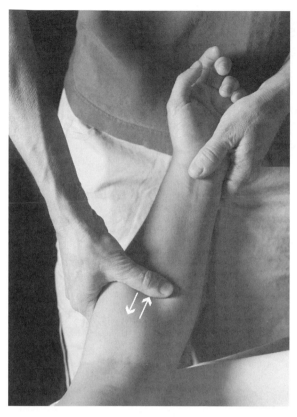

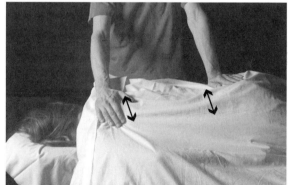

Figure 10.14g
Using the client's hand as a handle for shaking the hand or during petrissage and applying friction to the hand.

Figure 10.14f
Chucking the arm.

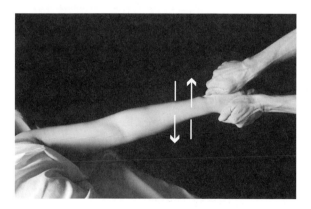

Figure 10.14h
Shaking applied to the arm.

Figure 10.14i
Rocking applied to the torso.

Rolling

Rolling is a rapid back-and-forth movement with the hands, in which the flesh is shaken and rolled around the axis, or the imaginary centerline of the body part. The intention of rolling is to warm and relax the tissue. Rolling encourages deep muscle relaxation (Figure 10.14a and b).

Chucking

The **chucking** movement is accomplished by grasping the flesh firmly in one or both hands and moving it up and down along the bone. It is a series of quick movements along the axis of the limb (Figure 10.14f).

rolling
is a rapid back-and-forth movement with the hands, in which the flesh is shaken and rolled around the axis of the body part.

chucking
involves the flesh being grasped firmly in one or both hands and moved up and down along the bone.

wringing
is a back-and-forth movement in which both hands are placed a short distance apart on either side of the limb and work in opposing directions.

Wringing

Wringing is a back-and-forth movement in which both of the practitioner's hands are placed a short distance apart on either side of the limb. It resembles wringing out a washcloth. The hands work in opposing directions, stretching and twisting the flesh against the bones in opposite directions. The practitioner's whole body is engaged in the movement. The hands make firm contact in both directions. Pressure is not so excessive as to cause pinching or burning (irritation) of the skin. Wringing gently stretches and warms the connective fascia.

shaking
allows for the release of tension by gently shaking a relaxed body part so that the flesh flops around the bone.

Shaking

Shaking is a movement that allows the client to release tension and at the same time indicates to the practitioner where the client may be storing tension in a part of the body. The relaxed body part is gently yet forcefully shaken laterally or horizontally so that the relaxed flesh flops around the bone. The practitioner observes where the body moves freely and where it seems to be stiff. Rigidness indicates body areas that are tense and require more attention. A type of bodywork known as Trager uses shaking and rocking extensively to locate and release tension.

jostling
involves grasping the entire muscle, lifting it slightly away from its position, and shaking it quickly across its axis.

Jostling

Jostling releases muscle tension, increases circulation, and relaxes muscles. It is most effective after muscles have exerted themselves, such as after a workout or competition. Jostling is done when the muscle is in a shortened and relaxed position. Grasp across the entire muscle, lift it slightly away from its position, and while the muscle remains relaxed, shake it quickly across its axis.

rocking
is a push-and-release movement applied to the client's body in either a side-to-side or an up-and-down direction.

Rocking

Rocking uses a push-and-release movement applied to the client's body in either a side-to-side or an up-and-down direction. The body is pushed away slightly and allowed to fully roll back and then pushed away again at a rhythmic rate that is unique to each individual. The practitioner is able to sense the client's rhythm within a few repetitions and then maintain that rhythm and apply it to other manipulations during the massage. Rocking is perhaps the most soothing and relaxing of all the massage manipulations.

vibration
is a continuous trembling or shaking movement delivered either by the practitioner or an electrical apparatus.

Vibration

Vibration is a continuous shaking or trembling movement transmitted from the practitioner's hand and arm or from an electrical appliance to a fixed point or along a selected area of the body. Vibration is often used to desensitize a point or area. Nerve trunks and centers are sometimes chosen as sites for the application of vibratory movements.

Manual contact vibration is usually done with the pads at the ends of the fingers or the soft touch of the palm of the hand. Light contact is made and the hand shaken back and forth as quickly as possible without moving over the skin where contact is being made.

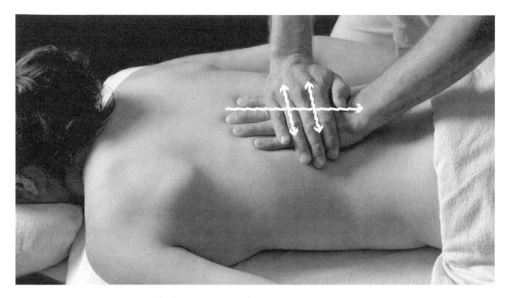

Figure 10.15
Vibrating over each vertebra.

The rate of vibration should be under the control of the massage practitioner. Manual vibrations usually range from 5 to 10 times per second; mechanical vibrations can be adjusted to give from 10 to 100 vibrations per second (Figure 10.15).

There are a variety of mechanical vibrators on the market. They can be classified by size. A popular small model straps on the back of the practitioner's hand. Another popular size is held (usually with two hands) by the practitioner and moved over the client's body. A larger floor-standing model unit uses a flexible applicator arm to deliver its therapeutic effects (Figure 10.16a to c).

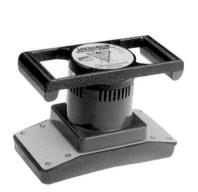

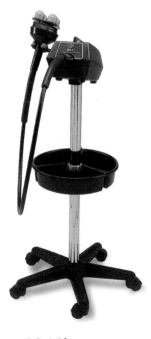

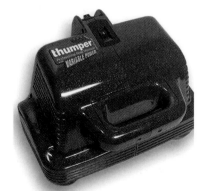

Figure 10.16a
Popular style of vibrator that uses an orbital movement. (Courtesy of Medi-Rub Corporation.)

Figure 10.16b
The floor-standing model has a flexible shaft and a variety of applicator heads. (Courtesy of General Physiotherapy, Inc.)

Figure 10.16c
Type of vibrator that uses a thumping action. (Courtesy of Thumper Massager Inc.)

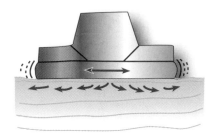

Figure 10.17a

Oscillating vibrators have a lineal back-and-forth action.

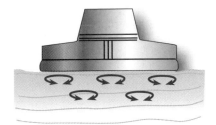

Figure 10.17b

Orbital vibrators have a circular action.

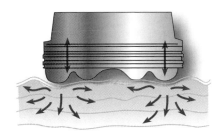

Figure 10.17c

"The Thumper"™ uses a percussion/compression action. Courtesy of Thumper, Inc.

Another way to classify mechanical vibrators is by the vibrating action they use. An oscillating vibrator has a back-and-forth movement. An orbital vibrator uses a circular motion. These vibrators produce a shaking movement when applied to the body. Another type of vibrator produces a "thumping" action. This rapid percussion/compression is directed into the tissues rather than laterally, along the surface. Using vibrators may enhance the effects of the massage and at the same time reduce the physical exertion of the practitioner (Figure 10.17a to c).

The effect of vibratory movements depends on the rate of vibration, the intensity of pressure, and the duration of the treatment. This form of massage is soothing and brings about relaxation and release of tension when applied lightly. It is stimulating when applied with pressure. A numbing effect is experienced when vibrations are applied for a prolonged period of time.

PERCUSSION MOVEMENTS

Percussion movements include quick, striking manipulations such as tapping, beating, and slapping, which are highly stimulating to the body. Percussion movements are executed with both hands simultaneously or alternately.

They do not use much force. Each blow to the body is a glancing contact wherein the practitioner's wrists remain very relaxed.

The general effects of percussion movements are to tone the muscles and impart a healthy glow to the part being massaged. With each striking movement, the muscles first contract and then relax as the fingers are removed from the body. In this way, muscles are toned. Percussion movements should never be applied directly over the spine or muscles that are abnormally contracted or over any sensitive area (Figure 10.18a to e). The movements may be done in the following ways:

1. Tapping with tips of the fingers

2. Slapping with flattened palm and fingers of the hand

3. Cupping with the cupped palm of the hand

4. Hacking with the ulnar border of the hand

5. Beating with a softly clenched hand

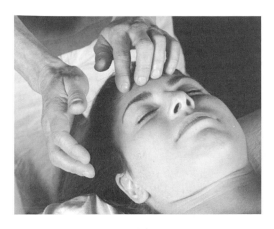

Figure 10.18a

Tapping with fingertips on the face.

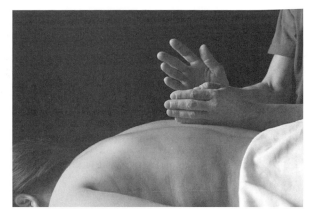

Figure 10.18b

Hacking movements on the back.

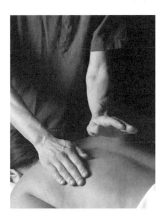

Figure 10.18c

Slapping movements on the back.

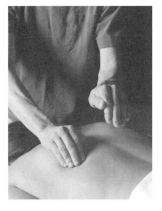

Figure 10.18d

Cupping movements on the thorax.

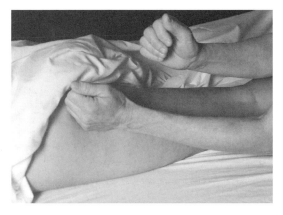

Figure 10.18e

Beating the thicker gluteal muscles.

Tapping

Tapping or **tapotement** is the lightest, most superficial of the percussion techniques. Tapping is used over delicate, sensitive areas such as the face. Only the fingertips are used for tapping. The fingers may be slightly flexed so that only the tips make contact, or, with the fingers held relatively straight, the pads perform a very superficial slapping technique.

Slapping

Slapping is very stimulating and must be used sparingly. Slapping encourages peripheral circulation and creates a "glow" to the area. It is applied with the palmar surface of the fingers and the hand. Slapping produces a crisp smacking sound when done correctly. As with all percussion strokes, the hands and wrists always remain loose and relaxed. Heavy pressure is avoided. Slapping uses a rhythmical, glancing contact with the body.

> **tapping**
> is the lightest, most superficial of the percussion techniques.

> **tapotement**
> movements include tapping, slapping, hacking, cupping, and beating.

> **slapping**
> uses a rhythmical, glancing contact with the body.

cupping

is a technique used by respiratory therapists to help break up lung congestion.

hacking

is a rapid striking movement that can be done with one or both hands.

beating

is the heaviest and deepest form of percussion and is done over the denser areas of the body.

passive joint movements

stretch the fibrous tissue and move the joint through its range of motion.

Cupping

Cupping is a technique often employed by respiratory therapists to help break up lung congestion. Cupping is most often employed over the rib cage. To perform cupping, form a cup by keeping the fingers together and slightly flexed and the thumb held close to the side of the palm. On each percussion, the perimeter of the hand contacts the body. The resulting sound is a hollow popping.

Hacking

Hacking, much like vibration, encourages relaxation and local circulation. Some theories claim that hacking stimulates the nerve responses in muscles and helps to firm the muscles. Hacking is a rapid striking movement that can be done with one or both hands. When both hands are used, the hands may strike alternately or together. A quick glancing strike is made with the little finger and the ulnar side of the hand. The wrist and fingers remain loose and relaxed, and the fingers are slightly spread apart. As the side of the hand strikes the body, the fingers come together causing a slight vibrating effect.

Beating

Beating is the heaviest and deepest form of percussion and is done over the thicker, denser, and fleshier areas of the body. The hands are held in a loose fist. Contact is made with the ulnar aspect of both hands either together or alternately. The wrists are relaxed so that the contact is the result of a rebounding, whiplike action of the hand and wrist. The force is never heavy or hard.

JOINT MOVEMENTS

There are a great variety of joint movements that can be used to manipulate any joint in the body, including joints of the toes, knees, hips, arms, the vertebrae, or even the less movable joints of the pelvis and cranium.

The basic classifications of joint movements are passive and active. **Passive joint movements (PJM)** are done while the client remains quietly relaxed and allow the practitioner to stretch and move the part of the body to be exercised. Passive joint movements can be used as an assessment tool to determine normal movement (full range of movement without restriction or pain). Passive joint movements gently stretch the fibrous connective tissue and move the joint through its range of motion. PJMs are used therapeutically to improve joint mobility and range of motion.

When performing PJMs, hold and support the limb so that the movement is directed toward the target joint. Move the limb in a normal movement pattern for that joint. Move the limb to the full extent of possible movement within the client's comfort level. If the movement is for assessment purposes, move only to the point of resistance and note the extent and quality of the movement. If the movement is therapeutic, challenge the range of movement by slightly extending or pushing into the end of the movement.

In **active joint movements,** the client actively participates in the exercise by contracting the muscles involved in the movement. In **active range-of-motion** movements, the client moves the limb or the joint without any intervention from the practitioner. This is a common assessment tool to determine what, if any, limitations may exist. The assessment may be done before and after treatment to note any changes. Active joint movements that involve the practitioner may be subdivided into two categories: active assistive and active resistive joint movements.

Active assistive joint movements are a therapeutic technique to restore mobility in a limb that has been injured. They are used when a client is not able to move a limb or move it through a full range of motion. When performing active assistive joint movements, the practitioner instructs the client to make a specific movement. This is best done by moving the limb passively through the desired movement. As the client attempts the movement, the therapist assists the limb through that movement as necessary. The movement is repeated several times.

Active resistive joint movements refer to a number of therapeutic techniques that improve mobility, flexibility, or strength, depending on how the technique is performed. As the name indicates, active resistive joint movements involve a movement that the client makes that is in some way resisted by the practitioner. The type and degree of the movement, the extent and direction of the resistance, the duration of the resistance, and the sequence of the actions all have an effect on the outcome of the procedure.

To perform active resistive joint movements to shoulder flexion, instruct the client on the movement by passively moving the arm from a neutral position next to the side to a position high over the head. Instruct the client to repeat the movement on your command. Place one hand on the wrist and the other just above the elbow. Instruct the client to move the arm. Resist the client's movement but allow the movement to take place. Repeat the movement several times, resisting a little more each time but always allowing the full movement to take place. This type of movement builds strength in the specific muscle groups being challenged. Active resistive joint movements can target any specific muscle group in the body.

Joint movements are used to help restore a client's mobility or increase flexibility in a joint. Often, passive and active joint movements will be combined. For example, to restore some mobility to a shoulder joint, the client is instructed to raise the arm to the point of discomfort (active unassisted movement). The therapist holds the arm in that position as the client is instructed to push against the therapist and attempt to continue the movement (active resistive joint movement). Then the client is instructed to relax as the therapist continues to move the client's arm (passive joint movement).

Passive and active joint movements have beneficial effects on the joint and the soft tissues associated with the joint. Most joint movements are applied to synovial joints.

active joint movements
are movements in which the client actively participates by contracting the muscles involved in the movement.

active range of motion
the client moves the limb or the joint without any intervention from the practitioner.

- The movements warm and lubricate the articulating surfaces within the joint capsule.

- Movements affect the proprioceptors and mechanoreceptors in the tissues surrounding the joint and in the associated muscles by manipulating the articulation through its full range of motion and introducing the limb to the possibility of new movement.

- The movements provide a stretch to the fascia of the associated muscles.

- Tendons and ligaments are flexed, stretched, and warmed to become more pliable.

- Lymph and venous blood circulation is stimulated due to the movement of the muscles.

Joint movements are most beneficial when performed through the full physiological range of motion. All joints have normal restrictions or barriers that limit the range of motion. These natural barriers can be classified as anatomical, physiological, or pathological.

Anatomical barriers limit movement due to the physical structure of the joint. Moving beyond an anatomical barrier would result in damage to the tissues involved.

The physiological barrier to a joint movement is encountered at the anatomical barrier, but usually before it is reached. The physiologic barrier may be due to bone-to-bone contact, such as the extension of the elbow where the movement is stopped when the olecranon of the ulna contacts the humerus. In healthy tissue, the physiologic barrier is usually due to soft tissue, either muscle or ligaments, limiting the movement at the end of a normal range of motion. The barrier may be due to soft tissue approximation, such as flexion of the elbow where the biceps presses against the forearm, restricting further movement. Sometimes the restriction is due to pull on ligaments as in the hyperextension of the hip. Most often, it is due to the pull of muscles that have reached the extent of their possible stretch.

A pathologic barrier is similar to the physiologic barrier, but it occurs either before the normal end of the range of motion is achieved or is accompanied by pain or discomfort that restricts the movement of the joint. Tense muscles, injured or scarred tissues, inflammation, or other pathological conditions may restrict the range of motion.

When performing joint movements on a client, the limb or joint should move easily and painlessly within its physiologic range of motion. It is beneficial for the practitioner to be familiar with the normal range of motion for the major synovial joints in the body. Keep in mind that normal range of motion may vary between individuals. As the practitioner moves a joint so that it approaches its physiologic barrier, the quality of the movement changes. The change in the quality of movement from the first sense of resistance to the extent of the physiologic or anatomic barrier is called **end feel.**

end feel
is the change in the quality of the feeling as the end of a movement is achieved.

End feel that results in bone-on-bone contact, such as the extension of the elbow, is termed **hard end feel.** Usually, however, the practitioner will feel a gradual tightening and springiness in the last few inches of the range of motion due to soft tissue approaching the extent of its possible stretch. This springy, rather painless limitation is termed **soft end feel.** On occasion, normal range of motion is restricted by muscle spasm or other conditions that cause pain during the movement. Abrupt restrictions to a joint movement before reaching the physiologic barrier due to pain is known as an **empty end feel.**

Joint movements have a great therapeutic benefit as an assessment tool and as a treatment to enhance function and mobility. The practitioner must be aware of the end feel of the joints and the reactions of the client when doing joint movements. Hard or soft end feel, free of pain and encountered at the physiologic barrier, indicates normal function of healthy tissue. Encountering a hard end feel before the normal physiologic barrier or a painful empty end feel indicate abnormal function. A soft end feel encountered before the normal physiologic barrier may indicate restrictions in the muscle's fascia or a neuromuscular guarding, shortening the functional length of an associated muscle. When a client exhibits restricted movement in certain joints, the practitioner may apply specific manipulations or movement to increase mobility (Figure 10.19a to j).

Joint movements are used extensively in soft tissue modalities such as proprioceptive neuromuscular facilitation (PNF), PNF stretching, muscle energy technique (MET), and position release. These modalities will be discussed in more detail in Chapters 13 and 18.

hard end feel
is a bone-against-bone feeling.

soft end feel
is a cushioned limitation where soft tissue prevents further movement, such as knee flexion.

empty end feel
is an abrupt restriction to a joint movement due to pain.

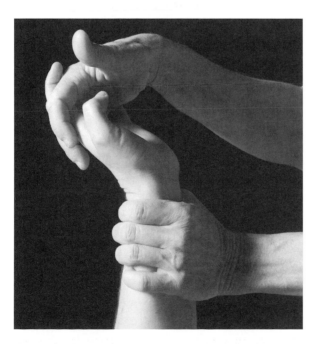

Figure 10.19a

Apply joint movements and rotation. Note the interlacing of the fingers.

continues

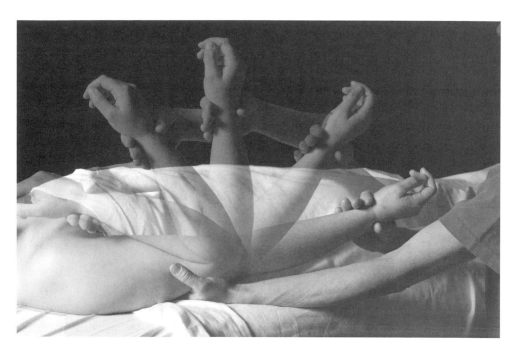

Figure 10.19b
Flexion and extension of the forearm.

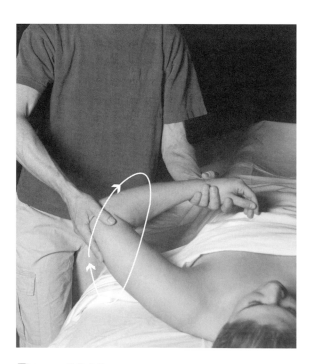

Figure 10.19c
Rotate the shoulder.

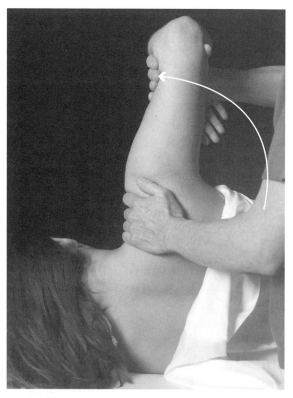

Figure 10.19d
Abduction of the arm. This is movement of a part away from the median line of the body.

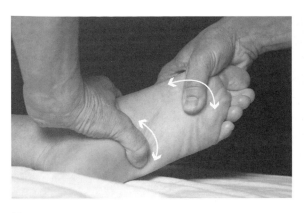

Figure 10.19e

Rotate and stretch the tarsals and metatarsals.

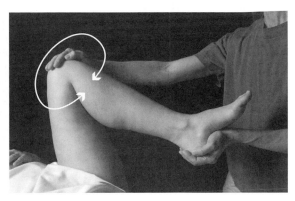

Figure 10.19f

Circumduction of the thigh.

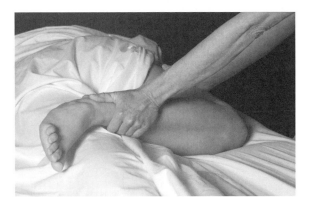

Figure 10.19g

Apply joint movements.

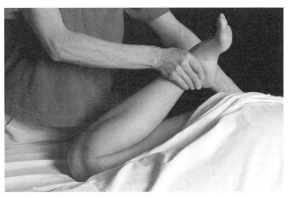

Figure 10.19h

Flexing the client's knee, pressing the heel against the gluteals.

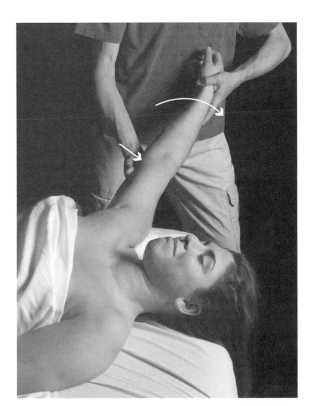

Figure 10.19i

Active assistive joint movement: The client tries to move her arm above her head as the therapist assists.

continues

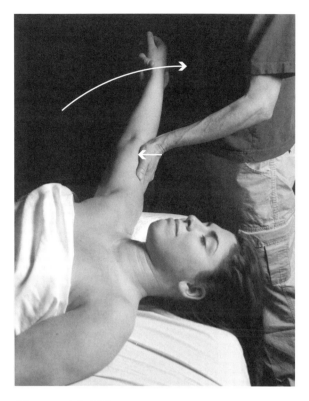

Figure 10.19j

Active resistive joint movement: The client
attempts to raise her arm as the therapist
resists the movement.

RHYTHM AND PRESSURE IN MASSAGE

People have individual vibrations and their own sense of rhythm. The
practitioner needs to remember that some people are high-strung
(tense), whereas others are very low-key (relaxed). It is important to
work with people according to their particular needs instead of following
a personal agenda and possibly working against the client's natural
rhythm. It is important to consider each individual situation when providing a therapeutic service. Usually someone coming for a massage is
seeking a relaxing, rejuvenating experience. The rhythm must be steady
and slightly slower than the client's pace in order to have a sedating effect. If the massage is part of an athletic training program, however, the
rhythm may be more upbeat. Practitioners can develop skills to tune in
to other people and work more effectively with them as individuals.
Clients will return to the practitioner who is not only well trained but
also sensitive and aware.

Breathing is a part of the body's natural rhythm and is important to
the practitioner's stamina and ability to move easily while giving massage.

The practitioner must develop an awareness of the right amount of
pressure to be used for various therapeutic situations and techniques. It
is important to begin to massage in an area of the body cautiously, gently, and lightly and then apply more pressure as you become aware of un-

derlying structures and the condition of tissues. This also helps you to note tension and stress buildup and determine how to proceed according to the client's body condition and sensitivity. The pressure varies with the technique used and according to the intended outcome. At no time should the pressure be so forceful as to cause injury to the tissues. The rule is to begin with a light and sensitive touch and increase the pressure as you work into an area. As tension in the area begins to dissipate and the muscles relax, the client will let you in even deeper. When it is time to leave the area, back out gradually, smoothing the way as you go.

One of the primary indications of tension or dysfunction in the muscles and soft tissue is pain. Massage therapy is one of the best methods of locating and treating these conditions. Many massage techniques directly manipulate the painful areas and therefore may be uncomfortable or even painful. People have different tolerances for pain. It is important not to work to a point that produces so much pain that the individual's pain threshold is crossed. Some deep tissue techniques advise that the most constructive therapy takes place at a depth and intensity that is barely tolerable to the client. When the pain threshold is violated, the client will tense up and the work will become less effective. Some bodywork does produce discomfort that is constructive; however, the pressure should never be so deep that it would hurt the client. Pain that hurts can not only damage the body, it can destroy the client's trust and ruin the therapeutic relationship. The first rule of massage and bodywork is: **Do no harm!**

QUESTIONS FOR DISCUSSION AND REVIEW

1. Name six basic classifications of movements used in massage.
2. What control should the practitioner have over the massage treatment?
3. Over which parts of the body are light movements applied?
4. Over which parts of the body are heavy movements applied?
5. In which direction is massage generally applied?
6. When are massage movements directed away from the heart?
7. What is the approximate duration of a full-body massage?
8. In terms of a massage technique, what is touch?
9. How is light touch administered, and what are its effects?
10. How is deep touch given, and when is it used?
11. How is aura stroking performed?
12. What is another name for feather stroking, and how is it used?
13. What is effleurage?
14. Which kind of effleurage requires the lightest possible touch?
15. Which kind of effleurage requires firm pressure?

16. What are the benefits of superficial gliding strokes?

17. What are the benefits of deep gliding strokes?

18. How is the kneading movement applied in massage?

19. What are the benefits of kneading?

20. What is the classical term that means the same as kneading?

21. For what part of the body is the fulling movement recommended?

22. What is the proper way to apply friction movements to the body?

23. What are the effects of friction on the connective tissue?

24. How is cross-fiber friction applied?

25. In what manner are compression movements applied to the body?

26. What are the benefits of compression movements?

27. What is the proper way to apply vibratory movements to the body?

28. What is a safe rate of vibration?

29. How can the practitioner control the effects produced by vibratory movements?

30. Why is excessive vibration harmful?

31. What is the proper way to apply percussion movements to the body?

32. Name the various forms of percussion movements.

33. What are the benefits of percussion movements?

34. To which parts of the body can joint movements be applied?

35. Name two types of joint movements.

36. Describe the difference between active assistive joint movements and active resistive joint movements.

37. What is range of motion?

38. Define end feel.

39. How is pressure regulated during a massage?

40. What is the significance of a pain threshold in the practice of massage?

Application of Massage Technique

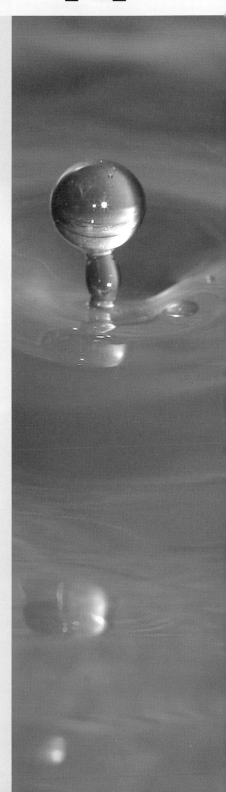

LEARNING OBJECTIVES

After you have mastered this chapter, you will be able to:

1. Demonstrate mastery of various hand exercises specifically for the benefit of massage practitioners.

2. Demonstrate correct standing posture and movements specifically for the benefit of massage practitioners.

3. Explain why it is necessary and desirable for the massage practitioner to develop coordination, balance, control, and stamina.

4. Explain why it is necessary and desirable for the massage practitioner to develop strong, flexible hands.

5. Describe the concepts of grounding and centering and how these practices benefit the massage practitioner.

INTRODUCTION

In recent times, the various movements used in body massage have been studied scientifically. Some movements are devised to induce relaxation, whereas others are meant to invigorate and stimulate the body. The massage practitioner is primarily concerned with manual movements that have beneficial effects on the client's body and how to apply these movements correctly and effectively. The correct application of the massage movements described in Chapter 10 requires more than the use of the practitioner's hands against the client's skin. When done correctly, the therapist's whole body is engaged in each movement. The feet are the foundation, the legs are the strength, the pelvis and torso supply the power, the heart supplies the love and compassion, and the arms and hands supply the intricate dexterity and communication with the client.

Massage is a physically demanding profession. The application of massage technique creates considerable stress on the practitioner's body. Improper posture, poor body alignment, and sloppy technique increase that stress and eventually result in injury or degenerative breakdown. Learning good body mechanics at the same time as learning massage techniques not only reduces fatigue and the chance of injury but also improves the delivery and outcome of the massage techniques.

The practice of massage requires the therapist to expend a tremendous amount of energy, not only physically but mentally and emotionally as well. If mental and emotional energy are not sustained, replenished, or increased, burnout eventually will result. It is important for the practitioner to be grounded, centered, and fully present during each massage session. In order for therapists to maintain the rigorous schedule necessary to make a living or even to supplement an income, they must be able to conserve, direct, and sustain their energy while performing daily massages.

This chapter focuses on techniques and exercises the practitioner may use to increase strength and endurance specific to the practice of massage. Exercises to improve mobility and posture are demonstrated and practiced. Finally, body mechanics to increase power, conserve energy, and reduce the chance of injury are studied and incorporated.

BUILDING STRENGTH AND FLEXIBILITY OF THE HANDS

The practitioner's hands are the most important tools used in massage. Hand mobility is important to maintain a regular rhythm and control when doing slow or fast movements. Flexible hands aid in working on the contours of the client's body and in controlling both speed and pressure. In addition to well-trained hands, the practitioner must have a good sense of balance and body control in order to move efficiently while applying various massage movements. Though the hands are the main implements delivering the manipulations to the client, the positioning and the strength of the entire body are essential to deliver effective massages over an extended period of time. The exercises shown here help develop strength, control, and flexibility of the hands (Figure 11.1a to h and Figure 11.2a to d).

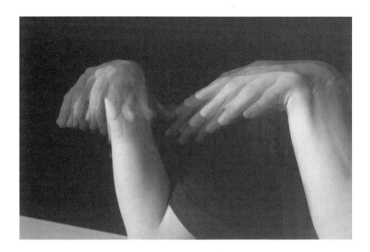

Figure 11.1a

Hold your hands at chest level and shake them vigorously for about 10 counts. This exercise warms and limbers the hands.

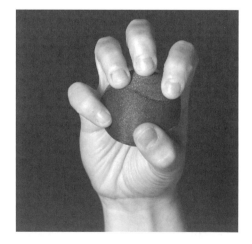

Figure 11.1b

Hold your hands at chest level. Use a small ball, *Therapuddy®*, or simply clinch your hands into tight fists. Squeeze the ball or fists as hard as you can and then release 10 times. Repeat this exercise several times. This exercise strengthens your hands and wrists.

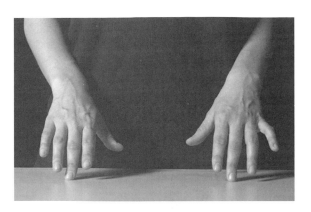

Figure 11.1c

Place both hands palm down on a flat surface. Begin with the thumbs and count each finger to the little finger and back to the thumbs by raising the digit off the surface as far as possible. This exercise is similar to playing a piano or typing. It is excellent for improving coordination and hand control.

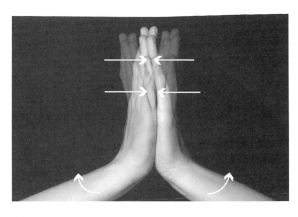

Figure 11.1d

Place your palms together at chest level. Press one hand against the other back and forth. This makes your wrists supple and strong. Repeat the presses about 10 times.

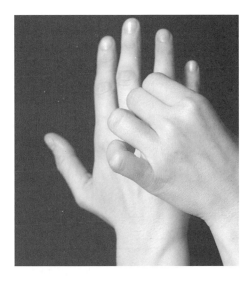

Figure 11.1e

Beginning with the thumb of the left hand, massage all the fingers of that hand by rubbing each finger from the knuckles of the hand to the tip of the finger. Repeat on the right hand. This exercise stimulates circulation and helps keep the hands supple.

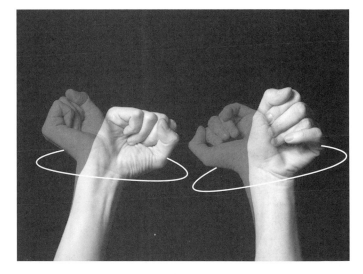

Figure 11.1f

Hold your hands in fists at chest level. Rotate both hands in circles forward 10 times, then reverse 10 times. This exercise strengthens and limbers the wrists.

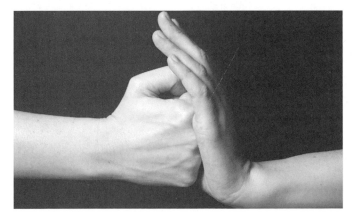

Figure 11.1g

Press the fist of one hand into the palm of the other, with each hand resisting the other. Do this 10 times on each hand. This exercise strengthens the entire arm and the hand.

continues

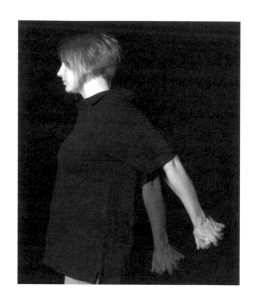

Figure 11.1h

Clasp your hands just below your waistline at the back of your body. Pull your arms upward while holding the tension for 10 counts. Pull your arms downward for 10 counts. This exercise strengthens the muscles of your arms, shoulders, and hands.

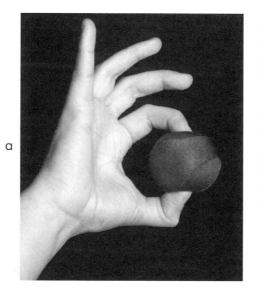

a

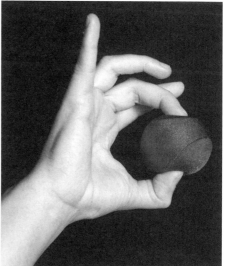

b

Figure 11.2a–11.2d

Hold a semisoft foam rubber ball between the thumb and first finger. Squeeze the ball as hard as possible, 10 times. Repeat, squeezing the ball with the second, third, and fourth fingers. Shake and massage that hand and repeat the exercise with the other hand.

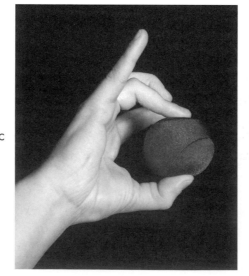

c

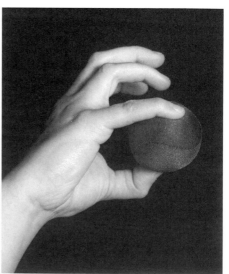

d

BODY MECHANICS

Even though the hands are the primary implement used to touch the client, all of the practitioner's body is used to deliver massage manipulations. Proper positioning of the feet, the strength of the legs, the position of the hips, back, shoulders, and head, and breathing all play an important role in the effective delivery of the massage, the level of fatigue, and the long-term health of the practitioner.

Body mechanics is the observation of body postures in relation to safe and efficient movement in daily living activities. Using good body mechanics increases the strength and power available in a movement while at the same time reducing the risk of potential injury to the practitioner.

Performing a full-body massage is a strenuous process. A professional massage therapist will perform five to eight massages a day four or five days a week. To do this, the practitioner must conserve energy.

Even though the hands are the point of contact during a massage, if the practitioner depends solely on the hands and arms to do the massage, the hands and arms will fatigue quickly. Tension in the hands and arms reflects into the shoulders and neck. Tension in the shoulders, arms, and hands or a consistent forward posture of the head often result in neck and shoulder pain. When the arms are overextended to perform long strokes or reach a distant body part, control, force, and pressure are compromised. Overreaching usually requires bending or twisting at the waist, which puts the back in a strained position.

The hands are the massage practitioner's most valuable tools. It is important to protect them. Avoid excessive wrist angles by staying behind the massage movements rather than on top of them. Avoid hyperextending the wrist and using the heel of the hand when applying compressive forces. Use the forearm and elbows when possible to apply deep pressure. When applying pressure with the fingers or thumb, use the cushioned palmar side of the thumb and fingers rather than the tips.

After years of practice, many massage therapists frequently experience fatigue, pain, and dysfunction in their hands and wrists, neck and shoulders, or lower back. Much of this discomfort can be avoided through the use of good body mechanics and movement. Keeping the head up, shoulders down and relaxed, and the arms and hands relaxed reduces the strain on the neck. By keeping the hands relatively close to the center of the body and the knees slightly flexed and feet apart, the practitioner uses the muscles in the legs and the movement of the whole body to deliver the strokes. When performing a manipulation that requires deep pressure or more force, the practitioner keeps the hand and arm in a stable position and leans the body into the movement. The practice of keeping the hands in good alignment and using body weight and leverage rather than muscle exertion of the upper body conserves energy and increases the power and strength when performing massage (Figure 11.3).

The risk of injury is directly proportionate to the amount of stress and the amount of biomechanical deviation. This is easy to observe in acute injuries such as a sprained ankle or a strained back. If a force is

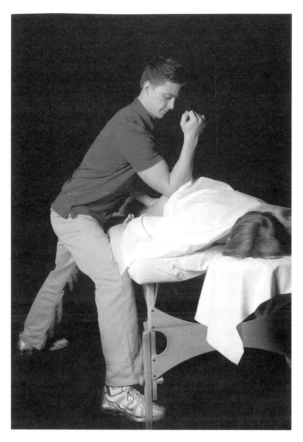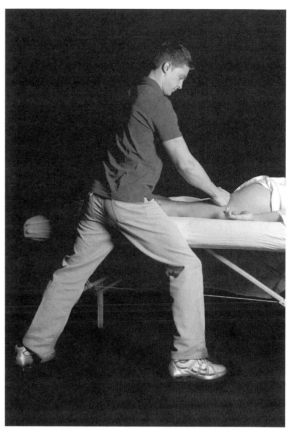

Figure 11.3

Use good body mechanics and lean into the movements to improve efficiency, power, and strength while reducing stress.

applied when the body is not in proper alignment, the result could be a torn ligament, tendon, muscle, or even a broken bone. Poor body mechanics practiced over a period of time become bad postural habits that cause structural (biomechanical) deviations. When the stress of muscular activity or even gravity is added to the biomechanically weak structure, dysfunction, pain, and injury will eventually result. This is precisely why many of your clients are seeking relief. It is important for the practitioner to avoid positions and practices that put undue stress on the back, neck, shoulders, arms, and hands.

As a massage therapist, you must develop good body mechanics. Using proper body positioning and posture will enable you to deliver powerful strokes and manipulations with a minimum of effort. Proper position and alignment of the back, shoulders, arms, wrists, and hands, especially when delivering forceful movements, will reduce the chance of overuse syndrome and injury.

The quality, effectiveness, and efficiency of nearly any massage manipulation are enhanced by incorporating body mechanics and movement. Engaging the body when applying stroking, kneading, and friction produces deeper, smoother, and more penetrating results with less effort and fatigue.

POSTURE AND STANCES

Correct posture and stances (foot positions) are important to the practitioner because they aid balance and allow the delivery of firmer, more powerful, more direct massage strokes. Proper stances allow the practitioner to lean into and out of the movements to deliver manipulations that penetrate with minimum effort and maximum effect. Correct posture is essential to conserve strength and prevent backache due to improper body mechanics that would put too much stress on the practitioner's arms and shoulders during the massage procedure. Good posture and body mechanics help sustain energy when it is necessary to work long hours, because they enable the practitioner to move around the table more freely and easily while maintaining the flow of movement and energy.

The most common stances are called the horse and the archer.

Horse Stance

In the horse stance, both feet are placed in line with the edge of the massage table. This is the most comfortable stance when doing petrissage on the legs or back. The knees are kept slightly flexed so that the therapist can apply firmer pressure to the manipulations by shifting weight side to side and leaning into the client, thereby preserving the strength in the arms. The back remains erect and relaxed. The shoulders are comfortably dropped and back. The breathing is deep and full (Figure 11.4a to c).

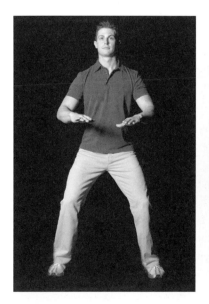
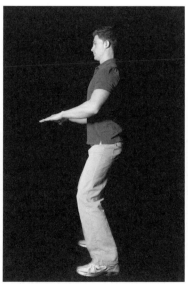
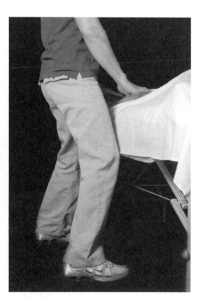

Figure 11.4a–c
Horse stance.

Archer Stance

The archer stance is the most commonly used position, especially when the practitioner's shoulders are at an angle (other than parallel) with the edge of the table or when the practitioner is stepping into a movement. For the archer stance, the feet are positioned so that an imaginary line drawn through the center of the back foot at the arch passes through the front foot at midheel and the third toe (Figure 11.5). The feet may be close together or a full stride apart. This foot position provides a solid, stable foundation for the therapist to lean into or pull back on a manipulation. By shifting weight from one foot to the other, the therapist can perform long rhythmic strokes without sacrificing good posture. This foot position also provides excellent mobility so that the therapist can step into or away from a movement smoothly and at the same time maintain contact and pressure. This eliminates the need to bend at the waist. The mobility allows the therapist's hands to remain close to his body, where they retain more control and strength. Mobility uses the muscles of the legs to provide much of the movement and strength for many of the manipulations. This, along with the practice of leaning and stepping into or away from the movement, provides a large portion of the energy needed to deliver massage treatments.

In either stance, the knees and ankles should be kept flexed slightly. Stiff, rigid knees contribute to fatigue, and locking the knees forces a posture that puts the back in danger of injury. The back remains relatively erect and stable. When it is necessary to lean over, the practitioner can step forward and bend from the hips, thereby maintaining the integrity of the spine.

Often, the tendency when performing massage is to tighten and raise the shoulders. The shoulders should remain relaxed and dropped to

Figure 11.5

In the archer stance, the forward foot is pointing in the direction of the movement.

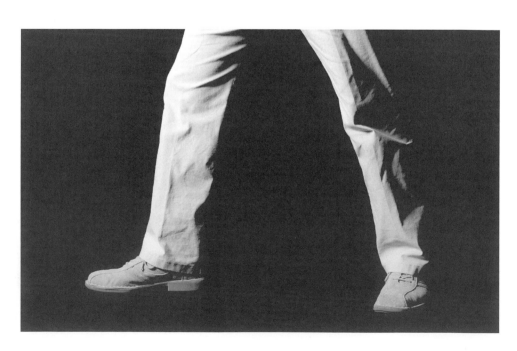

ensure optimum nerve and blood supply to the hands and arms. It is also important that the breathing be deep and full to supply plenty of oxygen and eliminate carbon dioxide.

Correct stances make it easier to shift weight from foot to foot so that movement is smooth, as in dancing. Correct stances give the practitioner more body power when leaning into the movements.

EXERCISES FOR STRENGTH, BALANCE, AND BODY CONTROL

Two techniques called **centering** and **grounding** are important to the practitioner because they provide a psychological, energetic, and physical base from which to work.

Centering: Centering is based on the concept that you have a geographical center in your body located about 2 inches below the navel in the pelvic area. The Chinese refer to this as the *tan tein* (don te-in). Many of the ancient writings about martial arts mention this concept. Having a sense of that center and moving from that center provide a quality of power, balance, and control.

Centering has both a physical and psychoemotional context. Emotionally, being centered refers to a certain confident sense of balance and self-assurance. Being centered means you feel self-assured and emotionally stable. Being uncentered means you feel insecure and unstable. Feeling centered (in control) is of value because it is important to be able to handle problems that arise without becoming frustrated or emotionally overwhelmed. Centering is accomplished by concentrating on the geographical center (*tan tein*) and on being self-assured (Figure 11.6).

Grounding: Grounding is based on the concept that you have a connection with the client and that you function as something of a grounding apparatus, helping the client to release unwanted tension and feelings of stress. Grounding is achieved by mentally visualizing yourself as having the ability to draw from a greater power or energy. By being grounded, you become a sort of conduit or conductor that allows the energies to pass through you. The negative energies can pass out of the client, and the positive energies can be directed into the client through you. Grounding allows these energy transfers to take place without you, the practitioner, being drained of your own energy or picking up any unwanted tension or stress from the client. Try thinking of yourself as a tree rooted to the ground.

centering
is based on the concept that you have a geographical center in your body about 2 inches below the navel.

grounding
is based on the concept that you have a connection with the client and that you function as a grounding apparatus in helping the client to release tension.

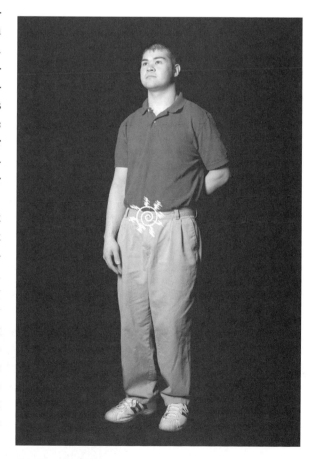

Figure 11.6

The *tan tein* is the geographical and energetic center of the body.

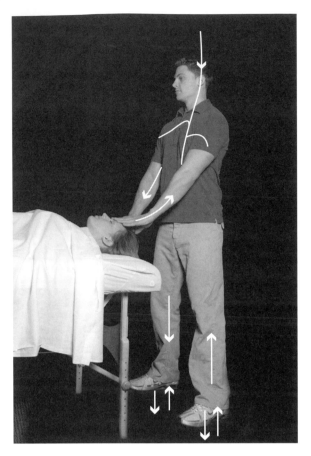

Figure 11.7

The practitioner's body serves as a conduit for positive energy to be transmitted into the client and negative energy to be grounded out of the client.

Controlled breathing is also helpful. The concepts of grounding and centering will become more clear as you master the following exercises (Figure 11.7).

Exercise 1—Grinding Corn

This exercise helps you reach the full length of the part of the client's body that is being worked on by being able to shift your weight easily from one foot to the other while maintaining good posture and balance. The exercise is called grinding corn because the movement is similar to using an old-fashioned hand corn grinder. You may also think of it as a movement similar to polishing a car. Use your imagination.

Procedure: Place your feet apart (about the width of your shoulders) and tilt your pelvis forward and upward. Bend your knees, and sink down until you are in a semi–knee bend. Do not go all the way down to a squatting position. Keep your back straight, and do not allow your head to jut forward. While maintaining this posture, hold your hands in front of your body (palms down) about the level of your waistline. Now begin to move both hands toward the right, forming a wide oval. This will look as if you are ready for a karate move.

After you get the feel of the standing position and hand movements, begin to move your right hand clockwise and your left hand counterclockwise. Shift your weight from foot to foot. Keep making the ovals (keeping your back straight) until you are comfortable with the movement. Lower your hands about 6 inches by bending your knees into a deeper knee bend. Continue practicing. As you continue the exercise, become aware of the centering concept previously described and allow your movements to be initiated from the pelvic area (about 2 inches below the navel), with the rest of your body following through. Remember, this is your geographical area or center that allows your entire body to move with balance and strength (Figure 11.8a to c).

This exercise can be performed while standing next to a massage table. As you practice the movement, glide your hands lightly over the surface of the table. Gradually increase the area your hands cover until you are able to reach from one end of the table to the other and from one side to the other. To do this, shift your weight from one foot to the other. Be conscious of your balance, and do not compromise your back by extending or leaning too far.

As you master these techniques and continue to practice them, your arms, hands, and shoulders will become less fatigued because of the support supplied by the rest of your body.

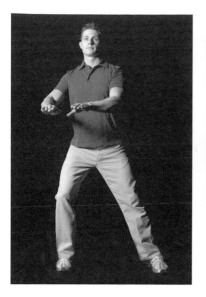

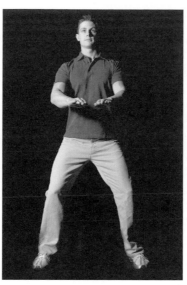

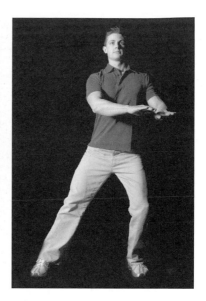

Figure 11.8a
Grinding corn: Move to the right, making large ovals with your hands and transferring your weight to the right foot.

Figure 11.8b
Grinding corn: Front view.

Figure 11.8c
Grinding corn builds strength in the legs as it teaches balance and coordination.

Exercise 2—The Wheel

Procedure: First, take a deep breath and exhale slowly. Repeat this several times. This exercise helps you to relax. Take a comfortable stance with your feet about 6 inches apart. Turn the left foot out at a 45° angle. Shift most of your weight to the left foot while bending your left knee slightly. With your left heel remaining on the floor, step forward with your right foot. Remember to keep your hips and shoulders facing forward and your knees bent. Your right foot should be forward about 15 to 20 inches. Shift your weight forward to the right foot then back again to the left, in a smooth motion, so that 90 percent of your weight shifts from one foot to the other. Once you have the feel of the stance, take a deep breath and exhale slowly while placing your hands about 6 inches apart with palms facing one another. Begin making circles with your hands while imagining that you are rotating a large wheel that is suspended in front of you. The top of the wheel is about shoulder level, and the bottom is at the level of your pubic bone. As you shift your weight forward, reach out and rotate the wheel up. Shift your weight back as you rotate the wheel back and down. Continue the movement and breathe deeply and slowly so that with each full revolution of the wheel, you take one full breath (inhale and exhale). Without breaking your rhythm, turn your right foot to a 45° angle and take one step forward. Repeat the exercise several times (Figure 11.9a to c).

To complete the exercise, bring your feet together so that your weight is distributed evenly. Turn your palms facing downward and allow your hands to float down to your sides. Stay in this position for a few seconds to experience the feeling. As you master this movement, you will

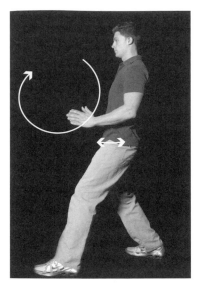

Figure 11.9a

The wheel is a good center-ing exercise that teaches deep breathing, balance, and moving from the center *(tan tein)*.

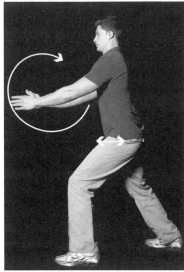

Figure 11.9b

The wheel: The body weight shifts forward and back from one foot to the other.

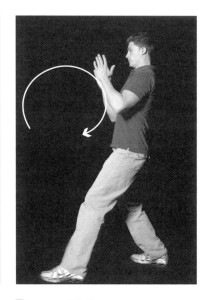

Figure 11.9c

The wheel: The hands de-scribe a large wheel. Each revolution of the wheel re-quires one full breath.

find that it is best accomplished by concentrating on originating the movement from the pelvic area (center or *tan tein*) and moving straight forward and backward while allowing the rest of your body to follow.

Exercise 3—Advance and Retreat

A variation of the wheel is a move that is valuable to the practice of mas-sage. As the name implies, advance and retreat involves a powerful for-ward movement followed by a controlled withdrawal.

Procedure: The position of the feet is essentially the same as for the wheel or the archer stance. The back foot is turned approximately 45° while the front foot is pointing in the direction of the movement. The distance the feet are apart determines the length and the power of the movement. Optimally, the feet should be between 16 and 32 inches apart. The knees remain flexed as 80 percent of the body weight moves from one foot to the other. The hands are positioned at about belt level and close to the side of the body. The primary movement is in the hips and pelvis as they move straight forward and back. The hips do not move up or down, just straight forward and back. The torso remains per-pendicular, and the hands accentuate the move only slightly. Change the position of the feet and the hands move to the other side of the body (Figure 11.10a and b).

Advance and retreat can be performed at the side of a massage table to illustrate the usefulness of the maneuver. Stand at the side of a massage table near one end, facing the other end. Turn the foot nearest the table

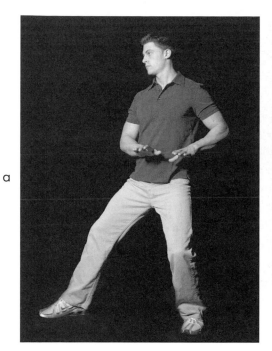

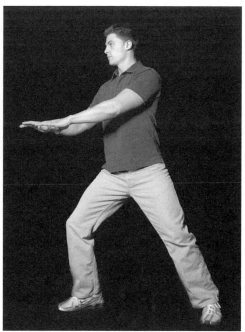

a

b

Figure 11.10

Advance and retreat: The hands are held at the same height as the *tan tein.* The feet are in a wide archer stance. (a) Retreat: Ninety percent of the weight is on the back foot. Hands are down to one side and upper body posture is erect. The body weight is shifted smoothly and powerfully forward. (b) Advance: Eighty percent of weight is shifted to the front leg. The arms are extended forward. The upper body maintains an erect posture.

45°. Step forward with the outside foot. Bend both knees slightly. Rest both hands on the table beside and slightly in front of you. (Your hands should be close to your body and about the level of the *tan tein.*) Shift your weight from one foot to the other. Notice how much of the length of the table you cover while moving your arms very little (Figure 11.11a and b).

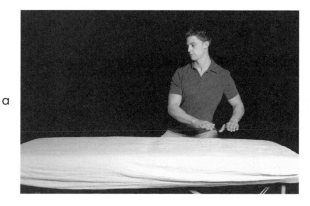

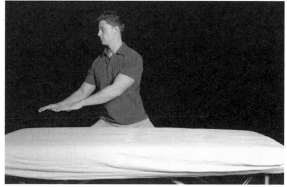

a

b

Figure 11.11

Using advance and retreat at the massage table allows the practitioner to move the length of the table in one stroke while maintaining good body mechanics.

Exercise 4—The Tree

This exercise emphasizes the importance of posture and concentration and is combined with centering, grounding, and correct breathing.

Procedure: Stand with your feet together, with your shoulders relaxed down and back. Pull your buttocks downward slightly. This will cause your pelvis to tilt upward. Take a deep breath and exhale slowly. Begin the exercise by turning your left foot out (bending the left knee) and shifting all your weight to your left foot. Keep your upper body erect. Move your right foot straight forward so that when your right leg is extended, the ball of your right foot rests lightly on the floor. Bring both arms up to about shoulder level to form a circle. This should look as if you are trying to reach around a large tree. Your fingers will be pointing toward each other, about 2 inches apart. Keep your head up, chin level, and gaze ahead. As you hold this pose, the leg bearing your weight may feel weak and begin to tremble. However, by maintaining the pose for about 3 minutes at a time and practicing your breathing exercises, you will soon experience a sense of renewed strength and power.

Change the pose to the left foot position (left foot forward) with your weight on your right foot, and continue to breathe deeply, exhaling slowly. Alternate the right and left feet, continuing to practice until you feel completely in control. To finish the exercise, bring your feet to a side-by-side position with your weight distributed evenly and your back straight. Allow your arms to float down to your sides. Take a moment to experience what is happening to your body (Figure 11.12).

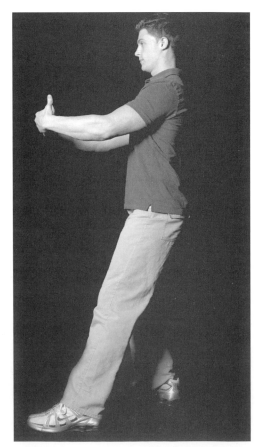

Figure 11.12

The tree exercise builds strength and endurance in your legs and shoulders as it encourages concentration and breathing.

Although you may find these exercises tiring and sometimes boring, remember that there is no easy way to accomplish erect posture, body strength, coordination, and proper breathing. Keep foremost in your mind that your goal is to be able to perform efficiently as a master of massage techniques. As you begin to do professional massage, you will see how these exercises increase your feeling of self-esteem.

PROFESSIONAL RULES TO REMEMBER

Knowledge of the restrictions and limitations of massage is as important as knowledge of its proper use. A well-trained practitioner knows when a massage treatment is indicated, how it can be modified for the greatest benefit to the client, and under what circumstances it should not be applied.

Before beginning the massage routines discussed in the next chapter, review the basic rules for safe and effective massage procedures.

1. Everything used in massage treatments should be clean and sanitary.

2. Wash your hands thoroughly with soap and hot water and rinse and dry them before and after each treatment.

3. Keep your nails short and smooth to avoid scratching the client's skin.

4. Avoid chilling the client by contact with cold hands or by having the temperature of the room too low for comfort.

5. Avoid massage immediately after the client has eaten a meal.

6. Avoid heavy, rapid, or jarring movements that might convey fear of injury to the client.

7. Never use any form of heavy stroking against the venous blood supply.

8. Never apply massage so vigorously that it causes fatigue in the client.

9. Allow the client to have a short rest period before and after the massage.

QUESTIONS FOR DISCUSSION AND REVIEW

1. Why is it necessary for the massage practitioner to develop strong, flexible hands?

2. What is body mechanics?

3. Why is it important for the massage practitioner to practice good body mechanics?

4. How can the practitioner increase the power and strength in a movement and at the same time conserve energy?

5. Why are good posture and the use of proper stances important to the massage practitioner?

Procedures for Complete Body Massages

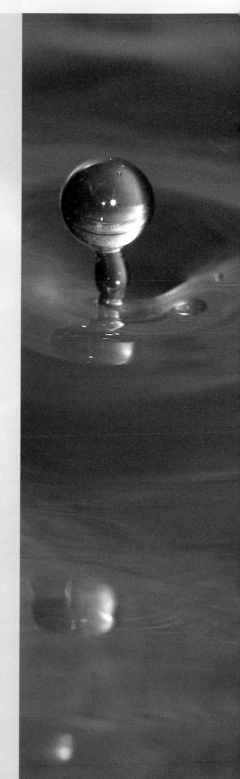

LEARNING OBJECTIVES

After you have mastered this chapter, you will be able to:

1. Demonstrate the steps in preparing a client for a massage session.
2. Demonstrate correct procedures for draping the client.
3. Explain the importance of assisting a client onto and off of a massage table.
4. Demonstrate a basic body massage (Massage 1).
5. Demonstrate massage variations (Massage 2).
6. Use correct anatomical terms when describing the part of the body being massaged.
7. Utilize correct posture and stances for the massage practitioner.
8. Demonstrate professional courtesies toward clients before, during, and after massage.
9. Understand when and where certain massage movements should and should not be applied.
10. Answer client questions concerning any aftereffects of massage.

INTRODUCTION

Massage procedure is the actual process of performing a massage therapy session. There are as many variations of doing a massage as there are therapists giving and clients receiving massages. Practitioners may adopt a general routine and practice it on every client they see with minor variations due to specific contraindications or client requests, or the therapist may provide therapeutic services tailored to the specific needs of a client on the day of her appointment. Regardless of the style and content of the massage treatment, guidelines should be followed to ensure that the services received by the client meet high professional standards and the client's expectations. Clients who receive courteous professional services will regard the treatment with respect. They will repeat business and refer others to your service.

PREPARING THE CLIENT FOR THE MASSAGE

When the preliminary interview is done and the client has completed any necessary forms, it is time to begin the actual massage. If this is the first time you have seen this client or if it is the client's first massage, an explanation of your services and clear instructions about what the client should do will eliminate false expectations and dispel much of the anxiety the client may have. It is at this time that the practitioner might obtain a signed informed consent document from the client. This document clearly states the services and qualifications of the therapist, that the client understands the scope of the services, and that the client understands or has received a copy of the therapist's policies. At the end of the preliminary consultation when the practitioner has ascertained that the client is free of any general contraindications and a strategy for the session has been formulated, briefly explain to the client what you will be doing and why. Show the client the facilities and explain the use of any equipment, such as steam baths or exercisers. Explain the dressing procedures and draping. Show the client the dressing room or area and explain the use of any wraps or drapes the client may use to get from the dressing area to the table.

Two commonly asked questions are "Do I have to take off my clothes?" and "How many of my clothes do I have to take off?" The most effective way to receive a massage is with all clothing removed. With proper draping, a client's modesty should never be compromised. However, many people (especially first timers) are not comfortable with all of their clothes removed. The client's comfort is of primary importance. Instruct the client that the best way to receive a thorough and complete massage is with all clothes removed and that draping will be used at all times to ensure modesty and that only the part of the body being massaged will be uncovered at any time. Explain that the genitals and breasts (private areas) will be carefully (modestly) covered at all times. Also give clients the option to leave on whatever they feel comfortable with. Many people will choose to wear their underwear, but even if they choose to remain fully clothed, it is possible to perform a massage through clothing. As time goes on and the client receives more massages, she may become more accustomed to the procedure and comfortable with her own body.

ASSISTING THE CLIENT ON AND OFF THE TABLE

For reasons of safety and liability, it is advisable that the practitioner is available to assist the client onto the table at the beginning of a massage and into a sitting position and off the table at the end of the massage.

The table may be too high for some clients, or various disabilities may prevent easy access to the table. A footstool is a useful item. It can be used as a step to assist some people onto the table and by the therapist to stand on for better leverage when performing some techniques.

The procedure you use may require the client to assume a specific position on the table. Careful instruction and physical guidance will ensure that the client ends up in the proper place. By keeping a hand on clients and guiding them as they sit down on the table and then as they lie down, you greatly reduce the possibility of injury, and clients are more likely to assume the position necessary to perform the massage. Maintaining contact as the client gets onto and off of the table also provides a feeling of comfort and security.

Draping procedures must include techniques that allow these movements to be accomplished while keeping the client modestly covered (Figure 12.1).

POSITIONING THE CLIENT ON THE MASSAGE TABLE

The client should assume a position on the massage table that is comfortable and allows access to the body in order to perform the massage. Once the client is sitting on the table, instruct and assist her to lie down either faceup, facedown, or a side-lying position, depending on the treatment to be given. When the client is lying down, she must be able to relax.

You may encounter a person who cannot comfortably lie on her back or facedown without support. In such cases, it is helpful to have foam cushions and bolsters in various shapes and sizes. These are made of fairly high-density foam and are covered with vinyl for easy cleaning.

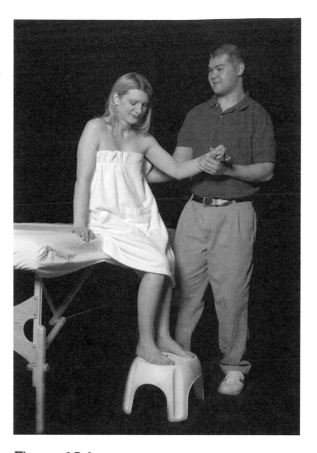

Figure 12.1

A stepstool may be used to help the client get onto the table. It is helpful for the therapist to lend a hand as the client gets onto and off of the table.

Bolsters as wide as the table and 4 to 8 inches in diameter can be used under the client's knees when the client is lying on her back. A bolster may be placed under the ankles when the client is lying facedown. Bolsters should be placed under the sheets or draping material so that they do not come in direct contact with the client's skin. Positioning with bolsters provides more comfort for the client who has reduced flexibility in the ankles, knees, or lower back. Firm bed pillows may also be used (Figure 12.2).

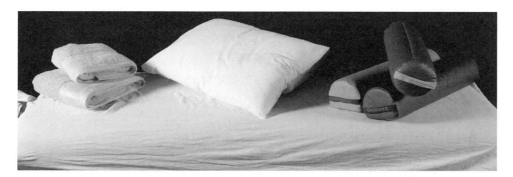

Figure 12.2

A variety of bolsters and pillows can be used to position the client for comfort.

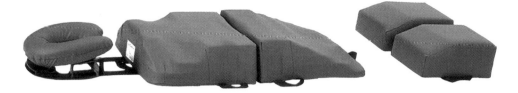

Figure 12.3a

Body Support Systems® provide comfortable whole body support.
(Courtesy of Body Support Systems, Inc.)

Another consideration when positioning the client facedown is to have a support to place under the client's chest to take the pressure off the cervical spine while in the prone position. This support should hold the chest 3 to 4 inches off the table while allowing the head to rest forward comfortably. Most modern massage tables have adjustable face cradles that provide comfortable head and neck support for the client in a facedown or prone position. Commercially manufactured Body Support Systems® consist of a number of specifically designed cushions that provide comfortable, full-body support when the client is in the prone position (Figure 12.3a).

Some people need support under the abdomen when they have severe low back discomfort. Elevating the midsection and abdomen 6 to 8 inches in this manner helps you work on the back more effectively. A person who is unable to lie back with the head resting on the table will need support for head and neck as well as the small of the back and behind the legs (Figure 12.3b to d).

A side-lying position has many advantages when a client is not comfortable in a supine or prone position. When a client is in the side-lying position, one pillow or cushion is placed under the head to keep the cervical spine straight. Another pillow or bolster is placed under the top leg, which is bent at the hip and the knee so that the pelvis is not torqued or twisted. Another pillow can be positioned under the top arm for the

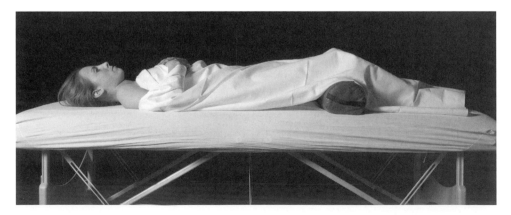

Figure 12.3b

In the supine position, a bolster behind the knees reduces tension in the back of the legs and the low back.

client to hug in order to maintain the arm and shoulder in a comfortable position.

The side-lying position works well for pregnant women in their second and third trimesters and for people with physical conditions that do not allow them to lie flat. This position also provides excellent access when working on the inside or outside of the thigh and on the side of the neck (Figure 12.3e).

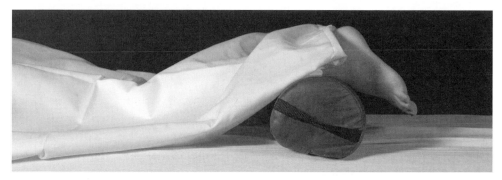

Figure 12.3c
In the prone position, a bolster under the ankles prevents hyperextension of the knee and ankle and relieves tension in the low back.

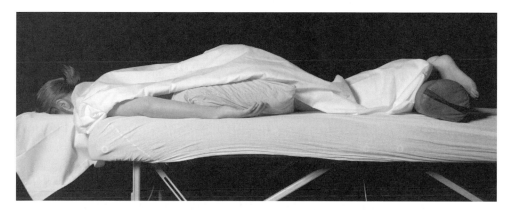

Figure 12.3d
Support under the abdomen relieves tension in the low back.

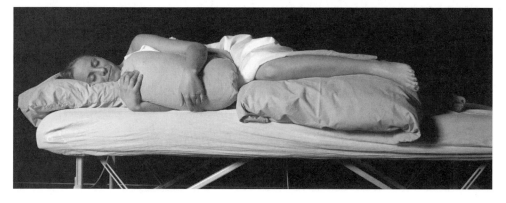

Figure 12.3e
In a side-lying position, pillows or bolsters are placed under the head and the upper leg. Another pillow is provided for the client to hug.

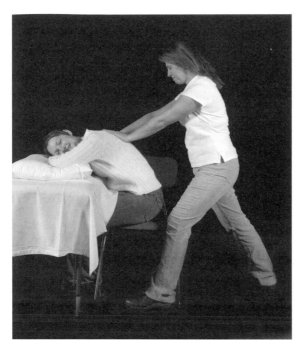

Figure 12.4a

If using a table is not practical, a supported seated massage is an alternative.

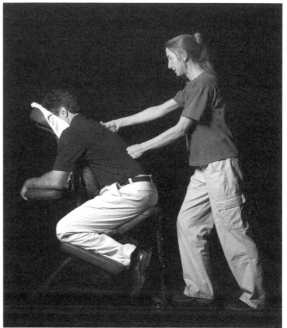

Figure 12.4b

Seated massage using a massage chair is usually done with the client fully clothed.

You may have clients coming to you for massage who will have different problems. Some clients will be unable to lie facedown, and others will not be able to lie flat on their backs without some kind of extra support. For this reason, extra supports should be a part of your professional equipment. For example, if a client is not able to get up on the massage table or lie down, you can use a chair and pillows to seat the person comfortably. You can then give a massage to the back quite easily (Fig. 12.4a).

A massage chair provides another alternative for a client to receive many of the benefits of an upper body massage in a seated position without removing clothing (Figure 12.4b).

Having a variety of supporting pillows or bolsters as part of your equipment will enable you to position and support your client when necessary. All bolsters and pillows that come in direct contact with the client must have removable cloth slipcovers. Fresh clean covers are used for each client. Bolsters and pillows can also be placed under the bottom sheet next to the table to avoid contact with the client's skin.

DRAPING PROCEDURES

draping
is the process of using linens to keep a client covered while receiving a massage.

The process of using linens to keep a client covered while performing a massage is called **draping.** This procedure allows for the client to be totally undressed and at the same time retain comfort, warmth, and modesty. It gives the practitioner the freedom to massage all parts of the body unencumbered by the client's clothing.

Proper draping ensures that the client stays warm and feels safe and comfortable. Perspiration, massage lubricant, and being in a reclining position all increase the rate at which the body loses heat. Massage stimulates the parasympathetic nervous system, affecting the basal body temperature, which results in the client becoming chilled more easily. The proper temperature for a massage room is between 72° F and 78° F. If the area is cooler than this, extra precautions should be taken to make sure the client remains warm. It is much easier for a person to get chilled than to warm up. If a person is chilled, it is nearly impossible for her to relax.

Two items to keep on hand to deal with chilling are a twin-size electric mattress pad to put on the table under the sheet and a flannel blanket or sheet to put over the client after she is on the massage table and is properly draped.

By using proper draping (uncovering only the portion of the body that is being massaged) and by always concealing the client's personal parts, the practitioner maintains a professional and ethical practice while preventing embarrassment to either the practitioner or the client.

There are several methods of draping. All methods consist of techniques of maintaining personal privacy while getting the client from the dressing area to the hydrotherapy area and/or the massage table; using adequate draping while the client receives the massage; and keeping the client well covered while she gets up from the massage table and returns to the dressing area.

METHODS OF DRAPING

There are several methods of draping that are easy and effective. In this chapter, we discuss two methods. Practice each of these until you are proficient. You may choose one style that works best for you, or you may combine portions of one method with another. While learning these various draping procedures, refer to the step-by-step directions and illustrations included in this chapter. The beginner should be careful to follow directions carefully and practice until able to drape a client smoothly and efficiently. It is also important to know how to instruct the client in how to change positions during the draping procedures.

Method 1—Top Cover Method

The top cover method uses a table covering along with a top covering that is large enough to cover the entire body. A large bath sheet towel or one half of a full or double sheet will serve this purpose well. The minimum size for the top cover is 72 inches long and 36 inches wide. It is possible to use two bath-sized towels as a top cover. When the client is lying on the table, the two towels are in a T configuration with the upper towel lying across the torso and the lower towel covering the lower extremities up to the hips. The lower towel is turned crossways over the central area of the body when it is time for the client to turn over.

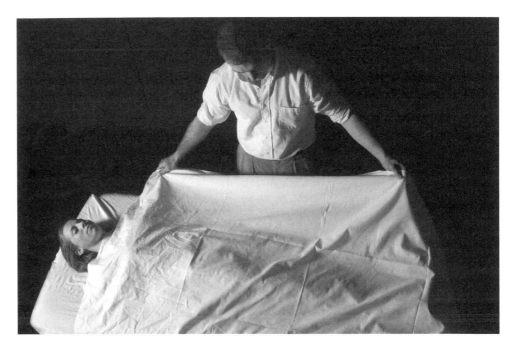

Figure 12.5

As the client takes her place on the massage table, situate the top cover lengthwise to cover all except her head. If the top cover is also used as a wrap, it is rearranged from across the client's body to a lengthwise position. If a terry wrap or towel is worn from the dressing area, the top cover can be laid in place and the wrap discreetly slipped from underneath.

The cover sheet may also serve as the wrap the client uses to get from the dressing area to the table.

The use of this type of draping ensures warmth and modesty while allowing easy access to each body part (Figure 12.5).

Method 2—Full Sheet Draping

Full sheet draping employs the use of a full-size double flat sheet (minimum width 80 inches) to cover the table and wrap the client. When working with a large client (200 pounds plus), it is necessary to use a queen-size sheet. When using this method, it is necessary to supply an additional wrap for the client to get from the dressing area to the table. After the client is on the table, the wrap is used to secure the sheet and to cover the client when she turns over and gets up after the massage (Figure 12.6).

The following items may be used in the draping process.

Sheets

- Full double flat sheets (minimum width 80 inches)
- Cot-size fitted sheets
- One half of full double sheets, cut and hemmed to use as a table covering or a cover sheet
- Disposable sheets to use as table coverings when laundry is a problem

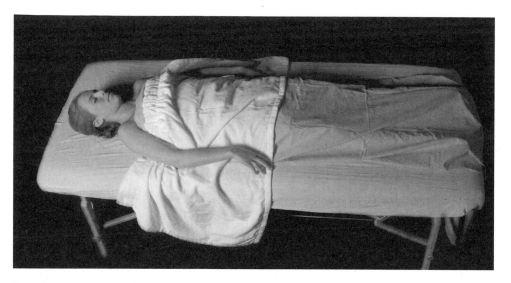

Figure 12.6

Full sheet draping covers the client securely in a cocoon-like wrap, and the client feels safe and warm.

Towels

- Bath-size towels for draping and for personal use after hydrotherapy
- Bath sheets for body covers
- Terry cloth wraps to wear to and from the dressing area

Miscellaneous

- Pillow cases for covering pillows and bolsters
- Washcloths, pillow covers, or specifically manufactured protectors to cover face cradles
- Flannel sheets to use when extra warmth is needed
- Twin-size electric mattress pad for use on the table when warmth is a problem, such as working in a home where it is too cool

Remember that any materials coming in contact with the client's skin must be freshly laundered and sanitary. Clean linens must be used for each client.

Draping from the Dressing Area to the Massage Table

The first step in the draping process requires some form of wrap to be worn from the dressing area to either the hydrotherapy area or the massage table. The method of draping during the massage as well as the size and gender of the client will determine the type of wrap that is used. In the cover sheet method, the cover sheet may be used. Terry cloth wraps can be provided instead of a towel for the client to wear in any method of draping. These wraps can be purchased in a department store or uniform department. The women's wrap fastens above the breasts; the men's wrap is a shorter version that wraps around and fastens at the waist. The length is usually just above the knees. These wraps are convenient because they secure and unfasten easily when the client is on the table, and they are easy to put back on after the massage. Wraps are available in small, large, and extra large sizes for men and women (Figures 12.7a and b).

When using a wrap or a towel, the client arranges it so that the open side is situated at the side of the body. As the client sits on the edge of the table, the wrap is lifted out of the way to avoid sitting on the wrap. The wrap is then unfastened as the client is instructed to lie down. As the client lies down, the wrap is smoothly slipped from under the body. In this way, the client is lying down on the table with the wrap covering the body, not underneath.

An alternative to this procedure is to have the client lie on the table and then unfasten the wrap. Have the client lift her body slightly as you carefully slip the wrap from underneath.

Having gotten the client on the table, lying down, and covered by the wrap, you are ready to proceed with the draping of your choice and the massage.

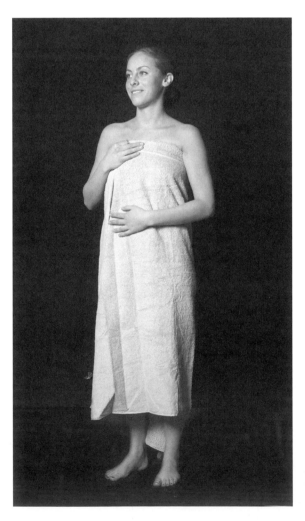

Figure 12.7a

The female wrap is long enough to cover the body and can be used as a top cover.

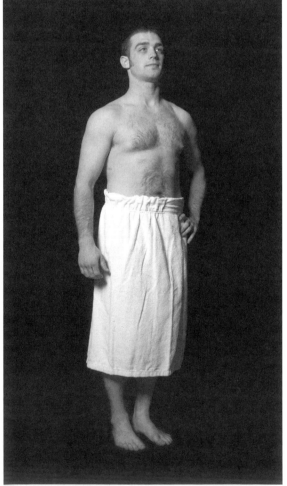

Figure 12.7b

The male wrap can be smaller but also must act as a modest covering.

When the massage has been completed and it is time for the client to get up and get dressed, a procedure must be followed that will maintain the client's privacy in a relaxed and efficient manner, while at the same time ensuring the client's safety. The procedure shown in Figure 12.8a to c will be helpful.

It is important to be courteous and attentive toward your clients from the time they enter your place of business until they leave. You should show concern for their safety and comfort at all times. Some clients will want and expect help when getting on or off the massage table; others will indicate that they prefer helping themselves. When in doubt, ask. For example you might say, "May I assist you?" or "Let me help you."

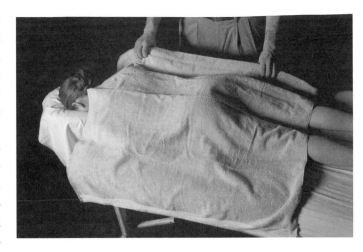

Figure 12.8a

When the massage is completed, the same wrap that the client wore from the dressing area to the massage table is used. The wrap is placed across the client's body, and other draping is removed. Instruct the client to lie on one side and arrange the wrap in such a way that it covers the back of the body with most of the wrap in front.

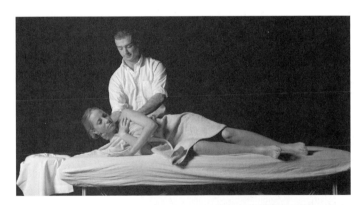

Figure 12.8b

From the side-lying position, the client draws her knees up so that her feet are just off the side of the table (women hold the wrap over the breasts) and the client uses her top hand and arm to push herself up while the practitioner assists her to a sitting position.

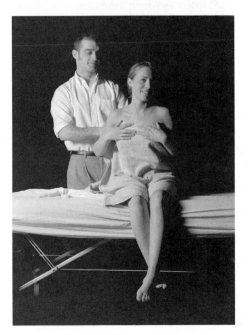

Figure 12.8c

At this point, the wrap is refastened while the client is given a chance to regain composure. After a moment or two, the client is instructed to stand and return to the dressing area. As the client stands, it is advisable for the practitioner to keep one hand on the client's arm for balance and the other hand on the table to prevent it from tipping.

Alternate Method

An optional and popular method to get the client undressed and onto the table is for the practitioner to instruct the client on the procedure and then leave the room, allowing the client privacy. The table is prepared with a table covering and a top sheet or large towel. The client is instructed to remove her clothing, lay on the table in the chosen position, and cover herself with the appropriate drape. The practitioner then leaves the room. The client disrobes, climbs on the table, and covers herself. It is important to give concise, yet simple, instructions so that the client is in the correct position and properly covered when the practitioner re-enters the massage room.

When the massage is complete, the practitioner may instruct the client to take a few minutes to relish the experience and then carefully get up and get dressed. The practitioner then exits the room and leaves the client on her own to get off the massage table and to get dressed. This method is considered by the author to be somewhat less professional because it increases the possibility that the client could be injured while getting onto or off of the massage table.

If there is any concern that the client may need some assistance getting up at the end of the session, the practitioner should remain in the massage room to assist the client to a sitting position and then off the table before leaving the room and allowing the client privacy to dress. Use proper draping techniques to ensure that the client remains modestly covered as she sits up and gets off the table.

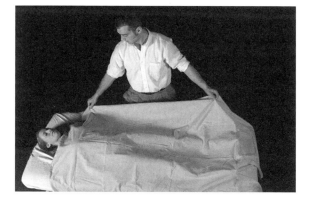

Figure 12.9a

As the client takes her place on the massage table, situate the top cover lengthwise to cover all except her head. If the top cover is also used as a wrap, it is rearranged from across the client's body to a lengthwise position. If a terry wrap or towel is worn from the dressing area, the top cover can be laid in place and the wrap discreetly slipped from underneath.

Method 1—The Top Cover Method

Follow the illustrations for the top cover method until you are able to remember how to do the entire procedure in a smooth and efficient manner (Figure 12.9a to h). Linens required for the top sheet method include a covering for the table, which could be a fitted cot or twin or flat sheet and a top cover. The top cover could be a large bath sheet (beach towel), a twin flat sheet, or half of a double flat sheet. Two bath towels could also be used as a top cover.

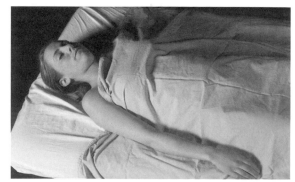

Figure 12.9b

As each arm is massaged, fold the top cover out of the way, exposing only the limb to be massaged.

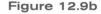

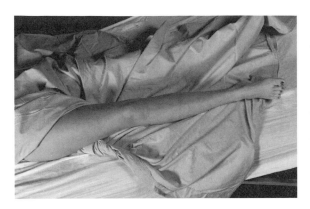

Figure 12.9c

To massage a leg, uncover that leg only. Lift the knee enough to reach under and pull the drape under the thigh and toward the buttock with one hand while positioning the cover snugly along the inguinal crease with your other hand.

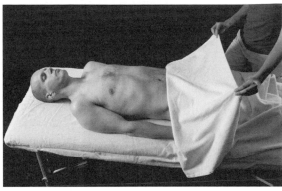

Figure 12.9d

To massage the chest and abdomen of a man, neatly fold the top cover to the level of the hips.

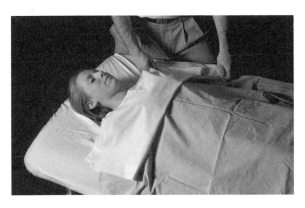

Figure 12.9e

To work on the abdomen of a woman, breast draping is needed. Fold another towel or pillow case to make a covering for the breasts and place it over the top cover.

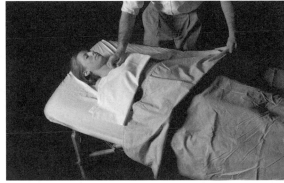

Figure 12.9f

Peel the top cover down while holding the folded towel or pillow case in place over the breasts.

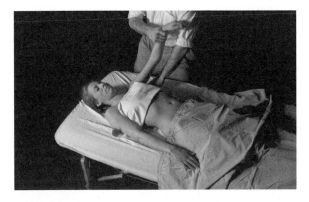

Figure 12.9g

Raise the client's arm and tuck the towel or pillow case used for the breast cover neatly under the scapula to hold the ends of the towel securely in place.

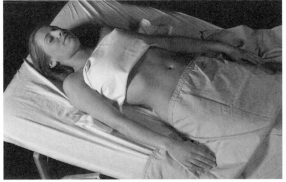

Figure 12.9h

Place the client's arm down. Tuck the other side of the towel or pillow case covering the breasts under the other scapula in the same manner. This draping method allows you to work on the abdomen, chest, and sides of the body without exposing the breasts.

When it is time for the client to turn over, a process is used so that the client stays discreetly covered and does not get tangled up in the drapes (see Figure 12.9i to k). The top cover is arranged to cover the client from the shoulders down with the edge of the cover nearest the practitioner draped slightly over the edge of the table. If the top drape is too narrow to overlap the edge of the table and still cover the client, the drape could be turned sidewise as long as it still covers the female client from the shoulders to mid-thigh. The practitioner leans against the side of the massage table to secure the table cover and the top drape with his thighs and reaches across the table to hold the top cover at the level of the shoulder with one hand and below the hips with the other. If the client is turning from supine to prone, the practitioner instructs the client, "Please roll over by turning to face me first, then on over to your stomach." If a face cradle is used, once the client is on her stomach, she is instructed to move (slide) up the table until her face is comfortably situated in the cradle. Ask whether the client is comfortable and make any adjustments necessary before beginning back massage.

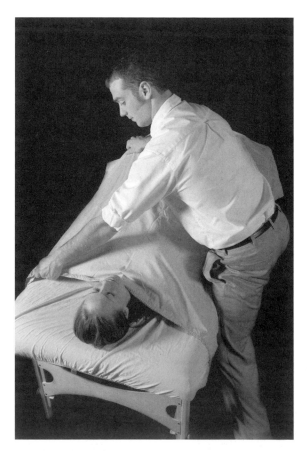

Figure 12.9i

When it is time to roll over, the drape is repositioned and held in place by the therapist leaning on the table and grasping the top cover at the level of the client's shoulders and hips.

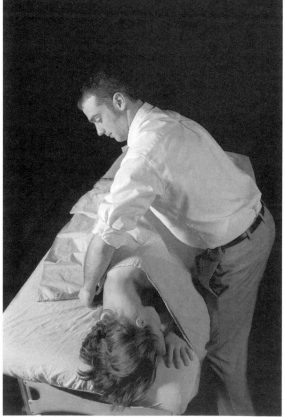

Figure 12.9j

When rolling from supine to prone, the client is instructed to roll first to face the therapist and then onto her stomach.

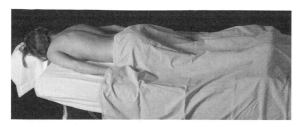

Figure 12.9k

To massage the back, neatly fold the top cover down to a level 2 inches below the beginning of the gluteal cleft.

If the client is turning from prone to supine, the practitioner positions and secures the drapes in the same manner and instructs the client to first turn away from the practitioner and then onto her back. As the client turns, the practitioner holds the top and bottom sheet in place by leaning against the table while reaching across the table and supporting the top drape at the level of the client's shoulders and upper thigh with his hands as the client turns over.

When the massage is complete and it is time for the client to return to the dressing area, use the top cover for a wrap by turning the cover sideways before having the client come to a sitting position. If you choose to use a separate wrap, put the wrap in place and, while holding it with one hand, peel the top cover from underneath the wrap.

Method 2—Full Sheet Draping

The following is a step-by-step description of the full sheet draping method (Figure. 12.10a to o). It incorporates the use of a double-size flat sheet and a separate wrap or towel. First, prepare the massage table by unfolding the double-size sheet and placing it on the massage table.

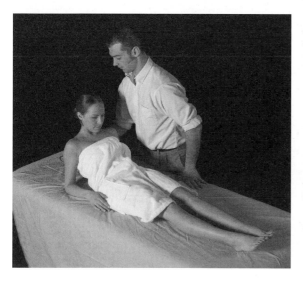

Figure 12.10a

Assist the client onto the table and into a supine (lying on her back) position. The wrap she wore to the table is used as a cover.

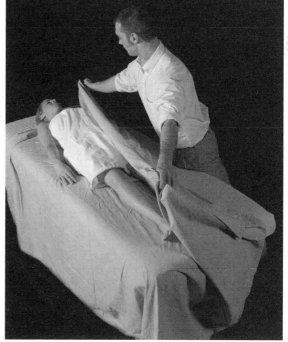

Figure 12.10b

Drape one side of the flat sheet over the client to cover her entire torso and one leg. The client may choose whether or not she wants her arms covered.

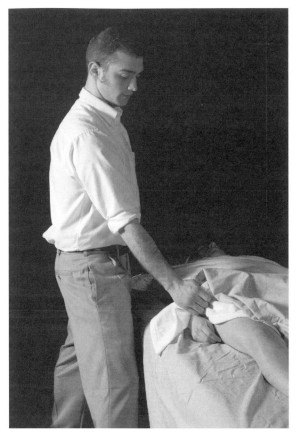

Figure 12.10c
Discreetly remove the wrap from underneath the draping.

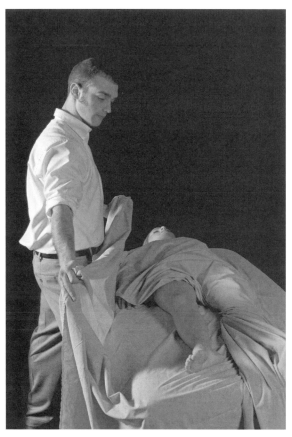

Figure 12.10d
Drape the other side of the flat sheet over the entire torso and the other leg.

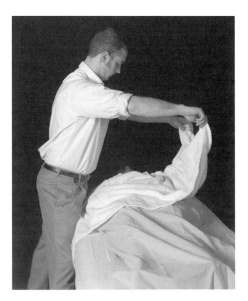

Figure 12.10e
Place the towel or wrap over the chest area to hold the drape in place. If it is not needed for this purpose, it may be placed aside for later use.

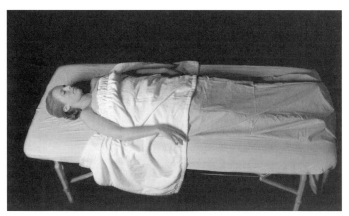

Figure 12.10f
If the client's arms are left outside the draping, there is no problem. (a) If the client prefers having her arms covered, then proceed with undraping them by holding the top of the draping, lifting it slightly, then reaching in with the other hand to grasp the client's wrist and lift her arm from beneath the drape. (b) After the arm has been massaged, the procedure is reversed, and the arm is placed back underneath the draping at the client's side.

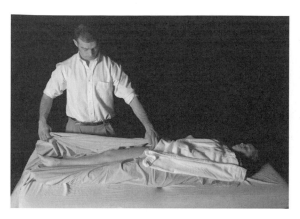

Figure 12.10g

Undrape the leg beginning at the foot. Peel the sheet upward all the way to the iliac crest (hipbone). Remember that when initially draping the client, each leg was draped independently and was covered by only one layer of the draping sheet.

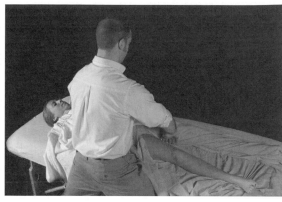

Figure 12.10h

Carefully tuck the drape covering the opposite leg under that thigh with one hand, while arranging the rest of the draping with the other hand across the torso and the genital area. This method assures that the client will be well covered when massaging upward to the hipbone and when performing leg stretches.

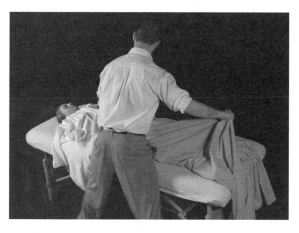

Figure 12.10i

Redrape the leg and the entire torso with the sheet on that side of the table, then proceed to the other leg in the same manner.

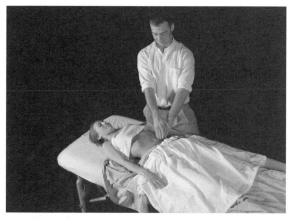

Figure 12.10j

Prepare to massage the upper part of the body by opening the draping to just above the pubic bone. When massaging a female client, fold the wrap (or towel) and use it as a breast covering. Use another towel to secure the draping at the level just above the pubic bone.

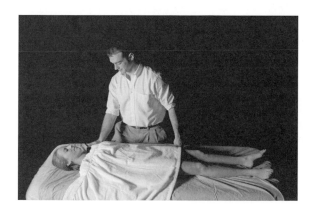

Figure 12.10k

When it is time for the client to turn over, use the wrap to cover the client from the shoulders to the knees.

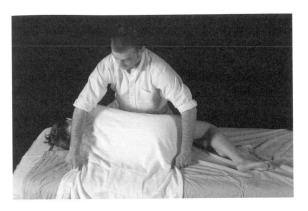

Figure 12.10l

Instruct the client to turn toward you by lifting her opposite shoulder first, then rolling onto her abdomen. Hold the wrap in place with your hands and the flat sheet in place by leaning against the table.

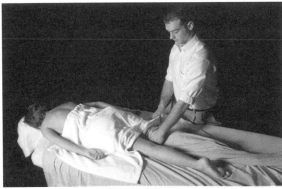

Figure 12.10m

With the client lying face down, place the wrap so that it covers the back down to the middle of the thighs. Drape the sheet over one leg and the back, then tuck it around under the same leg. Massage the other leg.

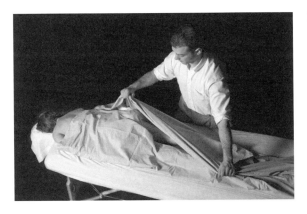

Figure 12.10n

Drape the leg after massaging it, and then undrape and massage the other leg in the same manner. Redrape the leg.

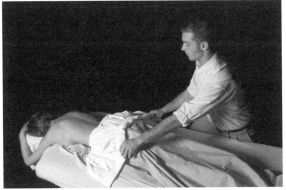

Figure 12.10o

Prepare to massage the back by peeling the wrap downward to expose the entire back. This method holds the leg draping in place and does not overly expose the gluteal area.

CONTACT WITH THE CLIENT AND QUALITY OF TOUCH

In administering a massage, there is much more to take into account than the application of strokes to various parts of the client's body. The practitioner must be aware of contact with the client, the quality of touch, and the constitution or composition of the massage itself.

From the time a client enters a massage establishment, the confidence and ability of the practitioner are communicated. The confidence shown through the initial contact instills a certain trust in the recipient that encourages relaxation. The success of that communication is largely dependent on the quality of touch of the therapist. Different individuals exhibit varying qualities in their touch just as there are vast differences in people's voices and the way they communicate. The quality of touch is a key to the way the client will respond to the therapist and the massage treatment.

Our intentions and attitudes are often communicated through our actions and physical contact with people as much as they are through the spoken word. The massage professional endeavors to promote a sense of relaxation and well-being. Massage is the touch profession. People who come for a massage usually come because they want to "let go" of something and literally put themselves into the hands of the practitioner. It is important that from the time clients enter the massage office until they leave, they are comfortable in the feeling that they are in good hands. The way that touch is administered to the client determines the success of the massage and is often the reason a client will return.

MAINTAINING CONTACT WITH THE CLIENT

Before beginning a professional body massage, it is important to "tune in" to the client.

The massage begins when the client is positioned on the massage table and you, the practitioner, come in contact with the client's body. After you undrape and apply massage lubricant to the part of the body to be massaged, you must remember to keep in contact with the client's body throughout the procedure. Try not to break the circuit of touch once it has been established between you and your client. Your goal is to maintain a constant flow without surges or breaks as long as contact is maintained. If the client is in a state of wakeful conversation with eyes open and is following you during the massage, then there is verbal and visual contact. However, if the client is in a state of relaxation with eyes closed, the sense of touch is the only communication. If contact is broken, there is an immediate reaction of concern on the part of the client, and relaxation may change to anxiety. It is important not to break contact until the massage is finished and the final strokes lightly feathered off.

When you maintain continuous contact, the client is constantly aware of your presence and activity and at the same time has a point of reference and an awareness of the parts of the body that are being massaged. As the various strokes are performed on the body part, the attention and awareness of the client follow. At some level of consciousness, clients are able to release the stress and tension in each part of their body at the same time that they tune out mental stress and tension. With their eyes closed, they float into a state of relaxation anchored only by the touch of your hands. If contact is broken, clients immediately lose that point of reference and wonder where you are, what you are doing, and what part of their body you are going to touch next. When contact is reestablished, it is as though attention is jolted to the new point of contact. If it is necessary to leave a client, this should be explained to the client. Explain that you must do something and will be right back. Recontact the client softly and inconspicuously.

Though continuous contact is important, it must be done in an efficient, unencumbered manner. There should be no element of surprise as the massage moves from one part of the body to another. This is accomplished through practice and the implementation of a logical massage sequence.

Sequence

sequence

refers to the pattern or design of a massage.

Sequence refers to the pattern or design of a massage. Developing a good sequence is especially important because it coordinates and organizes the massage so that there is smooth progression from one stroke to the next and from one body part to the next. Sequence provides a framework for a thought-out, logical progression and at the same time allows for flexibility and creativity. When doing a full-body massage, following a sequence ensures that each and every area of the body is massaged in some logical order.

There are numerous possibilities when formulating a full-body massage sequence depending on the style of the practitioner, the preferences and needs of the client, and the intentions of the session, among many other considerations. The sequence may begin with the client lying faceup, facedown, or on her side. The massage may begin at the head, at the feet, or somewhere in between. Generally, a Western or Swedish-style massage is designed so that the client will only need to change positions once or maybe twice. A relaxing, wellness massage sequence is designed so that each body area is thoroughly massaged in a logical order so that the entire body is included and the client feels balanced, complete, and relaxed. Some therapeutic applications may require the therapist to focus on specific areas of the client's body or to return to an area several times during a session but not even approach other areas of the body. In so doing, the therapist is following a sequence to efficiently address the specific needs of the client. Even in a relaxing full-body massage, the sequence is a guideline that is always flexible enough so that the individual needs of a client can be addressed.

Following a massage sequence on a particular body area provides a structure that you, the practitioner, can use to ensure a balanced and complete therapeutic application to that area. In the application of a massage, sequences are built within sequences and each body part is provided an equal experience. Even during the massage of a body part, there are conditions where adapting certain sequences proves to be both valuable and therapeutic.

There is a general massage rule to keep in mind: When doing massage, performing a stroke, or working on an area, work from general to specific, then back to general, AND from superficial to deep and back to superficial.

In working from general to specific, the entire area is relaxed and circulation is increased so that more specific massage can relieve congestion and spasm. Ischemic conditions also have a better chance of being relieved.

Following specific massage techniques with more generalized massage tends to normalize the area.

Likewise, by starting with more superficial strokes, the area is relaxed and the client's confidence is encouraged so that you are allowed to work more deeply into the tissues. Following deeper massage techniques, soothing superficial strokes dissipate the tension released from the target tissues and enhance a sense of relaxation.

This may be illustrated by doing a single stroke or a series of strokes—for instance, when doing gliding strokes over an area such as the calf of the leg. Begin with a very light stroke, repeat with a deeper stroke, and get increasingly deeper with each successive stroke until the maximum depth you want is achieved. Then the next few strokes are lighter until the final stroke is nearly as light as the first.

Another example may involve a variety of massage strokes that begin with general gliding strokes over an area. An area of tension is palpated. Kneading is followed by deeper kneading and deeper gliding. Next are a variety of friction techniques that address the tense tissue more directly and deeply. Deep pressure and transverse friction are applied directly to the tissue. This is followed by jostling, deep gliding, joint movements, gliding, and finally feather strokes.

Following a sequence when massaging particular conditions and areas provides a structure that allows for creativity and flexibility.

The sequence of the overall massage is designed in a logical progression that leaves the client with a feeling of completedness. Although a sequence may vary according to the situation, a pattern should be used that ensures that every part of the body is massaged properly and thoroughly.

Massage movements for adjacent areas as well as bilateral body parts should follow in sequence. For example, when beginning with the hand, the massage should progress to the arm and then to the shoulder. Then massage the other hand, arm, and shoulder, both shoulders, the neck, and the head. Finally, massage the chest, abdomen, one leg and foot, then the other leg and foot. This completes the massage for the front of the body.

Developing a sequence also ensures a thorough massage that is balanced between one body part and another. The following is an example of an effective sequence to be used on each body area when giving a relaxing, wellness massage.

1. Make contact with and undrape the body part to be massaged.

2. Apply massage lubricant with light effleurage.

3. Apply effleurage to accustom the body to your touch. Effleurage also flushes out the lymph and venous blood.

4. Apply petrissage, kneading the tissues to warm them. This also enables you to become aware of any areas of tension or congestion in the muscles.

5. Apply effleurage to flush the area.

6. Apply friction with any of the recommended friction techniques.

7. Apply effleurage to the entire area again, because this flushes the area while linking and integrating the segmented parts back into the whole.

8. Do joint movements to restore mobility by reinforcing the possibility of movement. At the same time, joint movements stretch the muscles and connective tissues and lubricate the joints.

9. Apply effleurage to flush out the loosened debris and to give a feeling of length to the body part.

10. Apply feather strokes. This stimulates the peripheral nervous system, smoothes the energy field, and says good-bye to that part of the body.

11. Redrape the part of the body that has been massaged, undrape the next part, and continue until the client has been given a thorough massage.

Contact While Applying Lubricant

When you are ready to apply the massage lubricant to the client's skin, lay the back of your hand lightly against the part of the body to be massaged. Put enough lubricant in the palm of your hand to apply a thin film over the body part on which you are to work. Do not apply lubricant directly from the container to the body surface because it will feel cold to the client and will cause discomfort. Rub your hands together to warm the lubricant to body temperature. This also makes it easier to spread the lubricant over the client's skin. Some practitioners prefer to use a massage lubricant holster that straps around the practitioner's waist and holds a lubricant bottle with a dispenser top. When more massage lubricant is needed, one hand maintains contact with the client while the other reaches for a couple squirts of lubricant. Once the lubricant is obtained, the practitioner briefly rubs his hands together to warm the lubricant before applying it to the client's body (Figure 12.11).

To apply lubricant efficiently, use long superficial strokes (effleurage) that cover the entire area to be massaged. As the lubricant is smoothed, strokes can become firmer. Effleurage is used to apply the lubricant and at the same time encourage the flow of body fluids toward the center of the body. Strokes should be continuous, pushing in the direction of the heart and then gliding back to the starting point. A good general rule is to keep the hand relaxed yet

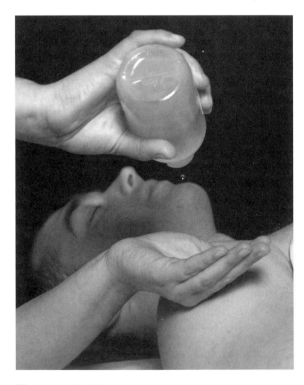

Figure 12.11

Before beginning massage movements, undrape the body part and apply the massage lubricant. With the back of your hands, maintain contact with the client's skin as you prepare to apply the massage lubricant.

firm, so that even when passing over an obstacle such as the knee or shoulder, the hand is in complete contact with the client's skin.

PROCEDURE FOR A GENERAL BODY MASSAGE

When a student is performing a massage, it is helpful to follow a routine to ensure that each area of the body is massaged in a cohesive manner. As the student gains experience, the routine is modified to meet the individual needs and goals of the client and the session. Ideally, each massage the student gives will be unique because every client is different.

The following two massage routines are generalized, full-body routines where the client begins in a supine position so that the front of the body is massaged and ends with the client in the prone position, concluding the full-body massage with a back massage.

The Massage 1 routine is flexible in that some steps can be omitted and others included. The student should follow the instructor's directions. The main objective is to give a beneficial and relaxing massage that is suited to the client's desires and needs.

1. **Preliminary steps:**

   a. Prepare the massage space by collecting all necessary supplies and arranging them as needed.

   b. Perform the consultation to determine the client's needs, determine any contraindications, and obtain informed consent.

   c. See that the client has all items needed to prepare for the massage.

   d. Direct the client to the dressing room and explain the preparation procedures.

2. **Hydrotherapy** (optional):

   a. Select the bath most suitable for the client.

   b. Adjust the bath equipment and accessories.

   c. Take the temperature of the bath.

   d. Assist the client as necessary during the bath. Give the client water to drink, and take the client's pulse if necessary.

   e. Assist the client as needed following the bath.

   f. Allow the client to rest for a short period following the bath.

3. **Preparation for body massage:**

   a. Wash and sanitize your hands.

   b. Assist the client onto the massage table and into a supine (faceup) position.

   c. Drape the client's body with sheet or towel, with the exception of the part to be massaged.

4. Order of treatment (overview):

The following procedure is suggested for a basic relaxing massage. However, it may be varied to suit the convenience of the practitioner and the needs of the client.

    a. Begin with the hands and arms, right then left.

    b. Proceed to front of the legs and feet, right then left.

    c. Continue movements over abdomen, chest, and neck.

    d. The client will turn over to assume a prone (facedown) position.

    e. Begin with the back of the legs, right then left.

    f. Finish the massage with the back of the body.

Following the massage, the client should be allowed to rest for a short period and then be assisted from the table.

Step-by-Step Procedures for Massage 1

The following step-by-step procedure helps you to learn basic massage techniques quickly. Draping is performed and all preliminary steps are observed.

General Arm Massage

1. Undrape an arm and apply the lubricant with a light, smooth effleurage stroke from the shoulder to the hand.
2. Apply effleurage to the arm three times.
3. Knead the arm from the shoulder to the elbow.
4. Apply effleurage to the arm from the elbow to the shoulder.
5. Bend the elbow and rest it on the table.
6. Knead the arm from the elbow to the wrist.
7. Apply effleurage to the arm from the wrist to the elbow.
8. Press the metacarpal bones back and forth.
9. Knead each finger and hand.
10. Rotate each finger.
11. Apply effleurage to the arm.
12. Roll the arm three times.
13. Apply joint movements to the arm.
14. Apply effleurage to the arm lightly three times.
15. Apply nerve strokes and redrape the arm.

Arm Movements for Body Massage

Depending on the client's requirements, the following movements may be included or omitted (Figure 12.12a to o).

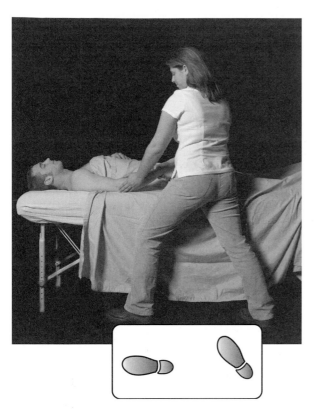

Figure 12.12a

Proper stance and posture are important. Proper posture reduces fatigue and proper stance allows mobility and power.

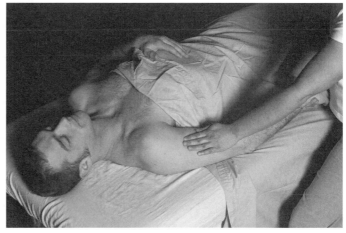

Figure 12.12b

Apply effleurage to the arm from the hand to the shoulder using firmer pressure. Maintain contact with the arm for the return stroke from the shoulder to the hand using lighter pressure.

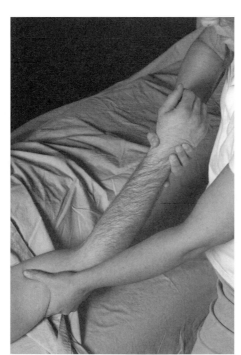

Figure 12.12c

Apply the same effleurage movement when massaging the back of the arm with firmer pressure on the upward stroke and lighter pressure on the return.

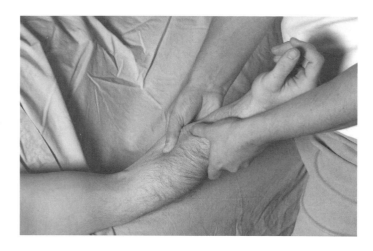

Figure 12.12d

Knead from the shoulder to the wrist.

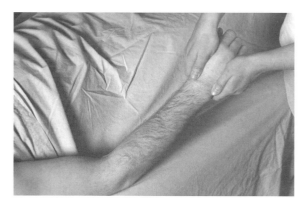

Figure 12.12e

Knead the carpals and metacarpals.

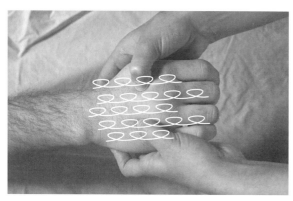

Figure 12.12f

Apply circular friction to the fingers and hand.

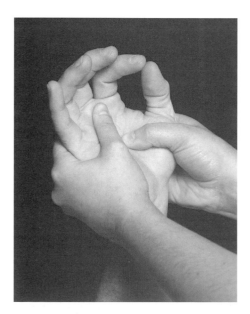

Figure 12.12g

While holding the client's hand, massage the palm, back of the hand, metacarpals, fingers, and upward over the wrist.

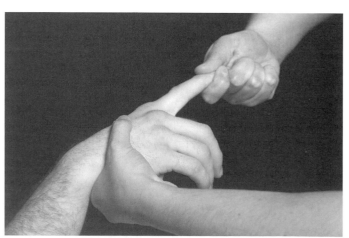

Figure 12.12h

Hold the forearm firmly. Rotate and circumduct the wrist. Knead and rotate each finger as you circumduct and apply traction.

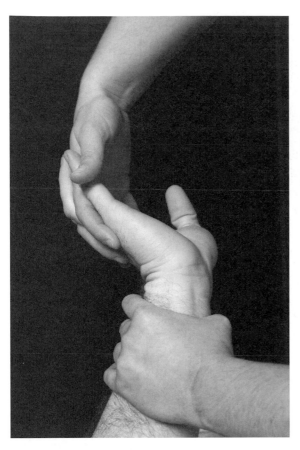

Figure 12.12i

Apply joint movements and rotation. Note the interlacing of the fingers.

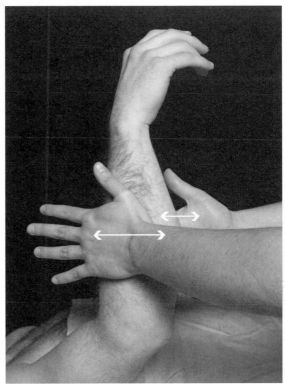

Figure 12.12j

Roll the arm.

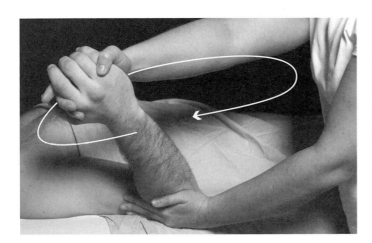

Figure 12.12k

Rotate the forearm. Note how the fingers are used to steady the client's elbow.

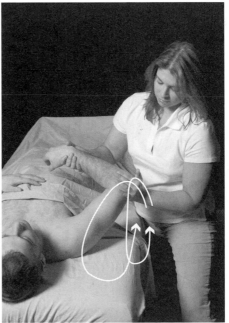

Figure 12.12l

Rotate the shoulder by moving the elbow. Note how the other hand supports the client's hand.

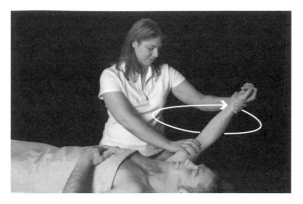

Figure 12.12m
Circumduct the shoulder.

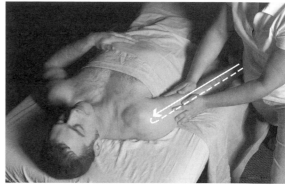

Figure 12.12n
Repeat gliding strokes to the lateral and medial aspects of the arm.

Figure 12.12o

Apply feather strokes (light effleurage) with your fingertips to complete the massage of the arm. Do the massage for the other arm using the same sequence of movements.

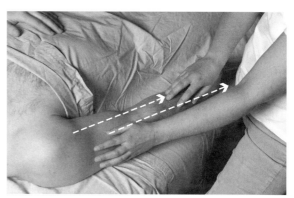

General Massage for the Foot and Leg

1. Undrape one leg and apply lubricant with a light, smooth effleurage stroke from the foot to the hip and back to the foot.

2. Apply effleurage to the leg three times.

3. Press metatarsal bones of the foot back and forth.

4. Knead each toe, around foot, ankle.

5. Rotate each toe three times.

6. Knead the leg three times.

7. Wring and roll the leg.

8. Apply effleurage to the leg three times.

9. Apply joint movements to the leg.

10. Apply effleurage to the leg lightly three times.

11. Apply nerve strokes and redrape the leg.

Massage for the Foot and Leg

Depending on the client's requirements, the following movements may be included or omitted (Figure 12.13a and b and Figure 12.14a to q).

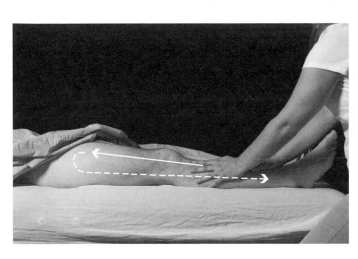

Figure 12.13a

Apply effleurage to the leg in long movements from the ankle to the hip. Apply more pressure on the stroke up the leg, and maintain light contact as your hands glide back to the starting point.

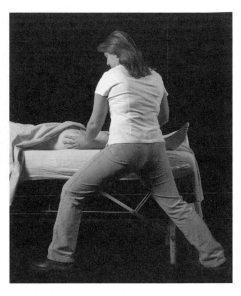

Figure 12.13b

Use good body mechanics. A wide archer stance allows the therapist to stroke the entire leg.

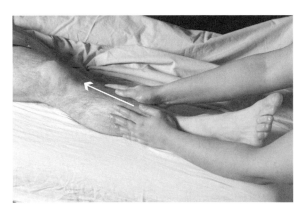

Figure 12.14a

Apply more pressure on the stroke in the direction of venous blood and lymph flow.

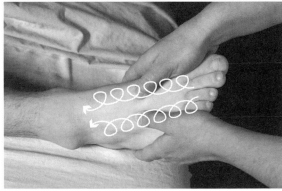

Figure 12.14b

Knead the top and bottom of the foot.

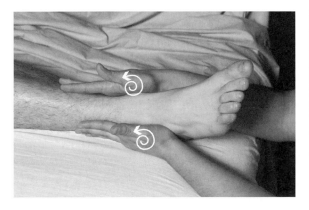

Figure 12.14c

Warm the foot and ankles with circular rubbing movements.

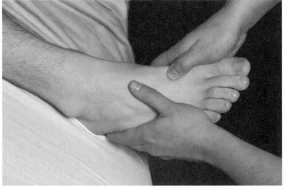

Figure 12.14d

Apply digital friction between the tendons and bones on all surfaces of the foot.

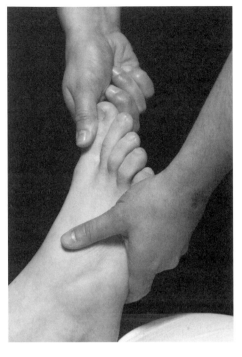

Figure 12.14e

Massage and rotate each digit.

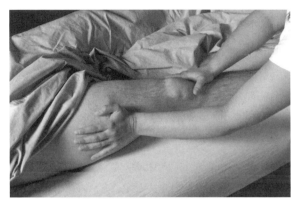

Figure 12.14f

Knead the leg and thigh in a circular motion.

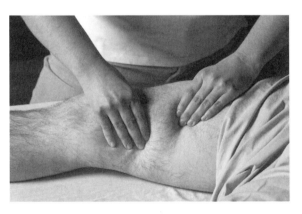

Figure 12.14g

Apply petrissage to the anterior thigh.

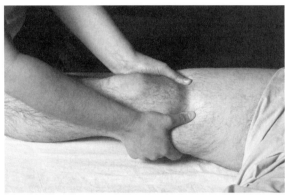

Figure 12.14h

Apply fulling (compression) movements.

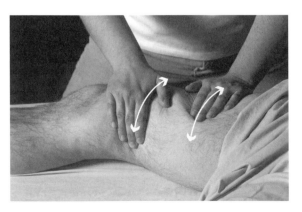

Figure 12.14i

Wring the muscles of the thigh.

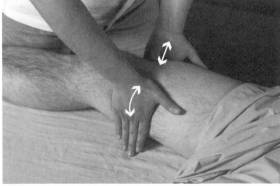

Figure 12.14j

Roll the muscles of the thigh.

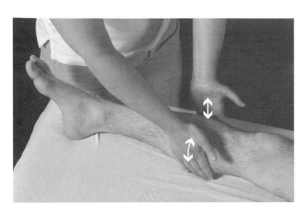

Figure 12.14k

Roll the muscles of the leg.

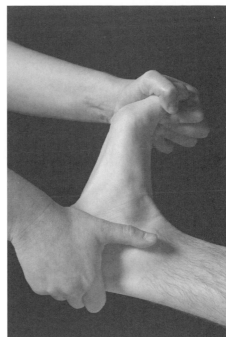

Figure 12.14l

Stretch the plantar surface of the foot and toes.

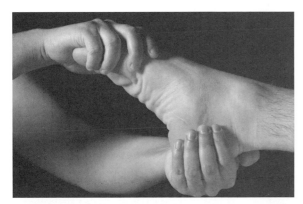

Figure 12.14m

Stretch the dorsal aspect of the foot and toes.

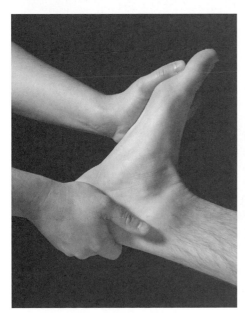

1

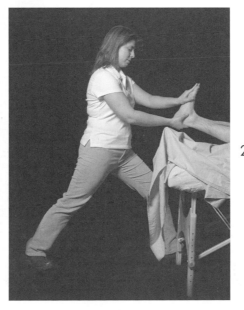

2

Figure 12.14n (1 and 2)

Stretch the Achilles' tendon. Note the position of the hands.

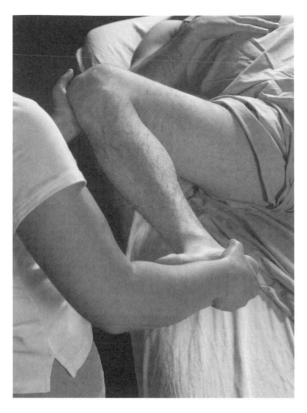

Figure 12.14o

Apply joint movements. Move the client's knee all the way to the chest. This position also may be used for joint rotations of the hip and knee in the range of motion. Note the position of the hands at the heel and knee.

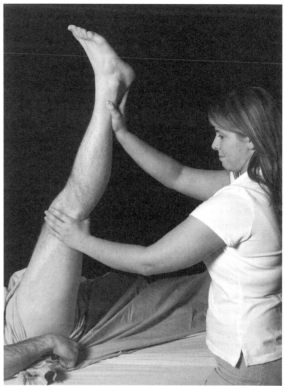

Figure 12.14p

Apply hamstring stretching movements.

Figure 12.14q

Complete the massage of the front of the leg with a nerve stroke, then redrape and continue to the next part.

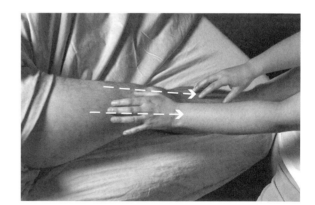

General Massage for the Chest and Neck

1. On a male client, undrape the torso to a level midway between the navel and the pubic bone to expose the abdomen. On a female, use breast draping. Some of the following strokes will be modified to accommodate the breast drape.

2. From the head of the table, stroke the back of the neck.

3. Knead back and sides of the neck and shoulders.

4. Stroke the chest three times. Stroke down the chest, around to the sides, coming up under each arm, and up and over the shoulders to the neck.

5. Apply deep gliding strokes along the ribs from the table toward the center of the chest.

6. Apply kneading to the pectoral muscles. (Avoid breast tissue on women.)

7. Repeat step #4.

Chest and Neck Movements

Depending on the client's requirements, the practitioner may include or omit any of the following movements (Figure 12.15a to h).

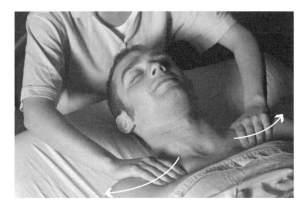

Figure 12.15a
Apply effleurage from the sternal notch and over the shoulders.

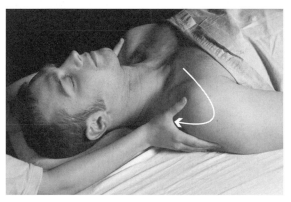

Figure 12.15b
Continue the movement across the shoulder and around the deltoid.

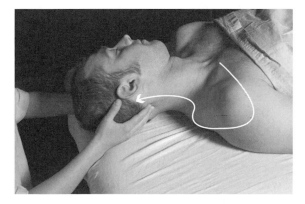

Figure 12.15c
Continue the movement up the trapezius to the occipital ridge.

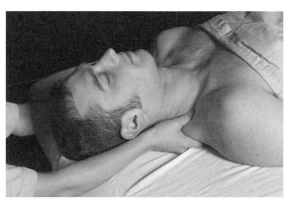

Figure 12.15d
Apply petrissage to the neck and shoulders.

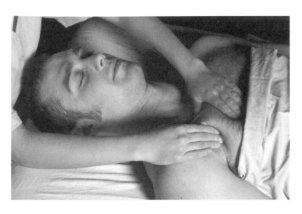

Figure 12.15e
Knead and apply friction to the pectoral muscles.

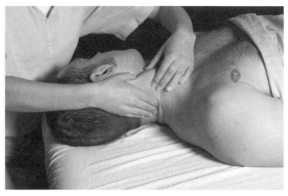

Figure 12.15f
Apply petrissage to back of neck and shoulder region.

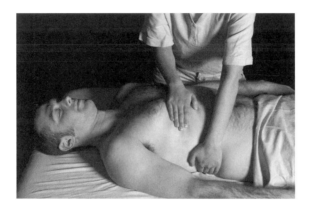

Figure 12.15g
Apply alternate hand stroking (shingles) from the axillary area to the hips.

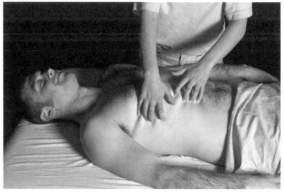

Figure 12.15h
Raking is done by flexing the tips of the fingers and stroking along the ribs from the table to the midline of the body.

Changing Position

The client turns over to a prone, facedown position. Maintain proper draping to prevent exposure while turning the client.

General Massage for the Back of the Legs

1. Undrape a leg and apply lubricant.
2. Move the leg closer to the edge of the table and apply effleurage from the heel to the hip three times.
3. Knead a foot from toe to heel.
4. Knead the leg from the heels to the hips.
5. Apply wringing and rolling.
6. Apply effleurage to each leg three times.
7. Apply nerve strokes and redrape.

Back of Leg Movements for Body Massage

Depending on the client's requirements, the following movements may be included or omitted (Figure 12.16a to g).

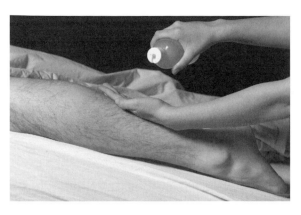

Figure 12.16a

Before beginning massage movements, prepare the posterior leg by draping and applying lubricant.

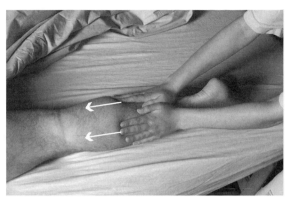

Figure 12.16b

Apply effleurage to the leg upward with both hands.

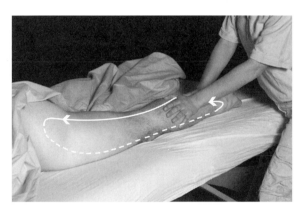

Figure 12.16c

Apply effleurage movements. Stroke toward the heart applying firmer pressure. *Note:* Place the leading hand on the lateral aspect of the leg in order to travel up and over the gluteal muscles and the iliac crest and back down the lateral side of the leg. At the same time, the medial hand travels up to the gluteal crease and back down the medial side of the leg. Both hands maintain contact, using much lighter pressure as they return to the starting point to repeat the stroke three or more times.

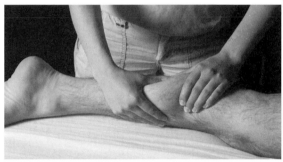

Figure 12.16d

Knead the calf muscles.

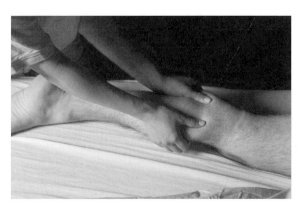

Figure 12.16e

Apply fulling or compression strokes to the entire leg.

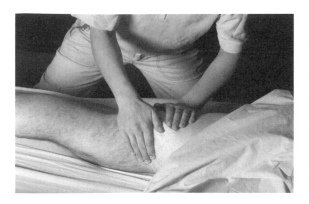

Figure 12.16f
Apply wringing to the back of the leg.

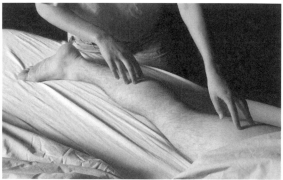

Figure 12.16g
Complete the massage of the posterior leg with several feather strokes (nerve stroke) from the hip to the foot.

General Massage for the Back of the Body

1. Undrape and apply lubricant to the back.

2. Standing at the side of the client, apply effluerage to the back five times up the spine and down on each side of the body.

3. Place the hands flat on each side of the spine, and stretch them outward toward the shoulders.

4. Continue step 3 to cover the entire back.

5. Vibrate along each side of the vertebral column from the neck to the sacrum.

6. Knead the entire back and each side of the torso.

7. Apply deep gliding strokes on the side of the torso from the table to the center of the back (shingles) from the hips to the shoulders.

8. From the head of the table, apply effleurage to the back three times. From the back of the neck, stroke down along the length of the spine, around to the side of the body, up the sides, around and over the shoulders, up to the neck, and repeat.

9. Apply light hacking movements along the spine, between the shoulders, over the gluteal muscles and the back of the legs. Avoid the kidney area.

10. Apply effleurage to the back lightly five times.

11. Apply nerve strokes to the entire back, redrape, and complete the massage.

Back Movements for Body Massage

Depending on the client's requirements, the following movements may be included or omitted (Figure 12.17a to l).

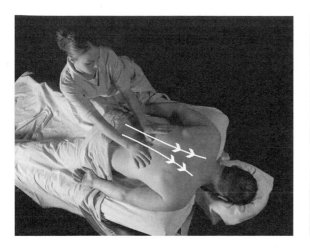

Figure 12.17a

Begin at the gluteal cleft and apply long strokes up along the muscles on each side of the spine.

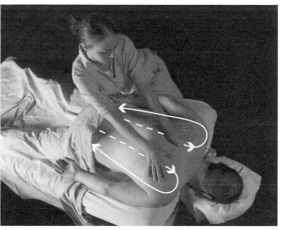

Figure 12.17b

Continue with effleurage strokes up the back and over the shoulders.

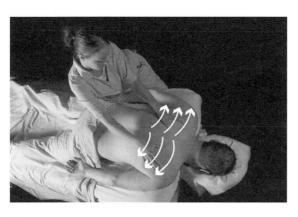

Figure 12.17c

Stroke the muscles of the back outward.

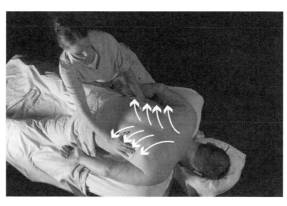

Figure 12.17d

Use fan stroking on the back.

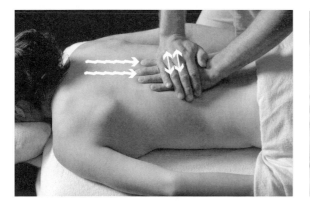

Figure 12.17e

Apply vibration movements along each vertebra by placing the fingers of one hand on each side of the spinous process and the other hand on top. Vibrate back and forth as you move down along the spine.

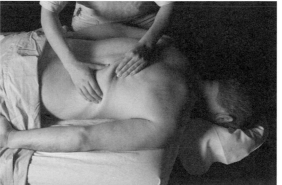

Figure 12.17f

Apply petrissage to the entire side that is opposite you. This takes several passes.

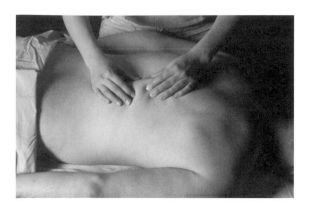

Figure 12.17g

Knead around the spine.

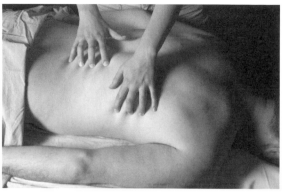

Figure 12.17h

Apply raking in alternate strokes so that the tips of the fingers glide between the ribs.

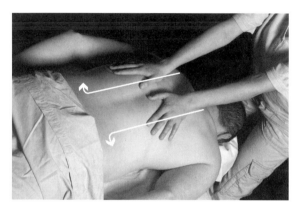

Figure 12.17i

Apply effleurage movements down the back, over and around the gluteal muscles, back up the sides, then over and around the shoulders to the nape of the neck.

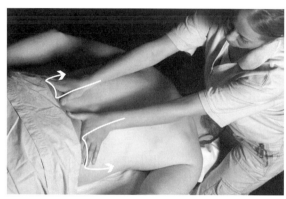

Figure 12.17j

Continue the caring stroke down the back and over the gluteal muscles.

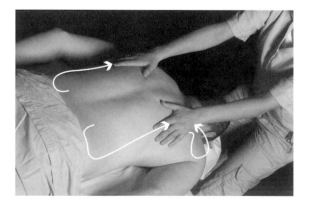

Figure 12.17k

The caring stroke is a continuous movement that proceeds up the side and around the shoulder to return to the starting point.

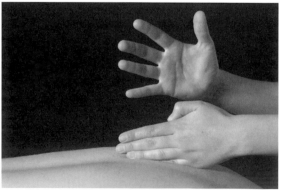

Figure 12.17l

Apply hacking movements to the back.

Completing the Treatment

1. After completing the final strokes, maintain light contact. Allow the client a few moments to savor the deep relaxation as he returns to a more conscious state. Adjust the draping and suggest that the client turn onto his side. Place a small pillow under his head, bend his knees, and allow him to rest a few minutes.

2. When it is time to get up, instruct the client to put his legs over the edge of the table and push himself into a sitting position with his upper arm. As he sits up, he can secure the wrap. You may assist the client by placing a hand under his shoulder and lifting him into a sitting position.

3. Suggest supplementary services and answer any questions the client may have.

4. When he is totally awake and reoriented, assist the client off the table and direct him to the dressing area.

5. After the client is dressed, collect your fees and set up the next appointment.

Final Considerations

1. Complete the client's record or SOAP notes.

2. Place supplies in their proper place; discard used items.

3. See that all equipment and items, including the massage table and bath, are properly prepared before the next client arrives.

PROCEDURE FOR PROFESSIONAL BODY MASSAGE

Massage 2

Massage, like any other skill, requires practice and patience to learn the basics, build speed, and develop new techniques. Each time you give a massage, you may find yourself becoming more innovative and more confident of your techniques. By the time you have learned Massage 1, you should be familiar with most of the terms for the various movements used in basic body massage. Massage 2 incorporates additional techniques to help you increase efficiency, remember the sequence of movements, and readily identify the movements and the parts of the anatomy by their proper names. While doing massage, pay attention to your hand positions and how you stand and move. Become more aware of the qualities of the tissues as you glide over and massage into each area of the body. Be sensitive to the different textures of the skin, the underlying fascia, and muscles. Begin to sense areas of tension and congestion where it might be appropriate to linger or provide additional techniques to the area.

Massage 2 enables you to review what you have learned and allows for even more creativity in varying massage routines. Before beginning the massage, concentrate on projecting the manner, attitude, and appearance of the professional massage practitioner. Read directions carefully for each step. After you have learned how to give a complete massage correctly and efficiently, you will not need to refer to your notes, illustrations, or written guides. Your aim is to be able to give the complete massage in a knowledgeable and professional manner.

Preliminary Steps

1. Prepare the facility and all products.

2. Before the client arrives, take a few quiet moments to prepare yourself with deep breathing, stretching, centering, and grounding.

3. If this is the client's first visit, be ready to greet the client on time and introduce yourself. In many places of business, the practitioner is addressed by the first name. For example, when introducing yourself to a new client, you might say, "Good morning, Mrs. Mason, I'm Carolyn. I'll be working with you today." You do not address the client by first name unless it is customary to do so or if the client has asked that you do so.

4. The first step with any client is the consultation or interview (see Chapter 9). Have the client fill out the information sheet first, and review it with the client to obtain more direct information. Discuss the client's needs and expectations and the kind of massage the client prefers. This is the time to be observant of the client's physical condition and determine what benefits should be derived from the massage or whether the client should be referred to another health care professional.

5. Put first-time clients at ease by showing the facility and explaining the services.

6. Explain to the client how to prepare for the massage. Show the client to the shower or hydrotherapy area, depending on which services that client has decided on. Provide proper draping for the client from the dressing area to the massage table.

7. Assist the client (as necessary) to the massage table and explain the position, either supine or prone, the client should assume. Drape the client appropriately and provide extra support (towels or bolster) under knees or head if necessary.

8. Attend to the client's comfort:

    a. Ask whether the client is warm enough. Adjust the room temperature or provide an extra blanket if necessary.

    b. Adjust pillows or bolsters so that the client is comfortable on the table.

    c. Encourage the client to speak up at any time the client feels discomfort of any kind so that adjustments can be made.

    d. Observe the client throughout the treatment for any signs of discomfort and ask for feedback if any such signs are noted.

There are many possibilities for varying massage techniques for different clients. Every massage will be unique according to the needs of the client and the practitioner's choices of the combination of massage techniques used during the session. The following massage procedure will help you to become more proficient and creative.

Breathing for Relaxation

When the client is on the table, relaxed and comfortable, encourage her to breathe fully and deeply. Many people have never done this and may need some basic coaching. Help the client by using some of the following suggestions:

Tell the client to breathe through the nose deeply so that the abdominal area expands first, followed by the chest. Hold for a few counts and then allow the breath to flow outward. Maintain the exhalation for a short time and repeat the exercise a few times. Observe the client's breathing and synchronize your own breathing. Have the client continue breathing freely for a few minutes to encourage relaxation and stress reduction.

Step-by-Step Procedure for Massage 2

The following procedure is a generalized massage routine designed as a relaxing full-body massage. It is only a guideline and may be varied or altered to fit the needs of each individual client and situation.

The client is positioned faceup (supine) on the massage table with a bolster under her knees to relieve any tension in her lower back. The head is resting on the table in a neutral position unless the client exhibits a severe head-forward position, in which case a folded towel or a small pillow can be placed under her head. The practitioner is standing or seated above the client's head facing the client.

Face massage may be done as the opening procedure of the massage, or for various reasons, massaging the face may be left out of the massage routine. If the client is wearing makeup, she may choose to not have a face massage, or to remove the makeup herself before the session, or to proceed with the massage over the makeup. When a face massage is included, it is usually at the beginning of the massage when the practitioner's hands have been freshly washed. Inform the client that very little lubricant will be used, if any at all.

(*Note:* Massaging a client's face, head, neck, and shoulders while positioned above her head may take several minutes. This is a good opportunity for the practitioner to get off her feet by sitting on a stool of a proper height that allows her to perform all manipulations while maintaining proper body mechanics.)

Massage the Face

1. If the massage begins with the face, once in place, the therapist may take a moment to quiet her thoughts, center and ground herself, and create intention before making initial contact with the client.

2. Initial contact is made by lightly placing the finger pads of both hands on the frontal eminence of the forehead and resting them there for several seconds. This is a good time to focus on the connection with the client. After a short time, a light pulse may be noted under the fingertips, indicating relaxation of the frontalis muscle and circulation in the area. The practitioner may prefer to make first contact by placing her hands on the client's shoulders if the face is not being massaged.

3. After a moment or when the pulse is noted, gently draw the fingers toward the hairline, gently stretching the frontalis muscle.

4. Place thumbs from both hands in the center of the forehead at the hairline. With slight pressure, glide the thumbs along the hairline to the temples and conclude with gentle circular friction at the temples. Return the thumb to the midline about a finger's width inferior to the first gliding stroke and repeat. Continue repeating the stroke at finger-width increments down the forehead to the eyebrows (see Figure 12.18a).

5. Beginning at one side of the forehead, do alternating diagonal gliding strokes from the eyebrows into the hairline. Begin with the pads of the fingers of one hand placed at the level of the eyebrow and glide those fingers in the direction of your corresponding shoulder. As soon as the stroke has progressed enough for the fingers of the other hand to be placed in the same place, do so and glide those fingers in the direction of the corresponding shoulder. Continue alternating diagonal strokes across the forehead and back again (see Figure 12.18b).

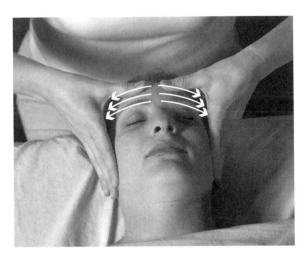

Figure 12.18a

Apply digital effleurage to the forehead from midline to hairline.

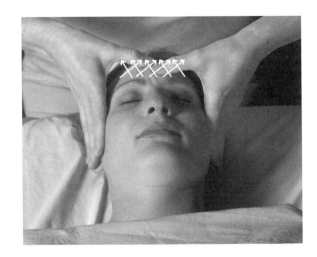

Figure 12.18b

Use a crisscross movement. Begin at one side of the forehead, making cross movements and then working back.

6. Grasp across the bridge of the nose with the thumb and finger and gently traction superiorly and away from the face (see Figure 12.18c).

7. Apply light gliding strokes from the nose to the side of the eye socket; first just superior to the supraorbital ridge, then just inferior to the supraorbital ridge, then just inferior to the infraorbital ridge, and finally over the infraorbital ridge. The muscle tissue around the eyes is perhaps the most delicate on the body, so massage movements likewise must be gentle (see Figure 12.18d). (*Caution:* Strokes around the eyes are avoided if the client is wearing contact lenses.)

8. Continue to massage with gentle circular friction, using the fingertips, beside the nose from the eyes to the mouth and laterally beneath the zygomatic arch. Gently press upward under the zygomatic arch with the fingertips. The medial portion of the zygomatic arch is the site of the origin of several mimetic muscles (muscles of expression). Though the friction massage is circular, the intention is to massage these muscles of expression in an upward direction. (See Figure 12.18e.)

9. Massage the masseter muscle with circular friction and gliding strokes with the thumb or fingers from the lateral aspect of the zygomatic arch to the ramus of the mandible. The parotid salivary gland is located over the posterior aspect of the masseter muscle and the TMJ. Pressure is avoided over the parotid gland and the TMJ.

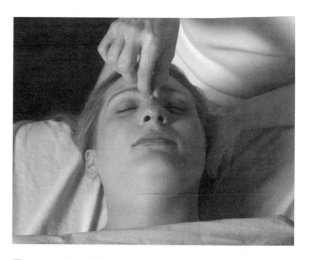

Figure 12.18c
Grasp the bridge of the nose and apply gentle traction.

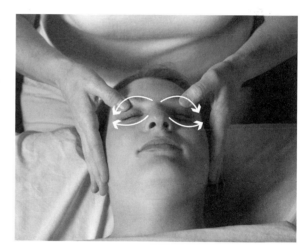

Figure 12.18d
Apply digital effleurage to the forehead and orbits. Do not put pressure on the eyeballs.

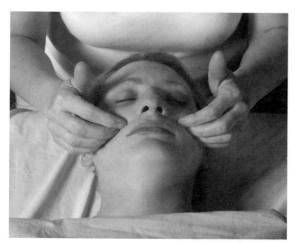

Figure 12.18e
Apply gentle friction from the nose to under the zygomatic arch bilaterally.

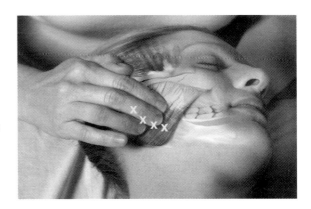

Figure 12.18f

Treat tender points or trigger points, which are common in the masseter muscle along the ramus of the jaw, with light digital compression.

10. Tender points or trigger points are common in the masseter muscle on the mandible. These may be addressed with gentle point compression for 6 to 10 seconds, repeated two or three times (see Figure 12.18f).

11. Continue to massage along the mandible from the tip of the chin to the ramus. The fingers apply gentle circular friction inferior to the mandible while the thumbs gently massage above the ridge. Gently massage under the chin with the fingertips while massaging the area from the lower lip to the chin with the thumbs. Finish with gliding strokes from the chin to the ear (see Figure 12.18g).

12. Repeat gliding strokes from the centerline of the face to the side of the head with an upward orientation in increments, starting at the chin, under the lips, above the lips, next to the nose, under the eyes, and over the eyes.

13. Complete the face massage by placing both hands lightly over the entire face, thenar eminence on the forehead and fingertips at the outer edge of the lips. Hold still for a moment, allowing the client to sink further into a relaxed state (see Figure 12.18h).

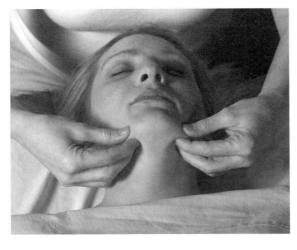

Figure 12.18g

Apply gentle circular friction inferior to the mandible with your fingers while your thumbs gently massage above the ridge.

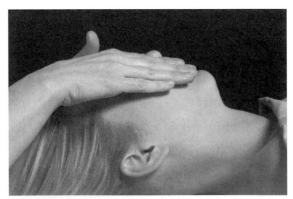

Figure 12.18h

Complete the face massage by placing both hands lightly over the entire face.

Massage the Scalp

To thoroughly massage the scalp, the therapist will turn the client's head first one way then the other, gently and securely supporting the client's head with one hand while massaging with the other (Figure 12.19).

In order to comfortably support the client's head, the therapist will place one hand on either side of the client's head so that the thumbs are positioned just in front of the ears and the fingers extend behind the ears just beyond the occipital ridge. The palms rest comfortably on the cranium so that the hand encircles the ear but is not covering it. Lift the head slightly and turn it on its axis so that it rests comfortably in the cradle of your hand. By using this cranial handle, the therapist should be able to easily and securely, gently rotate, extend, flex, and even apply gentle traction to the head and neck.

1. Without using lubricant and using the fingertips of the top hand, begin just inferior to the occipital ridge on the side of the head that is exposed and massage the scalp with small circular movements. Use moderate pressure, moving the scalp over the underlying tissues, being careful not to pull the hair. Massage thoroughly across the occipital region and continue the movements across and up the back of the head as you proceed toward the top of the head and above the ear. You may want to turn your hand around to continue the circular friction movements around the ear to cover the entire half of the scalp on the upward turned side of the head (see Figure 12.20).

2. Change the motion of the hand to a quick vibration with the fingers spread apart, starting at the front hairline and progressing toward the occiput, covering the exposed half of the head.

3. Smooth the hair and scalp by combing through the hair with the fingertips from the front hairline to the back.

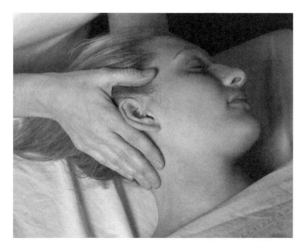

Figure 12.19
Note placement of the hands in the "handle" position supporting the head.

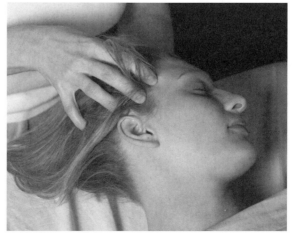

Figure 12.20
Massage the scalp by making rotating movements with the fingertips.

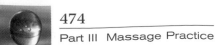

4. Lay the upper hand on the cranial "handle" and turn the head the other way and do the same procedure on the other side of the scalp. When the second side is completed, return the head to a neutral, forward-facing position.

Massage the Ear

The outer ears extend outward from the ear canal, which penetrates the auricular meatus to the delicate tissues of the inner ear. The outer ear is made up of cartilage and an abundance of nerves, so it is surprisingly sensitive. For this reason, some clients enjoy having their ears massaged, whereas others are uncomfortable with the practice. The French and Chinese have developed auricular therapies with the theory that points or areas of the outer ear are reflexively related to every area and organ in the body. Massaging the points in the ear may have stimulating, relaxing, or rejuvenating effects in areas of the body far removed from the ear (see Figure 12.21).

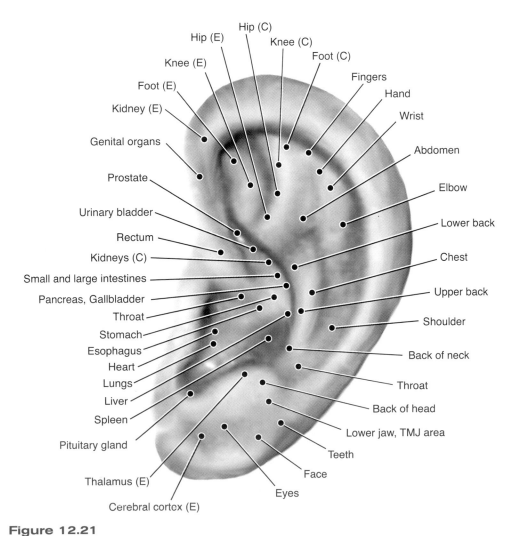

Figure 12.21

The Auricular Therapy Ear Chart shows areas in the ear as they relate to other areas of the body.

Both ears may be massaged simultaneously.

1. Begin by massaging the head all around the ear with circular friction.

2. Glide around the top and back of the ear where it joins to the head with the edge of your finger (two or three repetitions).

3. Beginning at the lower edge of the ear, using moderate pressure, unroll the outer edge of the ear between your thumb and fingers, applying a slight traction and working all the way around to the upper, anterior aspect of the ear (Figure 12.22a).

4. Starting at the top front of the ear, use a fingertip (well-trimmed fingernails, please) to carefully and with moderate pressure trace all the valleys and ridges of the ear. The thumb may be positioned behind the ear to provide a backing for the manipulation (see Figure 12.22b). If any crystals, crunchies, or other tissue abnormalities are encountered or if the client says there are tender points, spend a little extra time stimulating these points. These may be an indication of some condition in a related area of the body. You may want to make a note of the tender point for reference to the body area later in the massage or for the record for future treatments.

5. Beginning with the thumbs seated deeply in the center of the ear and the first finger at the base of the ear near the head, grip the ear firmly and slowly pull the ear at an angle away from the head. Massage the ear between the finger and thumb as you continue tractioning until you reach the outer periphery of the ear. Return the thumb to the center of the ear and repeat the sequence several times, each time in a slightly different direction—inferiorly, inferior-posteriorly, posteriorly, posterior-superiorly, superiorly.

6. Finish by gently tugging inferiorly on the ear lobes, gently grasping and unrolling the outer edges of the ears, and then using a gliding stroke with the finger, massage the attachment of the ear to the head.

From this point, the massage may continue to the jaw and face or to the neck.

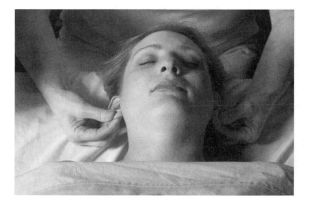

Figure 12.22a
Unroll the outer edge of the ear.

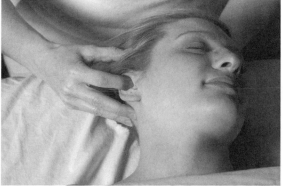

Figure 12.22b
Massage in and around the ears with light friction movement.

Massage the Neck

1. Apply lubricant with a bilateral-lateral effleurage stroke beginning at the sternal notch and continuing over the shoulders, up the trapezius and the back of the neck, to the occipital ridge (Figure 12.23a to c).

2. Turn the client's head to one side, supporting it with your hand. Continue effleurage strokes, leading with your little finger and beginning just inferior (below) the mastoid process (bony bump below and behind the ear). Continue down the lateral aspect of the neck, over the shoulder, and back up the trapezius to the occipital ridge. Repeat three to five times (Figure 12.24a to d).

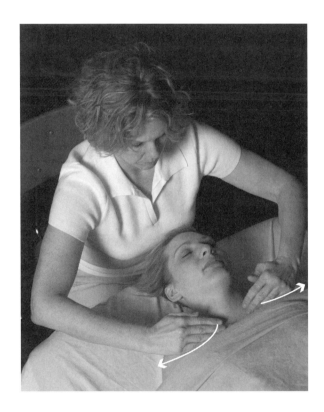

Figure 12.23a

Apply bilateral effleurage (beginning at the sternal notch). Use the hands simultaneously, leading with the little fingers.

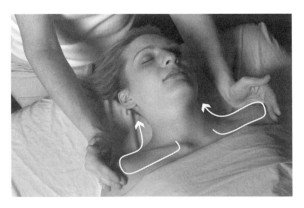

Figure 12.23b

Continue effleurage from the sternal notch, over the shoulders, and along the trapezius.

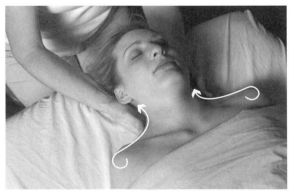

Figure 12.23c

Continue the movement up to the occipital ridge.

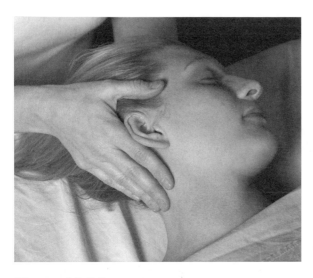

Figure 12.24a

Note placement of the hands in the "handle" position supporting the head.

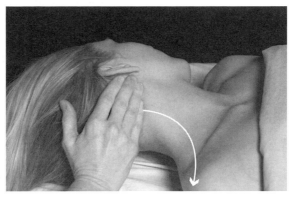

Figure 12.24b

Apply effleurage, leading with the little finger, just below the mastoid and continue down the neck.

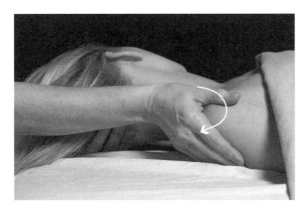

Figure 12.24c

Continue the movement across the shoulder and around the deltoid.

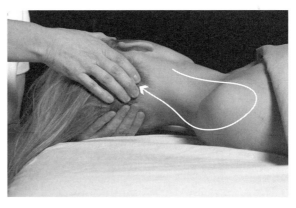

Figure 12.24d

Hand position at the completion of effleurage stroke.

3. Thoroughly knead that side of the neck, paying attention to any tight areas.

4. Repeat effleurage stroke on neck and shoulders.

5. Apply circular friction to any congested or tight areas.

6. Apply V-stroke effleurage to side and back of neck (Figure 12.25a to c).

7. Repeat effleurage.

8. Turn the client's head to the opposite side and repeat the movements as you did in steps 2 through 6.

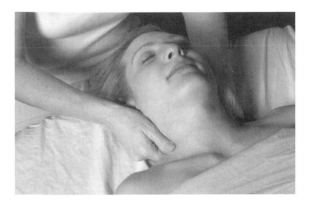

Figure 12.25a

Apply pertrissage to the neck and shoulders.

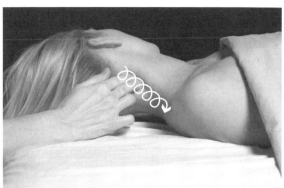

Figure 12.25b

Apply friction to the neck and shoulders.

Figure 12.25c

Apply V-stroke to the neck and shoulders.

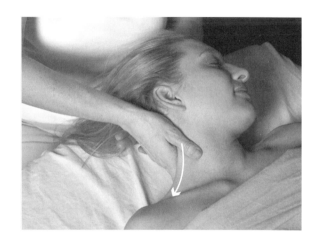

9. Return the client's head to the central position and apply bilateral-lateral petrissage and friction to the neck and shoulders.

10. Do the following joint movements: Tilt the head back with the chin up, then lower the chin down to the chest. Laterally flex the neck, moving the ear, first toward the right shoulder, then toward the left. Apply a slight traction as the head is returned to a neutral position. Rotate the head to its full range of motion (lateral rotation). The spine remains in a straight line. (*Note:* Joint movements of the neck are contraindicated in cases of osteoporosis.) (See Figure 12.26a to c.)

11. Hold the occiput in the palm of your hand or hook your fingers under the occiput and apply a slight traction to the neck.

12. Place one hand on each shoulder and gently alternately push them toward the feet, providing a gentle rocking motion (Figure 12.27a and b).

13. Repeat the stroking movement in step 1.

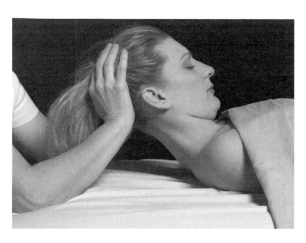

Figure 12.26a

Apply passive joint movements by rolling the head forward. Note placement of the hands on the client's head.

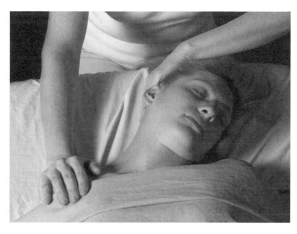

Figure 12.26b

Apply a passive stretch by supporting the head to the side with one hand and pushing the opposite shoulder toward the feet with the other.

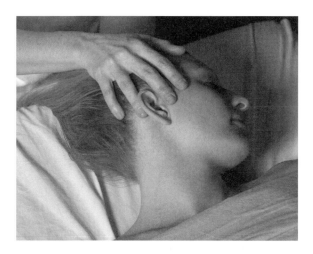

Figure 12.26c

Apply passive rotation to the neck, being careful to keep the cervical spine straight.

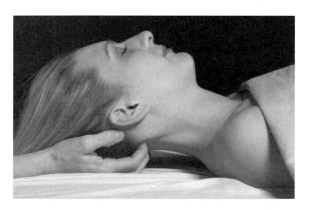

Figure 12.27a

Apply slight traction to the cervical spine by hooking the fingers under the occiput and pulling.

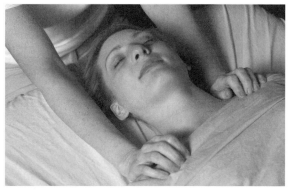

Figure 12.27b

Apply alternating pressure toward the feet to rock gently and stretch the shoulders.

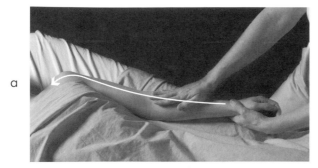
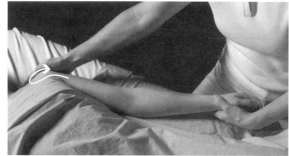
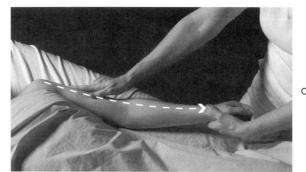

Figure 12.28a–c

Apply gliding strokes to the lateral aspect of the arm. Note the "handle" and hand position. The stroke is continuous from the wrist, up the arm, over the shoulder, and back to the wrist. Use more pressure on the stroke up to the shoulder and less pressure on the return.

Massage the Arms

1. Undrape one arm to make contact and apply lubricant to the client's arm from shoulder to wrist, using light effleurage.

2. Locate the handle at the wrist, and put the client's arm in slight traction by holding it with the wrist handle. Apply effleurage. Apply more pressure from wrist to neck, then lightly stroke as you return to the wrist. Hold the thumb side handle (the client's wrist) with the arm that is closest to the client. Begin from the wrist, up the arm, over the shoulder, and up to the back of the neck. Rotate your hand as it travels over the client's shoulder; at the same time, apply slight traction to the handle. Proceed up the back of the neck and then down under the shoulder (trapezius area); then glide back to the starting point at the wrist. Repeat three to five times (Figure 12.28a to c).

3. Change the handle to the ulnar side of the wrist. Apply effleurage with firmer pressure up the medial aspect of the arm over the shoulder, around and down into the axillary portion of the arm, then return to the wrist with lighter pressure. Do effleurage again three to five times (Figure 12.29a to c).

4. Using both hands, grasp the arm at shoulder level and apply petrissage, directing individual movements toward the shoulder while moving down the arm to the client's hand. On the upper arm, use both hands to alternately knead the biceps and triceps. On the lower arm, alternately knead the wrist flexors and extensors (Figure 12.30a and b).

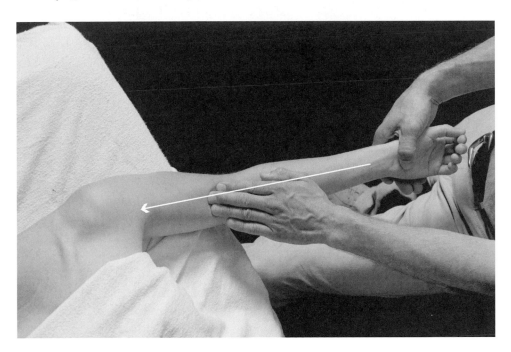

Figure 12.29a
Continue with effleurage movements on the medial aspect of the arm. Note "handle" and hand position.

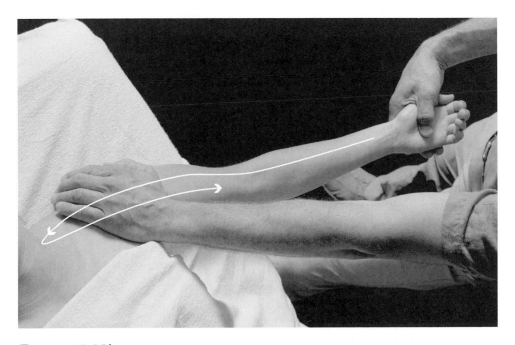

Figure 12.29b
Continue the effleurage movements up and over the shoulder, then back down the arm.

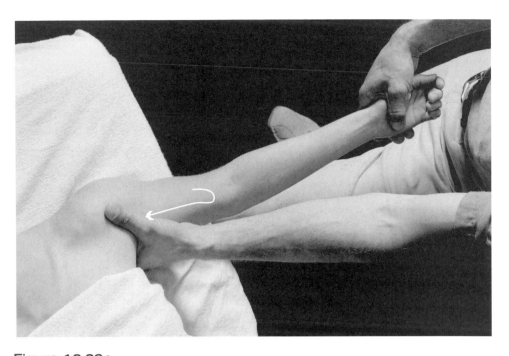

Figure 12.29c

Continue the effleurage movements up into the axillary area for a slight joint movement and stretch.

5. Wring and roll (using both hands) from the shoulder, moving down the arm and giving special attention to the muscles of the forearm (Figure 12.30a to e).

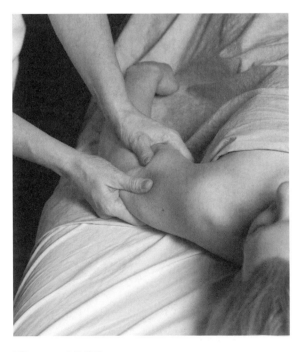

Figure 12.30a

Apply petrissage from the shoulder and continue down the arm.

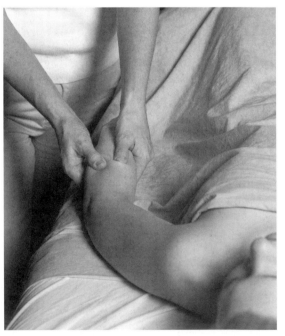

Figure 12.30b

Continue petrissage down the arm to the wrist.

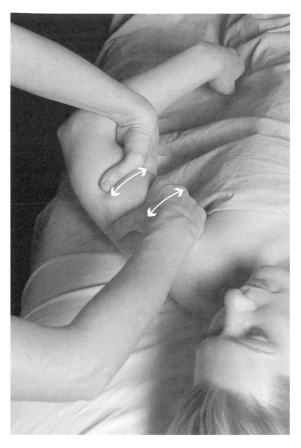

Figure 12.30c

Apply wringing movements from the shoulder to the wrist.

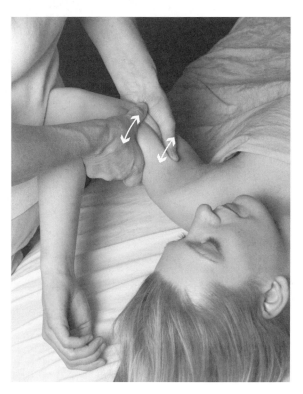

Figure 12.30d

An alternate position may be used for the wringing movements and kneading.

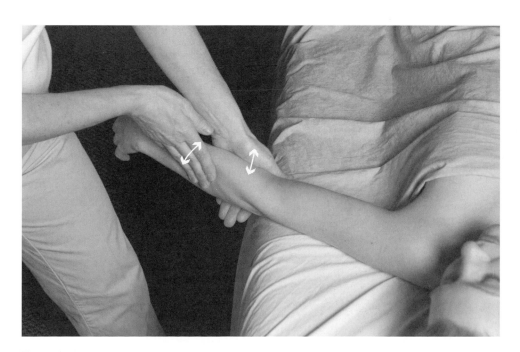

Figure 12.30e

Do rolling movements from the shoulder to the wrist.

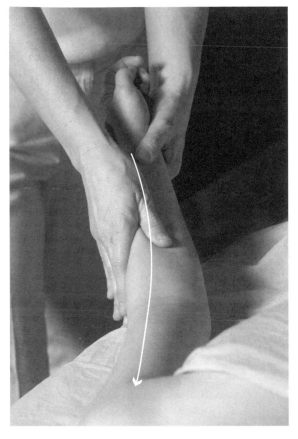

Figure 12.31a

Note the direction of V-stroke and position of the arm. Apply the same upward movement when massaging the back of the arm.

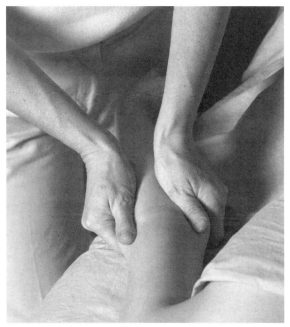

Figure 12.31b

Apply fulling to the arm.

6. Apply V-stroke effleurage from wrist to elbow on the medial and lateral sides of the forearm (Figure 12.31a).

7. Apply fulling to the forearm (Figure 12.31b).

8. Repeat effleurage to the medial and lateral side of the arm.

9. Massage the hand and then do joint movements on the arm and hand.

Massage the Hand

1. Apply petrissage to the palm of the client's hand.

2. Apply friction to the palm.

3. Apply petrissage to the back of the hand.

4. Apply friction to the back of the hand.

5. Do petrissage on each digit, including a joint movement (Figure 12.32a to f).

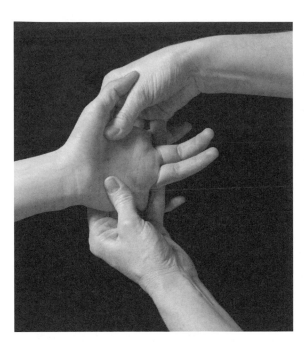

Figure 12.32a

Apply friction and petrissage to the palm of the hand, spreading the metacarpals.

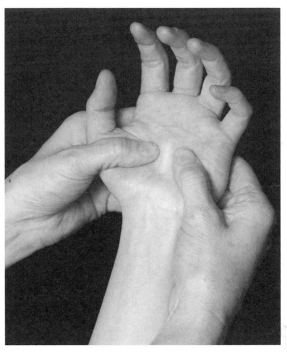

Figure 12.32b

With the client's elbow resting on the table, hold the hand upright and massage the palm of the hand with your thumbs, using circular movements in alternate directions. This relaxes the hand.

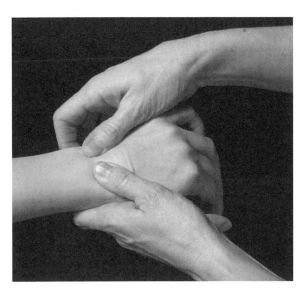

Figure 12.32c

Apply friction and petrissage to the wrist and muscles of the hand.

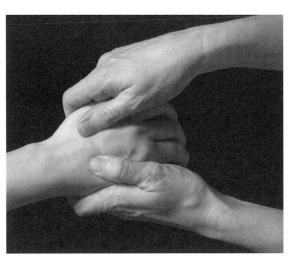

Figure 12.32d

Apply circular friction to the back of the hand.

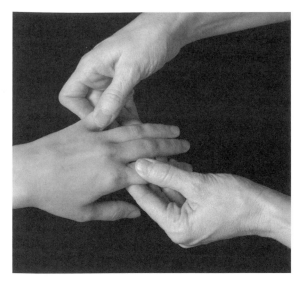

Figure 12.32e

Beginning at the base of each finger, apply friction and petrissage. Work downward to the tip of each finger.

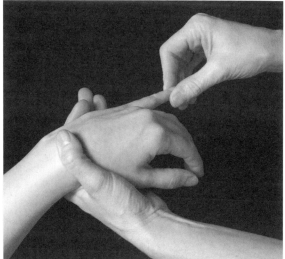

Figure 12.32f

Squeeze and gently twist each finger, beginning at the base and working toward the tip. Rotate each finger in large circles. Finish each finger with a gentle squeeze of the fingertip.

6. Apply joint movement. Support the client's hand and rotate all fingers clockwise and counterclockwise.

7. Extend, flex, and rotate the fingers, wrist, and elbow.

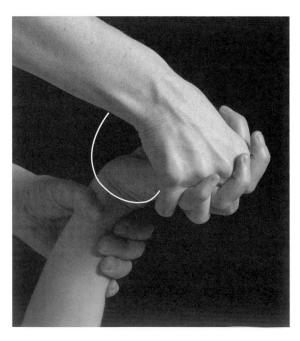

Figure 12.33a

Apply joint movements and rotation. Note the interlacing of the fingers.

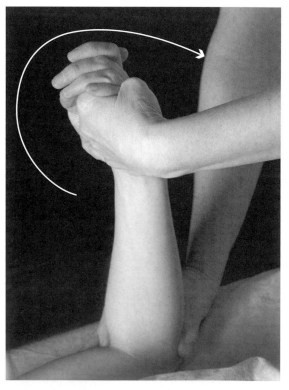

Figure 12.33b

Rotate the forearm. Note how the fingers are used to steady the client's elbow.

8. Rotate the shoulder joint clockwise and counterclockwise.

9. Extend the arm straight above the client's head to stretch the entire arm.

10. Apply effleurage from elbow past axillary area (Figure 12.33a to e).

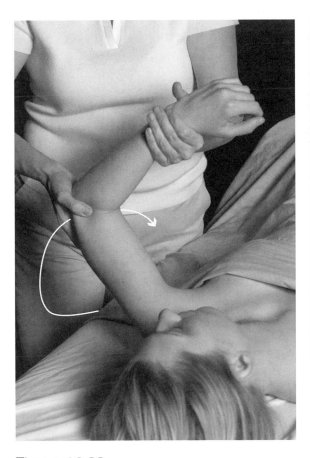

Figure 12.33c

Apply joint movements to the shoulder by moving the elbow in large circles. Note how the wrist is supported to prevent the client's hand from hitting her in the face.

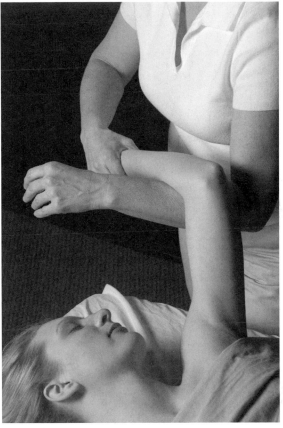

Figure 12.33d

Stretch the client's arm over your arm. A slight turn or stretch may be done with your hand holding the client's wrist.

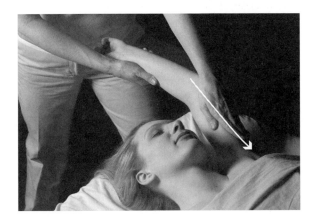

Figure 12.33e

Apply effleurage or compression to the axillary area.

11. Apply traction at the wrist while moving the arm from a position above the client's head and back down to the side.

12. Shake and vibrate the arm and hand (Figure 12.34a).

13. Apply a final effleurage of the arm and hand and rotate the shoulder.

14. Apply lateral effleurage; then feather downward with superficial strokes from the neck, down the arm, to the fingertips (Figure 12.34b).

15. Redrape the client as necessary, and repeat the arm and hand massage for the other arm and hand.

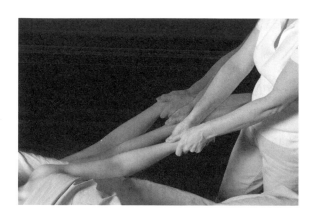

Figure 12.34a
Grasp the wrist securely, and vigorously shake the arm up and down.

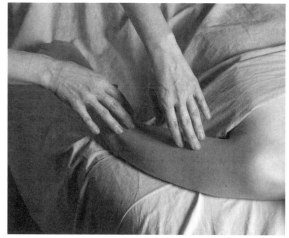

Figure 12.34b
Apply feather strokes (light effleurage) with your fingertips to complete the massage of the arm. Do the massage of the other arm using the same sequence of movements.

Massage the Feet

1. Move to the feet, maintaining contact by using a light brushing stroke down the side of the body. Pause momentarily to allow the client to sense where you are before you begin massaging the feet. Undrape one foot and leg up to the hip.

2. Use just enough lubricant to allow your hands to work smoothly. (One or two drops are usually enough. Sometimes no lubricant is needed on the feet.)

3. Apply effleurage to each aspect of the foot to strip out the venous fluid. Stroke from the toes up to and past the ankle on the top, side, and bottom of the foot.

4. Apply petrissage and friction to the bottom of the feet from the ball of the foot to the heel. Use a closed fist or heel of the hand to do deep gliding.

5. Apply kneading movements from the toes up to the ankles.

6. Apply small circular friction movements between each of the tendons on the top and sides of the foot.

7. Apply digital friction to each toe and between toes (Figure 12.35a to f).

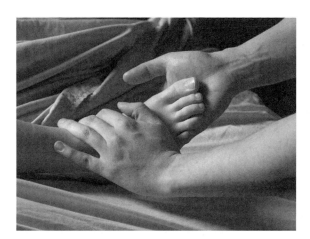

Figure 12.35a

Apply effleurage to both the top and bottom of the foot, working from the toes upward toward the heart.

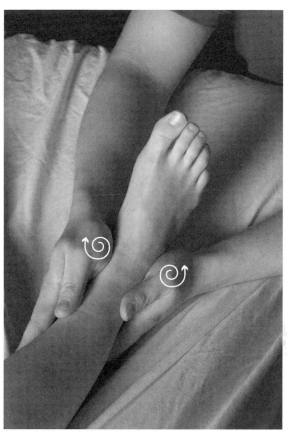

Figure 12.35b

Warm the foot and ankles with circular rubbing movements.

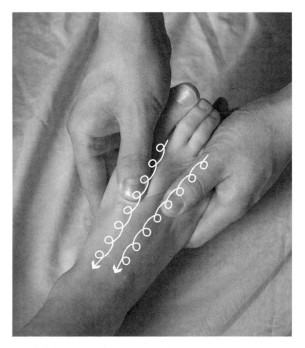

Figure 12.35c

Knead the foot using circular motions.

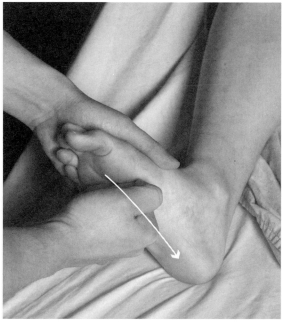

Figure 12.35d

Apply your knuckles to stroke down the plantar surface of the foot.

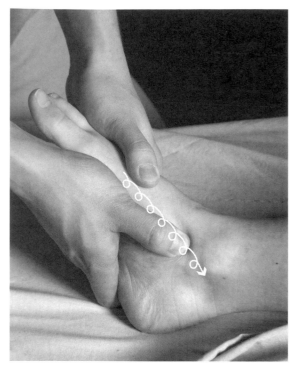

Figure 12.35e

Apply digital friction between the tendons and bones on all surfaces of the foot.

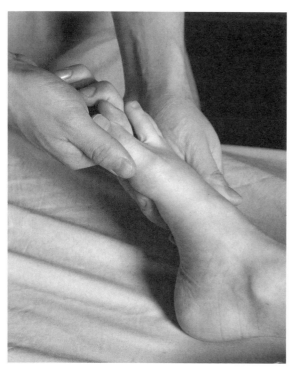

Figure 12.35f

Massage and rotate each digit.

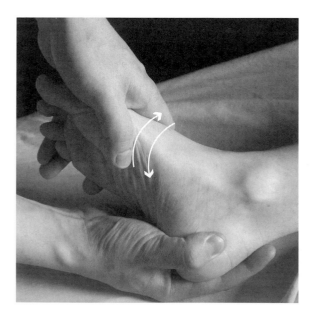

Figure 12.36a

Rotate and stretch the tarsus and metatarsus.

8. Beginning with the toes, incorporate joint movements, first individually, then together. Apply plantar and dorsal flexion of the toes, then to the entire foot. Rotate the foot and ankle, then separate the toes (phalanges) and wring and roll the foot (Figure 12.36a to e).

9. Repeat this entire procedure on the other foot.

Note: You may choose to work on adjacent parts of the body in sequence (from one part to the adjoining part) rather than interrupting the flow of movement. After working on the foot, proceed directly to the front of the leg. Then continue to the other foot and leg.

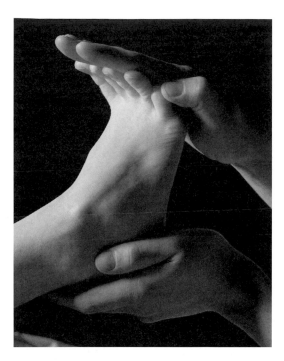

Figure 12.36b
Stretch the plantar surface of the foot and toes.

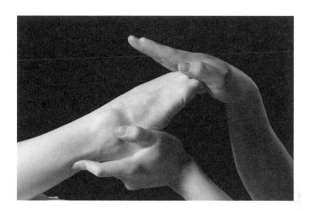

Figure 12.36c
Stretch the dorsal aspect of the foot and toes.

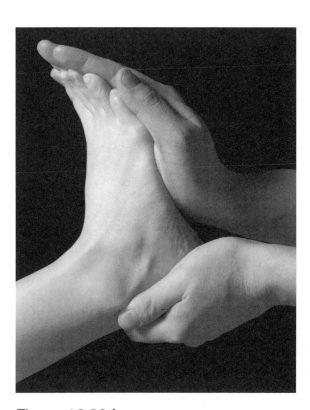

Figure 12.36d
Stretch the Achilles' tendon. Note the position of the hands.

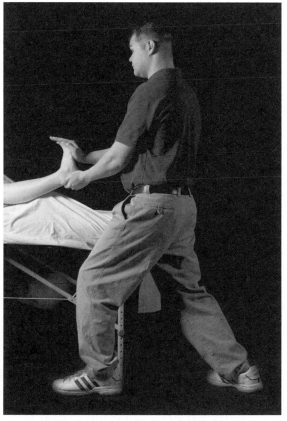

Figure 12.36e
As a practitioner, always be aware of using proper body mechanics.

Massage the Front of the Legs

1. Apply lubricant with light and continuous effleurage.

2. Apply effleurage with both hands, beginning at the ankle. Apply effleurage to the entire leg by leading with one hand on the lateral side of the leg and the other hand on the medial aspect of the leg. Your hands should span the entire front of the leg. Hand pressure may be increased with each effleurage stroke and feathered back to the starting point. The upward medial hand progresses to the groin and turns as it returns lightly along the medial aspect of the leg to the beginning point at the ankle. The lateral hand starts at the ankle, continues up the lateral aspect of the anterior leg, all the way to the anterior superior iliac spine (ASIS), along the iliac crest, and glides back to the starting point. Repeat these movements three to five times.

   Note: The leg is the longest part of the body. Be sure to use proper body mechanics and movement when applying long strokes to the leg (Figure 12.37a to d).

3. Apply petrissage, beginning at the ankle and proceeding up the leg along the fleshy parts along the side of the tibia to the knee. The thigh may require several passes up and down with this stroke because it is a large area.

4. Apply digital petrissage to the tendon areas around the patella.

5. Repeat effleurage (Figure 12.38a to d).

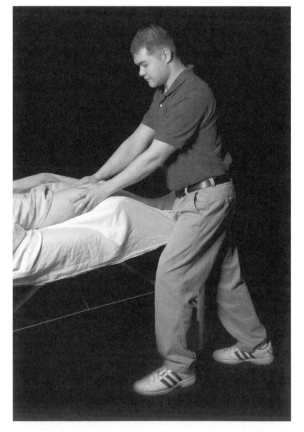

Figure 12.37a

Apply effleurage to the leg. Maintain good posture and stance, keep the back straight, flex the knees slightly.

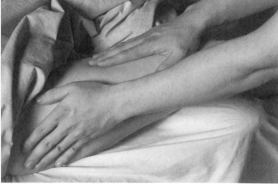

Figure 12.37b

The leading hand should be on the lateral side of the leg in order to travel up and over the ilium and return back to the starting point.

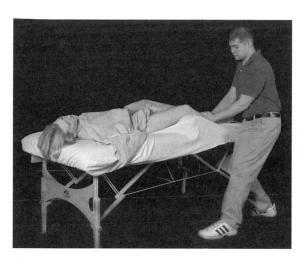

Figure 12.37c

Note the body position at the beginning of the gliding stroke on the anterior leg.

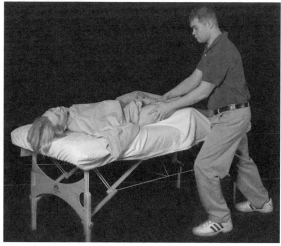

Figure 12.37d

Note the body position at the end of the gliding stroke on the anterior leg.

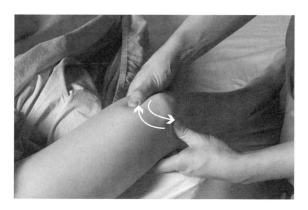

Figure 12.38a

Manipulate the patella by tracing circles with your thumb in opposite directions.

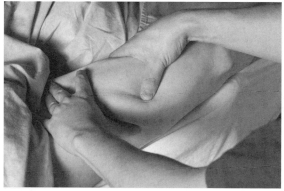

Figure 12.38b

Apply petrissage to the anterior leg.

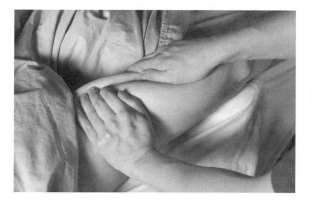

Figure 12.38c

Continue wringing movements to the thigh.

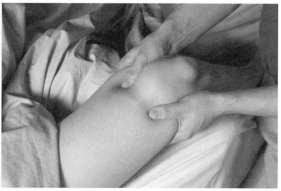

Figure 12.38d

Apply fulling (compression) movements.

Optional Position

(Bending the Knee) The following is an optional position for leg massage. In this position, the entire calf and thigh can be massaged easily. Position the client's foot flat on the table with the knee bent and the foot 16 to 18 inches from the buttocks. Wrap the foot with the drape and brace the leg either with your knee or by sitting on the table near the client's toes to keep the leg from sliding. Be sure the draping is intact to secure modesty of the pelvic area.

1. With the leg in the bent-knee position, apply effleurage from ankle to knee.

2. Apply petrissage from ankle to knee.

3. Repeat effleurage from ankle to knee.

4. While keeping the knee bent, apply a variety of friction techniques from ankle to knee. Pay special attention to areas that seem to be more congested or tight. Apply rolling, wringing, or cross-fiber friction in areas of tension.

5. Repeat effleurage from ankle to knee.

6. Keeping the leg in the bent-knee position, apply effleurage from knee to hip, groin, and gluteal crease.

7. Apply petrissage to the entire thigh. Make several passes to cover the entire circumference of the leg.

8. Apply wringing, rolling, and chucking.

9. Follow with effleurage to the entire leg (Figure 12.39a to e).

10. Apply joint movements. Grasp the ankle with one hand, and place the other hand just below the knee. Move the knee toward the chest

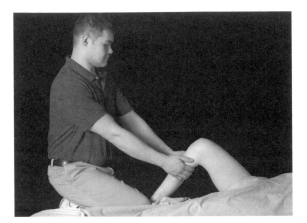

Figure 12.39a

Support the client's leg in a bent position using your knee (note the draping so that therapist's clothing does not touch client's skin).

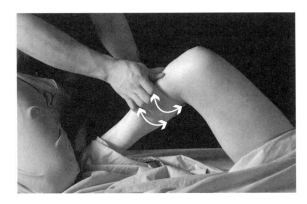

Figure 12.39b

In the bent-knee position, apply wringing and rolling movements to the calf.

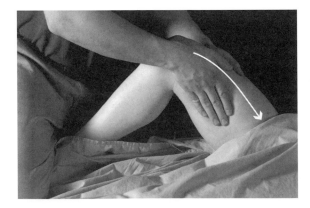

Figure 12.39c

With the client in the bent-knee position, apply effluerage to the thigh.

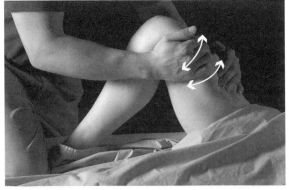

Figure 12.39d

Knead and wring the thigh in the bent-knee position.

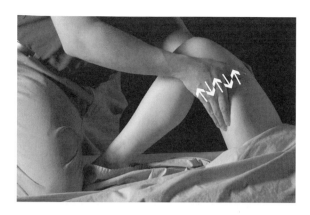

Figure 12.39e

Apply chucking to the thigh. With the client in the bent-knee position, manipulate soft tissue of the posterior aspect of the thigh and apply effluerage, petrissage, or rolling movements.

while flexing the knee and hips to the maximum. Pay attention to the degree of flexibility, and move the limbs firmly but not forcefully to their maximum range of movement. It is beneficial to have the client breathe deeply and then exhale as you apply downward pressure on the knee toward the chest.

11. Move your hand around to grasp the ankle at the level of the Achilles' tendon; then elevate the foot toward the ceiling to extend the leg and flex the hip. Flex the hip to its maximum range of movement by moving the foot toward the client's head.

12. Flex the client's knee by bringing it toward the chest; then rotate the bent leg laterally, retaining slight pressure on the knee to maintain full range of motion as the leg rotates outward. Return the leg to the table by continuing the hip rotation and slowly straightening the leg. Your hand should support the back of the leg to prevent hyperextension as the leg is returned to the table. Repeat this procedure two times (Figure 12.40a to e).

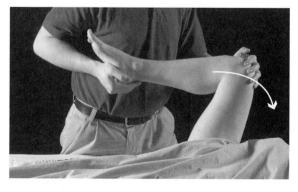

Figure 12.40a

Apply joint movements. The client's knee may be moved toward the chest, or this position may be used for joint rotations of the hip and knee within its normal range of motion. Note the position of the hands at the heel and the knee.

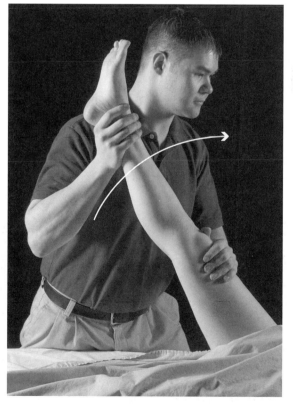

Figure 12.40b

Stretch the hamstrings by lifting the foot toward the ceiling and straightening the knee.

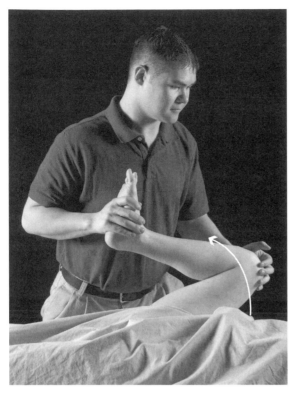

Figure 12.40c
Move the knee to the chest to stretch the hip and low back.

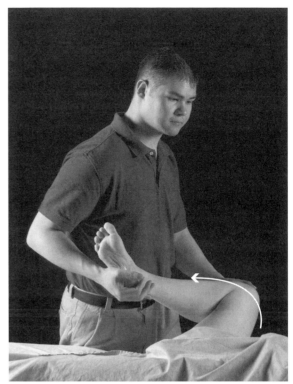

Figure 12.40d
Abduct, rotate, and circumduct the hip. Note the draping.

Figure 12.40e
Support the knee as you return the leg to the table.

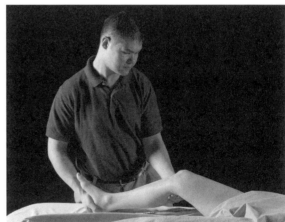

13. Move to the foot of the table and grasp the heel (handle) with the lateral hand (the one toward the outside of the leg you were working on). Rotate the foot and leg in the hip socket. This movement will be back and forth, and the foot movement will resemble that of a windshield wiper.

14. Dorsal flex and plantar flex the foot.

15. Place your other hand over the client's instep and apply slight traction. Shake the leg up and down. Keep the heel on the table to avoid hyperextension of the knee (Figure 12.41a to d).

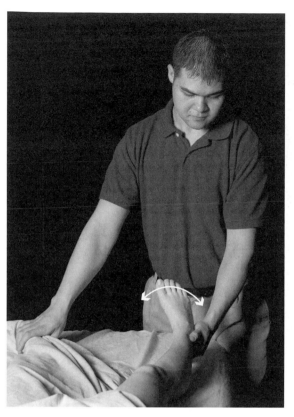

Figure 12.41a

Rotate the leg medially and laterally with a windshield wiper motion.

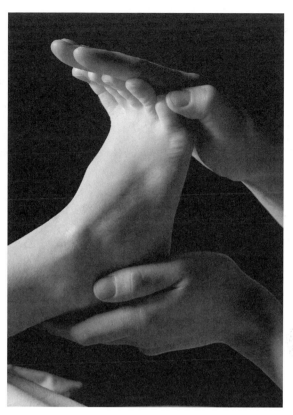

Figure 12.41b

Stretch the Achilles' tendon and calf muscles.

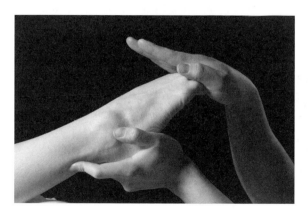

Figure 12.41c

Plantar flex the foot.

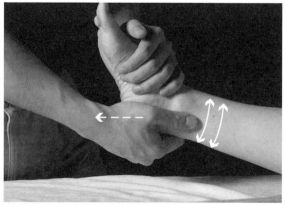

Figure 12.41d

Apply traction and shaking movements. This completes the sequence of movements for the anterior leg. Redrape the leg and proceed to massage the other leg.

16. Apply effleurage to the entire leg three to five times.

17. Apply feather (nerve) strokes from hip to toes, three to five times.

18. Redrape the leg and proceed to the other foot. Repeat the entire procedure on the other leg.

Massage the Abdomen and Chest

This part of the massage requires some special considerations. The need for draping varies when working with male and female clients. Breast draping is always used on female clients unless informed consent is given prior to the massage for specific procedures in which her breasts will be exposed. Professional standards recommend that draping procedures (as directed earlier in this chapter) be followed. When asked, some clients will opt not to have the abdomen or chest massaged.

The following massage description refers to techniques used on the fully exposed torso, with added comments when using breast draping.

In preparation for massage of the abdominal region, use a bolster or pillow to elevate the client's knees and support them so that the abdominal muscles will remain relaxed. Draping should be open enough to allow massaging down to the top of the pubic bone, and secure enough to avoid exposure of the genital area (Figure 12.42).

1. To begin, stand to the client's right to apply massage lubricant to the abdomen, chest, and sides of the body.

2. Do effleurage strokes on the abdomen and chest, over the shoulders, around and down the axillary areas, then down the sides of the crest of the ilium. Massage back to the center with a turn of your wrist and repeat the movements. When using breast draping, this stroke glides up as far as the drape will allow and then laterally over the ribs and down to the iliac crest. Massage should not be done directly over the sensitive area of the nipples on men or women.

3. Do circular effleurage on the abdomen in a clockwise direction following the path of the colon. On this stroke, one hand remains

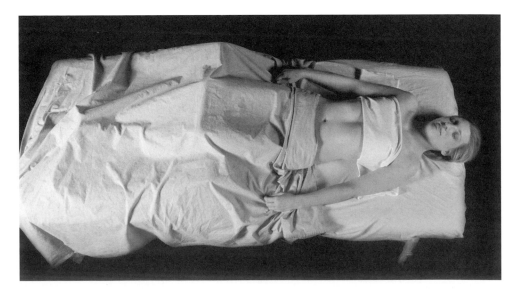

Figure 12.42

Note the correct position and draping for massage of the abdomen. Use a folded towel to cover the female client's breasts. Use a bolster to support the knees.

in constant contact doing circular massage. The other describes a semicircle beginning at the lower right of the client's abdomen, moving up the right side to the rib cage, across the abdomen just below the rib cage, then down the left side to an area just medial of the hipbone. Abdominal massage should always encourage the natural flow in the large intestines. Repeat the abdominal massage movements several times (see Figure 12.43a).

4. Knead the entire abdomen, massaging not only the abdominal muscles but also stimulating the action of the abdominal organs (Figure 12.43b).

5. To massage the large intestine more thoroughly, apply circular friction to its entire length. Begin in the area of the lower left part of the abdomen. The circles should be on an oblique (deviation to the vertical or horizontal line) plane of the surface of the abdomen so that pressure is increased and decreased repeatedly over an area about 2 inches square, and at the rate of about 100 circles per minute. This movement encourages the contents of the colon toward the rectum. Proceed slowly back along the course of the colon all the way to the cecum, the first portion of the colon (Figure 12.43c).

6. Grasp as much of the abdominal tissue as possible and gently lift and shake it (Figure 12-43d).

7. Do alternate hand strokes or shingles. Stand to one side of the client and reach over to the opposite side. Alternately pull your hands over the client's body toward you. As one hand nears

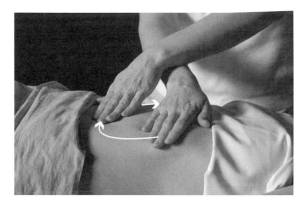

Figure 12.43a
Stroke the abdomen with deep circular movement in a clockwise direction.

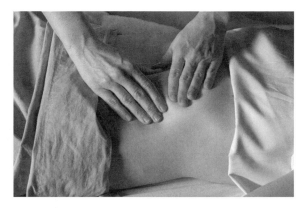

Figure 12.43b
Apply petrissage to the abdomen.

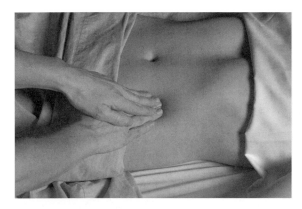

Figure 12.43c
Apply friction in small circles following the colon in reverse.

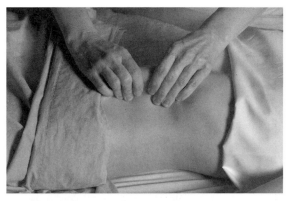

Figure 12.43d
Apply a shaking movement. Grasp the skin of the abdomen and shake it gently. This movement stimulates the action of the large and small intestines.

completion of the stroke, the other begins a stroke. This movement begins just below the crest of the ilium (hip bone) and may continue all the way over the shoulder and up the neck. When working with breast draping, it is necessary to adjust the drape to continue this movement up to the axillary area and back down to the hip. When massaging the area of the ribs, flex your fingers slightly and rake gently between the ribs with your fingertips (Figure 12.43e to h).

8. Move to the head of the table for the following stroke. This is referred to as the caring stroke and is a complete gliding stroke for the torso. This stroke can only be done when not using breast draping. Begin by placing your fingers (pointing toward each other) with palms flat on the client's skin at the uppermost aspect of the chest. Stroke downward over the chest and abdomen to the pubic bone. Rotate your hands over the client's hipbone, around the gluteus medius, around the sides, and back up to the axillary area. Rotate your hands as you continue upward, around the

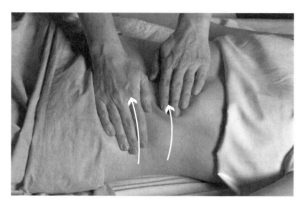

Figure 12.43e

Apply alternate-hand stroking movements (shingles) from the trochanter to the axilla. *Note:* Shingles is the name often used to describe alternate-hand effleurage in which one hand repeats the stroke as the other hand is about to complete the stroke.

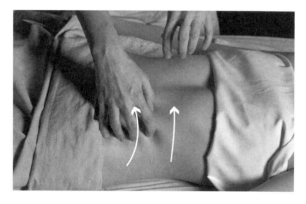

Figure 12.43f

Apply a raking movement several times across the ribs and abdomen using the tips of the fingers.

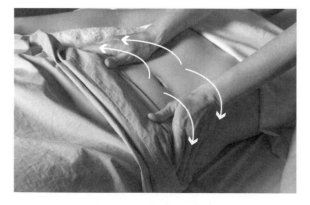

Figure 12.43g

Stretch the muscles of the stomach area and the abdominal region outward.

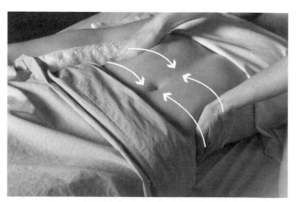

Figure 12.43h

Stretch the muscles over the stomach area and abdominal region inward.

shoulders, up the trapezius muscles to the back of the neck, ending at the occiput. Rotate your hands as you move them back down to the starting point. Repeat the movement several times. Beware of any residual tension your hands might perceive, and spend a few extra moments to work on those areas. Then repeat the caring stroke (Figure 12.44a to d).

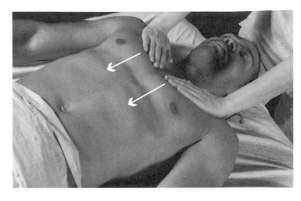

Figure 12.44a
Using the caring stroke, cover the entire front of the body and the neck. It is not possible to do the full caring stroke on women when they are using breast draping.

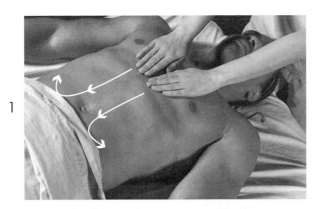

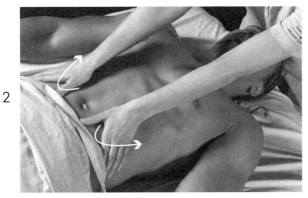
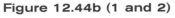

Figure 12.44b (1 and 2)
Note that the caring stroke begins at the clavicle with a stroke down the front of the body to the pubic bone.

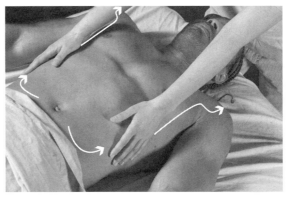

Figure 12.44c
Without losing contact with the client, rotate your hands to the sides of the client's body and stroke up to the axillary area.

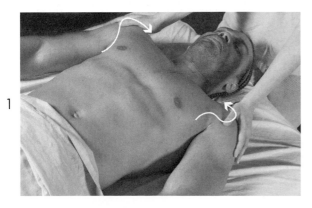

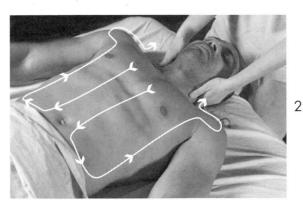

Figure 12.44d (1 and 2)
Stroke up, over, and around the shoulders and up the neck. Repeat the stroke several times.

This completes the massage of the front of the body.

At this point, reposition the top cover or wrap to cover the client, secure the cover, and ask the client to turn over to a prone (facedown) position. Be sure to follow proper draping procedures. Make the client comfortable by supplying a pillow or bolster to support the head, neck, back, chest, feet, or ankles as necessary.

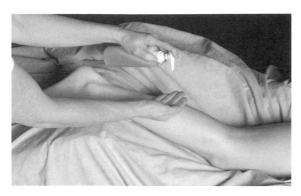

Figure 12.45a

Before beginning massage movements, prepare the posterior leg by undraping and applying lubricant. Keep the back of your hand against the client's skin while pouring the lubricant into your hand.

Massage the Back of the Legs

1. Undrape one leg. This massage is similar to the procedures for the front of the legs.

2. Make contact with the client's skin and apply the massage lubricant with light effleurage strokes.

3. Apply effleurage, leading with your lateral hand (medial hand following). Increase the pressure on the upward stroke with each pass. Maintain contact with much lighter pressure on the return stroke. Repeat three to five times.

4. Apply petrissage to the calf and thigh upward to the crest of the ilium (Figure 12.45a to g).

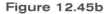

Figure 12.45b

Apply effleurage movements. Stroke toward the heart. *Note:* Place the leading hand on the lateral aspect of the leg in order to travel up and over the gluteal muscles and the iliac crest and back down the lateral side of the leg. At the same time, the medial hand travels up to the gluteal crease and then lightly down the medial side of the leg. Return both hands to the starting point to repeat the stroke three or more times.

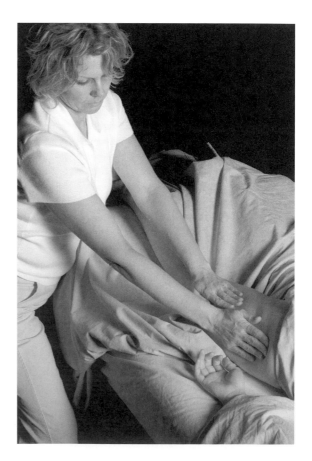

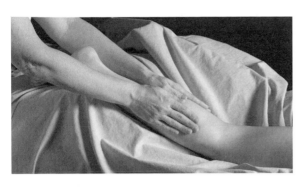

Figure 12.45c
Stroke the leg upward with both hands.

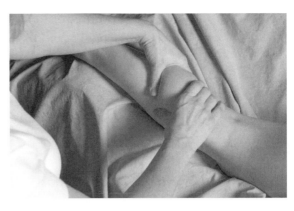

Figure 12.45d
Knead the calf muscles.

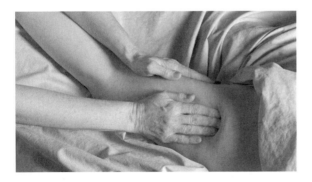

Figure 12.45e
Knead the muscles of the leg and thigh in a circular motion.

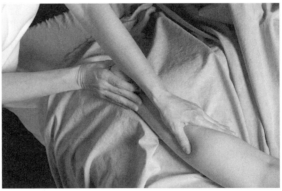

Figure 12.45f
Apply the V-stroke for deep stroking of the posterior leg.

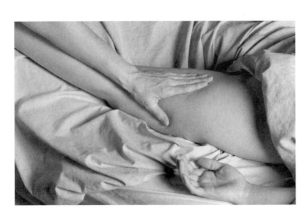

Figure 12.45g
Continue the V-stroke up the back of the thigh.

5. Repeat effleurage three to five times.

6. When there are particularly tight or tense areas, go over them with more specific friction movements such as compression, wringing, rolling, and deep friction. Using the heel of the hand or the elbow can be quite effective over the gluteal muscles and the hamstrings (Figure 12.46a to h).

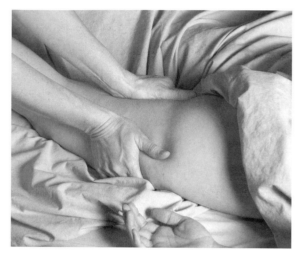

Figure 12.46a
Apply fulling strokes to the entire leg.

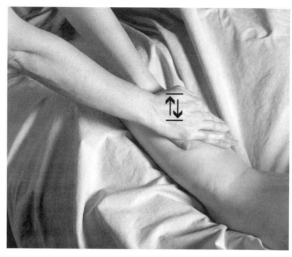

Figure 12.46b
Apply compression movements to the leg.

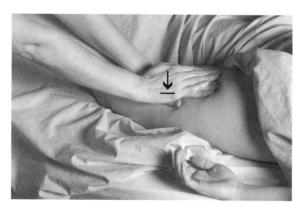

Figure 12.46c
Apply compression to the posterior thigh.

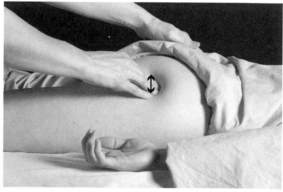

Figure 12.46d
Apply digital friction to the gluteal area.

Figure 12.46e
Using the heel of your hand, apply deep friction or deep pressure to the gluteal muscles.

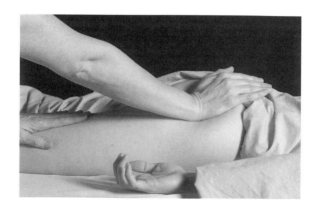

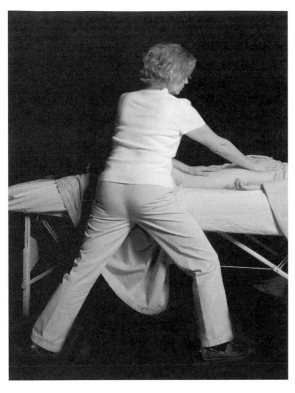

Figure 12.46f
When applying deep pressure, always use proper body mechanics.

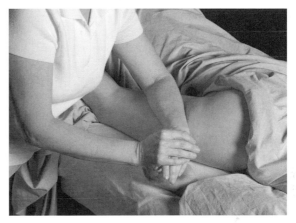

Figure 12.46g
Apply deep gliding to the muscles of the posterior leg using the elbow of the forearm.

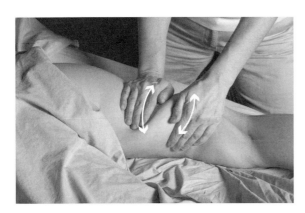

Figure 12.46h
Wring the back of the thigh.

7. Repeat effleurage.

8. Apply joint movements. Grasp the client's ankle and move the foot toward the buttocks with gentle pressure to flex the knee and to stretch the muscles on the front of the thigh. Continue by making increasingly larger circles with the ankle to rotate the hip joint. Return the foot to the table (Figure 12.47a to c).

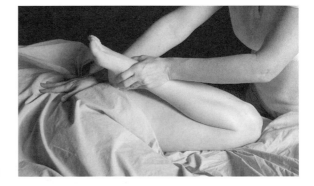

Figure 12.47a
Flex the client's knee, pressing the heel against the gluteal muscles.

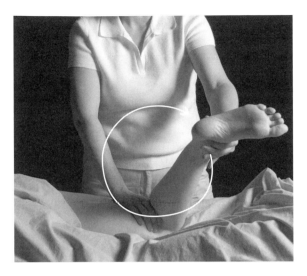

Figure 12.47b

Support the knee and circumduct the lower leg.

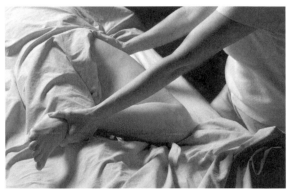

Figure 12.47c

Apply joint movements to flex the knee and laterally rotate the hip.

9. Apply percussion (optional) over the leg (Figure 12.48a and b).

10. Repeat effleurage as a finishing stroke, gently changing to feather (nerve) strokes.

11. Redrape the leg and repeat the entire procedure on the client's other leg.

Massage the Back

No massage is complete without a good back massage. It is important to give a good back massage because the client usually expects and looks forward to this part of the massage. There are hundreds of manipulations

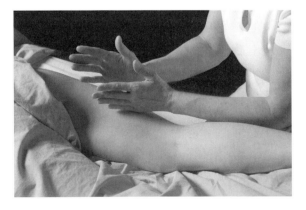

Figure 12.48a

Apply percussion to the posterior leg. The ulnar side of the hand aligns with the direction of muscle fibers.

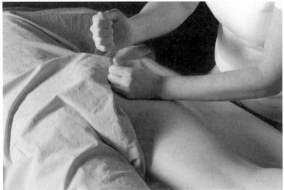

Figure 12.48b

Apply percussion (beating) to the gluteal area.

that may be done on the back. They range from extremely superficial stroking to deep tissue work using elbows and even knees when relieving tension around the spine, pelvis, and shoulders. The following is a basic soothing routine that is guaranteed to leave the recipient in a calm, relaxed state.

1. Follow proper draping procedures.

2. Stand to the side of the client. Apply massage lubricant with effleurage strokes.

3. Beginning at the top of the gluteal cleft, apply long effleurage strokes. Apply long gliding strokes up the spine to the nape of the neck.

4. Move your hands out and over the shoulders and down the sides to the hips. Rotate your hands and return to the starting point. Repeat the movement five to eight times. Use equal pressure on pulling and pushing strokes (Figure 12.49a to c).

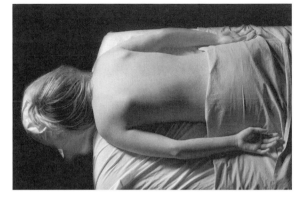

Figure 12.49a

Prepare for the massage of the back by adjusting the draping and applying lubricant with a light effleurage stroke.

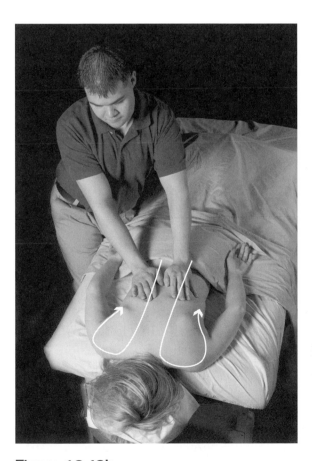

Figure 12.49b

Apply long strokes up the back beginning at the gluteal cleft. The ulnar side of the hand leads, with the fingers of one hand nearly touching the other at the midline of the back.

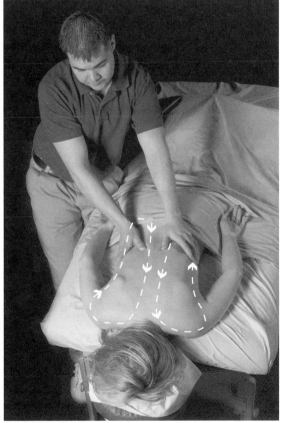

Figure 12.49c

Continue with effleurage strokes back down the sides, returning to the starting point. Pressure is consistent throughout the entire stroke.

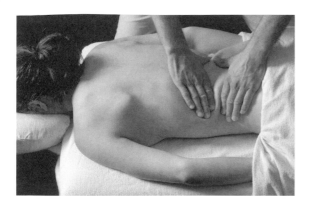

Figure 12.50a
Apply petrissage to the entire side that is opposite you. This takes several passes.

5. Apply petrissage. Begin with the gluteal region on the opposite side of the client from where you are standing. Knead the side of the body from below the hips up into the axillary area. Move hands to a position nearer to the spine (midway between the spine and extreme side of the body), then knead back down to the gluteal area. Work along the spine to include the trapezius muscles, the upper shoulders, and the neck.

6. Begin at the neck with alternate-hand strokes (shingles) from the side of the body to the spinal process. Move down to the top of the thigh and then back up to the top of the shoulder (Figure 12.50a to c).

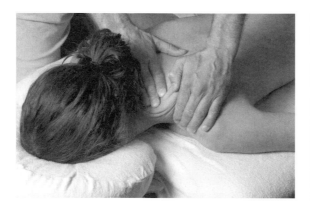

Figure 12.50b
Note that petrissage includes the trapezius muscles.

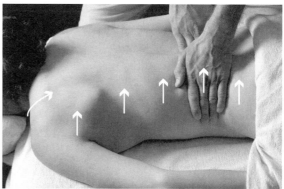

Figure 12.50c
Apply alternate-hand stroking movements (shingles) up and down the entire side.

7. Change sides and repeat steps 2 through 6.

8. Flex the client's elbow (closest to you), and place the client's hand on the table about 6 inches from the armpit. Some practitioners prefer to place the client's hand in the small of her back to abduct and elevate the scapula. In this position, a number of kneading and friction movements can easily be performed on all sides of the scapula. Special attention should be given to the teres, trapezius, the rhomboids, and the infraspinatus muscles.

9. Apply joint movement. With the client's hand still in position at the side, grasp the top of the shoulder with one hand. Place your fingers neatly into a notch near the coracoid process, and use this hold as a handle. Place the other hand just inferior to the scapula so the inferior angle of the scapula fits neatly into the V formed between your thumb and index finger. Lift and rotate the scapula away from the rib cage. Although this may seem unnecessary, it is

very effective in relieving a number of stress-related shoulder problems. Rotate the shoulder several times in both directions.

10. Abduct the elbow so the upper arm is at a square angle from the body and the forearm is relaxed at an angle from the upper arm. Support the arm with both of your hands just proximal to the elbow and gently swing the hand up and down, allowing the shoulder to rotate in a relaxed manner. Replace the hand and arm to the side of the body (Figure 12.51a to e).

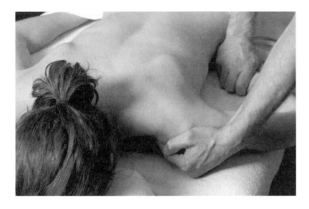

Figure 12.51a

Position the arm to elevate the scapula.

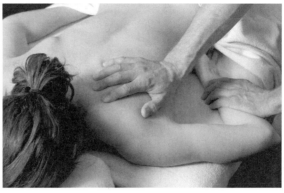

Figure 12.51b

Apply friction and compression movements to the muscles of the scapula.

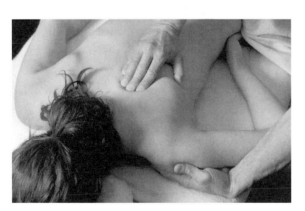

Figure 12.51c

Elevate the scapula and apply deep pressure and friction under the vertebral border.

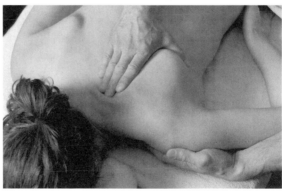

Figure 12.51d

Rotation of the shoulder is followed by stretching.

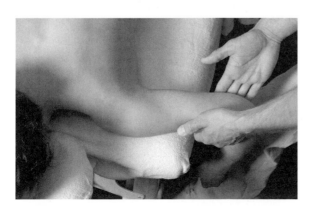

Figure 12.51e

Hold the arm at the elbow and rotate the shoulder by swinging the forearm back and forth.

11. Repeat all the movements, 8 through 10, on the other side of the back.

12. Apply deep kneading and friction to the gluteal area.

13. Repeat effleurage on the entire back area.

14. Apply wringing friction to the back, moving back and forth across the back and working all the way up the neck and back down.

15. Apply circular friction on each side of the spine on the erector spine muscles.

16. Do "hand walking" bilaterally along the spine. Begin at the base of the spine just above the sacrum. Use the full palm side of your hand to apply deep effleurage from the spine to the side of the body. This is almost a compression stroke that slides. Use considerable weight on the strokes as you walk your hands up the client's back. Less weight is used in the area of the kidneys and the 11th and 12th ribs. Proceed with the walking movements up the back all the way to the area of the first thoracic vertebrae and then back down to the sacrum.

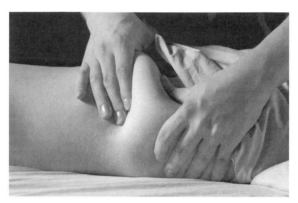

Figure 12.52a

Apply deep kneading over the gluteal region.

17. Do sacrospinalis vibration. Place the first two fingers of one hand to either side of the base of the client's spine, about 2 inches apart. Bend your fingers slightly so that they dig in on the medial edge of the sacrospinalis muscle and along each side of the spinus process.

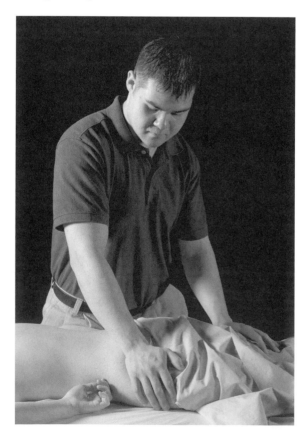

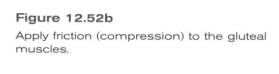

Figure 12.52b

Apply friction (compression) to the gluteal muscles.

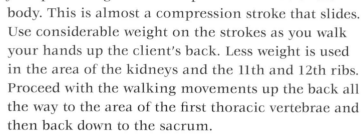

Place your other hand on the top of the hand resting on the client's back, and press down firmly while vibrating slowly (about 120 vibrations per minute) from side to side along the client's body. Slowly glide both hands up the spine, vibrating (jiggling) each spinal process back and forth about 3 to 10 times. Pay attention to any area along the spine that seems especially tense. These areas should be given extra attention. Work all the way up the spine to the seventh cervical vertebrae in this manner (Figure 12.52a to h).

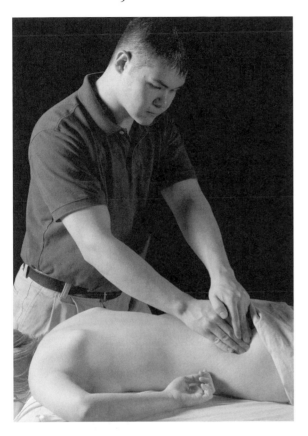

Figure 12.52c
Apply digital friction to the gluteal muscles.

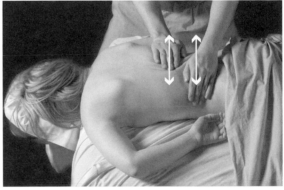

Figure 12.52d
Apply wringing movements up and down the entire back.

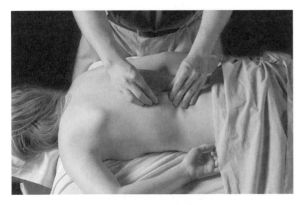

Figure 12.52e
Knead around the spine.

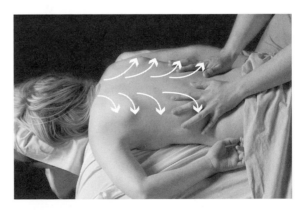

Figure 12.52f
Fan stroke the back.

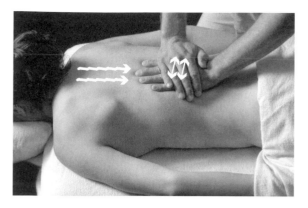

Figure 12.52g

Vibrate along the sacrospinalis.

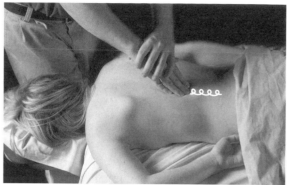

Figure 12.52h

Apply friction movements to the muscles along the spine with the fingertips of one hand braced with the other hand. Apply movements along both sides of the spine.

18. At this time, a number of percussion movements are optional. Hacking may be done lightly over the entire back, including the gluteals and the backs of the legs. (Avoid percussion over the area of the kidneys.) Beating movements may be applied over the thicker portions of the body. To end a stimulating massage, light slapping may be applied over the entire body (Figure 12.53a to d).

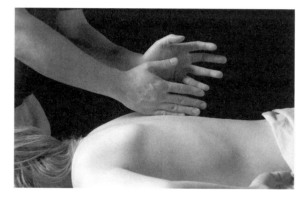

Figure 12.53a

Hacking movements on the back.

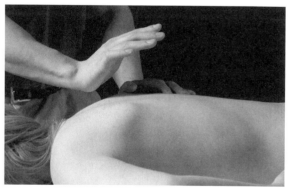

Figure 12.53b

Slapping movements on the back.

Figure 12.53c

Cupping along the back.

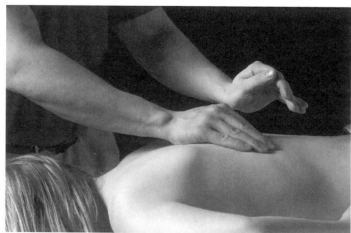

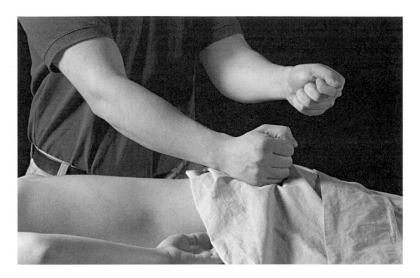

Figure 12.53d
Apply percussion with beating movements to the gluteal muscles.

19. A caring stroke completes the back massage. Remember that a caring stroke is an all-inclusive gliding stroke that is applied by standing at the head of the massage table. Place your hands on the upper back so that your fingers nearly touch in the area of the first and second thoracic vertebrae. Apply gliding strokes down the entire length of the spine. Your hands glide over the gluteals and return up the lateral portion of the torso to the axillary area, slide smoothly over the deltoids up the trapezius to the occiput, and return to the starting point. Repeat the movements several times (Figure 12.54a and b).

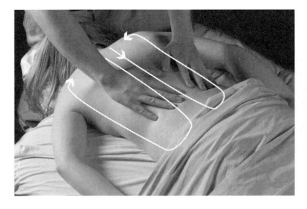

Figure 12.54a
Apply effleurage movements (caring strokes) from a position at the head of the client, beginning at the nape of the neck.

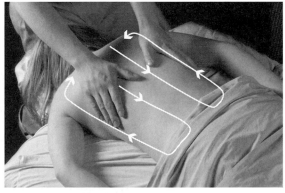

Figure 12.54b
Continue effleurage movements down the back, over and around the gluteal muscles, back up the sides, then over and around the shoulders to the nape of the neck.

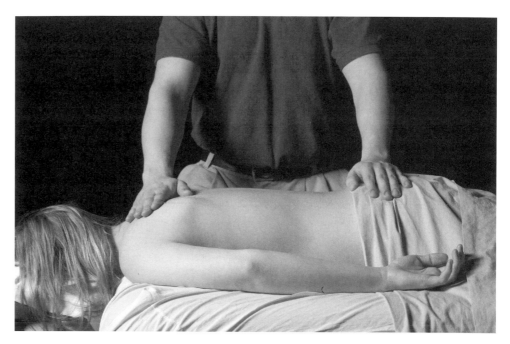

Figure 12.55

Say hello or good-bye to the client's body by applying a light touch to the base of the spine, the base of the neck, or the top of the head for a few moments.

A Finishing Touch

To complete the massage of the entire body, lightly place one hand on the sacrum and the other at the top of the spine and hold the position for several seconds. An option here is to apply a slight rocking motion (Figure 12.55).

The state of relaxation brought on by massage makes the client mentally receptive, as in hypnosis. When fully relaxed, the client can be guided by the practitioner through some mental or physical exercise to enhance or relieve a particular condition. For example, the practitioner may place his hands on the client and make suggestions such as "You feel rested and relaxed," or "You will sleep better tonight because you are free of tension," or "You feel more relaxed than you have for some time." This type of positive suggestion should be made just before the client is fully awake.

Allow the client to relax quietly without being disturbed for several minutes. Assist the client to a sitting position. Be sure that draping is properly placed and assist the client from the massage table as necessary. Show the client to the dressing area. After the client is dressed, take time to answer any questions or make recommendations.

Completion of the Massage

Following the massage, the client should be allowed to rest for a short while before going out to face the world again. This rest period is beneficial especially if you have done bodywork to the extent that some changes have taken place in the client's physical structure. A few moments of relaxation will help to integrate these changes into the client's psychological and neurological senses.

It is important to instruct the client in what to do and what to expect following the massage, especially clients who come to you for the first time. For example, when you ask the client to drink plenty of water to keep the system flushed out, explain that a massage, when done properly, can cause increased activity within the body tissues and that on the cellular level an increased rate of exchange of body fluids takes place. That increase means that some metabolic wastes have been expelled from the cells and have been put into the general systemic circulation. This waste material has to be dealt with because it puts an extra burden on the excretory system. An increase in the intake of water and other healthful fluids will assist in the process of elimination by supplying more fluids for the kidneys, the colon, the lungs, and for perspiration.

You will need to give some guidelines as to the amount of water the client should drink. It is difficult to suggest a certain amount, but usually 4 quarts a day is about right. If the treatment was given in the afternoon, the client should drink about 2 quarts of water that day and 4 quarts the following day.

Aftereffects of Massage

Some clients experience certain aftereffects following massage and should be told that this is no cause for alarm. Usually the effects are felt following the first or second massage. Some people complain of a slight headache, upset stomach and nausea, or the feeling they get with the onset of a cold. Such reactions are due to an increase in metabolic waste material in the circulatory system. The particular symptom the client experiences depends on the organs that are being overtaxed. The intensity of the massage movements should be limited until the client has built up more tolerance. The client will seldom have a symptom that lasts for any length of time; however, she should be told to call you if there is a problem.

Summary

In this chapter, you were introduced to procedures to safely get a client on and off the massage table, to position the client with pillows and bolsters to provide maximum comfort, and two methods of draping to provide warmth, modesty, and access to the body to apply massage. You were introduced to employing sequences into a massage routine. Guidelines when sequencing strokes include working from general to specific and back to general and working from superficial to deep and back to superficial. Similar sequences are used on each body part or area so that each area receives equitable treatment with other body areas. There is always latitude so that if a client indicates that she has extra tension or other related conditions in a particular part of her body, more attention and focus can be given to that area. In the overall massage, sequence is used to ensure that every area of the body receives massage in a logical order, resulting in a relaxing, whole body experience.

The effects of a massage manipulation may vary according to the intention, duration, depth, speed, excursion, or length of the massage manipulation. The effects of the overall massage are also determined by the intention, duration, speed, depth, choice of manipulations, and the sequence in which manipulations are applied.

The chapter contained two possible routines or guidelines for a relaxing, full-body massage. The routines are only a template for a non-specific full-body massage. As a student, it is helpful to follow a routine and become comfortable performing a complete massage. Be careful not to be stuck in the routine. Pay close attention to the tissues you are massaging and ask your client for feedback and adapt your techniques to best address your client's needs. As you gain experience, give yourself permission to experiment and improvise with combinations of techniques and manipulations you have learned. Create massage experiences that best suit your personal style and meet the needs and desires of your clients. The possibilities for orchestrating a full-body massage are nearly endless. Have fun and remember to organize the massage into a logical order, using a sequence of strokes on each body area and then connecting the areas together, ensuring that each part of the body receives a thorough massage in a manner that integrates into a whole body experience.

QUESTIONS FOR DISCUSSION AND REVIEW

1. How often should the practitioner wash hands with soap and water?
2. Why is it advisable to assist a client on and off the table?
3. How can the practitioner prevent the chilling of the client's body?
4. Briefly describe two methods of draping.
5. Besides draping, how can the therapist ensure that the client stays warm?
6. How can the practitioner avoid scratching the client's body?
7. Which massage movements should be avoided because they convey fear of injury to the client?
8. Is it better to massage the body before or after the client has eaten a meal?
9. What is the average duration of a massage?
10. In which conditions should massage never be applied?
11. What preliminaries require attention before body massage?
12. Which position does the client usually assume first for body massage?
13. What is the usual order of massage movements?
14. What are the final considerations after completing body massage?
15. What are some undesirable aftereffects of massage and why do they occur?
16. Why should the client be advised to drink plenty of water?

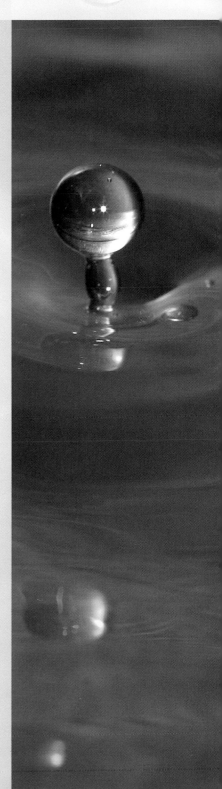

Therapeutic Procedure

LEARNING OBJECTIVES

After you have mastered this chapter, you will be able to:

1. Describe the four parts of the therapeutic procedure.

2. Demonstrate a client intake procedure for a therapeutic massage session.

3. Perform posture and gait assessment.

4. Demonstrate assessment by passive, active, and resisted movement.

5. Identify soft tissue barriers.

6. Palpate and differentiate tissue layers and textures.

7. Explain how assessment findings are used to develop session strategies.

8. Determine performance strategies specific to a client's needs.

9. Demonstrate how to identify and release constrictions in hypertonic tissue.

10. Explain the importance of evaluation.

INTRODUCTION

Chapter 12 described possible full-body massage routines. The therapist may choose from an endless number of possible routines for a full-body massage, or the massage may focus on a particular body area according to the client's request. People seeking massage for relaxation and stress relief benefit from relaxing full-body massages; however, when seeking relief from painful conditions or recovering from injury, more specific treatment regimes are better suited. Therapeutic massage may be modified in many ways to best fit the needs and desires of a client. Becoming competent in more sophisticated therapeutic applications requires more extensive training, practice, and expertise on the part of the therapist to determine through assessment where and what soft tissue components or body functions are involved and then provide appropriate therapeutic interventions. Chapter 13 now introduces therapeutic methodology to more specifically identify soft tissue conditions that respond to therapeutic soft

therapeutic procedure
is the process of acquiring a concise medical history, assessment procedures to determine constricted and painful conditions, developing treatment plans, performing appropriate treatment practices to more specifically address the conditions, and evaluating the results.

tissue interventions. **Therapeutic procedure**—which includes acquiring a concise medical history, assessment procedures to determine constricted and painful conditions, developing treatment plans, performing appropriate treatment practices to more specifically address the conditions, and evaluating the results is discussed here.

Therapeutic procedure involves four basic steps:

1. Assessment

2. Planning

3. Performance

4. Evaluation

Assessment involves reviewing any information available at the onset of the process to understand the present conditions. During the planning stage, the information gained from the assessment is used to determine strategies and select therapeutic techniques to address specific conditions found during the assessment. The performance is the actual application of the selected techniques. The evaluation examines the outcome of the session in regard to the effectiveness of the selected procedure for the condition.

All information must be carefully documented in the client's files. SOAP charts are well suited for recording information gained in each segment of the therapeutic procedure. (Refer to Chapter 9 for information about SOAP charts.)

The therapeutic process can be implemented in many ways in the course of a massage therapy program. It is valuable for long-range goal setting, short-range planning, and during an actual massage session. In long-range goal setting, the assessment might be extensive and the planning encompass a number of sessions (6 to 10). After the treatment strategy has been formulated and discussed and the treatments given, an evaluation is done to determine what progress has been made and what further therapy is needed.

Short-range planning may involve a single session. In this case, the assessment process may not be as extensive, but it may focus more on a specific complaint. The client's needs are considered, indications and contraindications are determined, and a treatment strategy is decided on. The session is performed, and at the conclusion, the outcome is evaluated as to the effectiveness of the session.

During the application of a therapeutic massage, the therapeutic procedure is constantly being applied. As the therapist proceeds through the massage, the hands are continuously assessing the condition of the tissues. The quality of the tissue, the constrictions in the tissue, or the movement of the limbs and the response from the client as different massage movements are being performed continuously provide information the therapist uses to plan the next movements. The evaluation process is also continuous as the therapist elicits feedback regarding the effectiveness throughout the treatment.

CLIENT INTAKE FOR THERAPEUTIC MASSAGE

Reasons for receiving massage vary widely. According to a 2002 survey conducted by the Opinion Research Corporation, 23 percent of the respondents who received massage did so to relax or reduce stress; 53 percent sought massage to improve some health concern; and 17 percent did so to pamper themselves. Primary concerns included pain relief, injury recovery, muscle soreness/stiffness, joint mobility, and other soft tissue dysfunction.

The preliminary client consultation was discussed in Chapter 9. A preliminary consultation for a therapeutic massage contains all the same elements as discussed earlier, plus more extensive assessment techniques and planning strategies are included to better determine what services can be provided to address the particular concerns of the client. A primary focus of the preliminary interview is to establish rapport between the therapist and client. The therapist must be receptive and show genuine interest for the client and at the same time be professional and confident. Mirroring the client with a similar voice tone and posture help to establish rapport. Establishing a good rapport enhances mutual respect, which strengthens the therapeutic relationship. Establish an environment for open communication. Clear communication is essential, especially in determining the client's needs and concerns. Practice good listening skills. Maintain eye contact when conversing. Paraphrase and repeat back to your clients what they have explained to be sure that you understand what is being said. Encourage feedback anytime—before, during, and after the session.

The extent of the intake process depends on the purpose of the client visit and the intent of the massage treatment. The client intake process for a therapeutic massage is more extensive than for a wellness/relaxing massage. The intake process begins when the client calls or makes the appointment and continues until there is agreement between the client and therapist to proceed and the massage treatment commences. The intake involves an exchange of information to determine the best course of action for the therapeutic relationship. Client intake includes several segments that may vary according to the individual situation. Some segments are:

- Setting the appointment—This may include an initial screening to determine the primary reason for the client visit and whether the practitioner's services match the client's needs.

- Initial greeting and consultation—Extra time may be scheduled for the first consultation to fill out intake forms (Figure 13-1) and exchange information such as reasons for the visit, policies, and procedures.

- Assessment—The assessment process consists of a client interview, history, observation, palpation, and special tests such as range of motion.

Client Intake Form

Name _____ Today's date _____

Address _____ Phone _____

City-State-ZIP _____ Email Address _____

Date of birth _____ Age _____ Sex _____ Social Security # _____

Occupation _____ Employer _____

Employer address _____ Business phone _____

Marital status _____ Spouse/partner's name _____

Children's name(s) and age(s) _____

Have you had massages before? _____ By whom? _____

How did you find out about our services? _____

Primary Health Care Provider _____ Phone # _____

Provider address _____ City _____ State ___ ZIP _____

May I have permission to consult your health provider? No ___ Yes ___ _____ (initial if yes)

List other health providers you use on the back of this page.

Insurance Company _____ Policy # _____

Name of policyholder _____

ID # _____ Group # _____ Claim # _____

Adjuster's Name _____

Adjuster's Address _____ City _____ ST ___ ZIP _____

Phone # _____ Time and date of verification _____

In case of emergency notify _____ Phone _____

Relationship _____

I understand that the massage services are designed to be a health aid and are in no way to take the place of a doctor's care when indicated. I am aware that the massage therapist does not diagnose disease nor prescribe medications. Information exchanged during any massage session is educational in nature and is intended to help me become more aware and conscious of my own health status and is to be used at my own discretion.

Client signature _____ Date _____

Figure 13.1

Client intake form.

- Treatment plan—When the relevant information has been collected during the assessment, a plan for the session or a number of sessions is devised.

- Informed consent—After the assessment findings and treatment plan are discussed between the therapist and the client and agreed upon, the client gives informed consent and the session commences.

ASSESSMENT TECHNIQUES

The successful practice of therapeutic massage depends on an accurate and thorough assessment. It is necessary for the therapist to understand as much about the client and his condition as possible to determine what massage procedures to perform on him or whether it is advisable to refer him to another health professional. The extent of the examination will depend on the intended therapy to be given. If a relaxing massage is the intent of the visit, only enough information needs to be exchanged to determine that there are no contraindications, informed consent is obtained and the session can commence. However, if the intent of the visit is to respond to specific concerns the client may have or to address some soft tissue dysfunction, a more extensive assessment will provide information to determine the nature of the dysfunction or pathology to help determine the best course of treatment. The assessment tools used will vary according to the modality of treatment. A common assessment protocol includes client and medical history (Figure 13.2), close observation, any number of functional assessments, and palpation of the suspected structures. The goal of the assessment is to—as specifically as possible—identify the dysfunctional tissues and, if possible, the conditions that caused the problem.

A concise client history provides a wealth of background information about social, physiological, and psychological elements related to the complaints of the client. Client information and medical history forms are filled out on the client's first visit. A client information form may include questions about the client's age, occupation, hobbies, and reason for seeking your services. These forms can be designed to provide extensive and vital information about the client's past and current physical condition and the client's expectations and concerns. The medical history form provides information regarding the client's past medical conditions, including major illnesses, medications, surgeries, traumas, and allergies. It should include contact information for doctors or other health care practitioners the client is seeing for any current conditions and a request for permission to contact those health care practitioners. Include questions about particular conditions the client has and the history of those conditions as well as a diagram of the body so that the client can illustrate areas of concern. The client will need to sign a separate "Release of Medical Information" form for you to share any of his personal information with other health professionals (Figure 13.3).

After the client has had an opportunity to fill out the intake and medical history forms and the practitioner has had a chance to review the forms, a consultation or interview between the client and practitioner provides an opportunity to further clarify the intentions for the session. This is the opportunity for the client to tell his story.

Information from the forms combined with a client interview clarifies the client's concerns, needs, and expectations. Reviewing the completed forms and questioning the client to clarify any information on the forms provides the therapist with preliminary information to make decisions on how to proceed, whether the client should be referred to another health professional, or whether the client's doctor should be contacted before going further. If in doubt, remain on the cautious side. Refer the client to an appropriate health professional for

---

Client Health History

Name _____ Today's date _____

Address _____ Home phone _____ Other phone _____

City-State-ZIP _____ Email address _____

Date of Birth _____ Age _____ Occupation _____

Who were you referred by or how did you find out about our services? _____

What is the reason for your visit to our office? _____
_____

What results would you like to achieve with our work? _____

Have you seen a doctor or another health practitioner regarding this or similar
conditions? _____

List their names and phone numbers. Do I have your permission to contact them? _____
_____

When did you first notice the condition and what started it? _____

What makes it worse? / better? _____

Please indicate any of the following conditions that apply to you. Mark any current
conditions with an "X" and past conditions with an "O."

__ Chronic pain, where   __ Asthma   __ Learning difficulties
_____   __ Fatigue   __ Depression
__ Joint pain, where   __ Frequent respiratory   __ Trouble sleeping
_____   illness   __ Trouble concentrating
__ Muscle pain, where   __ Lung or respiratory   __ Memory loss
_____   condition   __ Hearing problems
__ Other pain, where   __ Cold hands or feet   __ Vision problems
_____   __ Swollen ankles   __ Contacts
__ Headache   __ Varicose veins   __ Paralysis
__ Numbness, where   __ High blood pressure   __ Nervous system
_____   __ Low blood pressure   conditions
__ Broken bones, where,   __ Lymphedema   __ Allergies
   when _____   __ Heart condition   __ Rashes
__ Sprains/strains, where   __ Indigestion   __ Skin conditions
_____   __ Loss of appetite   __ Tumors/cancer
__ Arthritis   __ Diarrhea   __ Shingles/herpes
__ Osteoporosis   __ Constipation   __ Pregnancies
__ Bursitis   __ Gas/bloating   __ PMS
__ Tendonitis   __ Ulcers   __ Hysterectomy
__ Scoliosis   __ Digestive condition   __ Menopause
__ Bone disease   __ Bowel condition   __ Birth control
__ Dizziness   __ Eating disorders   __ Prostate
__ Difficulty breathing   __ Panic attacks/anxiety   __ Reproductive concerns
__ Sinus conditions   __ Hyperactivity

Explain any conditions noted above. _____
_____

continues

Figure 13.2

Client health history form.

---

more clarification about questionable conditions. Confer with or work
under the supervision of a medical doctor or other therapist in difficult
or questionable situations.

Information from the forms and interview provide information
about the nature of the complaint, what part or parts of the body are af-

Infectious and childhood diseases (list what and when) _____
Congenital or acquired disability (describe) _____
Surgeries (list what and when) _____
Injuries or accidents causing injury _____
List any other medical or health condition not listed _____
_____
List, including frequency of use, all medications, remedies, herbs, and supplements you
use. _____
_____
_____
Do you use any of the following? List frequency and amount.
Caffeine _____ Nicotine _____ Alcohol _____
Sugar _____ Recreational drugs _____
List stress-relieving activities you participate in. Include type and frequency; that is,
exercise, massage, hobbies, sports, etc. _____
_____
_____
List any other concerns or comments regarding you health status or well-being. _____
_____

On the above diagram, indicate any areas in which you experience pain with an X and
circle any other areas of concern.
To the best of my knowledge, I have disclosed all of my past and current health
conditions. I will inform the therapist of any changes in my health status.

Client signature _____ Date _____

Figure 13.2, *continued*
Client health history form.

fected, whether the condition is chronic or acute, and what makes it
worse or better. Find out when and how the condition started, what the
client has done about it, what treatments the client has received and by
whom, what has helped, what has made it worse, and so on. Was there
some incident that started the condition? Was the onset sudden or did it

---

Release of Medical Information Form

Client's name _____ Phone _____ _____
Address _____ City _____ State ___ ZIP _____
I hereby authorize _____(Practitioner's Name)_____ to release to any physician or health
care practitioner directly involved in my care any medical records or other personal
health information necessary for the purpose of receiving physician's recommendations
and approval, or sharing concerns regarding my health and well-being.
This authorization remains valid for the period of _____ to _____ or
for the time period that I am seeing the above-named practitioner.

Signed _____ Date _____

Figure 13.3
Release of medical information form.

come on slowly? What has been the progression of the condition? Where in the body did the client first notice it? Is this the first time the condition has happened? If not, how often, when was the last time, when was the first time? Questions should also ascertain how long the condition has persisted and whether it is constant or intermittent.

If it is a painful condition, determine the location of the pain. Can the client put a finger or hand on it? Does it radiate or has it traveled from its original location? What affects it? What makes it worse or better? Does the time of day or activity affect it? What is the intensity, the duration, and the frequency of the pain? Does it come and go? How often does it recur and what instigates its return? Describe the pain. Is it sharp? Dull? Radiating? Does the pain interfere with daily activities?

Question the client about his tolerance of the condition and what he has done to cope with and correct the problem. Learn about the client and his willingness to do something about the condition. Take notes on the answers and include them in the client files for future evaluations.

By this time, the therapist knows what the client's primary concerns are and whether her services will be of benefit. The therapist will also have a better idea of further assessments that will identify the involved structures, patterns, or causative factors related to the complaint.

Following the interview, the intake process may continue with various assessments that include observation or visual assessment, a variety of functional assessments, palpation, and specialized tests specific to the suspected condition or selected modalities. Information from the various assessments is gathered and analyzed to determine the best course of treatment. Results of the assessments and options of possible interventions or treatment modalities are discussed with the client, and a treatment plan or care plan is created and agreed upon between the therapist and the client. The client again provides informed consent by signing the care plan. This marks the end of the intake process, and the performance or application portion of the therapeutic procedure begins.

Subjective and Objective Findings

Information gained during the interview and assessment portion of the session will be both subjective and objective in nature. Subjective information will come from the client as he describes his experience of the situation. The client will answer questions as to what and where he feels the condition. When did it start? Is it constant or intermittent? What affects it, makes it better, makes it worse? During various tests, the client will describe the experience or how it feels.

The therapist, or another observer, determines objective information through observation, palpation, and specialized tests where the findings are quantifiable and usually measurable.

Pain Scale

A subjective pain scale is a useful tool to assess the relative discomfort a client is experiencing. The client is able to rate his pain as he describes a condition he has, guides the therapist as she performs a therapeutic technique, or assesses any improvement in his condition following a session. The pain scale provides the client the opportunity to describe the discomfort or pain being experienced on a scale of 0 to 10 (or 1 to 5) where 0 (or 1) is no discomfort and 10 (or 5) is unbearable, excruciating pain.

The pain scale may be used when a person is describing his discomfort during a preliminary assessment. At the end of the session, the client can again rate his discomfort to help determine the effectiveness of the session.

A pain scale is also used to determine appropriate amounts of pressure to be used during certain treatment modalities such as trigger point release or positional release. For instance, when applying pressure to a trigger point, ask the client to rate the discomfort and tell you when the rating is between 6 and 7. This is the ideal amount of pressure to have the greatest therapeutic value. If the discomfort rises above this level—that is, between 8 and 10—the client will become defensive, and any therapeutic gains and the trust of the client may be lost. Therapeutic uses of the pain scale will be discussed more in the trigger-point release and position release section of Chapter 18.

THE ARNDT-SCHULTZ LAW

The Arndt-Schultz law states that weak stimuli activate physiological processes, strong stimuli inhibit. If the therapeutic intervention (pressure on the muscle) is too strong, the nervous system will not respond to the intervention and will not shift its message from the spinal cord to the muscle. If there is too little pressure, the nervous system will not respond. At the level of 6 or 7 on a 10-point scale, the nervous system *will* respond to the intervention and shift the message that goes out the reflex arc to the muscle. Clients need to be trained that the old "grin and bear it" method is not the best way to shift their pain patterns.

OBSERVATION

Observation plays a major role in the assessment process. The observation portion of a client assessment should begin when the client walks in the door and continue until he leaves. The client's body language—that is, how the client holds himself, stands, moves, and sits—gives clues to where pain and tension are being held. Observing body language may also give some insight to the client's emotional makeup and self-esteem. Watch for guarded movements the client uses to avoid or mask any pain.

Through visual observation, the therapist can assess structural alignment and balance, bilateral discrepancies, and variations in skin color and integrity. Look for bilateral symmetry both structurally and in the way the client moves. Throughout the assessment, it is helpful to compare one side of the body with the other. When doing many of the comparisons, look at the good side first to get an idea of the personal norm for that individual, and then look at the affected side to assess the deviation from that norm. Note in the way a person moves whether he holds one side of the body tighter or higher. Is the gait (walking) balanced and normal? Does the client stand erect, list to one side, or stoop? Observation more formally comes into play when assessing posture and gait.

Posture Assessment

Assessing posture is observing how a person maintains an upright position in relation to gravitational forces. Posture is considered to be ideal when the body's mass is evenly distributed around its central axis that passes through the body's center of gravity (Figure 13.4 and Figure 13.5). When a client exhibits optimal posture, the postural muscles maintain a state of normal tonus. However, when postural balance becomes less than optimal, postural muscles must actively contract to redistribute the body mass in relation to the center of gravity and maintain that contraction, putting stress on joints and other connective tissue.

Observing posture gives many indications of muscular imbalance and structural deviation. Many postural discrepancies are due to agonist/antagonist imbalances. Posture is best observed from all four sides when the client is standing comfortably erect. Beginning at the feet, notice whether they are evenly angled and placed equal distance from the midline, and whether the arches are supporting the ankles. From the back, is the Achilles' tendon aligned perpendicular with the floor? Are the patellae pointing forward? Is the pelvis rotated or tilted, either side-to-side or front-to-back? The angle from the PSIS to the ASIS should be no more than 12 degrees from the horizontal. If a person has good posture, a plumb line will perfectly bisect the body when viewed from the front or back. From the side, the line would go through the ear, shoulder, elbow, acetabulum (as-e-**TAB**-yoo-lum), knee, and ankle. By extending the vertical plumb line forward, ideally the symphysis pubis, manibrium, and front of the zygomatic arch would be vertically aligned. When observing

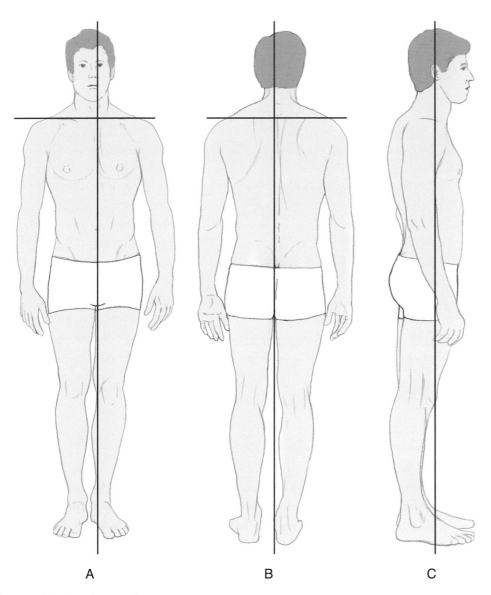

A   B   C

Figure 13.4 a, b, and c

Posture is observed from the (a) front, (b) back, and (c) side. A plumb line or grid is helpful to determine deviations in the posture.

a person, notice whether one side of the body is held higher than the other. Notice the hips, the shoulders at the AC joint, the hands, the ears, and the eyes to check whether they are level and even. Notice any rotation. Is there any rotation in the torso? Is either arm or leg rotated? Is the head rotated or tilted? The farther out of balance the body is, the more strain is placed on the postural muscles. As a body ages, the pull of gravity tends to increase the deviations.

When assessing posture, the therapist notes spinal curves, deviations from the coronal or sagittal plane, differences in elevation or rotation of postural (bony) landmarks, and any asymmetrical anatomical position. These findings are combined with information from other assessments to identify areas of possible somatic dysfunction.

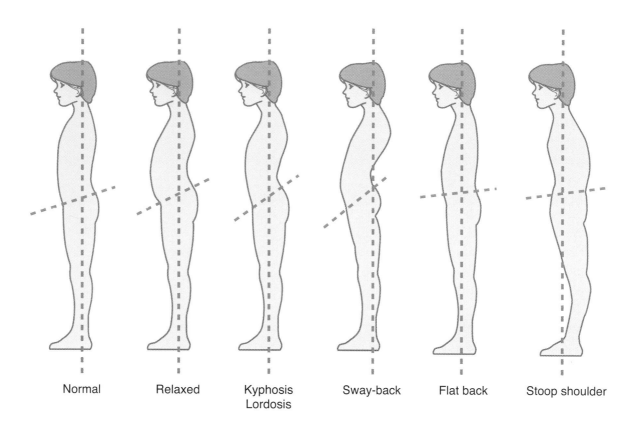

| Normal | Relaxed | Kyphosis Lordosis | Sway-back | Flat back | Stoop shoulder |

Figure 13.5

Normal posture (with plumb line).

When the client lies down on the table in the supine position and is comfortable, again notice any deviations from bilateral symmetry. Observe the contour of the body as well as structural and skeletal symmetry. Is the client straight? Is the head tilted or turned? Is one leg rotated at a different angle? Are the hips level? Most minor postural deviations are caused by muscular imbalance. There is either muscle weakness (flaccidity), muscle tension, or both. There is often an agonist/antagonist imbalance where one muscle is hypertonic and constricted while the opposing muscle is hypotonic and weak. Some forms of massage and soft tissue manipulation are very effective for relieving these imbalances.

Make note of abnormal marks, discoloration, varicosities, differences in skin texture, and scars. Check for skin conditions, redness, areas of increased heat, or swelling (signs of inflammation). Be aware of anything that might be a sign of former trauma or conditions that may indicate or contraindicate massage.

Postural distortion may result from a wide range of influences including physical or emotional trauma to poor work habits, pathologic conditions, or age. Through the process of compensation, a deviation in one area of the body may cause a shift in another in an attempt to reestablish an overall balance. Compensation usually results in increased tension on connective tissue and postural muscle. The farther out of balance the body is, the more the postural muscles are strained, resulting in increased pain and dysfunction.

Gait Assessment

Assessing **gait** is similar to assessing posture only with the body in motion. Methods of **gait assessment** have advanced with the use of computers, video cameras, and sophisticated measuring devices. For the purposes of massage therapy, the monitoring devices are the therapist's eyes. The client's gait should be viewed from front, back, and both sides to gain as much information as possible. The gait assessment is done as the client walks in a comfortable relaxed manner for several paces, back and forth in front of the therapist.

When walking, the steps should be even and smooth, with the heel of one foot making contact with the floor as the weight on the other foot transfers smoothly to the ball of the foot. The movement of the legs is in the direction of the line of motion with the knees and feet pointing in that direction. The steps are smooth and even. The torso is balanced above the body's center of gravity, and the pelvis shifts slightly at each step. The arms swing easily at the sides, opposite the legs. As the right foot moves forward, the left arm swings forward and vice versa. The hands are relaxed with the thumb forward, and the hands swing straight, forward and back. The head is balanced on the top of the spine, and the motion is fluid and smooth.

There are other considerations to observe. Is the gait initiated without undue pelvic tilt? Do the feet clear the ground with each step? Does the foot strike the ground in a heel-to-toe fashion? Is the step length symmetrical? Is the width of the stride symmetrical? Is there a straight alignment of the hip, knee, and ankle through the entire stride cycle? Is there ample extension in the hip to allow the step to roll off the ball of the foot and toe?

When assessing gait, the therapist notes any asymmetry, crossover or rotation of the feet or arms, or restrictions of free movement. Is there pain anywhere? The information gained during gait assessment may indicate body structures that are constricted. This information is combined with findings from other assessments to help determine areas of the body to focus on and to determine what interventions to use.

| **gait** |
| is a pattern or manner of walking. |

| **gait assessment** |
| is observing the manner in which a person walks to determine constrictions or related conditions. |

Assess Range of Motion

Observation is also important in tests such as **range of motion** to notice any restrictions in joint mobility, the quality of movement, and the client's reaction to the tests. Range of motion is the action of a joint through the entire extent of its movement. Assessing the extent and quality of that movement by testing the active, passive, and resisted (isometric) movement provides information about the tissues involved with the joint.

Dr. James Cyriax, an osteopath from England, has developed an extensive system of testing all the joints to isolate lesions in the hard and soft tissues. He has clarified and defined some terms and concepts that are invaluable when assessing range of motion. Those concepts include contractile tissue, inert tissue, end feel, and capsular patterns.

| **range of motion** |
| is the movement of a joint from one extreme of the articulation to the other. |

contractile tissues
are the fibrous tissues that have tensions placed on them during muscular contractions.

inert tissues
are the tissues that are not contractile such as bone, ligament, nerves.

end feel
is the change in the quality of the movement as the end of a movement is achieved.

capsular pattern
refers to the proportional limitation of any joint that is controlled by muscular contractions.

- **Contractile tissues** are the fibrous tissues that have tensions placed on them during muscular contractions and include muscle tissue, tendons, and the muscle attachments.
- **Inert tissues** are the tissues that are not contractile such as bone, ligament, bursa, blood vessels, nerves, nerve coverings, cartilage, and the like.
- **End feel** refers to the quality of the sensation the therapist feels as she passively moves a joint to the full extent of its possible range.
- **Capsular pattern** refers to the proportional limitation of any joint that is controlled by muscular contractions.

When assessing range of motion, test the good side first to help determine the individual's norm. First perform the active movements, then the passive, and finally the resisted movements. When testing, observe and record objective and subjective findings. Objective findings are things the therapist sees or feels such as muscle strength and degree of joint movement. Subjective findings include the amount of pain or discomfort the client feels and how he reacts to the pain. Objective findings generally can be measured, whereas subjective findings are usually felt or perceived.

Assess Active Movements

Assessing active movement indicates the client's ability and willingness to move a body part through a range of motion. The client is instructed to move through a particular range of motion. The client makes the movement totally unassisted. If the entire movement can be made smoothly and painlessly, chances are there is no problem with that joint or the associated soft tissue. Both contractile and inert tissues are involved during active movement, so if there is an obvious limitation, pain, or hesitation during the movement, a closer assessment is needed.

If there was any pain during the movement, the therapist should note when in the movement the pain occurred, the location of the pain on the client's body, the intensity of the pain, the quality of the pain, and the client's reaction to the pain. If there is limitation to the movement, note where the limitation occurred and whether or not it was accompanied by pain.

Assess Passive Movement

When assessing passive movement, the practitioner moves the client's joint through the full range of motion while the client remains relaxed. During passive movement, the practitioner determines the degree and quality of movement in a joint. The practitioner can sense whether the joint is hypermobile or hypomobile. The therapist also notes whether there are any catches, crepitus, or pain involved. The reactions of the client must also be observed. Any apprehensiveness or unwillingness must be considered and respected.

End feel plays a very important part in assessing passive movement. End feel is the feeling the therapist senses as she passively moves a limb to the limit of its range of motion. The quality of the end feel indicates the presence, type, and severity of lesions in the tissues associated with the joint.

There are three types of end feel considered normal: hard, soft, and springy.

- *Hard end feel* is a bone-against-bone feeling. This is an abrupt, painless limitation to further movement that happens at the normal end of the range of motion, such as knee or elbow extension.

- *Soft end feel* is a painless, cushioned limitation where soft tissue prevents further movement, such as knee or elbow flexion.

- *Springy end feel* is the most common. Limitation is due to the stretch of fibrous tissue as the joint reaches the extent of its range of motion, such as hip flexion or extension.

Normal end feel happens at the end of a normal range of motion and, unless carried to extremes, is painless. Pain or an observable limitation of movement indicates that some abnormal condition or lesion is present. If there is pain before reaching the end of the movement and there is no muscular resistance or spasm, bursitis or capsulitis might be involved. If the movement causes a sudden painful muscle reaction or spasm, the body may be protecting an injury in the area. Cyriax calls this an *"empty end feel."* The more acute and severe the injury, the more severe the pain and spasm. A medical referral and diagnosis should be recommended. Other abnormal patterns are similar to normal end feel, except that there is reduced movement or there is associated pain.

Passive movement assessment indicates the condition of the inert (non-contractile) tissues. Limitation of movement and pain are the indicators of dysfunction. Full, painless range of motion indicates that the joint and associated structures are healthy. Reduced range of motion that is limited with a painless, hard (bone-to-bone) end feel indicates osteoarthritis. Pain and limitation in all directions generally involve the whole joint and indicate capsulitis or arthritis. Pain or limitation in one direction and not another is usually due to stretching or compressing the involved tissue. More specific assessment must be done to isolate the involved tissue.

Assess Resisted Movement

Resisted or isometric movement is used to assess the condition of the contractile tissues (muscles, tendons, and attachments). This method is also known as muscle testing.

Indicators of lesions in the contractile tissue are weakness and pain. To perform resisted movement assessment or muscle testing, the therapist stabilizes a body part in a neutral position and instructs the client to move that body part in a specific direction. As the client contracts the muscle, the therapist applies pressure to move the body part in the opposite direction so that the limb does not move. Eliminating any joint movement minimizes reactions of the inert tissues and indicates the relative strength and condition of the contractile tissues. Positioning the body part and instructing the client to make specific movements isolate specific muscles to be tested.

When contractile tissues are involved, active movement and resisted movement will both give positive results. Passive movement will show nothing except at the end of the movement where the contractile tissue is stretched and will react with pain or spasm.

Muscle testing provides information as to the condition of the muscles involved in a specific movement. As with the other physical assessment tools, it is important to compare one side of the body with the other. Test the good side first for comparison. A muscle test that is strong and pain free indicates healthy muscle tissue. A strong and painful muscle test indicates a lesion in the contractile tissue such as a minor (first- or second-degree) muscle strain. A weak and painless muscle test indicates interference with the nerve supply, circulation, or energy to the muscle. No strength in the muscle may be due to a severed muscle or tendon (third-degree strain) or a loss of innervation. A very weak and painful muscle test indicates a severe lesion, possibly a torn ligament or fracture that should be referred to a doctor.

In general, the more severe the condition, the more severe the pain.

SOFT TISSUE BARRIERS

When assessing and treating soft tissue conditions, the therapist must recognize **soft tissue barriers.** These barriers represent the limits within which the tissues can be effectively manipulated. In developing sensitivity to soft tissue barriers, the therapist can better adjust the amount of pressure used to generate a therapeutic response from the tissues. Soft tissue barriers come under consideration when compressing the tissues, stretching the tissues, or mobilizing joints. For instance, when passively moving a healthy limb through its normal range of motion, the limb will move freely, without any resistance through the middle of the range. As the end of the range is approached, the therapist will notice the slightest resistance as the slack is taken out of the tissues and they begin to stretch. This is the beginning of the resistive barrier. The client may or may not sense the beginning of the **resistive barrier.** As the stretch is continued toward the end of the movement, more force is necessary until the tissues are stretched and the client feels like "that is about as far as it goes," which represents the **physiologic barrier.** With more force and possible discomfort to the client, the **anatomical barrier** is approached where the tissues would be maximally stretched; going any further may cause damage to the tissue.

Soft tissue barriers will vary according to the condition of the tissues. In healthy tissue, for instance, free and relatively painless movement may continue easily well into the physiologic barrier and approach

---

soft tissue barriers

are notable physiological changes in the quality of movement in soft tissue that represent the limits within which the tissues can be effectively manipulated.

---

resistive barrier

also known as the pathological barrier, is the first sign of resistance to a movement as tissue is moved and manipulated through its range of motion.

---

physiologic barrier

represents the extent of easy movement allowed during passive or active movements.

---

anatomical barrier

refers to the anatomical limit of motion of particular tissue. To move beyond the anatomic barrier would cause injury and disruption of tissues and supportive structures.

the anatomical barrier before any resistance is encountered. However, in damaged tissue or tissues that house latent or active trigger points or other injuries, restrictive and physiologic barriers may be encountered early in the movement.

Barriers are also taken into consideration when performing compression and fascial stretching manipulations. When using compression over a trigger point, the first contact with the nodule may be considered the restrictive barrier. The client may realize that you are on a tender spot, but there is no discomfort. As pressure is increased, the physiologic barrier is approached, and the client may express a response of discomfort often accompanied by pain in referral areas. The anatomical barrier should never be approached or passed in that doing so may cause damage to the tissues, injuring the motor endplates, bruising the tissue, or possibly activating latent trigger points.

As tissue is moved and manipulated through its range of motion, three types of barriers may be considered:

- The **freely flexible range of movement** refers to the pliable and easily movable range of the tissue.

- The resistive barrier or pathological barrier is the first sign of resistance to a movement and is important when assessing and treating soft tissue conditions.

- The *physiologic barrier* represents the extent of easy movement allowed during passive or active movements. The physiologic barrier is within the anatomic barrier and represents the comfortable end of soft tissue stretch in the range of motion.

- The *anatomical barrier* refers to the anatomical limit of motion of particular tissue. To move beyond the anatomic barrier would cause injury and disruption of tissues and supportive structures.

freely flexible range of movement

refers to the pliable and easily movable range of the tissue.

Physiologic and restrictive barriers are well within the anatomical limits of movement of the involved tissues. Approaching barriers that are abnormally restricted or painful that are within the normal range of motion may reflect a pathologic condition in the tissues. Restrictive and physiologic barriers reflect conditions of bind and ease related to contractile muscle tissue and fascia. When healthy tissue is manipulated or moved through its possible range, an ease of movement is sensed throughout the movement. As the tissue approaches the outer limits of possible movement, the first sense of bind is felt. The first encounter of bind represents contact with the resistive barrier in that direction. By using incrementally more force, movement can continue through the restrictive barrier into increased bind and resistance until the physiologic barrier is encountered. When contractile tissue is constricted or injured, the physiologic barrier is encountered before the end of the normal range of motion and well before the anatomical barrier. If more force were applied, movement could continue through the physiologic barrier into more bind until the anatomical barrier is approached. Movement beyond the physiological barrier usually causes excessive discomfort and

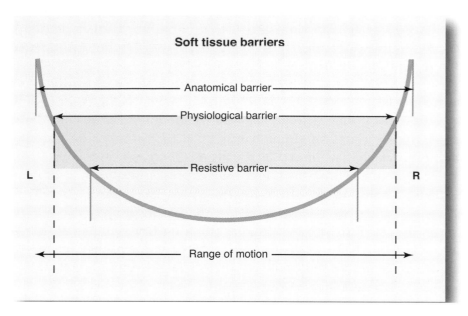

Figure 13.6
Soft tissue barriers.

possibly more trauma. Moving beyond the anatomical barrier would result in tissue damage. (Figure 13.6)

When addressing soft tissue conditions with less-than-healthy tissues, the amount of force used to approach barriers varies greatly and requires a developed sensitivity on the part of the therapist. The best therapeutic response is achieved applying forces that elicit responses between the restrictive and physiologic barriers.

PALPATION SKILLS

Many forms of bodywork disciplines require skill in sensing through touch the conditions and subtle changes that take place in the body's soft tissues. Acupuncture diagnosis reads the subtle differences in the deep and superficial pulses and palpates the exact locations of the acupuncture points. Acupressure, shiatsu, *Jin Shin Do,* and other touch modalities derived from the Asian model depend on the sense of touch to identify points on the body and monitor subtle changes in those points as they are treated. Craniosacral therapists monitor cranial rhythms and other subtle changes in the tissue as they palpate and treat body structures. In myofascial release, fascial preference and changes are monitored through palpation.

The sense of touch is one of the massage therapist's most powerful tools. It is what puts the therapist in close contact with the client. It is the means of communication between the therapist and the client's body. Developing palpation skills, sensing the difference in tissue quality and integrity, and responding with appropriate therapy techniques are marks of a good massage therapist.

Palpation is a skill and an art developed by the therapist that is a primary assessment tool allowing the therapist to listen to the client's body through the therapist's hands. Palpation skills are learned through experience. Palpation is an effective assessment tool because of the extreme sensitivity of the practitioner's hands and the ability to differentiate between subtle variations of temperature, texture, moisture, and density of the target tissues. The successful massage therapist will develop skills to differentiate between the feel of normal and abnormal soft tissue. The therapist should be able to identify with palpation bony structures, skeletal alignment, individual muscles, and various conditions of the soft tissue such as tight/loose conditions, constrictions, spasms, fibrosis, taut bands, and nodules or trigger points within the muscle.

Palpation is an assessment tool used during the preliminary assessment to identify and localize areas of concern, and it is also used extensively during the treatment phase to continuously identify target tissues and monitor changes in the soft tissue as the session progresses. The hands are the main vehicles to deliver manipulations to the soft tissue, and yet at the same time it is the hands that carefully monitor the underlying tissues for changes in response to the manipulations.

Although many massage therapists use palpation as the primary form of assessment, it is most accurate when used in conjunction with and after the aforementioned assessment skills. Especially in pain conditions where there is radiating or referred pain, observation and examination isolate the cause of the pain and then palpation pinpoints the source.

As with the other assessment techniques, it is important to make bilateral comparisons. Although many conditions affect both sides of the body, bilateral comparison helps establish what is normal for the individual and helps determine whether the tissue in question is involved in the dysfunctional condition.

Assessment by palpation is both objective and subjective. As the therapist's hands palpate the body's tissues, the therapist must pay close attention not only to the qualities of the tissue but also to the reactions of the client. The therapist begins lightly and proceeds to probe deeper into the tissues, noting any signs of tension, lesions, or pain.

Assessment using palpation can be done at many levels from superficial to deep. The most superficial level is just above the body, not quite touching the skin. Variations in temperature can be sensed. Warm areas may indicate increased activity or inflammation. Cooler areas may indicate congestion or reduced circulation. A subtle energy field may also be sensed at this level as a slight pressure against the palm of the hand, possibly indicating a highly active area, or as an empty feeling, indicating a depleted condition.

The next level of palpation is the skin surface. The temperature, texture, color, and moistness of the skin are noted. Increased temperature or surface moisture is indicative of conditions in deeper tissues. Remember, inflammation is a contraindication for local massage. The signs of inflammation are heat, redness, pain, and swelling. Palpation also detects

palpation
is a skill and an art developed by the therapist that is a primary assessment tool allowing the therapist to listen to the client's body through the therapist's hands.

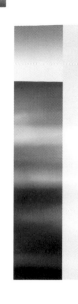

BOX 13.1 DESCRIPTIVE TERMS FOR LAYER PALPATORY EXAM

The texture and condition of the various tissues felt during palpatory examination may fall within one or more of following continuums of opposites:

superficial ~ deep	dry ~ moist
nonpainful ~ painful	soft ~ hard
cold ~ hot	compressible ~ rigid
hypomobile ~ hypermobile	flexible ~ stiff
smooth ~ rough	acute ~ chronic
thin ~ thick	circumscribed ~ diffuse

abnormal sensations the client may be experiencing such as lack of sensation or increased or diminished sensation.

The quality of the subcutaneous tissue or superficial fascia is the next level to be assessed by palpation. The superficial fascia connects the skin to the underlying muscle and other tissues while at the same time allowing for independent movement between them. Skin rolling is an important part of layer palpation; it gives the clinician information about the extensibility of the subcutaneous connective tissue. In skin rolling, the skin and superficial connective tissue are lifted up, away from the deeper tissues. The extensibility of the tissues, as well as the integrity of the tissues, may be palpated. A slight compression with the palm side of the fingers or hand should sense a springy cushion between the skin and the deeper tissues. The skin should also glide over the underlying tissues a short distance in every direction, though it will tend to have a preference to move one direction more freely that any of the others. Fascia that tends to be tight or stuck may indicate a deeper dysfunction.

Superficial fascia is also the site of superficial lymph nodes and blood vessels. The blood pulse can be felt by palpating superficial arteries. Lymph nodes feel like small nodules between the size of a small pea and a kidney bean. They can often be palpated along the side of the neck, in the axillary area, or along the inguinal area. Enlarged lymph nodes should be brought to the attention of your client and the client referred to his doctor so that the cause of the swollen nodules can be properly diagnosed.

The next level of palpation is the skeletal muscles and their related textures and structures. The deep palpatory exam includes compression, which is palpation through layers of tissue perpendicular to the tissue, and shear. Shear is movement of tissues between layers, moving parallel to the tissue. Muscle is comprised of contractile fibers that are organized and held in place by layers of connective tissues to form distinctive patterns that can be easily palpated. When palpating muscles, the therapist observes tissue consistency and texture. In a relaxed state, muscle is somewhat pliable and evenly grained with the fiber orientation easily identified. Normal qualities when palpating over a muscle would allow a moderate movement of the skin and subcutaneous tissue over the muscle tissue in all directions; an even, smooth grain when moving across the muscle fibers; a soft, yielding, painless firmness when pressing into the muscle. Abnormal qualities may include a restriction in the movement of the skin over the muscle sheaths and underlying structures, ropey or fibrous muscle tissue, tense or spasmed muscle tissue that is painful to the touch, or hypersensitive nodules that are painful when compressed. Constricted muscle feels denser or tighter, more restricted, more fibrous, and less pliable. A common palpable condition found in muscle that is usually associated with a lesion is a fibrous or taut band. Taut bands usually run the length of a muscle and feel like a hardened, fibrous bundle that you can actually pluck. Taut bands are usually associated with a previous injury, a strained muscle, or a habitually overstressed area. Often a taut band will harbor one or more hypersensitive points (trigger points). Palpation effectively locates other hypersensitive points and areas. Finding and reducing taut bands and trigger points is one of the most effective ways of treating soft tissue pain and dysfunction.

Toward the end of the muscle body, the connective tissue that separates and organizes the muscle fibers continues beyond the ends of the muscle fibers and becomes the muscle attachments in the form of rope-like tendons or wider tendon sheaths. This area, know as the musculo-tendinous junction, is a common area to palpate hypersensitive spots that indicate trigger points or microtrauma due to overexertion.

Tendons can be palpated from the ends of the muscle to the attachment to the bone, also known as the tenoperiosteal junction, where some tenderness may be noted if the muscle has been under excessive stress.

The massage therapist palpates bones as landmarks to identify muscle attachments or structural alignment. Palpating bony landmarks helps when observing structural discrepancies such as a tilted or rotated pelvis. Palpating the bony tissue around joints may indicate abnormal development or calcification. The position and regularity of the skeletal structure is also noted.

The next level to be palpated is the joints and the related ligaments. A joint is where two bones join together. Ligaments are tough, somewhat flexible connective tissue that connects the bones at the joints. They are slightly elastic and flexible enough to allow an appropriate amount of movement and at the same time are resilient enough to stabilize the joint. Excessive play in the joint or a painful response when palpating a ligament usually indicates a dysfunction.

Joints are usually palpated during active or passive joint movements. The quality of movement is assessed noting smooth, unrestricted, and painless movement through the range of motion. The end feel as the joint approaches the end of its range is also noted.

Another application of palpation is the visceral organs of the abdominal cavity. The liver and large intestine can easily be palpated. The body of the psoas muscle can be palpated and massaged through the abdominal muscles and viscera.

Structures that can be palpated

skin
subcutaneous fascia
blood vessels
lymph nodes
muscle sheaths
muscle bellies
musculotendinous junctions
tendons
deep fascia
ligaments
bone
joint spaces
abdominal viscera and structures

Figure 13.7
Structures that can be palpated.

---

acute

refers to a condition
with a sudden onset
and relatively short
duration.

---

chronic

refers to a lingering
or ongoing condition.

The therapist should be able to palpate in depth the location of the structures during the palpatory exam (see Figure 13.7). Is only the skin being palpated or is the subcutaneous fascia also being palpated? Is the muscle sheath being palpated or has the muscle belly been penetrated? Is the clinician palpating the musculotendinous junction or the tendon itself? Perfecting layer palpation requires development of tactile skills and includes the ability to detect tissue texture abnormalities. How is the tissue at that level different from surrounding tissues at the same level of depth or the tissue on the contralateral side? Palpating the soft tissues helps the therapist determine the feel of the individual client's normal soft tissue, detect anatomical anomalies, and detect soft tissue lesions or pathology.

Developing the skills of assessing the texture and condition of the tissues takes time and practice. The ability to accurately sense the tissues, together with the knowledge and skill to apply the appropriate therapeutic intervention to positively affect those tissues, provides the beneficial outcome to the client and is the hallmark of a good therapist.

ACUTE AND CHRONIC CONDITIONS

Acute and **chronic** are terms used to describe a condition, pain, or illness. Acute refers to a condition with a sudden onset and relatively short duration. Chronic refers to a lingering or ongoing condition. Acute pain is sharp, the symptom of an identifiable incident or illness, a warning to

---

BOX 13.2 TART

An assessment protocol that incorporates palpation and is used when addressing soft tissue dysfunction is represented by the acronym TART.

T = Texture of the superficial and deep tissues. Variations from normal include taut bands, adherent tissue, hypertonic or flaccid tissues.

A = Asymmetry in body structure as observed by a rotation, a curvature, or a bilateral inconsistency in the body structure. Asymmetry is also noted as bilateral difference in motion, tone, temperature, and the like.

R = Range of motion of a single or a number of related joints in an area of the body. Quality of movement, end feel, and restricted or excessive range are all noted.

T = Tenderness or pain in an area or in specific tissues. Pain may be evident in an area or excessive tenderness may be provoked when an area is palpated. Referred pain when pressure is applied to a point is an indication of an active myofascial trigger point.

take action. It is usually temporary. Chronic pain is persistent or intermittent over a long period of time, often dull, diffused, and many times without an identifiable cause or source.

An acute illness has a rapid onset and is relatively short lived. A chronic illness progresses slowly, is difficult or impossible to remedy, and may last weeks, months, years, or even be lifelong.

Acute Soft Tissue Injury

An acute injury is usually due to a trauma or abuse resulting in damage to the hard or soft tissue. When soft tissue is injured, whether at a cellular level or gross tissue damage, a natural process of healing and repair takes place. The process, known as the inflammatory response, is fairly predictable, with the focus being repair and reorganization of the damaged tissues. The stages of inflammation include the acute phase and the subacute phase, including the regenerative phase and the remodeling phase.

When tissue is injured, histamines are released that cause local vasodilation and increased vasopermeability resulting in swelling, heat, and increased tenderness at the site of the injury. During this early phase, local and systemic activity involves many biological processes that are working to reestablish homeostasis. Locally, the tissue is flooded with interstitial fluid as dead and damaged tissue is carried away while fibroblasts begin to lay down a random network of fibrin to secure the damaged tissue. During this initial period, which may last anywhere from a matter of hours to a week depending on the nature of the injury and the condition of the client, any treatment that might disrupt these delicate fibrin structures, including massage, is contraindicated. During this time, proper treatment would include rest, ice, compression, and elevation (RICE). An important benefit of RICE is that it reduces some of the swelling that would otherwise separate the ends of the injured tissue as well as the layers of fascia related to the injured tissue. Another advantage is that pain is greatly reduced.

During the regenerative phase, collagen fibers are produced that rather randomly create bridges to bind the tissues together, thereby creating not only scarring of the damaged tissue but also fibrous cross-linking between fascial sheaths. Stability of the tissue improves; however, if left unchecked, cross-linking in the fascia and scarring may negatively affect functionality. At this stage, tissues are very delicate, but gentle techniques may be employed that encourage alignment of the collagen network to restore stability as well as function. Techniques include mild tensioning or lengthening and light cross-fiber manipulations. Exercises may include gentle, passive range of motion that is well within the client's comfort level or pain tolerance. Non-weight bearing, active range of motion helps restore mobility and produce strong, pliable scar tissue. Techniques are applied to the surrounding tissues to help reduce spasms and splinting and to promote circulation, reducing ischemia and encouraging drainage.

Collagen production and cross-linking continue during the remodeling phase. Tensile strength of the tissue increases; however, pliability and functionality may be reduced because of the scarring and collagen crosshatching that effectively glue the involved layers of fascia together. Manipulations that slowly and deliberately lengthen the injured tissue to its full functional length, such as ROM, MET (using the antagonist), and gentle stretching exercises help reduce fibrosis and restore the tissue to full functionality. As flexibility is restored, gentle exercises can be initiated to regain strength and tone in the tissues.

A common physiological response to an acute injury is for spasms to occur in neighboring tissues, effectively splinting the injured tissue. It is not uncommon for these spasms to linger long after the injury has healed. Trigger points and ischemia develop, and what started as an acute injury becomes a long-standing chronic condition long after the injured tissue heals.

Treatment strategies for acute and chronic conditions are very different. Most acute conditions and injuries are a contraindication for most forms of massage and bodywork. Acute illnesses are often accompanied by fever and are contraindications for massage. Acute injury with tissue disruption is a contraindication for massage until the tissues have stabilized and infiltration and swelling have subsided. In the subacute stage of soft tissue injury, gentle lengthening and cross-fiber techniques may be employed. The sessions are rather short and quite frequent, sometimes daily or even twice a day. Sessions for more chronic conditions are usually of a longer duration and not as frequent.

USE ASSESSMENT INFORMATION TO PLAN SESSIONS

When the assessment has been completed, the therapist should have a clearer understanding of the client's reason for making the appointment. Information from the medical history, intake form, interview, observation, and various tests is combined and analyzed to better understand the conditions and concerns of the client. Information from movement assessments will note restrictions from pain and constriction and help determine what tissues and structures are involved. Careful palpation further identifies affected tissues. Using the assessment information, the therapist is better able to develop a treatment plan to best suit the needs of the client.

Part of developing a treatment plan is establishing goals for the session or a series of sessions (Figure 13.8). Goals must be realistic and attainable. The client's concerns and needs along with the assessment findings are considered when setting goals. Session strategies and therapeutic interventions are then chosen to work toward those goals. Following the implementation of those strategies, evaluation of the session helps determine whether those goals have been met or whether modification of the treatment plan is necessary to achieve those goals. Depending on the findings of the assessment and the chosen goals, a treatment plan may include the following:

- Referral to another health professional for further assessment
- Referral to another health professional for treatment in lieu of or in conjunction with massage
- The initial number and frequency of sessions to be given
- The estimated length of the treatments and whether they are full body or specific to the condition
- The use of other modalities such as heat, ice, or hydrotherapy
- What massage techniques will be used
- What results are expected and by when

Accurate assessment allows the therapist to design treatments with modalities and massage techniques and regimes that will best benefit the client. The modalities and techniques used will depend on the skills and knowledge of the therapist and techniques the therapist is qualified for and able to perform.

The assessment findings and treatment plan are discussed with the client so that he can be actively involved in the therapy process. Clients who actively participate in the therapy generally reap more benefits, respond to the therapy faster, and tend to follow through for a more lasting remedy. Discussing the assessment findings with clients teaches them about the functions of the body and the nature of the condition they have so that they can make educated choices as to what changes they can make to help correct the causes of the condition. Discussing optional therapy strategies enables clients to be involved and make choices about what they want to do about their condition. Discussing therapy strategies with clients gives them a clear idea of what the therapy will consist of and what they might expect during the actual sessions.

When discussing assessment findings and treatment plans with clients, use terminology the clients can understand. Some clients will be more interested than others. Be clear in describing assessment findings. Use diagrams and charts to illustrate physical conditions when possible. Describe the techniques you have chosen to use along with the expected benefits as well as the possible risks. Give enough information to inform clients without saturating them with unnecessary technicalities. Answer any questions the client may have about your findings and the chosen interventions. When the assessment findings and proposed treatment plan are understood and agreed upon, once again obtain

Goals for the performance of therapeutic massage

Help the body function more efficiently
Help increase client's self-awareness, balance, and fluidity
Relieve pain
Increase circulation
    Reduce ischemia
    Flush out toxins
Normalize soft tissue
    Release hypertonic muscle tissue
    Facilitate/strengthen hypotonic muscle tissue
    Lengthen constricted fascia
Improve flexibility and ROM
Reintegrate function into the whole
Relaxation/stress relief

Figure 13.8

Goals for the performance of therapeutic massage.

THE ROLE OF CONTINUING EDUCATION

In the current massage and bodywork profession, there are numerous modalities or systems of bodywork. (See Chapter 18 for a partial list of modalities.) Each modality has a different way of viewing the organism, assessing deviations from the optimum, and treating the body to encourage a return toward normalcy and balance. Some modalities work on different levels, such as the physical, mental, emotional, energetic, or spiritual. The serious student is encouraged to explore other modalities. Continuing education is a key for advanced learning, deeper understanding, additional skills, and greater appreciation of the human condition.

informed consent and proceed with the session. Always respect the client's right to modify or withdraw consent at any time while the session is in progress.

PERFORMANCE

In the performance portion of the therapeutic procedure, the therapist applies techniques and modalities to address the needs, concerns, and conditions discovered during the assessment with the intention of restoring normalcy, balance, and function.

When the preliminary assessment has been done and a treatment plan has been developed, it is time to begin the actual therapy. Depending on the chosen strategy, a number of modalities may proceed or follow the actual massage. Hot packs, ice packs, ice massage, hot baths, or hot showers can be used previous to massage therapy to enhance the desired therapeutic effects. Used with other therapy modalities, various types of electrical stimulation, ultrasound, and exercise can be incorporated to produce excellent results.

The assessment and planning stages of the therapeutic process provide a blueprint for the procedures performed during the actual therapeutic massage. By the time the therapist begins the massage portion of the session, she knows what the general conditions are and what approach and modalities she will use. It is not until the therapist begins to massage the client and her hands make contact and begin to manipulate the soft tissues that a continuous flow of information directs the intricate flow of the session. Even though a proposed outline for the massage session is followed, there is always room to alter the treatment according to the specific conditions encountered in the tissues during the actual session. Throughout the massage, the therapist continues the assessment as she works on each part of the body. As the therapist approaches an area of the body during the performance of a massage, a visual assessment will note body position, symmetry, and color of the area. The first contact will note temperature, texture of the skin, and surface moisture. Deeper contact will provide information about the connective and muscle tissue. These assessments during the performance of the massage help to continually formulate the session. Throughout the session, close attention is paid to the response of the client. Responses may be verbal, subtle movements, or changes in the actual tissue that is being manipulated. Many times nonverbal cues from the client such as facial expressions, sounds, or grimaces indicate pleasure or discomfort. The therapist continuously elicits feedback from the client and modifies the session to obtain the ultimate results. The assessment and evaluation continue to be intermingled throughout the actual performance of the massage, and although the plan for the massage is followed, adjustments and modifications to the plan may occur during the actual massage according to new information gained during the session.

Therapeutic massage is like an intense conversation. The therapist listens, observes, and examines the client to get an idea of the condition. Then the therapist's hands listen to the client's body and respond with manipulative touch. The body listens to the manipulations and responds. Hearing and feeling these responses, the therapist chooses the next delivery. Thus goes the close interaction of a therapeutic massage.

Massage Therapy for Soft Tissue Dysfunction

Musculoskeletal dysfunction is often characterized by postural deviation and/or movement restriction and is often accompanied by pain. Constrictions in soft tissue usually result from overuse, underuse, misuse, abuse, or trauma to the body. Soft tissue-related pain, myofascial pain, muscle pain or spasm, and ischemia all respond well to soft tissue interventions and therapeutic massage techniques. Tension, restricted movement, asymmetry, localized or referred pain, and stress are also indications for therapeutic massage. The intention of soft tissue intervention is reducing pain, restoring circulation, oxygenating tissue, releasing hypertonicity, improving functional range of motion, and integrating the restored area back into the whole.

To successfully restore the muscles to a healthier state when there has been dysfunction, pain, trauma, or compensation to an area of the body, proper rehabilitative steps ensure a longer-lasting recovery. After careful assessment to determine what tissues are involved and that there are no contraindications to treatment, the first step is to restore circulation and neuromuscular response to the tissues. The second step is to release any trigger points and fibrous restrictions in the muscle tissue and

BOX 13.3 CONDITIONS THAT RESPOND TO SOFT TISSUE INTERVENTION:

soft tissue pain

tension

asymmetry

restricted movement due to pain

restricted movement due to constricted muscle

hypertonic muscle

hypotonic muscle

fibrosis

scar tissue

old injury sites

hypersensitive points or areas

trigger points

taut bands in muscle

stress

restore flexibility. Follow that by rebuilding strength and endurance to the muscle. It is also important to, as far as possible, identify and remove the causative factors that initiated the dysfunction. In the case of acute, single-event onset conditions, this is fairly simple. In the case of chronic conditions, however, isolating the causative factors is more difficult, and eliminating them may mean changing habitual patterns or modifying workspaces. In either case, treatment does not begin and end in the office during the session and usually involves homework such as exercises or modifying some aspect of daily activity to alter the conditions that initiated the dysfunction.

Hypertonic and Hypotonic Muscles

Common structural body and postural imbalances generally involve muscles or groups of muscles that are constricted or hypertonic—that is, they seem tight, or result in a postural deviation or constriction in joint movement, or both. Constricted tissues could be the result of hypertonic musculature or, in cases of chronic conditions, constrictions or fibrosis in the fascia supporting the muscles. Examining the involved tissues with range of motion and palpation will reveal what tissues are involved. When examining and treating an area of the body, it is important to look beyond the specific site and include associated muscles in the treatment. When a muscle is constricted and overactive, it is common for the antagonist (the muscle responsible for the opposite movement) to be flaccid, weak, or hypotonic. By the same token, when a weak muscle is found, often the opposing muscle or possibly the synergistic muscles are found to be overactive, tight, or hypertonic. Many times in this type of circumstance, releasing the hypertonic or constricted tissues is the primary focus; however, stimulating and strengthening the hypotonic antagonist is also a major consideration in the treatment plan. If the target (constricted) muscle contains trigger points, it is important to relieve those and encourage the muscle to reestablish a normal resting length. At the same time, stimulating and strengthening the antagonist will have an inhibitory and balancing effect on its hypertonic partner. The overall result will be a more balanced structure.

MASSAGE TECHNIQUES TO ADDRESS SOFT TISSUE DYSFUNCTION

Abnormal and dysfunctional soft tissue conditions respond exceptionally well to systematically applied massage techniques directed specifically toward the affected tissues (Figure 13.9). Massage techniques affect the dysfunctional tissues either directly by manipulating the tissues or indirectly by influencing the neuromuscular mechanism in an attempt to restore a more normal function. Many effective techniques are similar to those used in wellness/relaxation massage but are directed toward the dysfunctional tissues. Other techniques are modified or combined for the specific effects they produce when applied to the body. Massage tech-

Effective techniques to address soft tissue conditions:

Directional Massage:
  Gliding techniques:

Superficial gliding	Introduces area to touch. Applies lubricant. Assesses superficial tissue quality. Improves circulation. Stimulates parasympathetic nervous system. Soothes and relaxes.
Deep gliding	Assess tissue quality. Increases circulation. Softens connective tissue. Separates adhesions.
J-Strokes	Stretches and aligns constricted fascia.

Cross-fiber techniques:

Digital or point specific	Assesses connective and contractile tissue. Softens connective tissue. Reduces scar tissue. Broadens fibrous tissue.
Broad Cross-Fiber Massage	Assesses contractile and connective tissue. Softens and reduces adhesions in soft tissue.

Trigger-Point Release:

	Ability to locate, assess, and reduce trigger-point activity.
Passive Positioning	Releases trigger points and taut bands. Resets neuromuscular feedback circuits.
Trigger Point Pressure Release Ischemic Compression	Reduces trigger-point activity.
MET	Restores flexibility and range of motion.

Passive and Active Joint Movements:

Passive Joint Movements	Restores length to constricted tissues. Mobilizes joints.
Passive Positioning or Position Release Techniques	Release hypertonic contractile tissues and help to reset pathophysiologic neuromuscular circuits.
Muscle Energy Techniques (MET)	Help muscles regain their normal resting length. Stimulate weak hypotonic muscles.

Figure 13.9

Effective techniques to address soft tissue conditions.

niques are used to identify abnormal tissues, normalize and restore function, and finally to reconnect and integrate the area with the whole.

Suspected areas of the body to be addressed are determined during the assessment and planning stages of the session. During the performance of the massage, the actual physical contact allows the therapist to identify the specific tissues involved. The therapist is able to palpate and identify the abnormal tissues with superficial gliding and light cross-fiber strokes. Massage techniques are then chosen to normalize the tissues. Trigger points are quieted with position release, ischemic compression, and Muscle Energy Technique. Fascial constriction is reduced with deep gliding, J-strokes, cross-fiber friction, and stretching. Hypotonic muscles are tonified with Muscle Energy Technique, J-strokes, and exercise. Finally, passive joint movements and superficial gliding help integrate and reconnect the tissues to the surrounding area and to the whole.

Directional Massage

Directional massage refers to a number of specifically directed massage strokes that target mostly the fascia and its related elements. Common directional massage strokes include superficial and deep gliding strokes, J-strokes, and cross-fiber strokes.

Gliding Strokes

Gliding strokes may be superficial or deep, depending on the intention with which they are preformed. Superficial gliding strokes are soothing techniques that introduce an area of the body to the therapist's touch, distribute massage lubricant, enhance local circulation, and prepare the area for deeper, more direct techniques. Superficial gliding is used to gather information about the quality of the tissue and identify palpable irregularities in tissue texture, density, and temperature. Superficial gliding is applied with the palm of the fingers and hand or the thumb (Figure 13.10a and b). Superficial gliding is often interspersed between deeper techniques and is used as a completion stroke to help ease the intensity of the therapy, integrate the effects of the techniques, and leave the area feeling complete and relaxed.

Deep gliding strokes are usually applied with the thumb, knuckles of a loose fist, the forearm, or the elbow, and they are applied in the direction of the underlying muscle fibers (Figure 13.11a to c). A minimal amount of lubricant is used to allow the movement to glide smoothly over the skin. The amount of pressure varies to engage, assess, and treat incrementally deeper layers of tissue beginning with lighter pressure on the skin and continuing with increased pressure as the movement is directed toward the deeper fascia and muscle tissue. The rate of motion or speed of the gliding stroke may vary according to the depth and intention for which the stroke is being applied. Sometimes referred to as muscle stripping, deep gliding follows the direction of the muscle fibers from one attachment to the other, usually distal to proximal. Occasionally, the direction is reversed, and sometimes it is applied across the muscle. Deep

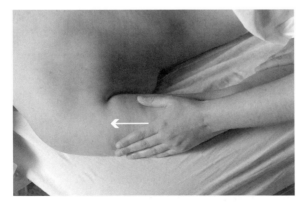

Figure 13.10a
Superficial gliding applied with the hand.

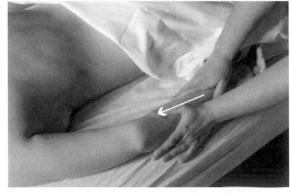

Figure 13.10b
Superficial gilding with the thumb.

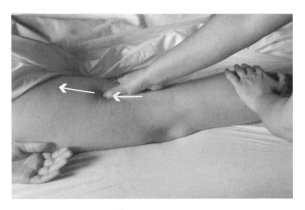

Figure 13.11a
Deep gliding applied with the thumb.

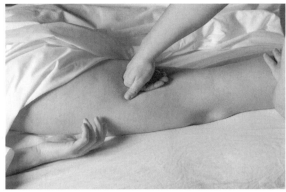

Figure 13.11b
Deep gliding applied with the knuckles of a soft fist.

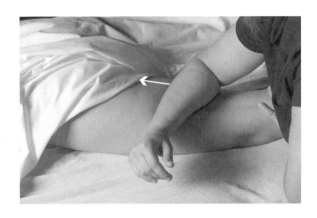

Figure 13.11c
Deep gliding applied with the forearm.

gliding is a technique that is used extensively in American-style neuro-muscular therapy. It is very useful in locating constricted, fibrous tissue; taut bands; and myofascial trigger points. As a treatment, it is used to flush out tissues, separate adhesions, and soften constricted contractile tissue and fascia.

The J-stroke

The J-stroke applies stresses to the fascia and is often directed toward the Golgi tendon apparatus or spindle cells. It can also be used to elongate contracted muscles or stretch, separate, and align constricted fascia.

The J-stroke is usually applied with one or both thumbs, but can also be done with the fingertips (see Figure 13.12a to c and Figure 13.13). It is a friction stroke that moves the superficial layers of tissue over the deeper layers. The side of the tip of the thumb makes light contact with the skin and pulls it slightly back in the opposite direction of the intended stroke and then moves deeper into the tissue to contact the fibrous tissue beneath. The thumb hooks and rotates as a deep stroke is then given in the intended direction, which is usually in line with the direction of the fibers of the underlying muscle or tendon. The stroke is as long as the superficial tissue movement will allow without the thumb gliding over the

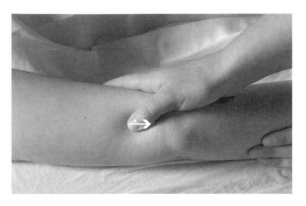

Figure 13.12a

The J-stroke begins by making contact with the skin.

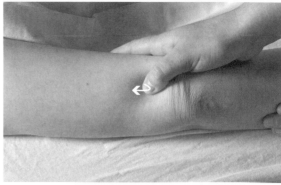

Figure 13.12b

Continue the J-stroke by drawing the superficial tissue back slightly.

Figure 13.12c

Complete by pressing into the deeper tissues and moving in the direction of the stroke as far as possible without sliding over the skin.

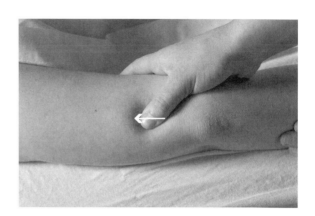

skin. The J-stroke may be repeated three to five times on the same spot, or may progress backward (in the opposite direction from the direction of the stroke) along the muscle being massaged.

To apply the J-stroke to a muscle, begin at the muscle attachment and do three to five strokes from the muscle toward the bony attachment, move toward the muscle body, and repeat two or three strokes so that they just barely overlap the previous position. Move back along the muscle and repeat the procedure. Continue until the whole muscle has been covered. The direction is usually toward the insertion, however, it may be reversed. Direction may be determined by palpating fascial preference of bind and ease and using the J-stroke to reduce fascial restrictions. Fascial preference may be determined by applying a slight pressure with the thumb or fingers into the tissue and moving first in one direction and then another to determine which direction moves easiest the farthest.

A J-stroke can be used to stimulate or sedate a muscle, depending on the muscle condition. To calm or sedate hypertonic muscle, directional massage would be directed toward the center of the muscle on the muscle body's contractile tissues (unloading the spindles). On the body of the muscle, both hands engage the muscle to shorten the muscle fibers and

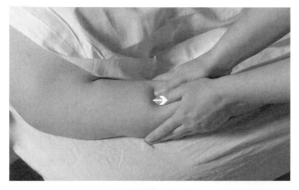

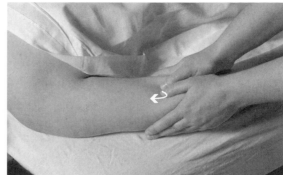

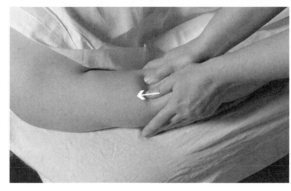

Figure 13.13
The J-stroke using two thumbs covers a wider area on the muscle.

crowd the spindle cells (Figure 13.14a). To stimulate a hypotonic muscle, the directions would reverse, massaging the muscle body away from the center, stretching the muscle fibers, activating the spindle cells, and encouraging the muscle to contract (Figure 13.14b).

Cross-Fiber Friction

As the name implies, cross-fiber or transverse friction massage is applied at a 90-degree angle to the fiber direction. When applied with light pressure, it is used as an assessment aid to locate taut bands associated

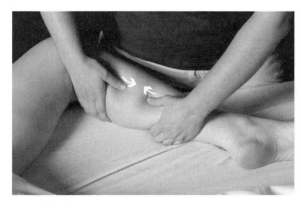

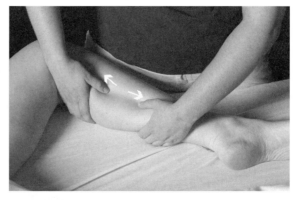

Figure 13.14a
To sedate a hypertonic or spasmed muscle, simultaneously apply J-strokes toward the center of the muscle.

Figure 13.14b
To stimulate a hypotonic muscle, simultaneously apply J-strokes away from the center of the muscle.

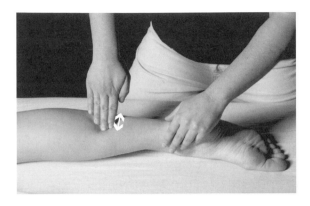

Figure 13.15a

Cross-fiber friction applied with the fingers.

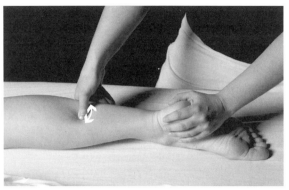

Figure 13.15b

Cross-fiber friction applied with the thumb.

with trigger points and constricted fibrous tissue. Cross-fiber friction, directed more specifically at deeper tissues, is a therapeutic modality to reduce fibrosis and separate fascial layers that have become stuck as a result of connective tissue gluing following local injury and inflammation. It is most effective when directed precisely toward a lesion in the muscle where adhesions interfere with the muscle's ability to contract and broaden painlessly or efficiently. Lesions may be in the muscle belly, the musculotendinous junction, or in the tendon, wherever trauma, microtrauma, or injury may occur. Cross-fiber friction helps reduce adhesions between fascial sheaths while at the same time encouraging the formation of a strong pliable scar tissue at the site of the injury.

Cross-fiber friction is generally applied with the flats of the fingertips (Figure 13.15a). However, the thumb can also be used (Figure 13.15b). Contact is made with the skin, and the skin and superficial tissues are moved back and forth over the deeper tissues in a direction perpendicular to the muscle or tendon fibers. The thumb or fingers move the superficial over the deeper tissues but do not slide over the skin. The length of the stroke is long enough to tease, roll, and separate the deeper fibers and short enough to not snap back and forth over the fibrous or taut bands. The depth is enough to compress and engage the deeper fibers and not so deep as to cause excessive discomfort or a flinching or retracting response from the client.

Broad cross-fiber strokes are less specific compression strokes, usually done with the palm of the hand (Figure 13.16). Pressure is applied against the muscle body toward the underlying bone structure with movements transverse to the fiber direction of the muscle. This is done with the intention of spreading and broadening the muscle tissue. Close attention is paid to the quality of the fibrous tissue as it moves under the hands for indications of taut bands or fibrosities that require more specific work.

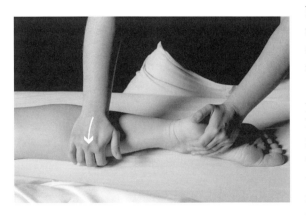

Figure 13.16

Broad cross-fiber friction is applied with the hand.

How Much Pressure Is Enough?

The right amount of pressure to use when doing bodywork varies greatly depending on the type of bodywork, the technique being applied, the condition of the client, and the condition of the target tissues. When doing manual lymph drainage, for instance, the pressure is very light, whereas in deep connective tissue therapies, such as deep gliding, cross-fiber friction, or ischemic compression, the pressure is considerably deeper. So the right amount of pressure to achieve the optimal therapeutic response is relative to the technique being used, the location and condition of the target tissue, and the intention of the manipulation. In most soft tissue techniques, the pressure is enough to engage the target tissues without causing an alarm response or damaging the target or surrounding tissues. Pressure is applied in a gradual manner where contact is made, and pressure is gradually increased so as to not invade the tissues or startle the client. When working deeply into an area, it is advantageous to enter slowly and occasionally pause and allow the tissues to open as they become more receptive to the pressure being applied. The amount of pressure will vary from one client to another and from one part of the body to another. Pressure will vary according to the texture and sensitivity of the target tissue in order to achieve a therapeutic response from the tissue.

The optimal therapeutic pressure would be that which would elicit the maximum therapeutic response without triggering an autonomic defensive reaction from the client. If the pressure is too abrupt or too intense, the client will respond with defense mechanisms that will negate any therapeutic gain, erode trust in the therapist/client relationship, and possibly cause injury to the tissues.

Dr. Arthur Pauls, the British osteopath who developed Orthobionomy, described *rebound* as a palpable tissue response to therapeutically applied pressure. Rebound refers to a springy, responsive, active feedback when a tissue is compressed or stretched just enough to engage the neuromuscular and proprioceptive reflexes. When compressing a point, as in ischemic compression, rebound is encountered between the resistive barrier and the anatomic barrier. To find it, make contact and slowly press into the point nearly to the level to elicit an "ouch" response from the client and then back off slightly. The pressure is enough to engage the point, to sort of float on the point, and to sense the dynamic changes in the tissue as the body responds to the therapeutic input. Likewise, when doing a joint movement, move the limb to the extent of possible movement and back off slightly and hold that position. Engaging the tissues in the rebound space is an optimal therapy zone where the body is most receptive to integrating the therapeutic input.

Trigger Points and Fibrosis

Trigger points are hypersensitive nodules that are usually located in hypertonic, dysfunctional, and often painful muscle tissue, although similar hypersensitive points are occasionally found in fascia, tendons, and even ligaments. Eliminating troublesome trigger points and restoring muscles to their normal resting length usually result in restoring pain-free function to the associated body area. Reducing fibrosis, eliminating trigger points, and restoring contractile muscle tissue to a normal resting length are three goals of therapeutic massage. Massage techniques that are effective at accomplishing these goals are passive positioning, directional massage techniques, and Muscle Energy Techniques. Trigger points, trigger-point release techniques, position release techniques, and Muscle Energy Techniques are discussed in Chapter 18.

REVIEW OUTCOME IN RELATION TO INTENT OF SESSION

Evaluation involves examining the outcome of the process in relation to the expected goals and objectives. Evaluation is important in that the client and therapist can gauge the effectiveness of the selected course of therapy according to the success in attaining the goals. Examining the outcome is important when deciding ongoing therapy. It provides a rationale for applying similar therapies for similar conditions in the future. Evaluation identifies the grounds for altering portions or all of the process to better achieve desired results. Finally, evaluation helps determine whether goals have been met and whether referral to another professional is warranted.

Evaluation is both subjective and objective. Much of the evaluation is based on how the client feels as a result of the therapy. Levels of posture, mobility, pain, and function can be reassessed to indicate the success of the treatment.

Evaluation is done at various times during the therapeutic process. After the assessment, an evaluation is done to decide how or whether to proceed. Evaluation occurs after a single session and during the performance of a session to determine the effectiveness of the chosen modalities and techniques. If the decision is made to do several sessions, evaluations after each session help to determine the continued course of therapy. The evaluation may carry over to the beginning of the following massage session to note more long-term improvements and effects of the chosen treatment and make adjustments to follow-up sessions. An evaluation at the end of the series helps to determine the course into the future.

QUESTIONS FOR DISCUSSION AND REVIEW

1. What are the four steps of a therapeutic procedure?

2. What is the purpose of each step of the therapeutic procedure?

3. How can the therapeutic procedure be implemented in therapeutic massage?

4. Name five important parts of the assessment process.

5. What is a pain scale and how is it used in the therapeutic process?

6. Name three types of movement tested when assessing range of motion.

7. Differentiate between the resistive barrier, the physiologic barrier, and the anatomical barrier.

8. List at least seven levels that soft tissue can be palpated.

9. According to Dr. James Cyriax, what is contractile tissue? Inert tissue? End feel?

10. Name three classifications of end feel considered to be normal.

11. What are the characteristics of abnormal end feel?

12. Differentiate between a chronic and an acute soft tissue condition.

13. What is the appropriate therapy in the initial stage of an acute soft tissue injury?

14. What information is used to develop a treatment plan?

15. Why are the assessment findings and treatment plan discussed with the client?

16. How is a therapeutic massage like an intense conversation?

17. Name three types of directional massage.

18. What are the important advantages of using the evaluation portion of the therapeutic process?

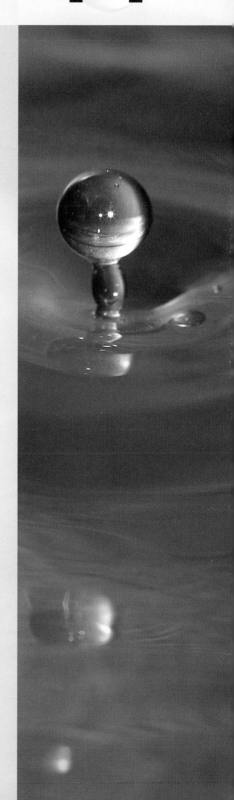

Hydrotherapy

LEARNING OBJECTIVES

After you have mastered this chapter, you will be able to:

1. Explain the use of heat and cold in body treatments.
2. Describe types of apparatus that may be approved for use by the massage practitioner.
3. Describe types of apparatus that may not be approved for use by the massage practitioner.
4. Describe at least five ways of applying heat to the body.
5. Define cryotherapy and demonstrate at least three ways to apply it.
6. Explain hydrotherapy as a therapeutic aid.
7. Explain the effects of different water temperatures on the body.
8. Describe the effects of various water treatments on the body.
9. Explain contraindications, safety rules, and time limits for various bath treatments.

INTRODUCTION

Although body massage is generally done by hand, there is a wide range of treatments that combine manual massage and the use of various other modalities. These treatments are designed to encourage circulation, improve the body's efficiency in eliminating toxins, and promote relaxation.

THE USE OF ELECTRICAL MODALITIES

A number of therapeutic methods that use electric stimulation have been found to be extremely beneficial in the treatment or rehabilitation of soft tissue or neurologic injuries. Examples include ultrasound, low- and medium-frequency electrical stimulation, electromagnetic stimulation, and others that use specific frequencies or pulses. Modalities requiring specific training should be performed only by qualified technicians under medical supervision. The use of most modalities using electricity is beyond the scope of therapeutic massage.

The practitioner must have sound knowledge of any procedure involving electrical equipment and its benefits as well as any contraindications of its use. Though no machine can replace the well-trained hands of the practitioner, machines can offer advantages when used in conjunction with manual massage. The machine is mainly used as a means to conserve the practitioner's energy and to increase the benefits of various treatments. All electrical equipment must be inspected regularly to ensure its safe operation.

One popular electrical apparatus used for body massage is the vibratory massager. It is used to produce either a relaxing or stimulating effect, depending on the method of application and the desired results. There are a variety of mechanical vibrators on the market. Using vibrators may enhance the effects of the massage and at the same time reduce the physical exertion of the practitioner. (Refer to Figure 10.16a to c).

THE USE AND EFFECTS OF HEAT AND COLD APPLICATIONS

The normal body temperature is 98.6°F. Physiologically, the body strives to maintain this temperature. When heat or cold is applied to the body, certain physiological changes occur. The nature and extent of those changes depend on the temperature and duration of the application and the size of the body area and thermal conductivity of the body part involved. The greater the temperature differentiation, the more dramatic the effect. If the temperature of the treatment is the same as the body temperature, there is little or no physiological reaction. Treatments of short duration may have different effects from longer treatments. For example, a short application of cold (2 to 5 seconds) has a stimulating effect, whereas an extended application (10 to 30 minutes) will depress metabolic activity. Local applications have specific local effects, whereas general applications have systemic effects. Some thermal applications will have both direct local effects and reflex effects. The physiological effects from the application of heat and cold are predictable, which makes the use of heat and cold a powerful therapeutic agent.

Treatments using extreme temperatures of both short or long duration should be avoided or be used under very close supervision. Using thermal treatments below freezing or above 115°F may damage tissues. Prolonged general treatments below 70°F may cause hypothermia. Prolonged general treatments above 110°F may cause hyperthermia. Either condition is potentially dangerous.

The application of heat causes a vasodilation and an increase of circulation in an attempt to dissipate the heat. A general application of heat will raise the body temperature, causing a feverlike reaction. There is profuse perspiration, the pulse rate increases, and the white blood cell count increases. A local application will cause local reddening (due to vasodilation), increased metabolism and leukocyte migration to the area, relaxation of local musculature, and a slight analgesia.

The quick, short application of cold is stimulating, whereas prolonged application of cold depresses metabolic activity. General application of cold reduces the body temperature (hypothermia). Although this has important therapeutic and medical advantages, it must only be done under strict medical supervision. Local applications of cold cause a reduction of nerve sensitivity, circulation, muscle spasms, and spasticity. They have a numbing, anesthetic, analgesic effect that makes them valuable in the relief of acute pain from bursitis, soft tissue injury, burns, and neuralgia.

APPLICATION OF HEAT

There are several sources for the application of heat. The choice of modality depends on the body part to be treated, its condition, and the objectives of the application. Modalities for the application of heat include:

- Dry heat
    Heating pad
    Infrared radiation
    Sauna
- Moist heat
    Immersion baths
    Spray (pulsating spray)
    Moist heat pack
    Steam baths
- Diathermy
    Shortwave
    Microwave

Heating Pads

Heating pads are plastic-covered pads that contain electric heating elements similar to electric blankets. A heating pad supplies a local source of dry heat and is easy to apply. The heating pad is useful for local applications on one part of the body while the therapist works on another. There are usually three heat level settings. Some heating pads are manufactured for application of moist heat. Manufacturers' instructions must be followed to prevent injury from burns or electrical shock.

Infrared Radiation

Infrared radiation may be produced from a bulb or an element. The warming effect of the sun is due to infrared radiation. As radiations are absorbed by the skin, heat is produced. The heat results in increased superficial circulation and sedation of sensory nerve endings. This results in the relaxation of tense or spasmed muscles, relief of pain, and increased availability of nutrients to the superficial tissues (Figure 14.1).

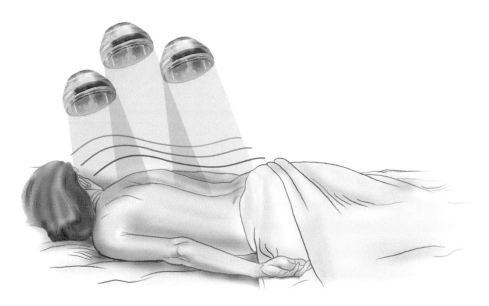

Figure 14.1
As infrared radiation is absorbed into the skin, heat is produced.

Immersion Baths

hydrotherapy
is the application of water in any of its three forms to the body for therapeutic purposes.

Whenever a body part is submerged in water, it is considered an immersion bath. Depending on the objective of the treatment, various areas may be treated and various temperatures may be used. The use of water for therapeutic purposes is **hydrotherapy.** Water is an effective medium for the application of thermal procedures (hot or cold) because it surrounds the body part and is an excellent conductor of heat or cold. Hydrotherapy will be discussed more thoroughly later in this chapter.

Spray (Pulsating Shower)

There are a variety of pulsating showerheads on the market today. The pulsating shower is an effective means of combining moist heat and mild compression. This combination calms sensory nerves and increases peripheral circulation. Increased circulation restores nutrients as it clears away metabolic wastes. Sedated nerves mean reduction of pain, relaxation of tense or spasmed muscles, and reduced stress.

Moist Heat Packs

Moist heat packs are generally chemical gel packs that are heated in a water bath, wrapped in a terry cloth cover, and placed on the body. A hydrocollator is used to heat and store the packs, which come in a variety of shapes, to conform to different areas of the body. The silica gel is formulated to retain heat and transfer it to the body part by means of conduction. Like heating pads, moist hot packs can be applied to one part of the body while the therapist works on another part (Figure 14.2).

Steam and Sauna Baths

Heat in a steam bath is produced by a steam generator. Heat in a sauna is produced by a dry heat source. The temperature in a stream bath is 120° to 130°F, whereas the temperature in a sauna may be 180° to 190°F. A steam bath may be a cabinet where the head remains outside of the heat or a steam room. Because the heat in a steam bath is supplied by steam, the air is supersaturated. This greatly reduces the body's ability to cool itself with perspiration. Saunas are always a room heated by dry heat. Evaporation of the body's perspiration has a cooling effect. This is why the sauna is so much hotter. Either one causes profuse sweating. Caution must be used to avoid overheating and to replace body fluids. Those with heart conditions, diabetes, and other conditions must consult their physician before using steam baths and saunas.

Diathermy

Diathermy (**DIE**-uh-thur-mee) is the application of oscillating electromagnetic fields to the tissue. The oscillating fields cause a distortion in the molecules and an ionic vibration that produces heat. Diathermy requires the use of specialized equipment and training and is beyond the scope of practice of massage therapy.

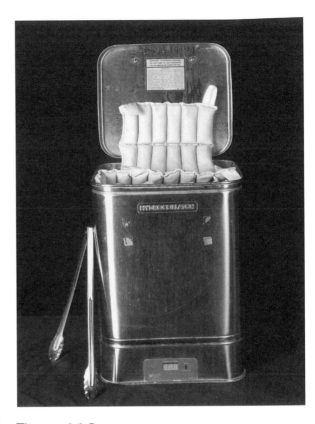

Figure 14.2

Moist heat packs are heated in water in a hydrocollator before being applied to the body.

diathermy
is the application of oscillating electromagnetic fields to the tissue.

cryotherapy
is the application of cold agents for therapeutic purposes.

CRYOTHERAPY

The application of cold agents for therapeutic purposes is known as **cryotherapy** (**KRIE**-o-ther-uh-pee). The primary goal of cryotherapy is to reduce the tissue temperature. As cold is applied to the body, heat is drawn from the tissues, causing cooling. The local application of cold is beneficial on painful, inflamed, and swollen areas. It acts as an analgesic to reduce pain and causes vasoconstriction to limit swelling.

The application of extreme cold should be of short duration to prevent injury to the tissue from freezing. The application of ice will cause a series of sensations that can act as an indicator of the duration of the application. The first sensation of the application of ice will naturally be cold. Following the cold sensation will be pain, aching, and sometimes burning. Next will be the cessation of pain (the analgesic effect). When the third stage is reached, application should be temporarily suspended. Treatment may be repeated as necessary as often as once an hour.

Ice is first aid for traumatic soft tissue injuries. When a soft tissue injury such as a sprain or strain occurs, the standard first aid treatment is to apply RICE, an acronym in which **R** = rest, **I** = ice, **C** = compression, and **E** = elevation. This reduces swelling, pain, and the secondary tissue damage that results from excessive swelling. As soon as swelling has subsided, limited massage therapy can proceed on the healing tissue.

Ice therapy can be used by itself or in conjunction with other modalities. In the case of swelling due to local inflammation, ice offers tremendous relief from the swelling and accompanying pain. One of the best ways to increase circulation to an area to promote healing is to alternate applications of heat and cold.

APPLICATION OF COLD

Sources for the local application of cold include:

- Immersion baths
- Ice packs
    Commercial ice bags
- Ice massage
- Compressor units with thermal packs and controls
- Vasocoolant sprays

Immersion Baths

The entire body or a body part can be immersed in cool or cold water. Cool and cold baths will be discussed later in this chapter. When working with an extremity, such as a foot, ankle, hand, wrist, or elbow, an immersion ice water bath can be used. Prepare a basin or tub of 60 percent ice and 40 percent water. Submerge the body part (foot, hand, forearm, or elbow) in the ice water until the feeling of cold or pain stops, then remove the body part from the bath and proceed with therapy.

Ice Pack

Ice packs are used for the local application of ice on a specific body part. They are effective in relieving pain, preventing swelling, and decreasing inflammation. They are indicated for the early treatment of sprains, strains, and other soft tissue injuries. They are effective in the treatment of acute joint and nerve inflammation.

Reusable commercial ice packs are available in a variety of types and sizes (Figure 14.3). These are usually a sealed plastic pack contain-

Figure 14.3

Commercially manufactured cold packs are available in a variety of shapes and sizes. They are stored in a freezer until needed.

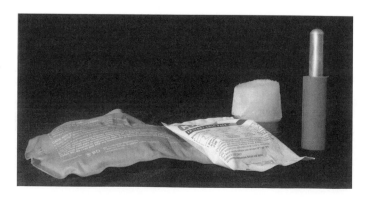

ing a chemical gel. The pack is stored in the freezer until needed. The pack is wrapped in a terry cloth to prevent direct contact with the skin. Direct contact is unsanitary and may result in injury from freezing the tissue. The chemical gel in the pack stays pliable at freezing temperatures so that the pack can conform to the area of the body to which it is applied (Figure 14.4).

When commercial ice packs are not available, ice in a plastic bag is just as effective. A Ziploc® bag or a plastic freezer bag makes an excellent ice pack. Be sure there are no leaks in the plastic bag. Fill it one third of the way with broken ice cubes or crushed ice, seal it closed, and apply it directly to the affected area. The ice bag may be held in place by an Ace bandage or towel wrap (Figure 14.5a to e).

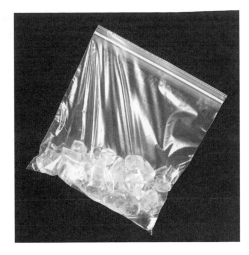

Figure 14.4

An inexpensive ice pack uses ice chips or cubes in a sealed plastic bag.

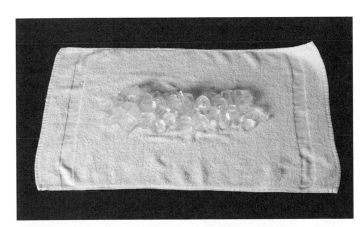

Figure 14.5a

Another alternative is to wrap ice in a towel and apply it to the affected area. Put crushed ice in the center of a towel.

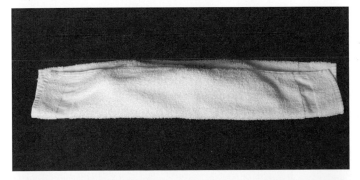

Figure 14.5b

Fold the sides of the towel over the ice.

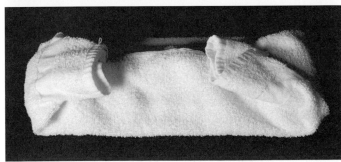

Figure 14.5c

Fold the ends of the towel.

continues

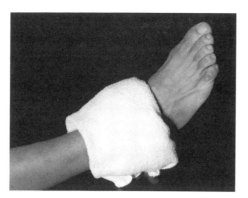

Figure 14.5d
Wrap the ice towel around the affected body part.

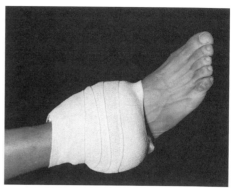

Figure 14.5e
Wrap the towel with an Ace bandage to secure it, and then apply compression.

Ice Massage

> **ice massage**
>
> is a local application of cold achieved by massaging a cube of ice over a small area such as a bursa, tendon, or small muscle.

Another way cryotherapy can be applied is **ice massage**. Ice massage is a local application of cold achieved by massaging a cube of ice over a small area such as a bursa, tendon, or small muscle. Commercial ice cups are available that are filled with water and stored in the freezer until needed. They provide a mold for the ice cube that includes a handle frozen into the cube so that the therapist can perform the ice massage without freezing his hand (Figure 14.6a to c). Another way this can be achieved is to freeze wa-

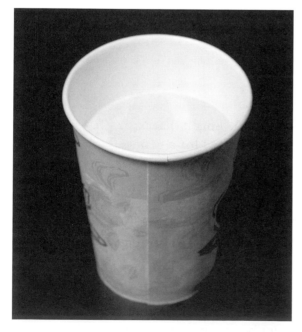

Figure 14.6a
Water frozen in a Styrofoam cup works well for ice massage.

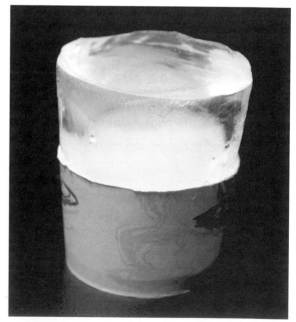

Figure 14.6b
When the water is frozen, peel the top half of the Styrofoam cup away to make an ice cup with an insulated handle.

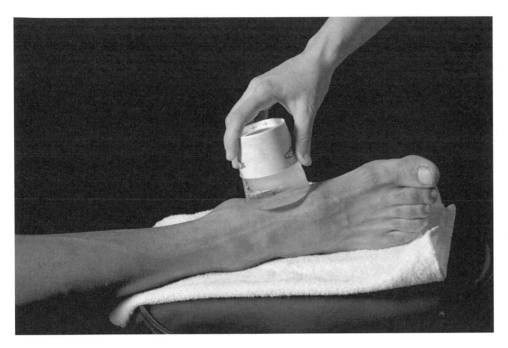

Figure 14.6c

Hold the bottom portion of the cup and apply ice massage.

ter in an 8-ounce Styrofoam cup. Remove the frozen cup from the freezer and cut the top half of the cup away. Use the base of the cup as a handle (Figure 14.7a to c). An ice lollipop can be made by freezing a tongue depressor into a cup of water. The ice pop is removed from the cup and held by the stick for application. Ice massage is effective for reducing local pain, inflammation, and swelling and stopping muscle spasms.

Compressor Units with Controls

Compressor units cool a fluid that is circulated through a pack that is applied to the body. The packs vary in size. A mat can be used for a general application. (These are employed for the control of high fever.) A smaller pack can be used for local application to an extremity. The temperature can be controlled by adjusting the controls on the unit. These units are relatively expensive and most commonly found in institutions that treat a large number of traumatic injuries.

Vapocoolant Sprays

Fluori-Methane is bottled under pressure and used as a vasocoolant spray. When sprayed on the skin, it evaporates very quickly, causing rapid cooling of the skin. It is an effective topical anesthetic used for trigger-point therapy and increasing the stretch in muscles. Caution must be used to avoid freezing the skin.

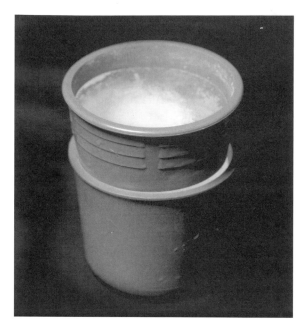

Figure 14.7a
Commercial ice cups are available.

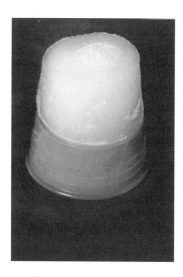

Figure 14.7b
When the ice is removed from the mold, a handle frozen into the ice protects the therapist's hand from the cold.

Figure 14.7c
Hold the bottom portion of the cup and apply ice massage.

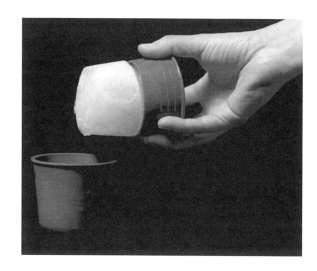

CONTRAST HEAT AND COLD

The alternating application of heat and cold is one of the most effective methods of increasing local circulation. Contrasting hot and cold cause an alternating vasodilation and vasoconstriction of the blood vessels in an area. Increased local circulation relieves stiffness and pain due to trauma and stimulates healing of injury and wounds.

Contrast baths require two tubs, one filled with hot water (105° to 110°F) and one with ice water. First, immerse the body part in the hot water for 3 to 5 minutes or until the client becomes accustomed to the hot water (until the water no longer feels hot). Remove the limb from the hot water and place it in the ice water for 30 seconds to 2 minutes or until the client becomes accustomed to the cold water. While the client is in the cold bath, add hot water to the hot bath to bring it back up to temperature. Repeat the procedure three to six times, finishing with a cold application. Always complete the treatment with a soak in the cold tub.

HYDROTHERAPY

Hydrotherapy (**HIGH**-dro-ther-uh-pee) is the application of water in any of its three forms (solid, liquid, vapor) to the body for therapeutic purposes. When properly used with body massage, hydrotherapy is an additional aid to the healthy functioning of the body.

Water has certain properties that make it a valuable therapeutic agent. It is readily available and relatively inexpensive to use. It has the ability to absorb and conduct heat. In its solid form as ice, it can be used as an effective cooling agent; in its vapor form, it can be used for facials and steam baths; and in its liquid state it can be used for sprays and immersion baths.

The temperature of water affects the body; therefore, it is important to understand how water temperature relates to body temperature. The normal temperature of the human body is 98.6°F or 37°C. The boiling point of water is 212°F or 100°C. The freezing point of water is 32°F or 0°C. Obviously we must not use water of too high or too low a temperature because it would be injurious to body tissues. Water temperatures above that of the body (98.6°F) are considered to be hot. Water that is slightly below normal body temperature is medium to warm (about 92° to 96°F). Water that is about 70° to 80°F is considered to be cool; and at 55°F and lower, it is considered cold.

Changes in the body as a result of hydrotherapy are classified as thermal, mechanical, and chemical. Thermal effects of water are produced by the application of water at temperatures above or below that of the body. This is done by way of baths, wraps, and packs that raise or lower the temperature of the body. Mechanical effects are produced by the pressure exerted on the surface of the body by sprays, whirlpool baths, and friction. Chemical effects are produced by drinking water as an aid to digestion and elimination.

To use hydrotherapy effectively, the following supplies and equipment are needed:

- Bathtubs and showers
- Running hot and cold water
- Spray attachments
- Bath thermometer
- Towels, bath blankets, bath brushes, sponges, loofahs, bath mitts, and the like
- A slab usually of marble or simulated material
- A resting couch and blanket or other covering
- A robe and slippers for the client

Bath Accessories

Soap, bath salts, oils, powders, and effervescent tablets are preparations that may be used during the bath. Soap is used for its cleansing action on

bath
is a practice where the body is surrounded by water or vapor.

sprays
are the projection of one or more streams of water against the body.

sponging
is the application of a liquid to the body by means of a sponge, cloth, or the hand.

tonic friction
is the application of friction to the body with cold water so as to produce a stimulating effect.

shampoo
is a cleansing measure accomplished with water and soap.

whirlpool
is a tub equipped with a powerful jet that causes the water to swirl around the occupant.

jacuzzi®
is a tub equipped with multiple jets that cause the water to move in multiple directions.

hot tub
is a tub with a heating device that may have jets and may or may not be large enough to accommodate several occupants.

the body. Bath salts increase the cleansing action of soap, especially in hard water. Bath oils also tend to increase the cleansing action of soap. Effervescent tablets produce bubbles of carbon dioxide gas that have a mild stimulating effect on the body. Dusting powders, body oils, and moisturizing lotions are used after the bath. Dusting powders impart fragrance and aid in drying the body. Body oils and moisturizing lotions help to lubricate the skin and replace natural oils lost during bathing.

Water Treatments

The various procedures used in hydrotherapy may be classified as follows:

1. **Baths:** Practices whereby the body is surrounded by water or vapor, such as in a whirlpool bath, tub bath, or steam bath

2. **Sprays:** The projection of one or more streams of water against the body, such as a shower or needle spray

3. **Sponging:** The application of a liquid to the body by means of a sponge, a cloth, or the hand

4. **Tonic friction:** The application of friction to the body with cold water so as to produce a stimulating or tonic effect

5. **Shampoos:** Cleansing measures accomplished with water and soap, such as a Swedish shampoo

6. **Whirlpool, Jacuzzi®, hot tubs:** These are usually large tubs equipped with jets or agitators that cause the water to flow in different directions. The main benefit derived from this type of bath or water treatment is relaxation

7. **Special water treatments:** The use of compresses, packs, and fomentations

Contraindications for Hydrotherapy

Water treatments that involve hot or cold applications should not be given when the client has cardiac impairment, diabetes, lung disease, kidney infection, extremely high or low blood pressure, or an infectious skin condition. The client's physician should be consulted when any questionable condition exists.

Body Reactions to Water Treatments

Water treatments are based on the simple physical property of water; namely, that heat, cold, or pressure can be conveyed to many blood vessels and nerves in the skin. The effects of water on the body vary according to the temperature and duration of the treatment and whether the application is general or local in character. The circulation of the blood and the sensations produced by the many nerve endings in the skin can be greatly influenced by skillfully applied water treatments.

special water treatments

use of compresses, packs, and fomentations.

The average temperature of the skin surface is about 92°F. Water approximating the temperature of the skin has no marked effect on the body. If water at a temperature different from that of the skin is applied, it will either transfer heat or absorb heat from the body. The difference in temperature has a stimulating effect on the vast network of blood vessels and nerves. The greater the difference between the temperature of water and that of the skin, the greater the stimulating effect of the treatment.

Each water application initiates a series of predictable reactions that are the result of the body accommodating itself to the new environment. The body reaction may be either stimulating or sedating to the circulatory system, the nervous system, and the eliminatory process. The practitioner who uses hydrotherapy should be familiar with the specific effects of cold, hot, and warm applications on the body.

Effects of Cold Water

The specific effects of water applications on the body are an immediate and temporary effect or a secondary and more lasting effect. Cold applications are valuable in improving the circulation, stimulating the nerves, and awakening the functional activity of body cells. The prolonged use of cold applications has a depressing effect on the body and must be used cautiously under strict supervision.

The immediate effects of cold water applications are manifested in the following ways:

1. The skin is chilled.

2. Surface blood vessels contract, and blood is driven to the interior of the body.

3. Nerve sensitivity is reduced.

4. The functional activity of body cells slows.

As soon as the cold application is discontinued, there is a secondary and more lasting effect on the body.

1. The skin becomes warmed and relaxed.

2. The surface blood vessels expand, bringing more blood to the skin.

3. Nerve sensitivity increases.

4. Adjacent body cells are stimulated in their functional activity.

Effects of Hot Water

The immediate effect of hot water applications is to draw the blood away from the interior and bring it to the surface temporarily. Local blood vessels dilate, and circulation increases. A secondary and more lasting effect occurs after the hot application is discontinued. Then the blood goes back to the interior of the body. Long and continued hot applications increase all skin functions and cause profuse sweating. Moderately warm applications have a relaxing effect on the blood vessels, muscles, and nerves and promote the functional activity of body cells.

Generally, the skin cannot tolerate hot water having a temperature in excess of 115°F. Above that temperature, water is injurious and may cause burns. However, the skin usually can tolerate steam vapor as high as 140°F. It is important to consider the client's sensitivity and tolerance to heat or cold.

A reliable bath thermometer is required to judge water temperature accurately. The temperature reading is obtained by moving the thermometer about in the water.

Kinds of Baths

The aim of all baths is the attainment of two objectives: external cleanliness and stimulation of bodily functions.

Depending on the temperature of water, the following kinds of baths are available for use:

1. Cold bath (40° to 65°F equal to 4.4° to 18.3°C)

2. Cool bath (67° to 75°F equal to 18.3° to 23.8°C)

3. Tepid bath (85° to 95°F equal to 29.4° to 35°C)

4. Saline (salt) bath (90° to 94°F equal to 32.2° to 35.5°C)

5. Warm bath (95° to 100°F equal to 35° to 37.7°C)

6. Hot bath (100° to 115°F equal to 37.7° to 43.3°C)

7. Sitz or hip bath (either hot or cold)

Cool Baths

Whether a cold bath is beneficial depends on its duration and the state of vitality and reserve strength of the client. If after a cold bath or shower the client comes out chilly, shivering, blue-lipped, or goose-fleshed, it indicates that her body reaction is not good. For the client who experiences a pleasant reaction and a feeling of warmth, the cold bath may be safely continued. A short cold bath or cold sponging of the body may be better tolerated if it is accompanied by friction and gentle rubbing with a rough towel.

The average time exposure for a cold bath or shower should be limited to between 3 to 5 minutes.

A cool bath provides a satisfactory temperature for all-around bathing, particularly during warm weather. A tepid (slightly warm) bath exerts a soothing and relaxing effect on the body and is recommended for nervous and excitable people.

Saline (Salt) Bath

A saline (salt) bath, at a temperature of 90° to 94°F, produces a marked tonic effect by stimulating the circulation. The effect is similar to natural bathing in sea water. The amount of common salt to use is 3 to 5 pounds to a tub of water. The client is left in the saline bath for 10 to 20 minutes.

Hot or Warm Baths

A warm or hot bath quiets tired nerves, soothes aching muscles, and helps to relieve insomnia. A cool shower should generally follow a warm bath because it forces some of the blood away from the skin, closes the pores, and leaves the body in a refreshed condition.

The warm or hot bath induces relaxation and relieves nervous tension. To accustom the body to the high temperature, first fill the tub with warm water. Have the client get in the warm tub, then gradually add hot water until the desired temperature is reached. The average time for hot baths or showers should range from 5 to 20 minutes. The following safety precautions should also be observed by the practitioner:

- Take the wrist pulse before and during the hot bath.
- Give the client water to drink during the hot bath.
- If the client complains of unpleasant reactions, place cold compresses over the forehead or on the back of the neck.

Very hot baths as well as very cold baths should be used only for clients who are in a healthy condition and who can withstand such treatments. For those clients whose health is not in the best condition, injurious effects may be produced. The hot bath or shower may give undue stimulation to the body and may overwork the heart. A cold bath or shower, on the other hand, is a tremendous shock to the nervous system.

Sitz or Hip Bath

The sitz or hip bath is applied only to the hips and pelvic region of the body, which is kept immersed in either hot, tepid, or cold water, or alternately hot and cold water. For a hot sitz bath, 5 to 10 minutes' contact is usually sufficient. The time for a cold sitz bath varies from 3 to 5 minutes. The effects of a sitz bath depend primarily on the temperature of the water and its length of contact with the body. Generally, the sitz bath is given as a stimulant to the pelvic region. The temperature of the hot sitz is usually 105° to 110°F.

Besides being effective in overcoming chronic constipation, sitz baths are also beneficial for the kidneys, bladder, and sex organs.

A large basin or bathtub is suitable for a sitz bath. The bath is prepared by filling the basin or tub with water (of the correct temperature) to about a depth of 6 inches or enough to immerse the client's buttocks comfortably. When using a basin (the feet outside), a blanket should be placed around the feet for warmth and a towel can be placed under the knees for added comfort. The client sits in such a manner that the buttocks and upper thighs are immersed.

Cabinet Bath

Bath cabinets are also known as vapor or steam cabinets. As used in body massage treatments, they are constructed in an upright or reclining position to accommodate the client's body while leaving the head exposed. When in operation, heat is generated, and warm, moist air surrounds the client's body. The heat, besides having a relaxing effect on the client, induces profuse perspiration. The intensity and duration of the heat can be controlled by a switch for low, medium, or high heat and by an automatic time clock. The manufacturer's instructions are the most reliable guide for the proper use and care of the bath cabinet.

Not all clients react the same way to the cabinet bath. Knowing the condition and tolerance of the client is of assistance in controlling the temperature and duration of this treatment. A client in a weakened or nervous condition should be given gentle treatments of short duration until improvement is shown. Always consult a physician before administering cabinet baths for a client with a systemic disorder such as heart trouble, high blood pressure, or any severe illness.

Length of Treatment

The exposure time in a cabinet bath ranges from 10 to 15 minutes. During this time, the practitioner should attend to the comfort and safety of the client and not to her reactions to the heat treatment. The client's heat tolerance will be greater if there is a gradual rise in the temperature of the bath cabinet. Postpone treatment if the client is ill, has an abnormal pulse or body temperature, and reacts unfavorably to the treatment.

The heat treatment induces profuse perspiration. To replace the fluids lost and to prevent body weakness, the practitioner should give the client water to drink at periodic intervals. If the client complains of a headache or a throbbing in the head during the treatment, cold compresses can be applied.

Following the cabinet bath, a mild tonic such as a tepid shower may be given. After this treatment, keep the client warmly wrapped to prevent chilling of the body (Figure 14.8).

WHIRLPOOL BATH

A whirlpool bath is a partial immersion bath in which the water is agitated to produce a slight pressure on the body. A whirlpool bath is beneficial to circulation, soothing to the muscles, and relaxing to the nerves. Whirlpool baths are often used by physicians as

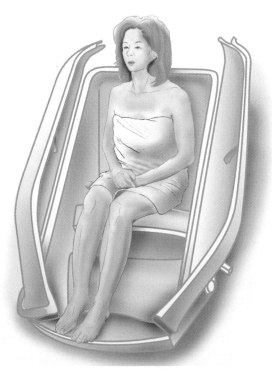

Figure 14.8
Client sitting in a vapor cabinet bath.

part of physical therapy for conditions such as arthritis, sprains, strained muscles, and relief of pain. The following supplies and equipment are needed:

1. Whirlpool tub

2. Bath mats and towels

3. Robe and sandals (disposable paper sandals)

4. Lotion or oil

5. Bath thermometer

6. Ice bag (optional)

7. Material for cold compress, if needed

8. Tank suits for women and trunks for men

Procedure

1. Fill the whirlpool tub to the recommended depth and test the temperature. Generally, the most desirable temperature is about 105° to 110°F, but the bath may be cooler.

2. Add the recommended antiseptic agents to the water.

3. Instruct the client in how to enter the tub safely.

4. The treatment time is usually about 15 to 30 minutes.

5. Instruct the client about rest period, showers, and drying off.

6. Complete the client's records noting benefits, reactions, effects, and the like.

7. Be sure the tub is sanitized thoroughly before it is used again.

RELAXING NEUTRAL TUB BATH

The neutral tub bath is basically for relaxation and has a sedative effect. The body is immersed in a tub of water at a neutral temperature (about 94° to 98°F) for about 15 to 25 minutes. The following supplies and equipment are needed:

1. Bathtub and bath thermometer

2. Bath towels and mat

3. Shower cap, robe, and slippers for client

4. Bath oil and lotion

5. Bath sheets

6. Compress cloth and basin of cool water

7. Air pillow and towel

Procedure

1. Check the room temperature to be sure it is comfortable for the client.

2. Instruct the client regarding bathing and dressing procedures.

3. Fill the tub to the appropriate level.

4. Test the temperature of the water to be sure it is comfortable. A recommended range is 94° to 98°F.

5. Assist the client into the tub, and place an air pillow or towel underneath her head.

6. Cover the client's body with a large towel or bath sheet.

7. Allow the client to relax for 15 to 25 minutes. Warm water may be added, if desired.

8. Assist the client out of the tub, and dry her body with a towel while applying light friction.

9. Supply the client with robe and slippers.

10. Allow the client time to rest. Complete the client's records, noting benefits of the bath or any adverse reactions. Be sure the tub is sanitized thoroughly before the next bath.

RUSSIAN BATH

The Russian bath is a full-body steam bath for the purpose of causing perspiration. The primary benefits are cleansing, relaxation, and improved metabolism. The following supplies and equipment are needed:

1. Steam room with a slab or bench for reclining

2. Padding and bath sheet for slab

3. Towels for neck and protection

4. Air pillow with a towel to cover

5. Shower cap to protect hair

6. Robe and slippers

7. Compress cloth and basin of cool water

8. Pitcher and glass of drinking water

9. Appropriate product to add to the bath

Procedure

1. Prepare the steam room for the desired temperature. Usually this is 110° to 140°F.

2. Take and record the client's pulse and temperature.

3. Have the client lie on the slab. Adjust the pillow underneath the client's head.

4. Cover the client with a large towel or bath sheet.

5. Apply a cool compress to the client's head, if desired.

6. Check the client's pulse as necessary.

7. Give client instructions about drinking water during treatment.

8. Allow the client to relax for 5 to 15 minutes.

9. Instruct the client to shower in a warm to cool shower following the steam bath.

10. Assist the client in drying off following the steam bath.

11. Allow the client to rest following the treatment.

QUESTIONS FOR DISCUSSION AND REVIEW

1. What precautions should be observed when using any electrical apparatus?

2. What are the effects of the application of heat?

3. Define *cryotherapy*.

4. What are the effects of the local application of ice?

5. What does the acronym RICE stand for and how is it used?

6. What is a contrast bath?

7. What is the main effect of a contrast bath?

8. Define *hydrotherapy*.

9. How are the effects of water treatments controlled?

10. What are the qualities of water that make it a valuable therapeutic tool?

11. Describe the three classifications of the effects hydrotherapy has on the body.

12. What are the contraindications for performing hydrotherapy?

13. In which three ways are cold applications beneficial?

14. When are cold applications undesirable?

15. What are the benefits of hot water applications?

16. How high a temperature can the skin safely tolerate?

17. What are the two objectives of baths?

18. What is the temperature of a warm bath? A hot bath?

19. What is the average duration of a cold bath, cold shower, or cold sitz bath?

20. What is the average duration of a hot saline or sitz bath?

21. What is the purpose of the cabinet bath?

22. What safety precautions should be observed during the operation of a bath cabinet?

23. What are the main benefits of a whirlpool bath?

24. What is a Russian bath and what are its benefits?

Massage in the Spa Setting
by Steve Capellini

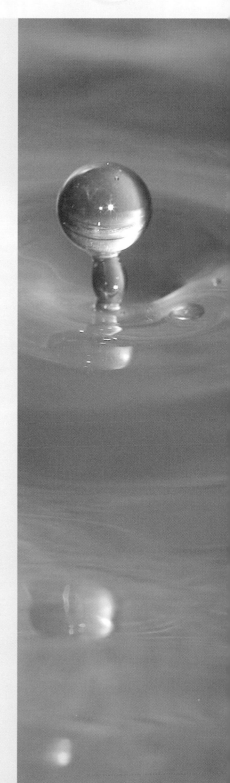

LEARNING OBJECTIVES

After you have mastered this chapter, you will be able to:

1. Describe the historical development of spas.

2. Describe the current state of the spa industry, including customer demographics and the various types of spas in which therapists work.

3. List and describe the most popular spa services performed by massage therapists.

4. Describe the most important attributes of an effective spa massage.

5. Demonstrate an ability to perform a spa exfoliation procedure and a spa body wrap procedure.

6. Describe the specialized hydrotherapy equipment and other apparatuses used in modern spas.

7. List and describe the qualities that make a massage therapist a good candidate for hiring by a spa, including customer service and other non–massage-related skills.

8. Describe the job potentials for massage therapists in spas, including possible career paths over time.

INTRODUCTION—WHAT IS SPA?

According to the International Spa Association (ISPA), a spa is a facility that is "devoted to enhancing overall well-being through a variety of professional services that encourage the renewal of mind, body and spirit." This official definition encapsulates much of what spa owners, operators, and employees attempt to do for their clients every day. Although some consumers continue to think of spas as places to indulge superficial pleasures and receive pampering services, and some spas continue to promote themselves as such, there is a growing trend toward recognizing the therapeutic and even life-changing value that spas can offer.

International Spa Association (ISPA)

is a professional organization consisting of member spas, owners, directors, technicians, consultants, writers, marketers, and suppliers of products and equipment who meet at conventions and roundtables to create standards, share information, and chart directions for the development of the spa industry worldwide. (ISPA, 2365 Harrodsburg Road, Suite A325, Lexington, KY 40504, (888) 651-4772, www.experienceispa.com)

Spas are as diverse as the people who run them. Some are rustic retreats situated in nature, with a heavy emphasis on diet, internal cleansing, and physical fitness (Figure 15.1). Others are chic, modern facilities located in the heart of urban centers, offering the latest in high-tech skin care (Figure 15.2). There are large spas, with hundreds of employees, and tiny spas operated by just one person. Some spas have hundreds of thousands of dollars worth of hydrotherapy equipment; others have no such equipment at all. There are spas that offer psychological counseling, medical screening, shamanic vision-questing, Watsu®, team building, Turkish bathing rituals, rock climbing, tennis clinics, cooking classes, weight loss, skiing, women's retreats, and much more.

In recent years, spas have become specialized, with certain facilities featuring specific offerings and catering to specific audiences. These will be explained later in "The State of the Spa Industry Today." All this specialization has made education a priority in the spa industry for two reasons. First, the public needs to be educated regarding spas in order to make the best choice for themselves when choosing a spa experience. Second, spa employees and potential employees need to be educated on the ever-growing number of modalities and special services available in order to perform them in a safe and effective manner.

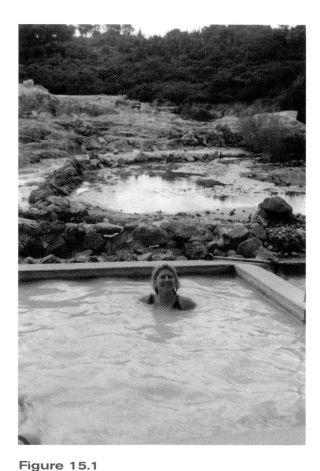

Figure 15.1

Some spas are rustic and natural like this one in Rotorua, New Zealand. (Reprinted with permission from Spas Research Fellowship.)

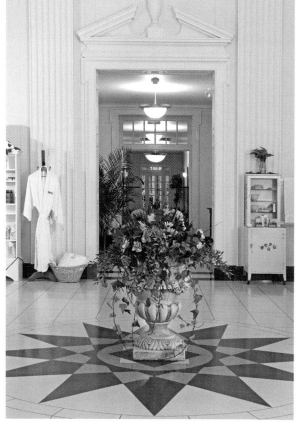

Figure 15.2

Some spas are modern and luxurious. (Courtesy of Roosevelt Baths, Saratoga Springs, NY.)

The underlying factor that ties such a diverse group of facilities together can be discovered in that ISPA definition: spas (and the people who work in them) are devoted to enhancing overall well-being through a variety of professional services. It takes both devotion and skill to perform the professional services expected in a spa. In this chapter, you learn about these skills, and you discover what will be expected of you if you embark upon a career in the spa industry. What will you need to know? Which services will you be expected to perform? How many massages will you be expected to do? What non-massage skills will be important to your success? How difficult is it to get a job in a spa, and how realistic is it for you to open your own spa some day?

Spas represent the modern incarnation of a long line of healing and wellness facilities used by humans for millennia. A good place to start your exploration of the spa world, then, is in its historical roots.

A BRIEF HISTORY OF SPA

The origins of the word *spa* itself offer clues to a very important aspect of the spa experience—water. Water is the essence of many spa services. It is the environment in which much of the healing and rejuvenation at spas takes place. We know from archaeological studies and written accounts that the earliest spas were often found at the source of a natural spring or, in the case of the ancient Romans, at sites to which such water was redirected via aqueducts. So what exactly does the word *spa* mean? By most accounts, it is an acronym, which is a word formed by putting together the first letters of other words. In this case, they are the Latin words *sanitas per aqua*. Several variations on the Latin have been cited, but they all mean the same thing, "health through water." The term might also have derived from the Latin verb *spagere,* which means to sprinkle or flow, like a fountain or spring.

Greek and Roman Roots

Both the ancient Athenian Greeks and Romans were, as a group, serious about bathing, and this is where much of the Western world's spa tradition began. During the height of the Roman empire, for instance, the average citizen used 300 gallons of water per day, compared with just 50 gallons per day for the modern American. The baths were very important, not just for cleansing, but for health, fitness, and as a social gathering place. The larger baths could accommodate thousands of people (Figure 15.3). Poetry was read in the baths; political discussions took place; and, of course, there was massage. Patrons progressed through a series of rooms warmed to different temperatures by a great fire kept raging below the stone floors of the building in a furnacelike room called the hypocaust.

These early baths were expensive to construct and maintain, but the rulers of the day, the Roman emperors, looked upon them as a way to impress the people with their generosity and greatness. The entry fee was

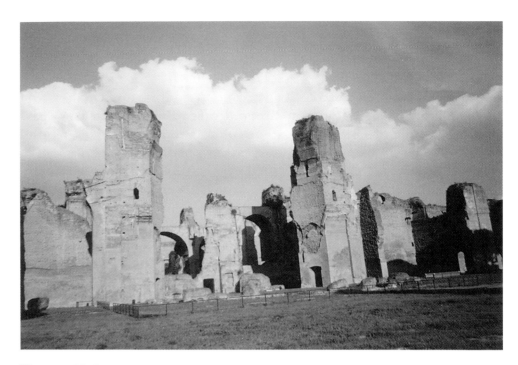

Figure 15.3

Ruins of the ancient Roman baths, or thermae, known as Caracalla. (Reprinted with permission from Spas Research Fellowship.)

kept very low, so almost all citizens could attend the baths. The labor, and even the massage, was provided by slaves.

As Roman civilization spread, so too did the use of the baths. Many Roman outposts were built at the site of a spring so that a bath could be constructed there, as occurred from northern Africa all the way to England. Many of these locations still feature spas today, and some, like Bath in England, have undergone extensive recent renovations.

Turkish Hammam

hammam
(also spelled hamam), a Turkish steam bath with elaborate cleansing, exfoliation, and massage rituals passed down for centuries, played an important role in Ottoman culture.

A descendant of the Roman thermae, **hammams** were a part of many mosques until they achieved an architectural and cultural significance of their own. Men and women bathe separately in the hammam, which, besides being a social center of the community, also holds spiritual significance. Often, the atmosphere inside the hot steamy main chamber where bathers are scrubbed and massaged seems more like a church than a spa, with diffused lighting and silence reigning. Some form of the hammam was incorporated by Arabic peoples for centuries. Mohammed himself, the founder of Islam, recommended sweat baths. He taught his followers that the heat in the hammam, which in Arabic means "spreader of warmth," improved fertility, and he wanted his flock to be fruitful and multiply.

Western nations, including England and the United States, have imported the concept of the hammam, which they called Turkish baths, with varying degrees of success. The concept has never become anywhere near as widespread as it is in Turkey and several other parts of the Islamic world, where it is interwoven with the daily lives of most people.

Asian Spa Roots

Through the centuries, people in Asia have given natural hot springs particular significance in their lives. Some cultures even considered them sacred, as in Japan, where the springs became known as **Onsen** and were used for communal bathing, personal renewal, and meditation. Onsen are always found in natural outdoor settings. They feature baths of varying temperature and treatments including massage and hydrotherapy. The Japanese treat them as more than a simple vacation; they regard them as spiritual retreats, where specific customs are to be observed.

In other Asian cultures, such as in Thailand, massage and herbal therapies have been used down through the ages, passed on from one generation to the next, until today when herbal spas exist side-by-side with modern European-inspired spas in resorts and hotels.

Onsen
are Japanese hot springs at the site of natural volcanic springwater, usually with massage and other relaxing therapies available.

bania
is a Russian-style communal steam bath.

European Spas

Europe has a long tradition of spas and spa therapy, beginning with the expansion of Roman culture as previously mentioned. Baden Baden and Bad Wörishofen in Germany, Montecatini and Terme di Saturnia in Italy, Bath in England, and the town of Spa in Belgium are all examples of centuries-old spas. Czechoslovakia, Hungary, Bulgaria, and several other European countries also have a history of spa culture. The locales where these spas operate are still known today as "spa towns" (Figure 15.4). They owe their existence to the water source and the therapies that were applied there. In addition, the Finns are famous for their saunas and the Russians for their **banias,** but these are not full-fledged spa facilities as we have come to think of them.

For many years, Europeans have gone to spas to "take the cure." In fact, the German word *kur* came to be synonymous with spa in the 1800s when Sebastian Kneipp christened his new healing system by that name. His techniques centered upon hydrotherapy

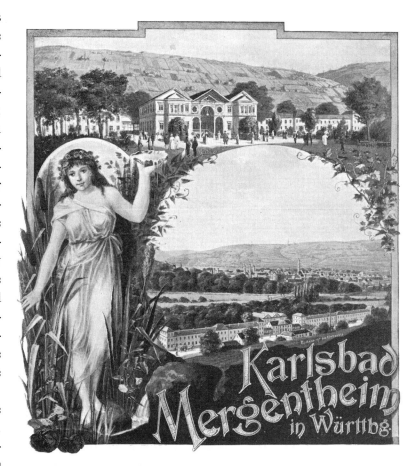

Figure 15.4

Advertisement for an early European spa in a typical spa town, Karlsbad, Germany. (Reprinted with permission from Spas Research Fellowship.)

using heat, cold, and immersions, plus herbs, exercise, and proper diet, which morphed over the years into some of our modern spa therapies and philosophies.

In Europe, spa philosophy always has been and continues to be more remedial and medically oriented than spa philosophy in the New World. Many European health plans pay for spa visits and spa treatments. Spa goers are likely to be prescribed a regime by medical personnel on staff at the spa. This regime may include multiple immersions in therapeutic waters and even the ingestion of mineral-laden springwaters in an attempt to improve physical conditions. More recently, some European spas have included the fitness and esthetic offerings of American spas, but at the same time, they have maintained their original dedication to medical treatments.

Early America

On the North American continent, hot springs have been revered as sacred healing retreats for centuries. Native Americans often set these places apart and agreed not to fight or hunt there. Native Americans also created their own early spas by pouring water over heated stones in small enclosures known as **sweat lodges** or **kivas.**

During the nineteenth and early twentieth centuries, spalike health retreats were built in many areas, most notably Hot Springs, Arkansas (Figure 15.5); White Sulphur Springs, West Virginia; and Saratoga, New

---

sweat lodge

is a Native American enclosure for sweating, cleansing, and purification, in which participants pour water over heated stones in ceremonial fashion to create heat while praying and chanting.

---

kiva

is an underground chamber used by the Pueblo tribe of Indians for ceremonial sweats and other rituals.

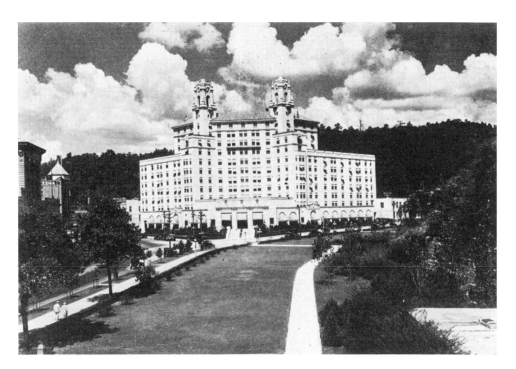

Figure 15.5

U.S. health spas or sanatoriums like the ones in Hot Springs, Arkansas, were popular early in the twentieth century and drew thousands of people to fancy new hotels like the Majestic. (Reprinted with permission from Spas Research Fellowship.)

York. John Harvey Kellogg also opened the Battle Creek Sanatorium in Michigan. Typical treatments administered at the early hot springs health spas always included a soak in the mineral pools (Figure 15.6), which became very popular. Saratoga Springs, for example, was first introduced in its natural state to white settlers by Native Americans in the 1700s, and by the early 1900s, it was accommodating thousands of visitors a day in extensive facilities.

Spa-going underwent a decline in popularity in the early to mid-twentieth century when most such activity was confined to weight loss visits to "fat farms." As the 1900s progressed, however, these facilities gave way to more modern spa ventures that focused on holistic health, fitness, diet, and overall well-being. The first such spa was the Golden Door in California, which opened in the late 1950s. Since that time, spas have continued to expand and modernize their offerings and facilities.

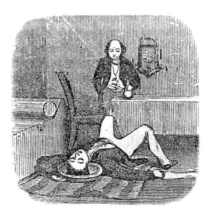

THE HEAD-BATH.

Figure 15.6

The head bath was used in sanatoriums to treat "all acute diseases about the head." (Reprinted with permission from Spas Research Fellowship.)

The State of the Spa Industry Today

The spa industry today is a dynamic and ever-changing segment of the economy that has seen tremendous growth over the past 20 years. Officially part of the **hospitality industry,** spas provide extremely specialized services that set them apart from other choices when consumers are deciding where to spend their discretionary income. More and more people are seeing the benefit of these services, as evidenced by the rising tide in spas and spa-going recently. The total number of U.S. spas almost quintupled from 1995 to 2004, rising from 2,674 to 12,102 (the statistics in this section are quoted from the International Spa Association's 2004 Spa Industry Profile). People paid a total of 136 million visits to spas in 2004, spending $11.2 billion. Of the spa body services performed, massage therapy remains by far the most popular, with about 60 percent of all spa guests receiving a massage treatment.

In 2003 and 2004, the spa industry experienced a leveling out of this quick expansion, and many experts now believe that it is entering a new phase of moderate growth. Though the number of facilities is still increasing, overall spa revenues and the total number of spa employees is not exploding any more. Spa owners and directors have begun to catch their collective breath and are now focusing on improving the quality of their workforce and their offerings for an increasingly experienced and demanding audience. Accordingly, the need for qualified, well-trained personnel continues to be strong.

Although spa customers come from many different backgrounds, certain groups are more likely to visit a spa than others. Over 70 percent of visitors, for example, are female. The average age is around 40, so the clientele tends to be mature, slightly older than the typical age for those who receive massage therapy outside the spa setting, which is around 30 years old. Income and education are also determining factors, with the average spa goer reporting an income of over $70,000 and over half of them holding college degrees.

> **hospitality industry**
>
> is the combined hotel, resort, restaurant, and entertainment industries that rely especially upon customer service and professional hospitality for their success.

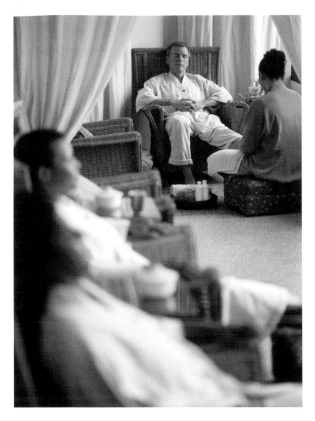

Figure 15.7

Spas are attracting an ever-growing number of male clients.

A number of trends continue to shape the character of the spa landscape. According to Susie Ellis, president of Spa Finders, in 2005 these trends included:

1. Weight loss: The number one reason that people list for making a spa visit is to get healthier and slim down.

2. Luxury: Spas represent the height of luxury, and people are willing to pay for a special luxurious experience at a spa, even if it is once in a lifetime.

3. Mother/daughter: People are looking for ways to include friends and loved ones in their spa experiences, and those spas that make it easy with special packages such as mother/daughter retreats can increase their business. Even children and teens are being taught the benefits of spa-going, and it is not unusual to encounter youthful clients in many spas that offer a family emphasis.

4. Men: Although spas are more popular with women, they are attracting an ever-growing number of men as well. Spas cater to a mere 30 percent male audience, but that still signifies over $3 billion in sales to men per year (Figure 15.7).

Types of Modern Spas

Spas encompass a wide array of businesses, offering their customers many choices, in much the same way that restaurants offer people choices in price, menu, service, and ambience. Although each spa is unique, spas can be categorized into six major types: destination spas, hotel/resort spas, day spas, club spas, medical/dental spas, and mineral spring spas. See Table 15.1 for more information about each type.

Spas in all these categories, of course, are "devoted to enhancing overall well-being through a variety of professional services that encourage the renewal of mind, body, and spirit." This is their commonality. Yet they attract a diverse clientele and present a wide range of philosophies and methods. The following two examples highlight the broad spectrum of offerings.

Canyon Ranch Spa: Many therapists would consider it a dream job to work for Canyon Ranch, one of the best known destination spas in the world. The spa was founded in 1979 by Mel Zuckerman, a businessman in Tucson, Arizona. He was successful but overweight and unhealthy, like so many people who lead sedentary, high-stress lifestyles. A trip to a California spa offered him and his wife a new vision, and they hoped to offer that same vision to guests at their new spa. The operation grew rapidly, expanded to a new location in Massachusetts in the 1980s,

Table 15.1

Types of Spas

TYPE OF SPA	APPROX. 2004 U.S. #	DESCRIPTION	LOCATION	CLIENTELE
Destination Spa	191	Facility with overnight accommodations catering exclusively to spa guests, often featuring advanced modalities and elaborate signature services in beautiful surroundings	Usually a separate building or compound with several buildings set apart from neighboring businesses or residences	High discretionary income individuals or couples willing to spend $2,500 to $6,000/week on health and wellness
Hotel/Resort Spa	1,662	Spa facilities located within a larger encompassing hotel, or resort, or cruise ship. The spa can be a main feature of the property or simply an amenity for guests to use at their leisure, offering a wide array of treatments, some rivaling those at destination spas	All major resorts and high-end hotels include spas with their new properties or add them to existing properties in order to compete effectively; spas rate high by consumers on list of requested hotel features	Families, couples; medium- to high-income range; either dedicated spa goers or casual vacationers; often one partner will spa while the other golfs, plays tennis, etc.
Day Spa	8,734	A spa where guests visit for a few hours or a day, with no sleepover accommodations available. These spas range from small one-person operations to full-blown centers offering treatments on a par with the large resorts	Often situated within a hair salon; can be a storefront, stand-alone building, a single multipurpose room, part of a massage clinic, in a shopping mall, or even in airports	Day spas cater to a wide array of individuals of many social classes, from low-medium to high-income levels who prize proximity, affordability, and personalized service
Club Spa	706	Spas that are part of a larger physical fitness facility, ranging from a minor addition to a major focus of the business	Many upscale urban fitness clubs consider it essential to include a spa, especially multipurpose lifestyle clubs	Physically active individuals who prize optimal performance and appearance; medium to medium-high income range
Medical/Dental Spa	471	Medical/dental spas are either dedicated spa facilities that operate in conjunction with a nearby medical practice or are incorporated into the actual practice, always under the supervision of a medical professional	Can be located at a wellness retreat center, at a resort, in a stand-alone building, or as part of an existing medical/dental practice	Ranging from high-income individuals willing to pay extra for personalized medical services in a comfortable environment to everyday patients at medical/dental offices given extra attention with or without spa services in a spalike setting
Mineral Springs Spa	338	Spas located at the actual source of mineral springs and incorporating these waters into their program and treatments	Can be a stand-alone destination-style spa or can be located within a resort built on the mineral spring property, often in rural settings, ranging from rustic to high end	A wide range, from weekend family vacationers at rustic spring sites to five-star hotel goers on gourmet retreats

opened its first SpaClub at the Venetian Resort in Las Vegas in the 1990s, and continues to grow rapidly today, with a Canyon Ranch spa aboard the *Queen Mary II* cruise ship, a healthy lifestyle community in Florida called Canyon Ranch Living, another resort spa near Orlando, and much more. The spa has become a global brand, attracting thousands of the most affluent and well-traveled people in the world. Its staff of medical doctors, psychologists, fitness experts, nutritionists, bodyworkers, chefs, and hospitality specialists cater to people who pay thousands of dollars a week. This is definitely the high end of what spas represent today.

Joy Spring Day Spa: Spas need not be grand ventures backed by multimillionaire investors. Tiny spas can offer the same level of service and therapeutic value as the large spas like Canyon Ranch. One such spa was Joy Spring. Owned and operated by just one woman, Joy Spring was situated in a trendy California coastal town for many years. The owner has since sold her spa to eventually open another location in Los Angeles, and her future is looking bright. The waiting room at Joy Spring consisted of two chairs and a single bookshelf in an area the size of a closet. But there was a little water fountain there, and a sense of calm. The small selection of books and gift items on the shelf was carefully chosen and arranged in an appealing way. Inside the treatment area was a steam cabinet, a massage table, and not too much else. When clients spent time in that room, however, they felt as if the rest of the world disappeared (Figure 15.8).

Both Canyon Ranch and Joy Spring have the right to call themselves spas, because spas

---

SPA MYTHS VERSUS SPA REALITY

Myth: You will be expected to do 10 massages in a row without a break.

Reality: Though a very small number of insensitive spa owners still try to force the maximum work out of their therapists, the trend today is to take care of therapists. A burned-out staff is not good for customer relations. Five or 6 services per day, often with a 10- to 15-minute break between sessions, is the normal maximum. Also, spa modalities such as body scrubs and wraps are not as hard on therapists' bodies.

continues

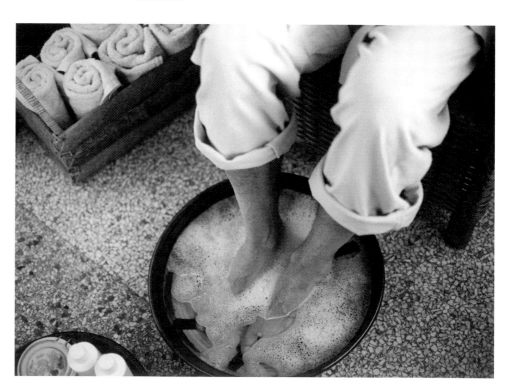

Figure 15.8

Even small spas can become luxurious using simple items such as a basin to soak the feet.

can be so many things for so many people. Regardless of the size of the operation or the breadth of offerings found there, a spa's success or failure will usually be determined by the quality of the therapeutic interaction between one guest and one therapist at a time. Canyon Ranch owner Mel Zuckerman was aware of this, and that is why he signed himself up for a massage and an herbal wrap every day during the first year of business in order to keep the emphasis where it belonged—on the treatments.

MASSAGE IN THE SPA INDUSTRY—FORMING REALISTIC EXPECTATIONS

The prospect of working in a spa, large or small, may seem daunting at first because there are so many variables involved, so many questions to ask. Through the influence of the media, gossip, or sheer lack of information, some students and beginning therapists form incomplete or misguided perceptions about what it is like to work in a spa. These perceptions spread through the massage community, making it nearly impossible to tell myth from reality. Some of the most common misperceptions circulating about the spa industry are listed in the accompanying sidebar "Spa Myths versus Spa Reality."

It is important to have a realistic set of expectations about the role of massage therapists working in spas. The most relevant information that is needed in this regard can be categorized into three main topics:

1. What you will be expected to do
2. What you will be expected to know
3. How you will be expected to act

The following sections explore these three essentials of spa work in order to help therapists envision their potential role in the industry.

SPA MYTHS VERSUS SPA REALITY—CONT'D

Myth: The only kind of massage done in spas is pampering massage.
Reality: Many spas offer advanced bodywork modalities on their menus, including craniosacral, neuromuscular, myofascial, and more. In some cases, training in these techniques is even provided and paid for by the spa.
Myth: Therapists are always poorly paid in spas.
Reality: Though it is true that spas have high overhead costs and must try to keep their expenses down, therapists still typically make $20 to $40/hour, with no overhead expenses of their own.
Myth: Only unmotivated or unskilled therapists work in spas.
Reality: Many highly motivated and skilled therapists work in spas. Some find it optimal to let the spa take care of business while they focus on therapy, content to remain in that relationship for many years. Others quickly move up to become supervisors, trainers, lead therapists, and directors. Some therapists pursue other goals while working in the spa, using it as a career stepping-stone.
Myth: You cannot perform in-depth work over a period of time in spas because the clientele is constantly changing.
Reality: Roughly three fourths of all locations are day spas or club spas with a local, repeat clientele. Even at resort and destination spas, therapists can work with clients repeatedly during their stay or even during return visits.

MASSAGE PRACTICE IN THE SPA SETTING

First and foremost in the spa come your duties as a massage therapist. Massage is what you have trained for and what you have been hired to do. Therefore, it is natural for a newly hired therapist to feel that all she need do to successfully fulfill her duties is to get behind that closed door as quickly as possible and begin the massage. When practicing massage in a spa, however, therapists need to remain aware that they are operating within a larger structure that encompasses and helps to define what it is they are doing in the treatment room.

Each spa has developed its own particular protocols and standards when it comes to implementing massage on their premises. In addition to massage, therapists may be required to perform several other spa modalities including body wraps; body scrubs; specialized rituals and exotic services such as **Ayurvedic** (eye-yur-VEY-dick), Indonesian, herbal detoxification treatments; and hydrotherapy baths and showers. It will be up to the therapist to master these protocols and follow them while on the job. The following points are important to keep in mind when practicing in a spa setting: scope of practice, intake procedures, optimal number of massages per day, timing of services, guest greetings, preparation, and cleanup.

Scope of Practice

The massage therapist in a spa setting is of course subject to all the same limitations to scope of practice as are massage therapists in any professional setting. Additional points to consider in a spa are these:

- Many spa guests are receiving their very first massage, and it is important to be sensitive to this. Often, it is appropriate to use extremely light pressure over the entire body at first, until a level of comfort and rapport can be established. Even if the therapist specializes in deep bodywork and is willing to share it with spa guests, the guests are often unprepared for it and may react adversely. Therapists should limit massage strokes to basic Swedish unless the guest has requested otherwise or after clear communication.

- Because people are often on a quest for better health while visiting a spa, they are especially open to suggestions about diet, nutrition, and lifestyle. It must be remembered that these are not massage therapists' areas of expertise.

- Some people visit spas in order to address long-term physical conditions, ranging from addictions to obesity to heart disease and many others. It is tempting to want to help people with these conditions, showing them how a combination of massage, detoxification, improved diet, and lifestyle offered at the spa will help heal many ills. However, it is important not to promise any benefits that cannot be substantiated or that are not sanctioned by the spa. In general, the benefits that therapists can rightfully claim for spa

---

ayurveda

is an ancient system of Indian medicine and healing; it has been modified in recent years for use in spa treatments such as body scrubs, face treatments, and massages.

services include those created by heat; special products such as herbs, clays, and seaweeds; and massage therapy (see page 694 for a list of those conditions generally relieved by massage).

● Because so many spa treatments involve the use of hot water, therapists must be thoroughly familiar with all contraindications for the use of heat.

Intake Procedures

Each spa has its own unique intake procedures. Some employ an extensive screening process that may even involve a doctor's visit, a stress test, and a thorough physical examination. Some have well-trained **intake specialists** who spend a half hour or more molding the guests' experience, recommending treatments, and gleaning much important information that therapists can use in their sessions. These facilities usually fall into the destination spa, medical spa, or mineral spa categories. Some resort and club spas have an extensive intake procedure as well. Other spas, however, have a bare-bones intake form that only asks for emergency contact information and the guest's reason for requesting massage. The majority of day spas require little screening and some require none at all.

> **intake specialists**
> also known as hospitality coordinators, spa concierges, and other titles, are spa employees who focus on pairing guests with appropriate treatments, therapists, services, and lifestyle choices during their stay at the spa.

As therapists study SOAP notes and charting during their massage education, they will no doubt see the value in these procedures, and the lack of such documentation in many spas may come as an unwelcome surprise. It is important, then, for therapists working in spas to use their own discretion when working with a guest for the first time. Whenever an intake form of any kind is available, it should be used to full advantage, and if the spa does not use one, it is permissible to ask the guest verbally about medical conditions and possible contraindications.

Some spas, especially hair and esthetics-based day spas, focus their intake questions on the skin rather than on overall health, because their main business consists of cosmetic procedures and the sale of cosmetic products. This paradigm works well for many spas. Some therapists new to the industry, however, perceive the lack of intake procedures at these spas as an insult to their therapeutic integrity, and this can lead to tension between management and massage staff. If this is the case, it is permissible for the therapist to suggest an intake procedure to spa management, but if one is not implemented, it is best for the therapist to either accept this or seek employment elsewhere rather than create ill will among the staff and guests.

Number of Massages

Because massage therapy is the most popular service in spas, it is often necessary for therapists to perform several sessions back-to-back. What this means differs from spa to spa, however. Many spas maintain a strict break of at least 15 minutes between treatments, with some going as high as 30 minutes. Other spas offer very little break at all, as little as 5 minutes, but these are increasingly rare because spa owners are seeing the benefit of keeping their employees healthy. It is not good for business to have therapists out of work and receiving worker's compensation due to carpal tunnel syndrome.

For the same reason, it is customary for spas to limit their therapists' total number of massage treatments each day. The number varies, but the norm is five massages per day. Many factors contribute to altering this number in particular spas. For example, some spas have therapists perform only two or three massages in a row, with less-taxing spa treatments interspersed throughout the day. Thus, a therapist can perform eight total treatments, but three of them may be body scrubs, wraps, or specialty services.

On-call therapists not employed full time by the spa are often called upon to perform more back-to-back services. When guest demand is at its peak, these therapists can sometimes perform eight massages or more. Attempting heroics by performing this number of full-hour sessions day after day is a sure way to cause injury. Though the lure of immediate income is strong, it is best to take a long-term point of view and pace oneself. Many therapists have enthusiastically entered the spa industry only to leave disillusioned a few short years later due to disability.

Spas that force therapists to perform too many massages, with no regard for their welfare, usually experience high turnover and lowered guest satisfaction. These spas are the least enjoyable to work for. Though there are no laws limiting the number of massages a spa can ask employees to perform, those spas that overwork their therapists soon build a poor reputation in the industry.

Over an extended period of employment at a spa, therapists find a rhythm that both satisfies guest demand and preserves their own health. This rhythm is different for each therapist, with some choosing to perform only 3 or 4 services of any kind on a given day or 20 in a given week. Others can perform several more as long as the massage services are interspersed with other spa treatments. There are a few—usually young—therapists capable of performing many massages a day for weeks on end.

Timing of Massage and Spa Services

Massage therapists sometimes find the strict time limitations imposed in the spa setting onerous. Constantly watching the clock, they feel, drains value from the massage, and the same massage given over and over again within a certain number of minutes becomes stale and rote. Therapists who work in spas need to overcome this challenge and find ways to make their work fresh within the confines of the spa's necessary structure. Meeting this challenge is the essence of giving a good **spa massage.**

Some therapists, wanting to give each guest the best service possible, habitually overrun the allotted time for each treatment, running in a per-

spa massage

is any massage given by a therapist within the structure and limitations of the spa setting, usually referring to the spa's basic Swedish massage, but also applicable to advanced modalities given in the spa.

petual state of slight delay. This can undermine the smooth running of the entire spa, from reservations to the front desk to the locker room—and, of course, it is not fair to the next guest who has arrived on time for his appointment. It is necessary to end the massage at least 5 minutes before the next treatment is scheduled to begin. Certain services such as body wraps and scrubs require more time to prepare than massage, and this needs to be taken into consideration.

If a guest arrives late to an appointment, it is the therapist's responsibility to inform him that the treatment needs to end on time and will necessarily be curtailed. If the spa allows it and no appointment is scheduled afterwards, the therapist may perform the full service. Even if both therapist and client have free time directly after the scheduled service, it is usually not a good idea to run over or intentionally give a longer treatment because guests given an extra long massage or spa service may tell other guests and cause jealousy.

Spas usually prescribe the length of each massage and spa service on their menu, and guests expect that this time will not include preparation and cleanup. Thus, a 75-minute massage is scheduled on the books in a 90-minute block, allowing for time before and after the actual hands-on treatment. The typical time frame for a full-body massage is 50 minutes at most spas, with a 75-minute extended option. It is rare for a spa to offer a 20- or 25-minute massage, unless it is localized and confined to one area, such as the neck and shoulders or the feet.

Most spas have a cancellation policy in effect and will charge guests fully or partially for skipped services. In this case, the therapist may or may not be compensated, depending upon the compensation structure and internal policies of the spa. If the therapist is paid for her time, it is her responsibility to find some productive work in the spa to fill the hour, such as stocking and tidying the treatment room, working on client notes, or cleaning.

Guest Greetings

Massage therapists generally greet their clients in a cordial manner, regardless of the setting, whether the massage takes place in a clinic, in an office, or in the client's home. Spa directors, though, expect extra cordiality from their therapists, above and beyond that rendered in other venues. Spas create high expectations among their guests, and therapists need to be aware that their actions are reflecting upon the entire operation. Some spas have a script for the greeting process, designating exactly what to say and do when meeting a guest, escorting him to the treatment room, explaining the treatment, especially draping, conversation during the treatment, and then saying good-bye. Therapists who work in one of these spas will need to memorize this script and adhere to it for the most part. More often, though, spas leave the details up to the therapist.

The following are general guidelines that apply in most spas when greeting guests:

- Shake hands firmly when first meeting, giving the guest confidence in your touch.

- Look the guest directly in the eyes for a moment to establish contact and trust.

- Speak slowly and clearly, introducing yourself with word such as, "Hello, Mrs. Reed, my name is Elaine, and I will be performing your Balinese Ritual for you today."

- Lead the way to the treatment area because the guest may be uncertain where to go.

- Explain the treatment clearly and thoroughly, including draping concerns, as many spa guests are modest and somewhat apprehensive at this stage of their spa experience.

- Do not solicit feedback from the client during the treatment other than asking about pressure and comfort.

- After the treatment, offer water, tea, or some other healthy refreshment, if the spa allows.

- Usher the guest back to the locker room or rest area, making sure he is reoriented.

- Do not solicit tips. Although tips are accepted in most spas, therapists should never directly ask for them.

Preparation and Cleanup

Massage therapists in the spa setting do not have much time to clean their treatment room after each session and prepare it for the next. Therefore, it is necessary to learn effective planning and economy of movement. The room itself should be well stocked, utilizing as much shelf space, under-table space, counter space, and cabinet space as possible in order to avoid unnecessary trips to the supply room down the hall. Also, the limited time between treatments must be used judiciously to attend to personal needs.

Therapists need to make sure that all traces of the previous client have been cleaned up before ushering the next guest into the room. This may be difficult after certain spa treatments, which require the use of multiple towels and products. A hamper, bag, or other receptacle either in the room or nearby is helpful to deal with the quantity of soiled linens generated in the spa treatment room.

Therapists need to arrive early enough beforehand to prepare for certain spa treatments that entail extensive lead time, such as the herbal wrap, for example, which requires 5 minutes for wringing of the sheets.

It is important to keep all surfaces and equipment sanitary before, between, and after all treatments, and especially at the end of the day. Some spas hire spa technicians, locker room attendants, and after-hours cleaning crews to do the bulk of this cleaning, but hygiene in the treatment room during the day is ultimately the therapist's responsibility, as it may directly impact the health of the client. Read more about sanitation in "Specialized Spa Equipment," later in this chapter.

Common Advanced Bodywork Techniques in Spas

There are certain advanced bodywork modalities that have found great favor in spas recently. They can be found on the treatment menus at large destination spas and small day spas alike. Many spa guests have become conversant in bodywork terminology and will come to a spa seeking "deep work" or "Thai massage" or "craniosacral." Others, seeking adventure, will try something new as long as it is offered in the safe environment of the spa. Every advanced modality in existence is available in at least one spa, but there are several that are most popular. These are listed in Table 15.2. Aromatherapy applications and stone massage are not listed in this table because they are so common in spas today. No longer considered advanced, aromatherapy and stone massage are almost essential for spas of any size to offer on their menus. They are discussed further later in this chapter.

Often, spa management will pay for the advanced education necessary for their therapists to become proficient in advanced techniques. Sometimes management will invite instructors in to offer training at the spa itself. This creates loyalty among the staff and is sometimes extended only to those therapists who have been employed by the spa for a certain period of time, usually one year. It is one of the major benefits for working at an established spa with an emphasis on training.

SPA MASSAGE

Taking into account the wide variety of bodywork administered in spas, it is difficult to arrive at one simple definition for spa massage. However, when people use this term, they most often mean a spa's basic massage offering, which is commonly Swedish massage or relaxation massage (see the sidebar "The Real Meaning of 'Relaxation Massage'"). The term *spa massage* can have a negative connotation, as some believe it is less effective compared to a therapeutic massage. This distinction is unnecessary and unhelpful. A massage session executed in a spa can be as therapeutic as one executed elsewhere.

It is challenging, however, for many therapists working in spas to give high-quality therapeutic massage sessions consistently. This is true for three main reasons:

1. **Low expectations:** Many spa guests arrive with no particular complaints or pains, and they do not expect the massage therapy session to help them very much beyond simple relaxation.

2. **Time constraints:** It is difficult for therapists to retain enthusiasm and high energy levels when doing many massages each day or week, all within the same time guidelines.

3. **Inexperienced clients:** Many spa guests are first-time massage recipients or casual recipients who have not formed an appreciation for bodywork and need to be educated about its effects and benefits.

Table 15.2

Advanced Massage Techniques Typically Offered in Spas

ADVANCED TECHNIQUE	PURPOSE	POPULARITY
Ayurveda	Meaning "knowledge of life," Ayurveda is an ancient Indian system of medicine recently adapted for application in modern spas where its main purpose is to rebalance the body's skin and internal organs through application of herbs, oils, creams, massage, and exfoliation	Very popular in destination and resort spas, many spas having a menu of several Ayurvedic services available
Craniosacral	Craniosacral therapy treats the bones and membranes surrounding the brain and spinal cord in order to free restrictions in the flow of cerebral spinal fluid, increasing overall health and relieving pain and stress	One of the more popular advanced modalities in many spas, guests enjoy the delicacy of the touch as well as the effective therapy
Deep tissue	Spas use this term to refer to a wide range of techniques, including connective tissue, neuromuscular, trigger-point, even sports massage	Quite popular among spa guests who like deep pressure but are unfamiliar or unconcerned with specific terms and techniques
Manual lymph drainage	This gentle massage uses light, rhythmical, spiral-like movements to accelerate the movement of lymphatic fluids in the body	Somewhat popular in spas, especially medical spas and spas with advanced esthetics programs
Myofascial	A gentle stretching and elongation of the connective tissues in and around the muscles, especially at trigger points, this therapy restores balance, health, and elasticity while relieving pain	Not as popular as craniosacral therapy in spas, this therapy is nonetheless prized for its gentle effectiveness
Neuromuscular	A method for addressing soft-tissue abnormalities to reduce tightness, pain, and pathologic dysfunction	Somewhat popular in spas, especially among guests with specific pains or complaints
Reiki	A system of treatment that channels universal healing energy through the practitioners into and around the client's body, sometimes without direct hands-on application	Though unproven scientifically, Reiki is quite popular in spas; some guests enjoy the esoteric and non-threatening nature of the treatment
Shiatsu	Focusing on a series of specific points along energy pathways or meridians, this technique from Japan uses finger pressure to invigorate the body and allow healing energies to flow more freely	Many Asian therapies and themes are very popular in spas today, and shiatsu is one of the most popular of all
Structural alignment	Any of several modalities that focus on realigning the body's connective tissues in a more balanced and healthy way	Not very popular in spas, as it features a series of treatments; guests prefer clinics or private practice settings for ongoing treatment series
Thai massage	An ancient system of massage that includes stimulation of pressure points, energy work, and yogalike stretching to improve health and well-being; several training programs exist in Thailand and the West, and some spas offer training on-site	Spa guests love the stretching in this technique, which is gaining rapidly in popularity; remaining clothed makes it more accessible for modest guests
Watsu	Meaning water-Shiatsu, this treatment is given with both guest and therapist submerged in warm (90° to 98°F), chest-deep water; the therapist floats, stretches, and massages the guest to open joints, improve mobility, and open energy pathways to promote healing	Becoming more and more popular in spas, it is only limited by the extensive infrastructure requirements (a special warm pool is needed to perform the treatments)

With these constraints in mind, it is still possible for spa therapists to make their massage sessions fresh and effective, giving each client a customized experience in spite of the fact that many of the massage moves and timing may be the same from massage to massage. This requires discipline and enhanced skill on the part of the spa therapist. Far from being easier to perform than massage administered in other venues, spa massage can be, in a certain fashion, more challenging, and therapists who master it can rightfully feel proud. In order to achieve this, therapists working in spas profit by paying particularly close attention to three special concerns while applying the massage techniques learned in this book: timing, transitions, and uniqueness.

Timing of the Spa Massage

One of the biggest challenges of a spa massage is to create a sense of time-lessness within the very strict time structure imposed in the spa setting. There are three main ways to do this:

1. *Slow down.* Paradoxically, when therapists slow down movements during a massage and perform fewer maneuvers with greater concentration and focus, from the client's point of view, the massage actually seems longer and more luxurious. Rushing to get in many massage moves actually makes the massage seem shorter. Therapists can choose three or four key techniques on each area, then focus on them in a slow, methodical manner.

2. *Internalize timing.* A spa massage should be a well-paced 50-minute session that is soothing and relaxing but at the same time has specific therapeutic goals. To achieve this, spa therapists need to develop a heightened awareness of their own (as well as their clients') internal sense of rhythm. Instead of watching the clock constantly, feeling the deadline of the 50-minute time frame looming ever closer, it is possible to end the massage right on time yet rarely, if ever, glance at the clock. After performing hundreds of massages within the spa's tight time frame, the therapist's mind becomes accustomed to the time needed for each area and knows spontaneously when to move on. Learn to trust this inner clock.

3. *Focus on the moment.* Therapists need to think about what they are doing, not about what they are going to be doing next. Once the spa massage routine becomes second nature, it is easy to think in terms of the next step instead of the step presently being performed. Several times throughout the massage, therapists should remind themselves to focus on the tissues beneath their fingers, and let that guide them to a new next step, which may come as a surprise. With this surprise, therapists become more in tune with the client, who will experience a longer lasting, more thorough massage.

Transitions during Spa Massage

In the same way that the moments of silence between musical notes help define the music, the movements between massage strokes, between segments, and between treatments are as important as the massage itself, especially when working within the limited parameters of a spa massage.

Between Strokes

Pay particular attention to and spend more time on maintaining physical contact with the client and developing a creative sequence during a spa massage. Focus on those movements that connect the separate strokes during a massage, making them flow and become part of a graceful whole rather than disjointed, which is especially important in the time-pressed environment of a spa.

Between Segments

By focusing on graceful transitions from one part of the body to the next, the therapist can avoid creating a hurried sensation while covering the entire body in a shorter time frame. Make the first stroke and the last on each area especially relaxing. Even while adjusting the drapes, use slow, deliberate movements to augment the client's sense of ease and timelessness.

Between Treatments

Between treatments is the one time when it is better to speed up. Refresh yourself. Get the blood flowing. Move around. Rapidly clean the treatment room and set up for the next client so that you will not be rushing once it is time to start again.

Making a Spa Massage Unique

In the spa setting, it is important to remember that each client is unique, even though they all may have similar expectations and even though the

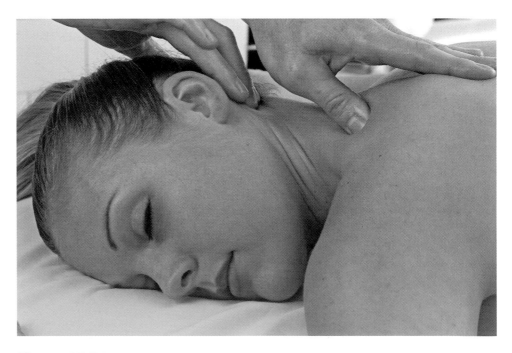

Figure 15.9

Spa massage can incorporate energy work along with other modalities and be every bit as therapeutic as therapeutic massage.

setting, protocols, and routine are the same for each. All clients on a given day may be receiving the same massage, yet each treatment should be slightly different and geared to that client's needs.

Target Problem Areas

A relaxing spa massage is made even better when the therapist applies targeted work to those areas holding tension. Using trigger-point and other therapies (see pages 544 and 741), problem areas can be identified and techniques applied to relieve tension and holding patterns. These will be different for each client. After focusing on such areas, move on seamlessly to the next step of the spa massage routine.

Focus on the Client's Breath

Therapists can use the breath as a guide to tune into each client's unique tension-release patterns. Do not make your own breath too conspicuous; rather just focus on the client's breath. Observe. Make subtle adjustments when you notice a change in rhythm or depth.

Avoid Burnout

Therapists need to take care of themselves physically and mentally so that they are fresh enough to offer each client a unique experience. This means receiving periodic bodywork themselves, getting adequate rest, taking time off, and practicing moderation.

STONE MASSAGE

Stone massage has become extremely popular in spas (Figure 15.10). Displayed on the menu at many facilities, stone massage goes by many names, including Stone Massage, Hot Rock Therapy, Hot Stone Massage, and LaStone Therapy; as well as many regionalized terms, such as Hotter'n Texas Summer Rock Massage, and terms personalized to particular spas, such as Satori Wellness Spa

THE REAL MEANING OF RELAXATION MASSAGE

The literature at many spas refers to something known as a *relaxation massage,* which sounds relatively benign, if not bland, but what exactly is it? The standard response to this question is that a relaxation massage is a Swedish massage (as compared to one of the advanced modalities), but as you are no doubt learning in school now, a Swedish massage can also be invigorating, stimulating, therapeutic, and downright intense (Figure 15.9). Is "relaxation" simply a code word for "fluffy spa-type with no therapeutic value"? Are spas doomed forever to suffer from this stigma as places where relaxation equals substandard?

Seen from another angle, all massage should be relaxation massage, should it not? Even deep structural integration, which may be intense in the moment, leads eventually to a relaxation of tissues and holding patterns in the body.

The problem here is that we are looking at the terminology from a massage therapist's point of view. The real meaning of the term *relaxation* as it is used in terms of spa massage is correctly understood when seen from the client's point of view, as it probably has more to do with easing clients' fear than anything else. It is a way to let spa guests know that they are not going to be mauled by a rough Russian or Turkish character like the ones depicted in certain old-time movies. By default, over the years, the term has ended up applying to any massage that is nonthreatening, though unfairly so, because Swedish massage is actually much more than simply relaxing.

Heated Stone Experience. Regardless of the name, these treatments all share certain common elements:

1. **Stones:** Several types of stone are used for treatments, the most common being basalt, which is volcanic in origin. Typically, practitioners utilize stones of several shapes and sizes appropriate to different parts of the body. These stones are heated in hot water, usually in a roaster, and then either placed on the body or used by the practitioner to apply massage techniques. Also, other types of stones, usually marble, are cooled in a refrigerator or freezer and applied to the skin to complement the effects of the heat.

2. **Massage:** Although it may consist primarily of energy work and not involve extensive Swedish-style massage techniques, stone massage is, in the end, massage. The official definition of massage in most state and local laws includes the use of heat, cold, and therapeutic instruments in the treatment of soft tissue. Stones, in this sense, can be construed as therapeutic instruments.

3. **Heat and cold:** One of the most important effects of stone massage derives from its use of contrast therapy. Alternating hot and cold stones are applied, creating a stimulating effect on the circulation that pumps more blood to the tissues being treated (see page 564 for more on this pumping effect of contrast therapy).

These common elements (stones, massage, and temperature) can be modified with any number of specific techniques or products to make the stone treatment unique. For instance, some spas incorporate the use of

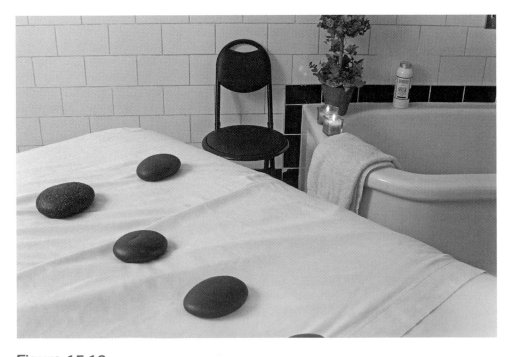

Figure 15.10

Many guests look forward to stone massage, which is one of the most popular modalities in spas.

essential oils with the stones, some specialize in treating the face with small stones, some spas use the stones primarily as instruments in deep tissue massage, and others create an entire stone theme for their spa such as the Stone Spa in New York City.

Rocks and stones have been used therapeutically for hundreds of years by Native Americans to create heat for their sweat lodge ceremonies. The temperatures at which they are used for that purpose, however, are much too high for direct application to the body. Other cultures have used heated stones to aid healing, warm living spaces, make beds more comfortable during the winter, and heat special chambers such as the famous Finnish sauna. In the 1990s, a new systemized method of applying hot and cold stones as part of a massage session was first devised by Mary Nelson of Tucson, Arizona. She is given credit for developing the technique called LaStone Therapy.

Some therapists claim that the effectiveness of stone therapy derives from the energy of the stones themselves. Because the stones were formed millions of years ago and are a fundamental part of planet Earth, they are believed to emanate vibrations that connect the recipients of stone massage directly to the nature of the planet and ultimately to their own bodies. Therapists should exercise discretion when speaking in these terms with clients, as some spa guests prefer a more scientific explanation of the benefits of the therapies they receive. Whether or not the esoteric benefits of stone massage really exist is a matter of debate, but the therapeutic benefits of massage plus temperature therapy are undeniable.

Modern stone massage offers spas a simple way to add something exotic to the menu and put clients back in touch with a piece of the natural world. A stone massage program is easy to set up, requiring only a heating unit, a refrigerator or freezer, and the stones themselves. However, caution must be exercised when practicing stone massage.

Safety and Sanitation

The application of hard, hot objects to the skin and tissues beneath is inherently hazardous. It follows that students must be trained adequately before using stones on clients. When applying stone massage, certain safety considerations must be kept in mind.

Water Temperature

Water in the heating container must be kept at the correct temperature, which is between 110° and 140°F. Temperatures below 110°F do not generate sufficient warmth for therapeutic application, and temperatures above 140°F make it difficult to handle the stones. Stones heated beyond this temperature may also cause discomfort for the client or even damage tissue if applied directly to the skin.

Client Protection

Stones may be placed directly on the skin, but the therapist must exercise caution when doing so. Often, it is preferable to place sheets, pillowcases, or towels between the rocks and the skin in order to protect the client from possible harm or discomfort. The thickness of these protective layers may be adjusted during the course of the treatment as the temperature of the stones changes.

Cleaning Stones and Implements

Proper sanitation is crucial in order to ensure a safe experience for the client. The stones should be cleansed with fresh water after each use and before being placed back in the heating unit. If the stones are sticky from lubricant, they can be cleansed with alcohol. The water in the heating unit should be changed daily. A sterilizing solution can be added to the heating unit each day to ensure a sanitary treatment.

Depth of Pressure with Stones

When using stones as tools during deep tissue massage, some therapists tend to apply excessive pressure as they strive for therapeutic effects. It must be remembered that stones penetrate the tissues much more forcefully than therapist's fingers or thumbs do. Extreme caution must be exercised in order not to cause damage.

SPA MODALITIES

Therapists hired by a spa are often, though not always, required to perform a number of modalities in addition to their massage duties. These can include body wraps, **exfoliation,** foot treatments, back treatments, scalp treatments, face treatments, herbal detoxification treatments, hydrotherapy baths, therapeutic showers, cellulite treatments, aromatherapy, **parafango,** and clay, mud, and seaweed treatments (Figure 15.11).

exfoliation
is any of a number of spa treatments whose primary purpose is to cleanse the body of dead skin cells, thus softening the skin, helping the body to eliminate better through the skin, and preparing the skin for better absorption of other therapeutic products.

parafango
is a combination of paraffin wax and fango mud used in spa wraps and localized applications to soften, moisten, and purify the skin while warming and relaxing the muscles.

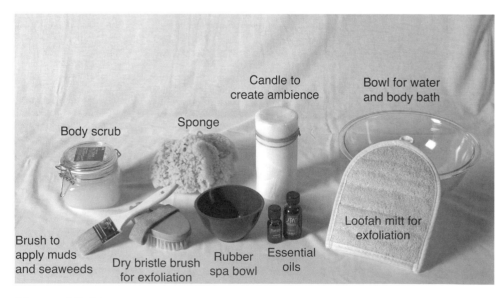

Figure 15-11

Popular items found in a spa therapist's treatment room: (a) body scrub, (b) brush to apply muds and seaweeds, (c) dry bristle brush for exfoliation, (d) sponge, (e) rubber spa bowl, (f) candle to create ambience, (g) essential oils, (h) loofah mitt for exfoliation, (i) bowl for water and body bath.

These modalities are listed in Table 15.3. Some spas also offer advanced treatments such as the *Rasul* and Balinese *Lulur* rituals that incorporate basic modalities but use specialized equipment and ingredients. Each individual spa offers some kind of training for newly hired therapists, ranging from a cursory introduction to an elaborate multiday hands-on workshop. Generally speaking, those spas with the best reputations offer the most extensive training. Spa managers and directors appreciate therapists who come to the job already knowing the basic procedures involved with spa modalities but who are open to learning the specific protocols practiced at each spa.

Table 15.3

Spa Modalities That Therapists Typically Perform

SPA MODALITIES	DESCRIPTION	BENEFITS/ USES	CONTRA- INDICATIONS
Back treatment	Also called a back facial, this treatment cleanses and draws impurities from the back area with mud and partial body wrapping	Especially appropriate for modest clients who want a partial body wrap	Sensitivity to heat; excessive open acne on the back
Bust treatment	Not very popular except in some beauty-oriented day spas, this treatment uses creams and serums to firm the skin and subcutaneous tissues of the breast area	Imparts a more elastic and glowing appearance to the skin	Many clients are too modest for a bust treatment; local laws on draping and appropriate touch must be consulted and followed
Cellulite treatment	Often including underwater massage in a hydrotherapy tub, this treatment features vigorous massage, wrapping, and special products (usually seaweed-based) to promote an improved appearance to affected areas	Drains superficial tissues; noninvasive way to improve appearance in a comfortable spa setting	Allergies to iodine; claustrophobia
Exfoliation	Includes dry brushing, body polish, sea salt glow, and any number of procedures involving exfoliants (nut shell meal, seeds, etc.) to cleanse the skin	Prepares skin to absorb spa products; cleanses away dead cells; imparts healthy glow	Open sores; cuts; abrasions; communicable skin conditions; psoriasis; aggravated acute acne
Face treatment	A face treatment including cleansing, exfoliation, and nutritive mask that therapists can perform within their scope of practice in the spa setting	Cleanses, balances, and imparts a glow to the skin of the face	Open sores; cuts; communicable skin conditions; acute acne; and recent peels
Foot treatment	Can include exfoliation, soaking, mud/seaweed application, wrapping, massage, and reflexology, in addition to pedicure if therapist is qualified	Reflex benefits for the entire body, in addition to product benefits; softens tough feet; deeply relaxing	Open sores; cuts or abrasions on feet; athlete's foot
Herbal wrap	Hot herb-infused sheets are wrapped around the client to induce a false-fever state, promoting detoxification through the pores	Spa guests often receive a series of herbal wraps to aid detoxification and cessation of smoking, caffeine, etc.	Heart disease, high or low blood pressure, pregnancy, diabetes, claustrophobia, allergies to specific herbs
Mud/clay wrap	Most common types are black Baltic and fango (volcanic-based) muds, applied to skin prior to wrap	Nourishes and exfoliates skin; humic acids also help draw out impurities	None for non-heated mud; slight contraindications for warmed mud include high blood pressure, heart disease

continues

Table 15.3, cont'd

Spa Modalities That Therapists Typically Perform

SPA MODALITIES	DESCRIPTION	BENEFITS/ USES	CONTRA-INDICATIONS
Mud Immersions	Clients are completely immersed in warmed therapeutic muds, or they cover themselves head to foot in clay amd then lie in the sun	Deeply drawing and purifying of the entire body; nourishing for the skin	Done only in specially equipped spas, usually near mud/clay source, with proper sanitation
Hydrotherapy bath (Figure 15.12)	The use of water's percussive, thermal, and chemical properties in a specialized tub; when the water's mineral and gas contents are used therapeutically, it is called **balneotherapy**	To warm client prior to treatment, open pores, encourage detoxification, soothe muscles	Hypertension, dizziness, fever, communicable skin conditions
Parafango	A blend of paraffin wax and fango (mud from a volcanic source) that is smoothed onto a part or the whole body while warm; then a wrap is applied	Effects created by heat penetrate to warm joints, relieve pain and heal; softens skin	Acute arthritis, blood clots, acute skin conditions; also high blood pressure for full-body parafango
Sauna/steam bath	Dry or steam heat is applied in a special chamber usually in the spa's common area	Excellent for relaxing muscles prior to treatment; cleansing; strengthens circulatory system	High blood pressure, hypertension, heart disease, diabetes, pregnancy
Scalp treatment	A cleansing of the scalp and hair, often with an oil or mud application and wrap, plus massage	Promotes circulation to the scalp; cleanses; gives body and luster	Extremely oily hair
Scotch hose	A high pressure hose that sprays the standing client (sometimes with seawater)	Highly invigorating, stimulates circulation	More popular in European-style spas, less so in others; too stimulating for some clients; spray should be aimed away from sensitive areas
Sea salt treatment	A specialized treatment that adds the benefits of the sea and seawater (remineralizing, rejuvenating) to those listed previously for general exfoliation	Softens and smoothes skin; removes dead skin cells	Open sores, cuts, abrasions; communicable skin conditions; aggravated acute acne; recently shaved legs
Seaweed wrap (Figure 15.13)	A blend of reconstituted seaweed and essential oils is applied to the skin after exfoliation, then the client is wrapped; massage often follows	Seaweed remineralizes the entire body as ingredients soak into pores; rejuvenates skin	Allergies to iodine, which is found in many seaweeds
Swiss shower (Figure 15.14)	Multiple shower heads in stall aimed at client from all directions; water temperature is often adjusted by therapist/technician for contrast therapy	Used to effectively wash off spa products and stimulate circulation; invigorating	Fine high-powered water stream may be too intense for some clients
Thalassotherapy	The use of seawater or sea products (oils, extracts, powders, seaweeds) in baths or other spa treatments	Remineralizes; promotes detoxification; supplies sea nutrients through pores	Allergies to iodine
Vichy shower	Multiple showerheads on a long arm suspended above the treatment table apply water pressure, sometimes including contrast therapy	Relaxing; washes away spa products such as mud, salt, seaweed	None

Some spa therapists do not have to perform these other modalities, either as a result of their own choice or the spa's policies. Quite often these therapists are on call and are used by the spa only when guest demand for massage surges. The therapists who stay busiest, and therefore earn the most money, are those who master as many of the spa's modal-

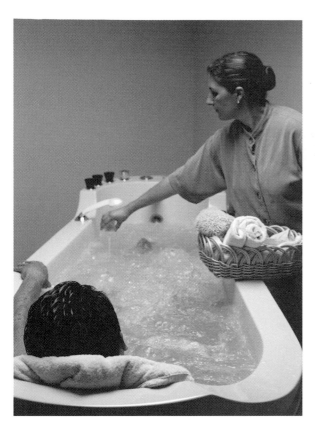

Figure 15.12

Hydrotherapy tubs, popular in larger spas, have multiple therapist-controlled jets, an underwater massage wand, and can incorporate thalassotherapy and aromatherapy.

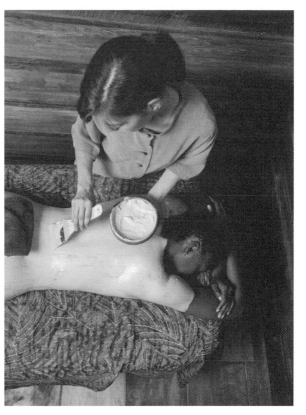

Figure 15.13

Body wraps employ the use of muds, seaweeds, clays, and other ingredients to nourish the skin and affect the entire body.

ities as possible. It is therefore in the therapist's best interest to train extensively on general spa modalities before joining a spa team and then to continue training on specific modalities whenever the opportunity arises during employment. Therapists who do not wish to perform these modalities may lessen their chances for advancement and for getting preferred schedules. Spa directors appreciate those therapists who are proficient in a wide range of treatments so that they can cover as many guest requests as possible.

The rules and laws vary widely from state to state regarding what a massage therapist can and cannot do in the spa setting. For example, in some states, the law requires massage therapists to perform body wraps and exfoliation treatments, whereas in others, the law allows untrained **spa technicians** to perform these treatments. In most cases, it is more appropriate for massage therapists to perform these services because they have been trained extensively in proper procedures for dealing with draping, health concerns, contraindications, precautions, anatomy, and hydrotherapy. Massage therapy associations have hired lawyers and lobbyists to work on legislation regarding these matters, but because it is a state issue, some irregularities still arise. The best spas, however, usually have trained therapists apply most, if not all, modalities.

> **spa technicians**
>
> are employees who assist therapists and estheticians in setting up treatment areas, keeping areas clean, preparing treatments, and in some cases, performing certain modalities such as wraps and body scrubs.

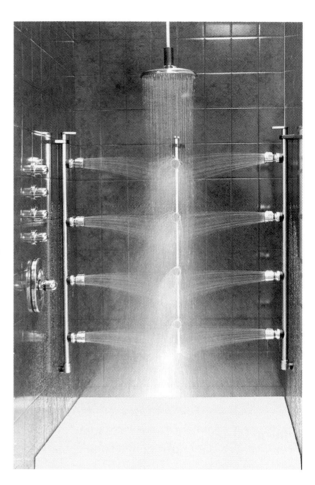

Figure 15.14

The Swiss shower, with its multiple heads, is a stimulating treatment that is also used to remove spa products after body wraps and exfoliation services. (Courtesy of HydroCo USA: www.hydroco.com.)

AROMATHERAPY

aromatherapy
is the use of essential oils processed from herbs, flowers, fruits, stems, spices, and roots in massage, inhalation, or other modalities to affect mood and improve health and well-being.

diffusers
are devices using fans, heat, or steam dispersion to release the aromas of essential oils into a room for therapeutic and/or esthetic purposes.

Aromatherapy is commonly used in almost all spas in one form or another. In the spa industry, it can be defined as the use of essential oils processed from herbs, flowers, fruits, spices, stems, bark, and roots in massage, inhalation, or other modalities to affect mood and improve health and well-being. Some spas offer extensive aromatherapy treatment options on their menus, whereas others list just a basic aromatherapy massage, but it is rare for a spa to offer no aromatherapy treatments at all. At the very least, in small spas, aromatherapy candles or **diffusers** are used to impart some of the benefits of aromatherapy to guests even if no aromatherapy treatments are offered.

Essential oils and plant extracts have been used for many years in many lands, from the ancient Greek, Indian, and Egyptian cultures to the present day. They are used to treat ailments, promote beauty, and bolster well-being. The word *aromatherapy* itself was first used in the 1920s by Rene Gattfosse, a French perfumer.

When using essential oils, it is important to remember that they are powerfully concentrated substances, and as such should be treated with caution. When used improperly, some oils can overstimulate the body, and because very little of these substances (just a few drops) is needed to create an effect, it is usually recommended not to use them full strength or **neat,** but in combination with a **carrier oil** or other medium. Some common carrier oils are apricot kernel oil, avocado oil, grapeseed oil, jojoba oil, sesame oil, sweet almond oil, and wheat germ oil.

A wide range of essential oils are available for use by the spa therapist, with an equally wide array of possible benefits. These include, but are certainly not limited to, mood uplifting, mood calming, accelerating wound healing, antibacterial and antifungal cleansing, hormonal balancing, pain reduction, easing of nasal and bronchial congestion, and enhancing circulation.

If they are kept out of direct sunlight in tightly capped, dark-colored bottles and stored in a cool dry place, essential oils can have a shelf life of several years. Dozens of companies offer hundreds of essential oils for use in spas, and many of them are high quality. Some oils are more expensive than others because they require a very large amount of initial product to produce a small amount of the oil. For example, 8,000 individual jasmine blossoms are needed to produce one gram of jasmine oil. It is only natural, then, that spas can charge a premium for massage and other services that include aromatherapy.

Ten Common Essential Oils

Each spa chooses a brand of aromatherapy oils and a range of oils within that brand to use in its treatments. Essential oils can be placed into one of three categories for easy description. "Top notes" are stimulating and uplifting, and their fragrance lasts just a few hours once it is out of the bottle. "Middle notes" last longer and are potent in their therapeutic effects on the body, but they do not have as strong a fragrance. "Base notes" last the longest and are often sweet-smelling and calming. Table 15.4 lists 10 popular oils used in many spas, with their effects.

Aromatherapy Massage

Aromatherapy massage is the most popular aromatherapy modality used in spas. A few spas hire highly trained aromatherapy experts to administer these massages, but the majority of spas require that all the massage therapists on staff, or at least a significant number, perform aromatherapy massage. The step-by-step procedure for an aromatherapy massage is similar to that for a typical Swedish spa massage, with a few notable distinctions.

- Before the treatment, the therapist must check the guest's intake form for sensitivities to aromas or, if no form is used, ask the guest verbally.
- Before the treatment, the therapist should explain to the client the therapeutic outcomes desired through the choice of essential oils.
- The massage strokes are predominantly light and flowing, similar to an **Esalen massage** style.
- Time is allowed for the client to experience the aromas. For example, at the beginning of a sequence over the face, the therapist cups

neat

refers to the application of an essential oil at its full, undiluted strength.

carrier oil

is massage lubricant into which essential oils are blended for aromatherapy applications.

Esalen massage

is a style of massage developed at Esalen Institute in northern California that features long, flowing strokes that connect all parts of the body into a whole.

Table 15.4

Common Essential Oils Used in Spas

ESSENTIAL OIL	DERIVATION	EFFECT/ NOTE	USES	CONTRA-INDICATIONS
Chamomile	Flowers	Calming middle note	Useful for premenstrual pain/tension, indigestion, as an anti-inflammatory	May cause minor skin irritation
Eucalyptus	Leaves	Stimulating and antiseptic/top note	Useful for coughs and colds, bronchitis, viral infections, muscular aches, cuts	Can irritate skin in high doses; harmful if ingested
Geranium	Flowers/leaves	Mildly astringent/ middle note	Useful for cuts, sores, fungal infections; as an insect repellant; for soothing skin problems, eczema, bruises; mildly diuretic; antidepressant	May cause irritation to very sensitive skin
Jasmine	Flowers	Antidepressant/ base note	Useful for depression, postnatal depression; strengthening contractions during labor; as an aphrodisiac	May cause headaches in some people
Lavender	Flowers	Mildly analgesic/ middle note	Useful for headaches, wounds, bruises, antiseptic, insect bites, oily skin, acne, swelling, calming insomnia, mild depression	None
Lemongrass	Leaf	Refreshing/top note	Useful to fight stress, fatigue, indigestion, muscle soreness; stimulates appetite; acts as an antidepressant, antiseptic, diuretic	Can be irritating to sensitive skin
Neroli	Rind	Relaxing/top note	Useful for insomnia, anxiety, nervous depression; mildly warming; improving circulation, acne, premenstrual tension/pain, backache	Photosensitive, should not be applied before exposure to sun
Rose	Flowers	Relaxing/middle/ base note	Useful for sore throat and sinus, congestion, puffiness, mild sedative, insomnia, premenstrual tension/pain, menopause	None

her hands a few inches away from the client's face and asks the client to inhale the oil for its therapeutic benefits. This can be done through the face cradle when the client is prone.

- It is especially important to make sure that blankets and/or an infrared heating lamp are in place to keep the client warm, if necessary, because spa guests often experience a chill during this treatment, either as an effect of certain oils or because the overall treatment is so calming and sedating.

Blending the Oils

Many spas offer standardized aromatherapy massage treatments on the menu. The essential oils for these treatments have been preblended into a carrier oil for ready use, and guests do not have a choice regarding the oil in their treatment. An example of this would be an "Uplifting Citrus Aromatherapy Treatment," using essential oils of orange, lemon, and neroli. For a customized aromatherapy massage, on the other hand, the therapist must consult with the client before the massage regarding his preferences and desired outcomes for the treatment. Then the essential oil drops are blended into the carrier oil in the presence of the guest directly prior to beginning the treatment.

It is necessary to add the essential oils to the carrier oil drop by drop in order to achieve the correct strength. This process is facilitated by aromatherapy bottles themselves, most of which are outfitted with tops that allow one drop at a time to escape when upturned. The correct number of drops is 12 to 15 for each ounce of carrier oil. Thus, for a preblended mixture, a therapist could use approximately 96 to 120 drops for an 8-ounce bottle of carrier oil. Many companies sell preblended aromatherapy products, which eliminates the need for measuring and blending.

Essential oils can also be blended into massage lotions and creams. Certain of these do not readily absorb the oils and must be warmed appropriately to create an **emulsion** that will work for massage. In all cases, stir or gently swirl the drops of essential oil into the medium rather than shaking.

> **emulsion**
> is a uniform mixture of two or more liquids, such as an essential oil and a massage lotion.

Aromatherapy Wrap

An aromatherapy wrap uses essential oils, a carrier oil or lotion, and wrapping layers like *muslin* sheets and blankets to create a cocoon experience for the client. Some spas prefer to use preblended products, whereas others customize the treatment, blending the oils according to the client's preference. The treatment is quite gentle and meditative, focusing on the client's mood and state of mind more than any musculoskeletal problems that may be apparent. In fact, the therapist will often forego massage entirely during an aromatherapy wrap and instead simply apply the product with long, superficial gliding strokes over the entire body. Some spas offer a choice between this simple application and a more comprehensive aromatherapy wrap with massage included.

To start the treatment, the therapist places a drop of essential oil blend on her fingertip, then touches it to several energy points, corresponding to shiatsu points, along the body. After this, the blend is applied to the body in long strokes, and the client is covered immediately to ensure warmth. The client turns over, and the procedure is repeated on the front of the body before wrapping the client in layers of muslin and blankets. A bolster is placed beneath the knees, the lights are turned low, and the client is left wrapped for 20 minutes on average in most spas. During this time, the therapist often applies a light noninvasive therapy such as craniosacral to the head and neck area.

Aromatherapy Bath

Aromatherapy baths are popular in many spas. They can be defined as any bath that incorporates the use of aromatherapy essential oils. In this sense, many hydrotherapy baths on a spa's menu may in fact be aromatherapy baths, although they are not labeled as such, as essential oils are routinely added to hydrotherapy tubs to enhance guests' experience. Popular essential oil choices for aromatherapy baths include chamomile, lavender, rose, and rosemary. Certain especially cooling or highly stimulating oils such as peppermint, ginger, or juniper should be avoided for aromatherapy baths.

Only 5 to 10 drops of essential oil are added as the bath is filling. These drops may be blended with a carrier oil beforehand if a more silky texture is desired for the bath. The warm water, usually 100° to 104°F, helps release the aroma of the oil, so the benefits of inhalation are increased.

Aromatherapy Diffusers

Aromatherapy diffusers disperse the oils into the air of a room, spreading the beneficial effects over a wide area and enhancing the overall ambience of a space. They are used extensively in spas, especially those that specialize in aromatherapy. Often, they are used by smaller spas as a cost-effective way to add atmosphere and therapeutic value without a large investment.

Diffusers come in many forms:

- *Atomizers* are for the more advanced user. These turn the liquid oils into an extremely fine mist that fills the area with scent. They offer the highest concentration of oil in the air.

- *Fan diffusers* are extremely simple to operate and are inexpensive. Dabs of essential oil are placed on a piece of cotton or cloth and placed inside a small unit behind a fan that takes air in through the oils and disperses it into the room.

- *Clay/candle diffusers* come with a small tea candle or votive candle that warms essential oils placed in a clay or ceramic receptacle.

- *Lightbulb rings* are small rings that are placed on top of lightbulbs. When lit, the heat from the bulbs gradually burns away essential oils placed in the ring, filling the room with aroma.

BODY WRAPS

Spas offer many types of body wraps for various purposes. Some are for heating the body and detoxification, such as the herbal wrap. Some are meant primarily to relax and improve mood and well-being, such as the aromatherapy wrap. Some are meant to nourish, cleanse, and improve the superficial contour of the skin, such as cellulite wraps. Mud and clay wraps have multiple effects, such as purging and drawing impurities out through the pores, softening the skin, and improving joint elasticity when heated. Seaweed wraps remineralize the skin and entire body as the micronutrients and seaborne minerals soak in through the pores. Less frequently in spas, weight-loss or inch-loss wraps are applied for purely cosmetic purposes.

Spa body wraps can be categorized into two main types: those that apply heat to the body and those that do not. Heat is a necessary ingredient for some types of purging wraps, such as the herbal wrap. As with all heat treatments, it is important to remember the main contraindications for heated body wraps: high blood pressure, heart diseases, and pregnancy. Nonheated wraps include the aromatherapy wrap and many seaweed and mud wraps, which rely upon the body's own heat to keep the client warm during the treatment.

Body wraps can be further differentiated as either loose or tight, partial or whole. Thus, a therapist could perform a loose torso wrap with mud for purification, or a tight full-body wrap with seaweed for remineralization. Partial wraps include leg wraps, foot wraps, hand wraps, and torso wraps. There are also treatments, such as the back facial, that do not actually wrap around the entire body or body part but still involve the use of blankets or other coverings to retain heat and can therefore be considered a type of wrap (refer to Table 15.3 for more information on the back facial).

Though the purpose for each type of body wrap varies, they all have certain characteristics in common:

- *Comfort and security:* People generally experience a sense of safety and of being protected when they are wrapped up. It is a comforting sensation that is not generally available to adults except in the spa environment.

- *Warmth:* Whether applied externally or created as a process of body heat, warmth is an integral part of all body wraps, offering a sense of nurturing and engendering deep relaxation.

- *Enclosed environment* The enclosed warm environment of body wraps offer ideal conditions for a wide variety of spa products to act upon the body in an effective manner, absorbing through the pores rather than dissipating into the air.

General Body Wrap Protocols

All body wraps are similar in that they envelop the client inside various layers while products are acting upon the skin. Each wrap is unique, however, in the particular manner in which it is applied. Some, for example, call for multiple layers of blankets, sheets, and towels to be wrapped around the client. Others, such as the aromatherapy wrap, may call for only one blanket and one sheet. Still others, such as the drying clay wrap, require only a thin layer of gauze on the skin that is heated by an infrared lamp. As stated earlier, some wraps are tight, whereas some are applied more loosely. Regardless of the wrap being performed, certain general protocols apply:

- *Exercise caution:* All wraps, especially heat wraps, can cause certain clients to feel claustrophobic. Therefore, the therapist should reassure the client about this issue, instructing her to leave her arms unwrapped over her head in order to be more comfortable. With heat wraps, it is important not to apply any overly hot sheets or products, to avoid burning sensitive skin. The mouth and nose, of course, must remain unwrapped at all times. Always check for allergies or sensitivities to products before applying a wrap.

- *Communicate:* It is important to communicate verbally with the client about the nature of the wrap. Clients sometimes complain that they are unsure what to do while the wrap is being performed or while they are lying in the room, alone, wrapped up. Always let the client know that you are available, even while out of the room. Inform clients how long the wrap will last and what they might expect to experience during it. Offer water, a cold compress for heat wraps, and anything else that can make the client more comfortable.

- *Always use a bolster:* Because of the extra weight on the legs created by most wraps, it is important to always place a bolster under the knees so that the client's lower back does not become hyperextended (Figure 15.15).

Seaweed Body Wrap Procedure

Preparation

Prepare the table with the following layers: a double- or queen-size blanket on the table, a **thermal blanket** over that, a large bath towel or bath sheet, then a layer of **plastic body wrap** (Figure 15-16a). Another bath towel is used on top of the client for draping. Warm the seaweed mixture prior to use in a hydrocollator or other heating unit, avoiding microwaves. Seaweed products are usually mixed with an essential oil blend to improve effectiveness and aroma.

---

thermal blanket

also known as a space blanket. This thin polyethylene and metallic-coated sheet that retains heat during spa body wraps and aromatherapy.

---

plastic body wrap

is a thin, transparent, disposable plastic sheet used to wrap directly around the client's skin during mud, clay, and seaweed body wraps.

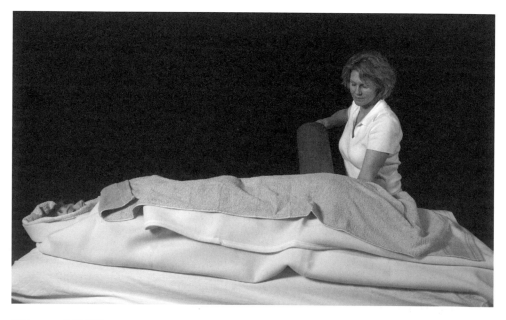

Figure 15.15

It is especially important to place a bolster under the knees of a wrapped client.

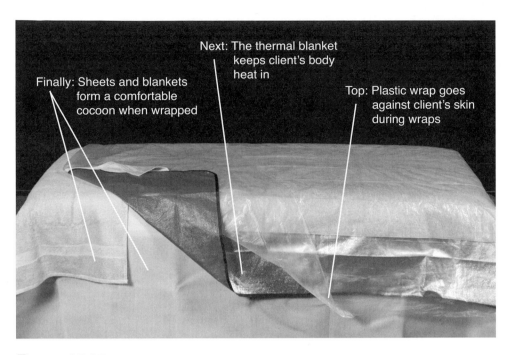

Finally: Sheets and blankets form a comfortable cocoon when wrapped

Next: The thermal blanket keeps client's body heat in

Top: Plastic wrap goes against client's skin during wraps

Figure 15.16a

For a mud- or seaweed-based body wrap, the table is layered with a blanket, thermal blanket, towel, and plastic wrap.

If the treatment is given in a dry room, four hot, moist hand towels are needed to remove the product. These can be stored in a roaster or insulated cooler.

The treatment is prefaced with an exfoliation of the skin. This can be a brief body-brushing or dry-loofah brushing, or a complete sea salt scrub or body polish added on as a separate treatment before the wrap.

Application

At the beginning of the treatment, the therapist should let the client know the special benefits of the products being applied. This is both to educate the client and to improve chances for sales of home care products from the spa after the treatment.

1. The client lays down supine under the drape. Fold the drape down and away from the client's upper body, inserting a breast and pelvic towel as appropriate (Figure 15.16b). Exfoliate the body for 2 minutes with a dry bristle brush or dry loofah.

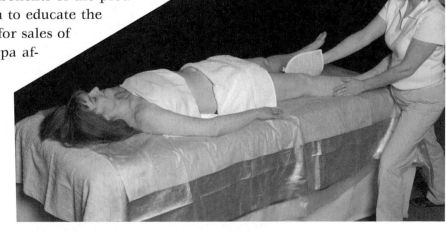

Figure 15.16b

The client lies on the plastic and is draped appropriately. The treatment is prefaced with an exfoliation of the skin.

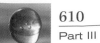

2. Instruct the client to roll to one side while applying warmed seaweed to the back and the back of the upper leg and buttocks in a thin even layer with your hand or natural bristle brush (Figure 15.16c).

3. Help the client roll over to the other side and repeat the procedure.

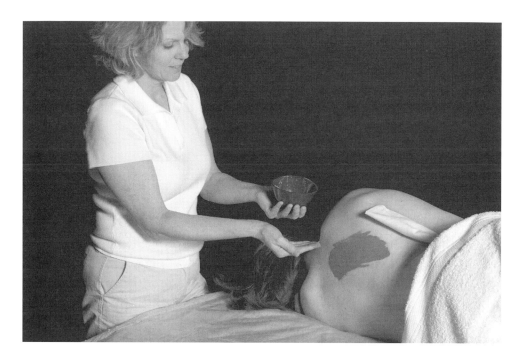

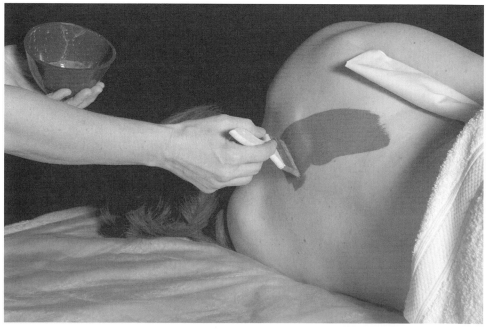

Figure 15.16c
The application begins using hands or a natural bristle brush. The back can be reached as the client rolls slightly to one side.

4. Moving quickly to avoid seaweed cooling, apply in an even layer over the front the client's body starting with the legs. Wrap each area in plastic after the application, especially if the room is cool (Figure 15.16d). Avoid the feet if reflexology will be applied during the wrap. Move to the abdomen, and the area around and between the breasts. Finish with the arms and **décolletage.**

> **décolletage**
> is the area of the upper chest above the breasts and onto the front of the neck.

Wrapping

1. When the client is completely covered with seaweed, wrap the body with plastic first, then a thermal blanket, then a blanket. Lay a bath sheet over this cocoon to seal in body heat and place an eye-pillow over the client's eyes (Figure 15.16e and f).

2. Place a bolster beneath the knees.

3. Allow the client to rest for 25 minutes.

4. Perform a gentle foot reflexology routine or scalp massage during this time. Or, if the client prefers, you may leave the room to let her rest (Figure 15.16g).

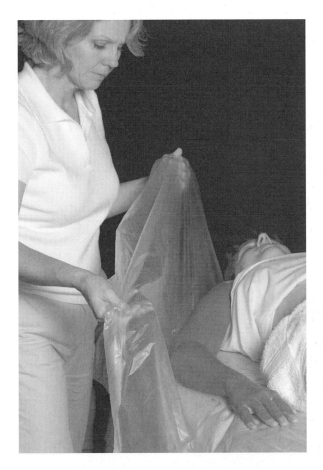

Figure 15.16d

The therapist moves quickly to avoid cooling the client, and each part of the body can be covered with the plastic wrap as the application to the area is completed.

continues

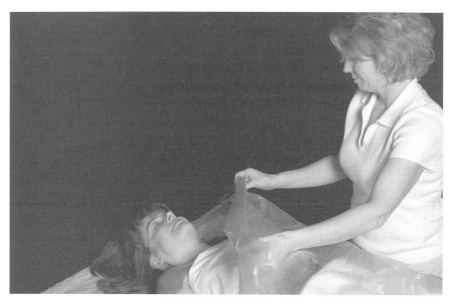

Figure 15.16e

When the client is completely covered with seaweed, wrap the body with plastic first, then a thermal blanket, then a blanket.

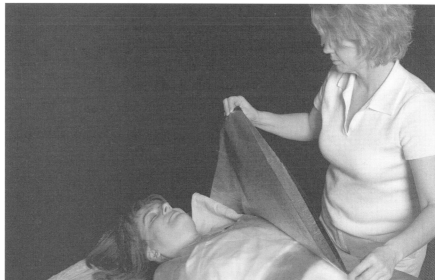

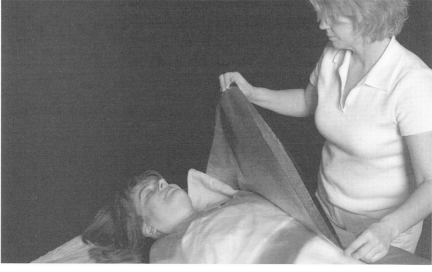

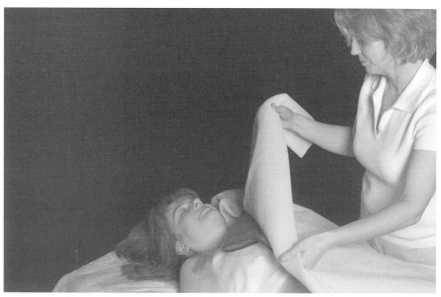

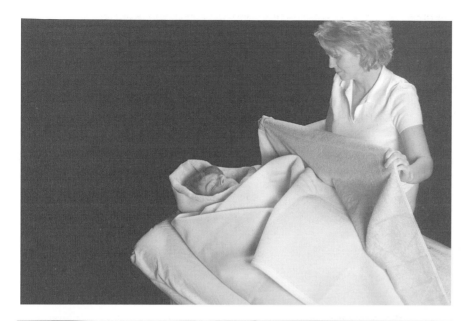

Figure 15.16f
Lay a bath sheet over the client to create a cocoon to seal in body heat, an eye pillow over the eyes, and a bolster beneath the knees. The client rests for 25 minutes.

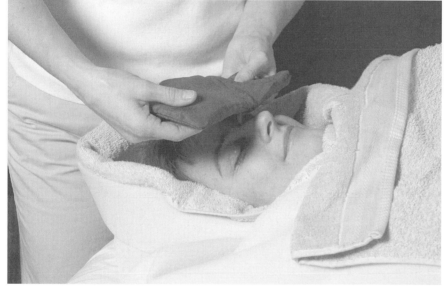

Unwrapping/Cleaning

Note: This procedure is for a dry room body wrap. In a spa wet room, the client proceeds at this point into the shower while the therapist cleans and prepares the table.

1. Having a folded warm moist towel ready, peel away the plastic from the upper body while rolling the plastic down toward the table. Remove the seaweed from the stomach with the towel.

2. Remove the seaweed from the décolletage and arms (Figure 15.16h).

3. Assist the client to sit up. With a fresh warm, moist hand towel, press the towel lengthwise along the back to moisten the seaweed. Then remove the remaining seaweed from the back.

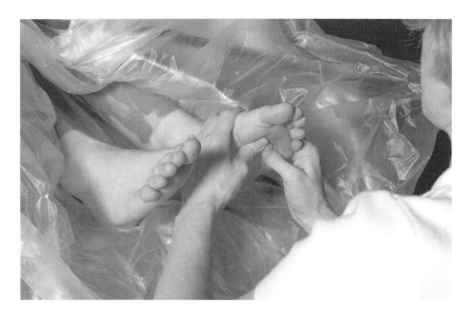

Figure 15.16g

Perform a gentle foot reflexology routine or scalp massage during this time.

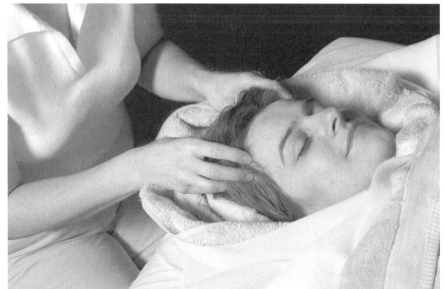

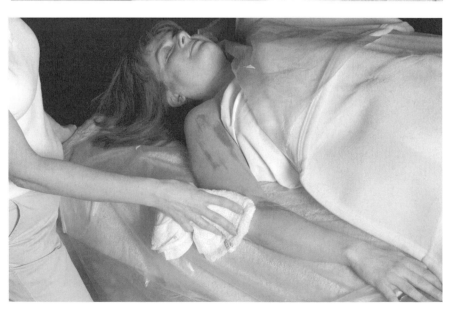

Figure 15.16h

Unwrap the client and re-move the seaweed with four hot, wet towels, peel-ing away layers one area at a time.

4. Prior to the client's lying back down, roll the plastic and thermal blanket toward her buttocks. Have the client lie down and cover her upper body with a bath sheet.

5. Peel back the plastic from the client's right leg, then remove the seaweed with a separate, fresh, moist hand towel. As the leg is cleansed, have the client lift her hip and roll/fold the plastic and thermal blanket from under the body.

6. Repeat on the client's left leg. Remove the plastic/thermal blanket from the table entirely. Cover the client with a bath sheet to prevent chilling.

Finishing

1. At this point in the treatment, you can finish with a 5- to 10-minute application of a hydrating lotion or proceed with a particular massage therapy service.

2. If proceeding with a massage, instruct the client to lie faceup on top of a fitted sheet. Drape appropriately. Incorporate a massage to expand the procedure, making it a full 1½- hour treatment.

3. Or, for a simple application, undrape and redrape the client as appropriate while you apply a finishing lotion or body butter. Start with the right leg, then the left leg, then move to the stomach and décolletage, left arm, then right (Figure 15.16i).

4. When applying lotion to the stomach, use a breast towel to cover the client.

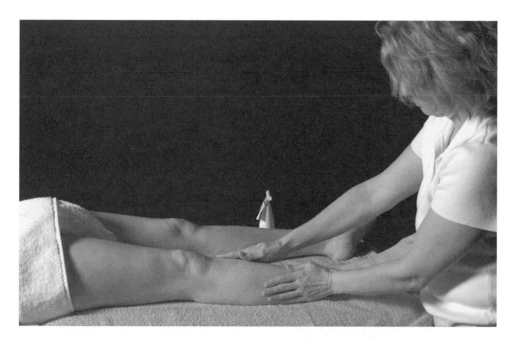

Figure 15.16i

Finish with a 5- to 10-minute application of a hydrating lotion or proceed with a massage therapy service.

5. When finished with the front side, hold up the upper bath sheet between you and the client and have the client turn over onto her stomach. Apply lubricant, starting with the left leg, then the right leg, and finishing with the upper back. When the treatment is complete, leave the room and let the client rest until she is ready to get dressed.

EXFOLIATION

thermae
are hot springs or baths, especially the baths of ancient Rome.

strigil
is a curved, usually metallic, instrument used in ancient Greece and Rome to scrape dead skin cells, oil, and dirt from bathers' skin.

Exfoliation has been practiced in many cultures for thousands of years. Back in the days of the great Roman baths, or **thermae**, citizens would have their personal massage therapists (who were slaves) scour them with instruments known as **strigils** (curved, metallic tool for scraping the skin) after taking their hot baths. Participants in athletic games would cover themselves with olive oil to protect their skin and then scrape it off with strigils, too.

The root of the word exfoliation comes from the Latin *ex* (to take away) and *folium* (leaf). So, exfoliation can be construed as meaning "taking away leaves," and you would see why if you were to look through a microscope at the upper layer of dead skin cells on your body, the stratum corneum, which looks like millions of tiny leaves (refer to Figure 5.14). These leaves are sometimes visible floating in the air in enclosed spaces.

The main benefits of exfoliation include the following:

● It assists the skin's own regenerative processes.

● It aids in the absorption of spa products applied afterward.

● It thoroughly cleanses and promotes overall hygiene.

● It creates a healthy glow and radiant shine to the skin.

Though there are no contraindications for receiving exfoliation services more often, spa guests typically receive only one full exfoliation treatment per stay, but they may receive several shorter exfoliations as part of other spa services. For example, the skin is often exfoliated for 5 minutes before the application of a body mud or seaweed. Female guests should be warned not to shave their legs 24 hours before a salt-based exfoliation service, as it would cause discomfort and irritation. The room in which the exfoliation is given must be at least 80°F, because clients cool down quickly when water is applied to their skin.

Exfoliation services go by many names in spas (see Table 15.5), and many exotic scrubbing ingredients are used to lure clients into the exfoliation room. Some common products used to scrub the body include: fruit seeds, crushed nut shells, cornmeal, salt (often from the Dead Sea), sugar, oatmeal, enzymes, jojoba wax beads, polyethylene balls, crushed pearls, pumice, and ground rice grains, among others. Additional products are added to the primary scrubbing agents in order to enhance the treatment or make it even more exotic. These can include, among many

Table 15.5

Exfoliation Services Offered in Spas

EXFOLIATION SERVICE	DESCRIPTION
Body scrub	This generic term refers to a wide range of exfoliation services and can even include salt rubs
Body polish	This name usually refers to a more refined and gentler exfoliation service using smaller and perhaps softer particles of exfoliant; the polish is suitable for more sensitive skin types
Sea salt glow	Using sea salts, the body is thoroughly exfoliated in this service, which is sometimes too abrasive for people with sensitive skin or those who have recently shaved their legs; the most popular salts for this service come from the Dead Sea in Israel, which are high in minerals
Salt glow/salt rub/salt scrub	An abbreviated name for the sea salt glow, though the name can sometimes signify that the salts are NOT from the Dead Sea
Body gommage	This term is popular, especially in European-inspired spas, and means, roughly translated, a "gumming" of the skin using familiar exfoliating agents
Dry brush massage	Using a dry bristle body brush, the therapist sweeps the skin clean for a full half-hour service; this is known to be especially therapeutic for the lymphatic system and is used during internal detoxification programs as well as to cleanse the skin
Swedish shampoo	This term is used infrequently in spas today—it refers to a body scrub technique using a bath brush or mitt and soapy water; it is similar to a body polish or body scrub
Loofah scrub	A somewhat rare spa service in which the therapist uses only a loofah to exfoliate the skin; it can be quite abrasive, depending upon the texture of the loofah

others, such ingredients as lime, lemon, orange, ginger, coconut, milk, honey, lavender, pomegranate, and chamomile.

The principal maneuver for all exfoliation techniques is a circular scrubbing action to avoid stretching the delicate connective tissues of the skin too far in any one direction. Massage therapists need to remember that they are not giving a massage service during exfoliation. Exfoliation maneuvers are distinct and have different intents (Figure 15.17).

Wet Room versus Dry Room Exfoliation

In some spas, the client reclines on a **wet table,** which is a specially constructed waterproof treatment table with built-in drainage used for exfoliation and body wrap services. Products are washed from the body with a shower hose or a built-in **Vichy shower** above the table. This type of treatment area is called a **wet room.** In spas without the infrastructure or budget necessary for a room with plumbing and a wet table, a regular massage table can be used with a vinyl drape or thermal blanket over it for protection. This is called a **dry room** spa setup.

Regardless of the products used, the procedure for many body scrubs is the same. First, the client's skin is moistened, either with a hot wet towel in a dry room or a shower in a wet room, then the exfoliant is ap-

> **wet table**
> is a specially constructed waterproof treatment table with built-in drainage used in spas for exfoliation and body wrap services.

> **Vichy shower**
> is a multihead inline shower extending out over a treatment table under which clients recline on a wet table to receive spa services.

Figure 15.17

Exfoliation maneuvers are circular. Although they may involve pressure, the primary action is on the body's surface, not its inner structures.

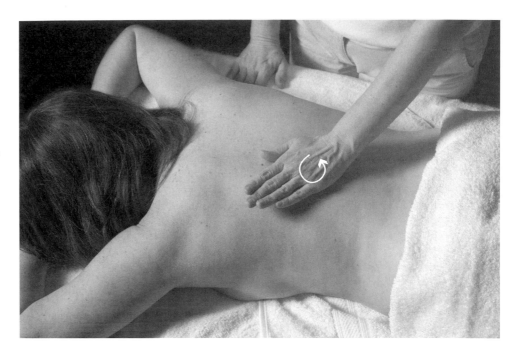

wet room
is a tiled treatment room with plumbing that contains one or more of the following: wet table, shower, Vichy shower, hydrotherapy tub, Swiss shower.

dry room
is a massage room used for spa treatments performed without the use of showers and baths.

plied. The therapist works the exfoliant into the skin, then cleanses it off. Some exfoliations include washing with a body bath or soap. Finally, a moisturizer or massage oil is applied.

Exfoliation Procedure

This procedure is for a dry room exfoliation using hot wet towels instead of a shower. The term *exfoliant* here refers to any chosen scrubbing agent except for salt. See the slightly different Salt Glow protocol later in the chapter. *Body bath* refers to any liquid type soap. In spas, the choice of liquid soaps for this purpose is usually aromatic, often with essential oils added.

Preparation

Rinse and wring out four hand towels and keep them hot in a towel cabinet or insulated container. Warm the exfoliant so that it will not shock the client during application. Fill a large bowl with hot water and place a loofah mitt or pad in the water. Prepare a massage table with a vinyl drape or a thermal blanket to protect the table from moisture. Then layer a large bath towel or bath sheet on top of this for the client to lie on (Figure 15.18a). Drape the client normally with a bath towel, or diaper drape. Keep in mind that this drape may become quite damp in a wet room but will remain mostly dry using the hot towel method in a dry room.

Exfoliating the Back and Back of Legs

1. First, moisten the back and back of the legs with the fabric side of the loofah pad or a sponge (Figure 15.18b).

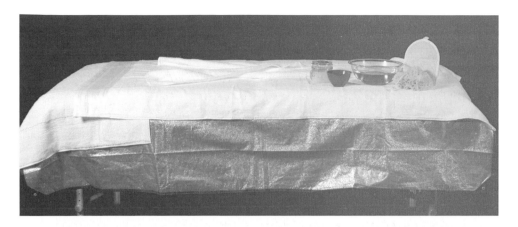

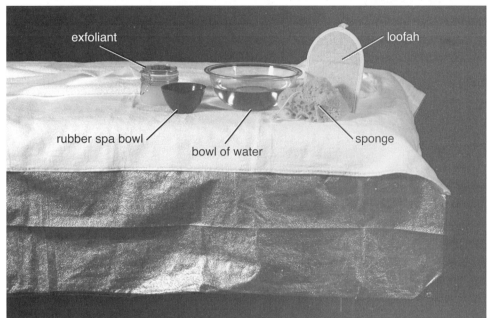

exfoliant

loofah

rubber spa bowl

bowl of water

sponge

Figure 15.18a

Prepare a massage table with a vinyl drape or a space blanket. Then layer a large bath towel or bath sheet on top of this for the client to lie on.

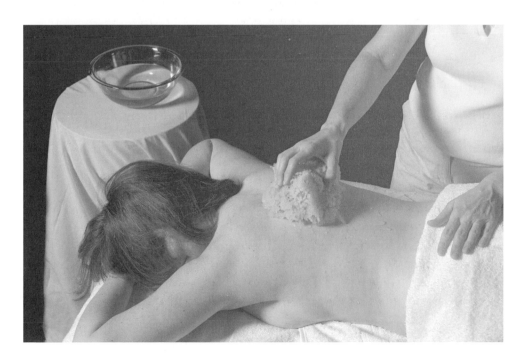

Figure 15.18b

The first step in an exfoliation treatment is moistening the skin.

2. Place a quarter-sized dab of exfoliant in your palm and rub into the back first, using the circular exfoliating movement (Figure 15.18c).

3. Apply more exfoliant as needed, move down to the right foot, and work up over the right leg to the buttock.

4. Repeat on the left leg.

5. Spend 5 minutes on this entire part of the procedure, and then use the first hot wet towel to wipe away the exfoliant from the back and the back of the legs (Figure 15.18d).

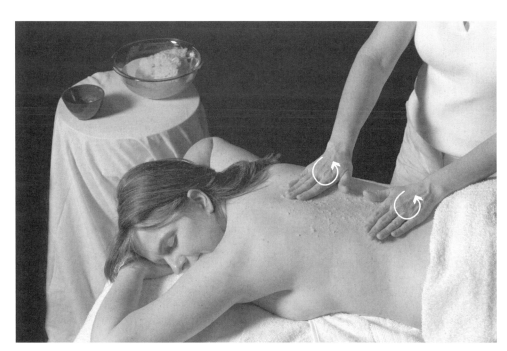

Figure 15.18c

The therapist applies the exfoliant to one part of the body at a time using circular movements, starting with the back, then continuing with the back of the legs.

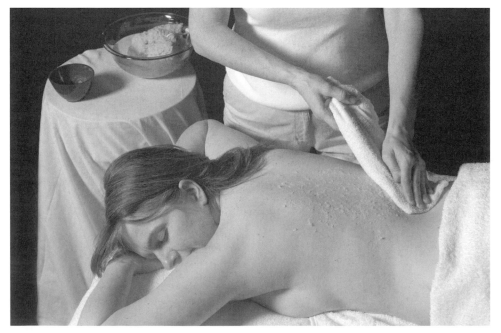

Figure 15.18d

When the back is finished, the therapist wipes excess exfoliant away with hot, wet towels.

Cleansing the Back and Back of the Legs

1. Dip the loofah pad in the bowl of hot water, place a quarter-sized dab of body bath on the scrubbing surface, and use it to cleanse the back and the back of the legs, using circular exfoliating movements (Figure 15.18e).

2. After 5 minutes, use the second hot, wet towel to wipe off the excess soap (Figure 15.18f).

3. Spend 5 minutes on this part of the procedure, then ask the client to roll over, keeping the drape covering intact.

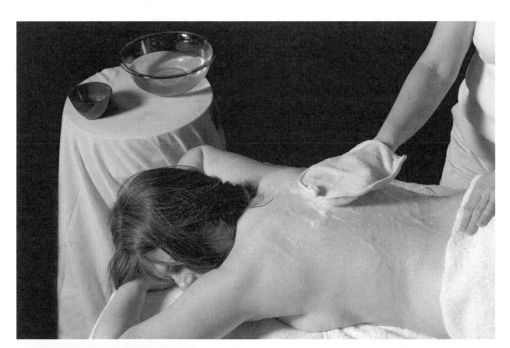

Figure 15.18e
The therapist uses a sponge or loofah with body bath to cleanse the back, then the back of the legs.

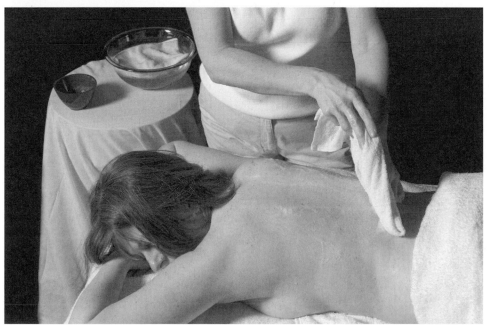

Figure 15.18f
Then wipe soap off the body with another hot, moist towel.

Exfoliating the Front of the Body

1. The exfoliating steps are repeated here (Figure 15.18g to i), using a quarter-sized dab of exfoliant to start on the feet, legs, abdomen, sides, arms, and décolletage.

2. Wipe off the exfoliant with the third hot, wet towel. This part of the procedure takes 5 minutes.

Figure 15.18g

The client rolls over and the process is repeated on the front of the body. First, the therapist moistens the skin.

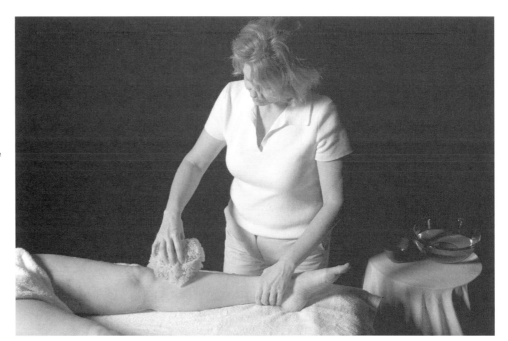

Figure 15.18h

The therapist exfoliates the front of the legs, torso, arms, and chest. Females must be covered with a breast drape.

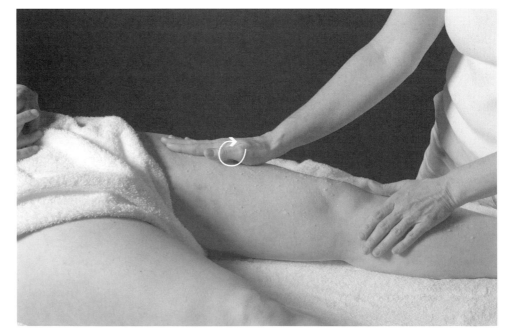

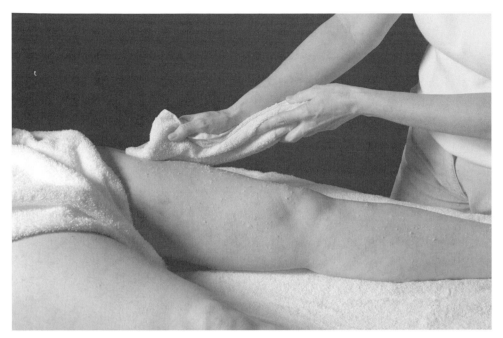

Figure 15.18i
The exfoliant is wiped away with a hot, wet towel.

Cleansing the Front of the Body

1. Apply body bath to the loofah pad soaked in hot water and use it to cleanse the front of the body (Figure 15.18j).

2. Wipe off soap with the last hot, wet towel (Figure 15.18k).

3. Use a dry towel to wipe away any excess moisture. This part of the procedure also lasts 5 minutes.

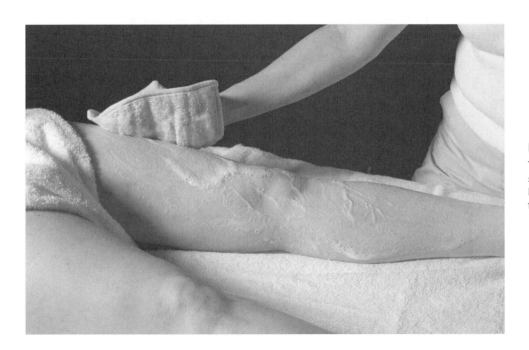

Figure 15.18j
The therapist uses a sponge or loofah with body bath to cleanse the front of the body.

continues

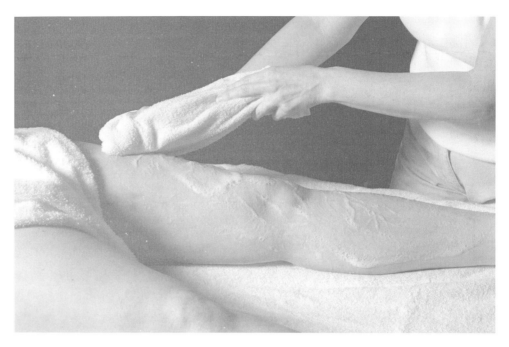

Figure 15.18k

The therapist uses a final hot, wet towel to wipe away excess soap and any leftover exfoliant.

Application of Moisturizer

1. Apply moisturizing lotion or massage oil to the front of the body. This can also be the start of a longer massage, creating a combination exfoliation/massage service (Figure 15.18l).

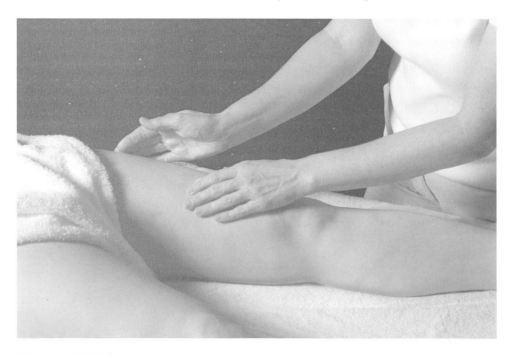

Figure 15.18l

A lotion or oil is briefly applied to moisturize the skin. This can also be the beginning of a massage, extending the service to an hour or hour and a half.

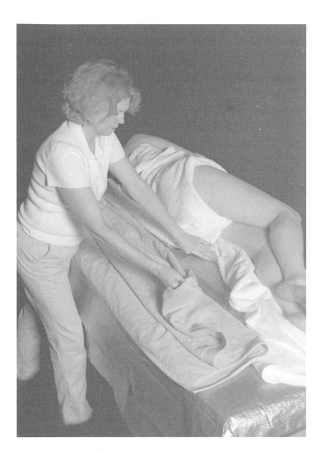

Figure 15.18m
The client rolls over as the therapist changes the towel beneath her.

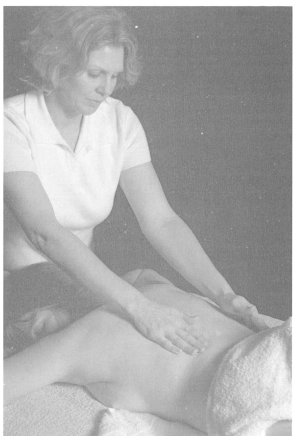

Figure 15.18n
The treatment ends with an application of moisturizer to the back and the back of the legs.

2. Ask the client to roll over. Change the bottom towel while the client rolls, pushing it to one side, then slipping it out from beneath the client while sliding a new towel underneath (Figure 15.18m). This is so that the client does not lie in damp exfoliant and soap residue.

3. Finish the treatment with an application of moisturizing lotion or massage oil to the back (Figure 15.18n). The entire application to the front and the back of the body lasts 5 minutes, for 25-minute total treatment time with 5 minutes left to prepare for the next client.

Sea Salt Glow Procedure

The sea salt glow often utilizes salts from the Dead Sea, which are high in magnesium, potassium, calcium, bromine, and other minerals. The procedure is somewhat messier than a body scrub or body polish, but it can still be performed in a dry room, as the following procedure indicates.

Preparation

Rinse and wring out four hand towels and keep them hot in a towel cabinet or insulated container. Mix approximately one-half cup of salts with a small amount of water, teaspoon by teaspoon, until a paste is formed. Six to eight drops of essential oil may be added to this to improve the aroma and add to the effect. Warm the salt so that it will not shock the client during application. Prepare a massage table and draping as for the exfoliation procedure described previously.

Salt Glow to the Back and the Back of the Legs

1. First, moisten the back and the back of the legs with a washcloth.

2. Place a quarter- to a half-dollar-sized dab of salt in your palm and rub it into the back first, using the circular exfoliating movement.

3. Move down to the right foot and work up over the right leg to the buttock.

4. Repeat on the left leg.

5. Spend 10 minutes on this entire part of the procedure, and then use two hot, wet towels to wipe away the salt from the back and the back of the legs.

6. Ask the client to roll over. Help keep the drape intact during the roll.

Salt Glow to the Front of the Body

1. Moisten the feet and front of the legs with a washcloth.

2. Using the sea salt mixture, start exfoliating the feet first, paying special attention to the heels.

3. Move up the front of the right leg, then the left.

4. Exfoliate the abdomen, sides, décolletage, and arms.

5. Wipe off the exfoliant with two more hot, wet towels. This entire part of the procedure takes approximately 10 minutes.

Application of Moisturizer

1. Apply moisturizing lotion or massage oil to the front of the body. This can also be the start of a longer massage, creating a combination exfoliation/massage service.

2. Ask the client to roll over. Change the bottom towel while the client rolls, pushing it to one side, then slipping it out from beneath the client while sliding a new towel underneath. This is so that the client does not lie in damp salt granules.

3. Finish the treatment with an application of moisturizing lotion or massage oil to the back and back of the legs. The entire application to the front and the back of the body lasts 5 minutes, for 25-minute total treatment time with 5 minutes left to prepare for the next client.

SPA COMPANY POLICIES AND PHILOSOPHY

In addition to performing massage and other modalities, spa therapists also need to interact with fellow employees and learn to thrive within the larger structure of the spa. Some therapists find that working for a company is the most challenging aspect of spa work because it means that they are not as independent as they would perhaps like to be. In order to work successfully at a spa, however, therapists need to know, accept, and adhere to company policies. These policies cover a range of employee issues, including time concerns, appearance, attitude, professional development, and physical attributes.

- *Time concerns:* punctuality; amount of time per service; amount of time between services; time spent on tasks other than massage; time spent charting, logging, and filling out intake forms
- *Appearance:* uniform, hair length, beard/mustaches, body piercing, visible tattoos, makeup, weight, cigarette smoking, neatness
- *Attitude:* team player, responsible, mature, communicative, positive, calm under pressure, trustworthy, humble, attentive, able to follow instructions
- *Professional development:* desire for continuous improvement, ongoing skill building through advanced education, passion for the work, development of customer service skills, development of sales skills, longevity in spa positions
- *Physical attributes:* healthy lifestyle, endurance, strength

Before accepting a position in a spa, therapists should ask themselves whether they are willing to accept an employer's guidelines regarding these issues. It is important to thoroughly read a copy of the spa's employment policies, usually found in a company employee manual or handbook, prior to beginning work. If any spa policies seem unacceptable, they should be discussed with spa management.

Professional Career Management

Perhaps the most common issue that causes tension between therapists and spa management is compensation. Some therapists resent working in spas because the spa takes a large percentage of the income from each treatment. This resentment is unproductive for all involved. It reduces the quality of the guests' experience, poisons the atmosphere of the spa, frustrates spa management, and may result in the dismissal of the therapist.

The percentage of total treatment cost kept by the spa is not the most important issue. Rather, it must be remembered that the spa is performing a valuable service for the therapist. This service can be called "professional career management." The spa, in exchange for a percentage of the price of each treatment, offers therapists many benefits, including a built-in clientele, marketing, advertising, appointment booking, billing, payroll, supplies, equipment, training, support staff, and a clean facility. Everything down to laundry services is taken care of for the therapist, and the high cost of this support must be taken into account.

Product and Treatment Knowledge

In addition to knowing the spa's policies and procedures, therapists must also possess a thorough knowledge of spa products and treatments. Often, this information is provided by the vendors who manufacture and sell the products to the spa. These vendors naturally have a bias in favor of their own products and procedures, and therefore it is beneficial for the therapist to seek additional information beyond what the vendors provide. The spa may offer a treatment guidebook, which should be studied diligently. In case the spa does not offer such a guidebook, the therapist should take the time to study on her own. The following are the main topics to study regarding spa product and treatment knowledge:

- *Benefits/effects:* What are the benefits of the product or service? Which systems of the body do they work on? Is the procedure effective used just once or are repeated applications required?

- *Contraindications:* What are the conditions that should not be treated with the products or procedure? How might they adversely affect people with specific conditions?

- *Background:* What is the history of the product or treatment in spas? Is there any folklore associated with it? What information is scientific and what is anecdotal? Is the treatment performed differently in different spas or different areas of the world? Were the products or treatment originally developed as part of any indigenous culture?

- *Integration:* Can spa guests integrate the benefits of the treatment into their lives via a home care regime? If so, how? What retail products are associated with the treatment? Can the guest adopt certain lifestyle activities to help integrate the intended outcomes of the treatment?

SPECIALIZED SPA EQUIPMENT

Modern spas utilize many specialized pieces of equipment to create their advanced services (Figure 15.19). Each spa offers some degree of training on this equipment, but it is important to have a grasp of general equipment knowledge before arriving for work at a spa. It is also important to be familiar with the precautions and sanitation requirements for each item. The equipment in Table 15.6 can be found in many spas throughout the world.

CUSTOMER SERVICE

Spa customers expect a high level of customer service, and it is vital that the spa therapist learn those techniques and skills that will add to the spa's ability to provide it. In order to excel in this area, therapists must first of all understand precisely what customer service entails. Customer

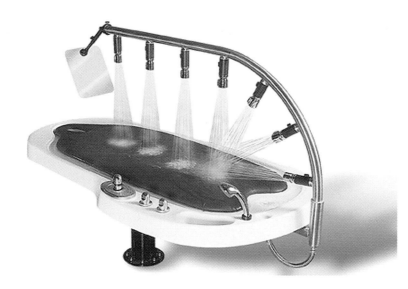

Figure 15.19

Vichy shower with wet table.
(Courtesy of HydroCo USA:
www.hydroco.com.)

Table 15.6
Specialized Spa Equipment

EQUIPMENT	DESCRIPTION	USES	WHERE FOUND	PRECAUTIONS	COST
Endermologie	Computerized massage device using rollers and suction to stretch and tone superficial subcutaneous connective tissue	Used in spas mainly as an anticellulite treatment, though also used for sports and therapeutic applications for athletes, burn victims, and others	Somewhat popular in U.S. spas, though more so in Europe and Asia; has spawned numerous competing devices for similar use	On strongest settings can be overstimulating to skin	$30,000 to $35,000
Hydrotherapy tub	One-person tub with multiple therapist-controlled jets aimed at specific body zones; most also have a "wand" for high-powered underwater massage	Used for baths, immersions, soaks, cellulite treatments, and other modalities, often in combination with a massage or body scrub; relaxes muscles, opens pores, relieves tension	Popular in larger spas with extensive menus; often underutilized in smaller spas, where these tubs can become a financial drain and are often sold at a loss	Care taken when clients enter/exit tub; heat may cause dizziness; must be cleaned with disinfectant after every use; many tubs have a built-in cleaning cycle	$9,000 to $20,000+
Scotch hose	A high-pressure spray (sometimes using sea water) aimed at a standing client	Extremely invigorating; stimulates circulation; used for bracing and toning effects, especially if cold/hot contrast therapy used	Most popular in older European-style spas and spas modeled after that style	Clients need to be forewarned about intensity of spray; area needs to be cleaned and disinfected after use	$500 to $5,000
Swiss shower	A shower stall with heads aimed at the client from all sides and above, usually controlled by therapist outside of stall	Used for washing off muds, seaweeds, and exfoliants and for stimulating percussive and thermal effects, often with contrasting hot and cold	Usually constructed only in larger spas; popularity is waning as newer spas opt for Vichy showers over Swiss	Same as regular shower stall; some clients find the spray too intense (it is called a "needle shower" by some)	$1,500 to $5,000
Vichy shower	A long horizontally aligned pipe with multiple heads aimed down to spray a client's body while she reclines on a wet table	Used primarily for exfoliations and wrap services to wash off product; also adds luxurious feel to specialty massages beneath heavy spray; provides hot/cold benefits	Very popular, although somewhat expensive to install	Table beneath shower must be cleaned after use; pooled water should be wiped away; spray must be directed away from the client's face	$3,000 to $6,000

service can be defined as the ability of an organization or individual to take care of the needs, wishes, questions, requests, and complaints of its clientele. Excellent customer service consists of doing these things consistently, to a very high standard of satisfaction, and in a largely transparent manner, which means that the customer often does not even notice the efforts being made on her behalf.

Therapists new to the spa industry often make the mistake of thinking that it is their hands-on skills alone that determines their value in the workplace. Spa directors and owners, however, think otherwise. They consistently rank customer service skills at the top of the list and often omit massage skills entirely when speaking about what they seek in new employees. A certain level of technical skill is taken for granted; customer service skills are cherished. Two of the main customer service skills therapists need in the spa setting are retail skills and teamwork skills.

Retail Skills

Therapists employed in spas sometimes complain if they are expected to recommend products for spa guests to buy or to perform any sales-related activities whatsoever. However, it is important to realize the importance of retail sales for the success of the spa. Most spas depend upon retail profits to keep the business operational. Without these profits, many spas would close and many therapists would be out of a job. It is therefore in spa therapists' best interests to help with retail sales, as long as these sales are executed with integrity, honesty, and skill.

Sales Integrity

When selling products in the spa, therapists need to believe in their hearts that the products involved will make a real difference in clients' lives. It is preferable, in fact, that the therapist has used the products at home and can vouch personally for their effectiveness. There is no need to become a professional salesperson. Sales flow naturally from a discussion about the benefits of the treatment. Products simply extend those benefits into the home. For this reason, it is important to look at spa products as part of a home care regime, not as just an indulgence.

Some spas offer their therapists a commission on the products sold. Even if this commission is of no interest to the therapist, the sale is still important for the success of the spa and the satisfaction of the client. If therapists feel uncomfortable taking commissions for sales, they can offer this extra money to the front desk staff or even donate it to a charity.

Therapists need to know that selling products to a client is not against the ethical code of any massage association. Selling is not against the law. It is not against the rules. What it does run counter to is some therapists' view of themselves as quasi-medical practitioners. Medically oriented massage usually does not involve retail sales, although some practitioners of this modality offer their clients medicinal herbs, exercise equipment, stretching devices, and other allied items for sale. Spa massage, it must be remembered, is not medical massage, and it is completely permissible to offer spa clients the opportunity to take home the benefits of the products they have had applied in the spa. Therapists need to know that this is a normal, acceptable part of their duties at many spas. In fact, therapists who are comfortable with selling are highly regarded by spa owners and directors.

Sales Honesty

Therapists should never make false or misleading claims about the effectiveness of the products for sale in the spa. Instead, they should state only that which has been verified through long experience. Vague, general claims should be avoided. The spa world has been the subject of much scrutiny from the media and the public regarding false claims, and in order to counter this, the best policy is to assert only that which can be proven. Exfoliating products do indeed rid the body of dead cells. Seaweed does indeed penetrate the pores and add minerals to the body. Hot herbal wraps do indeed help leach impurities out through the pores. If no fantastic promises are made, and clients are given realistic expectations regarding the use of spa products, sales in the spa can benefit everyone— the spa, the client, and the therapist.

Therapists should always let clients know before the treatment begins that they will be recommending home care products for purchase after the service is over. This is so that clients do not feel unfairly taken advantage of when they are relaxed and their guards are lowered after the treatment. The fact that products are available should be stated before, during, and after the treatment. The statement should be matter-of-fact and informational.

Sales Skill

In order for therapists to sell skillfully, they must posses a thorough knowledge of the product (see "Product and Treatment Knowledge," earlier in this chapter), a certain level of enthusiasm about the results to be gained from using the product, and at least some degree of comfort with the act of selling itself. It is helpful, in this regard, to observe the skill and ease with which many estheticians offer products to their clientele. They expect the client to want to purchase products to continue the effects of the treatment at home. They are confident that clients will be happy with the results, so they are not squeamish about suggesting that the client make the purchase.

When the therapist is comfortable in a selling situation, certain skills come easily, making the transaction a natural part of the therapeutic offering (Figure 15.20). Three basic techniques may help the therapist sell spa products tactfully and successfully:

- *Self-observation:* When attempting to sell something in the spa, therapists need to gauge their own feelings and reactions to the process. Often, clients will react more to the nonverbal message and body language of the spa employee, rather than the words she is speaking. The most important thing is to be comfortable, not slick.

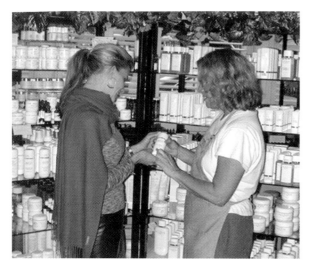

Figure 15-20

A therapist is assisting a guest to choose products in a spa store. Although it is not a spa therapist's primary responsibility, retail sales are an important part of the job description. (Courtesy of Preston Wynne, Inc.)

● *Closing:* At the same time, it is also important to actually ask for the sale. Some therapists who find selling uncomfortable beat around the bush and never state outright their request that the client buy something. A simple "Would you like to purchase this product and make it part of your home care routine?" is sufficient.

● *Detachment:* No matter the response from the client, therapists should not take it personally. In fact, the more detached and serene about the transaction the therapist is, the more comfortable the client will feel, and the better the chance is for a sale.

Teamwork Skills

Massage therapists, unlike most other professionals, have the ability to work for the most part independently and free of support. The moment a therapist walks through the door of a spa for the first day on the job, however, that independence is taken away. Therapists who work in the spa industry are irrevocably part of a team, sometimes a large team. It is important to remember this.

As anyone who works at the front desk or in management at a spa knows, a team-oriented attitude on the part of the massage and spa treatment staff is absolutely essential for the overall functioning of the spa. Everything therapists do and say behind closed doors during that vast amount of quality time spent with the guests reflects mightily on the perception guests have of the spa. Spa therapists are in a real sense setting the underlying tone of the entire operation.

The main teamwork skills required to work successfully in a spa include:

● *Ability to follow direction:* Spa therapists need to follow the guidance handed down from spa management. Although this may prove difficult for independent-minded practitioners, it is absolutely essential in order for the team to work together as a unit. All teams have a leader. Spas are no exception.

● *Anticipating others' needs:* Spa therapists should constantly be looking out for ways that they can help guests before the guests even know they need help. Offer directions to other areas of the spa. Bring water or tea before it is requested. Suggest ways to improve guests' experience.

● *Presenting a united front:* Therapists should refrain from speaking to guests about the internal operations of the spa, especially problems with management or other employees. Every business operation has its share of conflicts. Therapists need to leave these conflicts outside the treatment room, or the level of service of the entire spa will suffer.

- *Pitching in:* Even if a particular task, such as picking up dirty towels or cleaning a bathroom counter, is not on a massage therapist's job description, it should still be executed diligently and with a positive attitude in order to ensure the smooth, seamless running of the spa. If no one else is available at the moment, the rule is "pitch in."

EMPLOYMENT OPPORTUNITIES IN THE SPA INDUSTRY

The contact between service providers and customers is perhaps greater in spas than in any other industry, thus making the hiring and training of quality personnel especially important as owners and directors continue to seek well-qualified therapists with the proper attitudes to fill many positions in spas all over the world. Spas employ nearly 300,000 people in the United States alone, and by far, the largest percentage of pay goes to the hands-on staff. Therapists and estheticians are the backbone of the industry. On the other hand, spas are currently the largest source of jobs for therapists and the single largest employer of new massage school graduates. Spas need therapists. Therapists need spas. This synergy creates a most promising job market in a wide range of possible workspaces.

Today, therapists can find work not only in the traditional spa settings described in Table 15.1 but also in many unique environments. Many therapists seek the adventure of working aboard a cruise ship, for example. Spas can be found in airport terminals, and some airlines have begun offering massage and spa services to passengers on transatlantic flights. Safari spas can be found in the wilds of Africa, soul-stirring spas in the Himalayan highlands, thermal spas in outback Chile, adventure spas in Australian rain forests, exotic spas in Thai jungles, wine-themed spas in Napa Valley, and thousands of local spas right around the corner in every city and in most towns.

So how, exactly, does one go about finding and securing the right job in this vast industry? Therapists are understandably confused when first setting out to seek a position. Should they just walk in the front door and ask for a job? Should they get a recommendation from somebody first? To whom should they present it? Is a résumé important? Which spas are more likely to be hiring? When is the best time to apply?

Realistic Expectations

Therapists need to follow certain practical steps as they begin to carve out a career for themselves in the spa industry. First, it is important to create a résumé that includes vital statistics, school history and training, job experience, and personal achievements. Even therapists new to the job market will present themselves more professionally if they have a well-prepared résumé, with proper spelling, full dates, past work history, and schools attended.

Recommendations are not necessary in order to get an interview at a spa; however, a therapist's chances at landing the job will not be hurt if she comes to the interview highly recommended by somebody who knows the spa director or owner personally. Written recommendations are best, but a phone call can help too.

Timing is important when applying for a spa job. Many spas operate on a seasonal basis, meaning that they have busy times of the year and slow times. Therapists will be more successful in their job searches if they time applications to coincide with the beginning of the busy season, when spas are looking for personnel. These times vary widely according to location. Spas in ski resort towns will be looking to hire in November, for example, whereas beach spas will hire more therapists in May. It is also important to time any job application to occur at a quiet time during the spa's daily operations. Mornings when the spa first opens are usually the best time.

Spas advertise their need for therapists in a number of ways: through magazines, mailings, classifieds, job postings in massage schools, and word of mouth. Therapists seeking their first spa position should be prepared to work "on call," which means they will not at first be a part of the spa's permanent staff. This position is usually temporary, and as the therapist shows responsibility and skill, she can move to a full-time position. The key to success in a spa position is to be willing to do whatever is necessary for the overall success of the spa. To do this, therapists need to think of the business as their own, even if they are working part time. Those therapists who maintain an outsider's attitude and do not help co-create success for the spa business as a whole stand a much lower chance of progressing in the industry, no matter how skilled they are in the treatment room.

Interviewing for Spa Positions

In the larger spas, especially in the resort sector, it is usually necessary to pass through the human resources department on the way to a therapist position. In smaller facilities, interviews are conducted directly with the spa director or manager. Also, some spas use peer interviews, which means that prospective therapists are screened by members of the massage staff.

When interviewing with any of these gatekeepers, therapists should emphasize the customer service and teamwork skills discussed in previous sections in this chapter. Spas are wary of therapists who present themselves as "job junkies" who move quickly from position to position, leaving because of poor relationships with management. They watch for patterns of past injury on the job, as this may point to improper work habits. They also pay attention to the reputation of the massage school attended by the therapist. One other important point is flexibility in scheduling. Therapists who can work any shift, including evenings, weekends, and holidays, are given preference because the spa industry requires these hours of its employees.

Therapists should come to the interview prepared to talk about how they chose massage as a career, past work situations, attitude toward clients, and how they would deal with problems on the job. In addition, they should have some knowledge of the spa where they are applying and be able to explain why they want to work at that particular facility. Research helps with this.

Test Massages

Perhaps one of the most feared hurdles therapists must leap on the way to a spa position is that of the test massage. For many people, it is nerve wracking to perform under such conditions, but it is usually a necessary step if the spa is going to get a good idea of a candidate's skill. The test massage involves giving a full treatment to somebody on the spa's staff, most often a supervisor, manager, owner, or director. Both participants in this process know that the therapist is being judged, which does not make for a relaxing treatment much of the time.

Therapists can overcome some of the anxiety that attends these test massages by practicing on as many people as possible before applying for the position, ideally with several of these practice treatments given back-to-back, as this is the way many spas are now operating test massage interviews. In order to simulate the real-world conditions of a spa, applicants are often asked to give two or three massages in a row to see how well they hold up under the pressure and the strain.

It must be remembered that the test massage is not just about massage. Applicants are also being screened for certain invisible, yet crucial, attributes that can make or break a therapist's chances at getting a job. (See the accompanying sidebar, "Top Behavioral Characteristics of a Successful Spa Therapist".) Although newly graduated therapists are rightfully proud of their technical skills, it is not massage talent alone that can get them that coveted position at an exciting spa, but rather character, personality, presence, and attitude.

TOP BEHAVIORAL CHARACTERISTICS OF A SUCCESSFUL SPA THERAPIST

A group of 12 spa directors from top U.S. spas were gathered at a symposium and asked what were the top characteristics on which they judged massage therapy job candidates. These directors had their own views on the importance of various qualities, so none could be ranked as more important than another. These, in random order, were their responses:

- **Team player**
- **Responsible**
- **Caring and open-hearted**
- **Open-minded**
- **Mature**
- **Good communicator**
- **Positive**
- **Calm under pressure**
- **Honest/trustworthy**
- **Able to follow instructions**
- **Passionate about doing spa work and massage**
- **Healthy/leading a healthy lifestyle**
- **Customer-service oriented**
- **Sales-oriented**
- **Common sense**
- **Ability to accept change**
- **Humility**
- **Desire for continuous improvement (how many classes have they taken?)**
- **History of success/longevity in previous positions**
- **Neatness/tidiness**

ADVANCING YOUR SPA CAREER

Because the spa industry has been growing so quickly, it has afforded many opportunities for employees to move up through the ranks. Often these employees are massage therapists. There are no precise statistics on this matter, but therapists now hold a large number of upper management spa positions, including supervisor, trainer, manager, director, and even owner.

SPA RESOURCES FOR THE BEGINNING PRACTITIONER

There are many resources available for massage therapists who are interested in pursuing a career in the spa industry. It is wise to familiarize yourself with these resources prior to making a final decision regarding your career path. The resources included here are spa magazines, spa books, spa associations, spa trade shows, and spa Web sites.

Spa Magazines

- *American Spa:* a "pro-sumer" (targeting both professionals and consumers) magazine with industry information and spa profiles; www.americanspamag.com
- *Day Spa Magazine:* a trade magazine dealing with day spa issues; www.dayspamag.com
- *PULSE:* the official magazine of the International Spa Association (ISPA); www.experienceispa.com
- *Spa Finders:* A magazine offering a huge amount of information on spas worldwide, plus much industry information; www.spafinders.com
- *Spa Magazine:* a consumer magazine focusing on the benefits of the spa lifestyle; www.spamagazine.com
- *Spa Management Magazine:* A magazine focusing on issues pertinent to spa managers, directors , and staff; www.spamanagement.com

Moving up the corporate ladder has advantages and disadvantages. On the one hand, therapists who move up can achieve more security and make higher salaries. However, some therapists who move up find that the money does not compensate for the increased paperwork and managerial responsibilities. In fact, the per-hour wage for performing massage in a spa is often higher than that received by many managers because managers have to work so many more hours. So, in this sense, professional advancement within the spa industry is a trade-off. Therapists trade their hands-on work and extensive interactions with clients for more involvement in spa operations, more prestige perhaps, more opportunities for travel, and sometimes more pay. Therapists who work in other capacities within the spa industry also find that they can save their bodies from the symptoms of overuse that plague some practitioners.

If, after careful consideration, a therapist decides that she would like to move up within the spa industry, there are several points to keep in mind:

- *Laying a foundation:* Some therapists jump the gun when it comes to promoting themselves in the industry. It is important to learn the job from the ground up, becoming thoroughly familiar with all aspects of daily operations before moving on to supervising others. This is a particular strength of massage therapists, as compared to managers who come to the industry from outside. Those who take their time to climb the ladder often do better once they have scaled it.

● *Becoming active:* Therapists who expect to move into higher positions need to get involved with the overall operations of the spa at an early stage, even before making a career advancement. There are always opportunities for volunteer work, assisting the manager, learning the systems, and more. This must be done in unobtrusive and helpful ways. Therapists can also show a willingness to help in other departments outside their own, as this is expected of managers as well.

● *Learning from others:* Therapists should watch how managers and supervisors conduct business, learning the protocols and routines of the spa. They should ask questions of people in other departments, even those considered below the rank of therapist such as locker-room attendants. Everyone who knows the spa has a key to some area of the operation that can be useful.

Therapists can also find opportunities to become trainers or consultants in the spa industry. Much room for growth exists in this sector, and to pursue it, therapists should focus on learning as much as they can about the business of spas as well as the treatments. This can be achieved by attending spa conferences and taking advantage of the educational offerings provided there. Also, therapists should learn as many modalities as possible in order to attain a broad understanding of all spa offerings. This, along with plenty of on-the-job experience in the spa, will prepare therapists to make the leap to training and consulting. Often, this leap is facilitated through extensive networking in the industry, and this only happens over an extended period of time.

Opening Your Own Spa

The ultimate dream of many therapists who enter the spa sector is to one day open their own spa facility. Plenty of therapists have done so, some with more success than others.

SPA RESOURCES FOR THE BEGINNING PRACTITIONER

Spa Books

- *100 Best Spas of the World,* by Bernard Burt (Globe Pequot Press): top spas reviewed
- *Day Spa Techniques,* by Erica Miller (Milady): hands-on information for the spa therapist on a number of popular techniques
- *Day Spa Operations,* by Erica Miller (Milady): instructions and insight into opening and operating a day spa
- *Fodor's Healthy Escapes,* by Bernard Burt: a travel guide to spas around the world, with information about program, price, orientation, and so on.
- *Spa Work: A Massage Therapist's Guide to Success in the Spa Industry,* by Steve Capellini (available 2007): all facets of spa work discussed and clarified
- *The Spa Encyclopedia,* by Hannelore Leavy and Reinhard Bergel (Milady): instructions on how to apply dozens of spa treatments

Spa Associations

- International Spa Association (ISPA): the most comprehensive, worldwide spa association, originated in 1991; great networking and educational opportunities; www.experienceispa.com
- Day Spa Association: works in conjunction with the Medical Spa Association; focused primarily on smaller facilities; www.dayspaassociation.com
- Medical Spa Association: works in conjunction with the Day Spa Association, focused on medical/wellness spas; www.medicalspaassociation.org
- Spa Canada: the latest information about the growing spa industry in Canada; www.spacanada.com

continues

One most important point to keep in mind is that spas are first and foremost a business. Though spas are often run by professional therapists, estheticians, doctors, and other professionals who are passionate about what they do and treat their spas as very personal projects, spas must also be run as businesses—by the numbers—and someone involved with the operation must be willing to take a dispassionate look at the enterprise.

Each therapist is familiar with her own strengths and weaknesses. If, as is often the case, the therapist who is passionate about opening a spa is not strong in business or accounting, it is appropriate to partner with somebody who is. Therapists can also learn about business via books, seminars, and school programs. If, after considering the challenges, a therapist decides to pursue the opening of a spa, certain initial steps should be taken to maximize the potential for success:

- *Start slowly:* Therapists often feel rushed as they pursue their spa dreams. They want to move forward quickly because they perceive competition moving in and windows of opportunity closing. In addition, their enthusiasm propels them forward, sometimes too quickly. It is best to take an ordered, measured approach to any plans that are being made and not rush into a project that may fail later due to lack of foresight.

- *Assess limitations:* Therapists need to stay within their own limits. Undercapitalization is the number one reason that new spas fail, and this simply means that not enough funds have been put aside to start and sustain the new business through its early phases before the clientele builds and income increases. It is best to start out small, even if it means simply adding spa services to a one-room massage therapy practice.

- *Enlist allies:* Most spa projects above a one-room operation require the skills and energies of more than one person in order to materialize. Therapists should not be shy about asking for help and creating ways to share responsibilities and profits in a new venture.

SPA RESOURCES FOR THE BEGINNING PRACTITIONER

Spa Trade Shows

- **American Spa Expo: held in New York City in the spring, with much emphasis on medical spas, cosmetic applications, and business building ideas; www.americanspaexpo.com**
- **Esthétique SPA International: with shows in Vancouver, Halifax, and Toronto; for more information, see www.spa-show.com**
- **International Congress of Esthetics: a focus on esthetics, with shows in Long Beach, Philadelphia, Dallas, and Miami; www.dermascope.com**
- **International Cosmetics, Esthetics, and Spa Show (ICESS): held in Las Vegas each spring and Orlando each fall, this show draws attendees from the salon, day spa, and resort spa industries; Las Vegas is the more well-attended show; www.magda.com**
- **International Spa Association (ISPA) Annual Convention: alternating between Dallas and Las Vegas, in the fall, a gathering of industry leaders from around the world; the most spa-intensive of all the trade shows; www.experienceispa.com**
- **Spa & Resort Expo & Conference/Medical Spa Expo & Conference: with three venues to choose from (Miami, New York, and Los Angeles), this conference allows practitioners from many regions to attend; www.spaandresortexpo.com**

continues

- *Keep learning:* Running a spa business requires extensive knowledge of many areas of expertise, including bookkeeping, management, retail, housekeeping, human resources, equipment maintenance, and customer relations, and this list does not even include the main reason most therapists want to open their own spa in the first place, which is to create a space where they can use their skills to help improve their clients' lives.

Keeping the previous warnings in mind, therapists should still know that it is entirely possible to start a successful spa business. Many therapists have, and many will continue to do so. A large segment of the public is open to receiving massage in the spa setting, and it is a powerful way to reach out to a wider audience than ever before, allowing people to experience the benefits of touch therapy and natural, therapeutic spa products.

CONCLUSION

The conclusion to the 2004 ISPA spa industry study stated:

> The rapid growth of the industry has created significant competition for scarce qualified resources at all levels. The problem in the industry has shifted away from the size of the labor pool to the quality of the labor pool. In a one-on-one service industry, the image of a business is a direct reflection of the image of its staff. It is critical that spa industry human resources be properly trained and developed into qualified professionals to uphold a sterling image for the industry.

This quote highlights how important it is for therapists to become well trained and highly qualified if they are to fulfill their role in the booming spa market. Massage therapists truly are the most vital resources in spas, the key to any spa's success, and a growing force in the creation of the industry as a whole. Through education, diligence, and good working relations with professionals from allied fields, therapists will continue to find their opportunities for success in the spa world expanding exponentially.

SPA RESOURCES FOR THE BEGINNING PRACTITIONER

WEB SITES

- www.royaltreatment.com: the Web site of spa trainer and author Steve Capellini
- www.spafinders.com: a spa-specific travel and education site to make bookings and discover new information, along with much industry news and updates
- www.spagoer.com: the insider's guide to the spa industry, with people, names, places, jobs, gossip, and more, by the author of *100 Best Spas of the World*
- www.spamailinglist.com: an extensive review of many spas with contact information, plus much information for the professional
- www.spas.about.com: a clearinghouse of every type of information about the spa industry, for both consumers and professionals
- www.pwsuccesssystems.com: a successful spa owner and business developer has created multiple-day trainings for therapists and others who are serious about starting their own spa businesses, including information on hiring, compensation, budgets, demographics, customer service, and more

QUESTIONS FOR DISCUSSION AND REVIEW

1. What are the origins of the word *spa?*

2. What were the names of the early spas or baths developed in Rome, Turkey, and Japan?

3. How big was the U.S. spa market in 2004?

4. Name the major categories of spas.

5. Name some of the spa modalities in addition to massage that therapists might be required to perform.

6. Which points are most important to keep in mind when practicing massage in a spa setting?

7. What are the major challenges to consistently giving high-quality therapeutic massage in the spa setting, and what three aspects of a spa massage should therapists pay attention to in order to overcome them?

8. By law, can only massage therapists perform body wraps and scrubs in a spa setting?

9. What is the definition of a spa cellulite treatment?

10. What is the definition of a spa parafango treatment?

11. How can aromatherapy be defined in the spa industry?

12. What are some carrier oils commonly used for aromatherapy massage?

13. What are some distinctions that make an aromatherapy massage different from a Swedish massage?

14. What are some of the purposes body wraps are used for in the spa?

15. What are the main benefits of exfoliation?

16. What is the principle maneuver for all exfoliation techniques?

17. What employee issues, defined in a spa's company policies, should be known, accepted, and adhered to by spa therapists?

18. Define professional career management as it applies to massage therapists working in a spa setting.

19. What is a Vichy shower and what is it used for?

20. What is a wet table?

21. Define customer service as it can be applied in the spa.

22. Why are retail sales important in the spa?

23. What are the main teamwork skills required to work successfully in a spa?

24. What should therapists be prepared to talk about when going on a spa job interview?

25. What steps should therapists take if they are considering opening a spa?

Athletic/Sports Massage

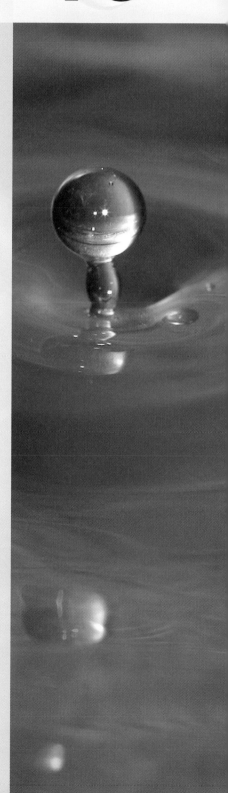

LEARNING OBJECTIVES

After you have mastered this chapter, you will be able to:

1. Define athletic/sports massage.

2. Explain the purposes of athletic massage.

3. Explain the causes of muscle fatigue.

4. Explain the major benefits of athletic massage.

5. Explain contraindications for athletic massage.

6. Locate the major stress points of the body.

7. Explain the importance of warm-up exercises and massage to the athlete's performance.

8. Explain the relationship of certain athletic or sports activities to possible injuries.

9. Describe the four basic applications of athletic massage and the goals of each.

10. Demonstrate massage techniques commonly used in athletic massage.

11. Identify the presence of soft tissue injury.

INTRODUCTION

As far back as antiquity, massage was used to restore and to rejuvenate war-torn and weary soldiers as they returned to Rome. The Roman athletes enjoyed the benefits of restorative massage and baths.

For many years, the great athletes of the European and Soviet countries included massage as part of their intensive and continuous training schedules. In 1972, Lasse Viren, sometimes called the Flying Finn, credited daily deep friction massage with his ability to train hard enough to win gold medals in the 5,000 and 10,000 meters at the Olympic games. In 1980, Jack Meagher and Pat Boughton published the first book in the United States on the subject entitled *Sportsmassage*.

In the United States, massage is recognized as a valuable asset to improve the athlete's ability to perform better with fewer physical ill effects from maximum effort. In 1984, for the first time, massage was made available for all athletes competing in the summer Olympic games in Los Angeles. Since then, massage areas have become a common sight at many athletic events across the country. Many athletes participate in regular massage as part of their training regimen. For many athletes and trainers, massage has become the therapy of choice in the rehabilitation of minor sports injuries.

Throughout the 1980s, sports massage was instrumental in opening the door for the recognition of massage as a viable treatment for soft tissue injury, dysfunction, and pain. Many massage techniques used and developed for sports massage are just as applicable for soft tissue lesions and injuries suffered in the practices of day-to-day living.

PURPOSE OF ATHLETIC MASSAGE

Athletic massage, also called sports massage, is the application of massage techniques that combine sound anatomical and physiological knowledge, an understanding of strength training and conditioning, and specific massage skills to enhance athletic performance. Athletic massage enables athletes to attain their highest potential by accelerating the body's natural restorative processes, enabling the athlete to participate more often in rigorous physical training and conditioning. Massage helps to reduce the chance of injury by identifying and eliminating conditions in the soft tissue that are at potential risk of injury. When injury has occurred, massage helps to restore mobility and flexibility to injured muscle tissue, while reducing recovery time. Athletic massage, when done correctly, can improve the athlete's ability to perform while reducing the incidence of lost time due to injury and fatigue. Receiving sports massage on a regular basis may extend the athlete's career.

Adaptive sports massage (or sports massage for athletes with disabilities) is a specialty that requires additional knowledge and training regarding the disabilities being worked with. This may include mental disabilities (such as experienced by Special Olympians) or physical disabilities (such as those experienced by amputees, people in wheelchairs, or those who are sight or hearing impaired). Although athletes with disabilities do not get the recognition and media attention they deserve, their need for massage therapy and athletic training is just as important as for any other athlete. At the present time, there are no books in publication specific to adaptive sports massage, but articles have been published, and there are a few therapists around the country who specialize and teach workshops on this topic. (Contact the American Massage Therapy Association for resources.)

The sports massage techniques are the same for athletes with disabilities, although they may be used at different times. For instance, a pre-event massage done on a sprinter with cerebral palsy would be very relaxing instead of invigorating. Although most athletes are very agile at getting around, there may also be times that lifting or using a transfer board is necessary. But like all people, the person who knows what is needed to give peak performance is the person living in the body.

Athletic massage is not reserved just for the highly competitive athlete. The same techniques are effective on any active individual for assessing and working on soft tissue conditions.

The Athletic/Sports Massage Therapist

To be an effective athletic (sports) massage therapist, a person should have a thorough understanding of anatomy, physiology, kinesiology, biomechanics, and massage technique. The massage therapist should have a sound knowledge of anatomy and be familiar with the various structures of the body. Of particular interest are the skeletal system and the muscular system. It is important also to understand the circulatory system and the nervous system, especially the neuromuscular functions. An understanding of kinesiology, which is the study of body movement, helps the therapist recognize what structures are involved in the movements of particular sports, especially when pain is present. The therapist must also understand which muscles and muscle groups the athlete is using in a particular sport.

Biomechanics refers to the integrated movement of the entire body. For instance, the manner in which the foot is placed affects what the knees, hip, back, shoulders, and head do. Tension in a particular body area also indicates tension or misalignment in other areas of the body. Because the body is used in a particular way, specific areas are going to be stressed. A deviation in the structure of one area of the body will be reflected throughout the body. Deviations often appear as patterns of structural imbalance. These deviations, when stressed, often result in injury. The more severe the deviation, the sooner an injury may occur.

Physiology is important in understanding the role each system plays in supporting the others so that they function as a whole organism. The better the therapist understands the body's response to exercise, strain, and injury, the better she will be able to offer massage services that will benefit the athlete.

An accepted principle in sports physiology is that in order to improve either strength or endurance, appropriate stresses must be applied to **overload** the system, forcing the body to adapt to the heavier load. Proper conditioning involves overloading the system an acceptable amount, and then allowing the system time to recuperate and adapt to a new level of ability. If the intensity of the training exceeds the body's ability to recuperate, injury or breakdown will probably result.

overload
states that the participant in an exercise program applies stresses to the body that are greater than what it is accustomed to.

During intense training, competition, and sometimes in everyday life, muscle strength and endurance are pushed to the limits and beyond. The result may include:

- Increased metabolic waste buildup in the tissues.
- Strains in the muscle or connective tissue. These may range from microscopic trauma to major injury.
- Inflammation and associated fibrosis.
- Spasms and pain that restrict movement.

These are negative effects of exercise. Skillfully applied athletic massage effectively counteracts each of these conditions. It normally takes a muscle that has been stressed to a point of fatigue 48 to 72 hours to rest, adapt, and recuperate. Athletic massage can reduce the recuperation time by as much as 50 percent.

Beneficial Effects of Athletic Massage

The goal of athletic massage is to enhance the athlete's performance. Performance is regulated by the efficiency, precision, and freedom with which the athlete is able to move. Efficiency is dependent on training and conditioning. Athletic massage allows for more intense training. Restrictions from pain, spasms, and tension inhibit freedom of movement. Without freedom of movement, precision is adversely affected. Athletic massage reduces many of the restrictions.

The following are beneficial effects of athletic massage:

1. It causes hyperemia, making more oxygen and nutrients necessary for growth and repair available to the body area being massaged.
2. It stimulates circulation and lymph drainage to flush out metabolic wastes of exertion quickly. It is three to five times more effective in combating fatigue than resting.
3. It stretches and broadens muscles, tendons, and ligaments.
4. It reduces muscle spasm.
5. It identifies possible trouble areas and helps to eliminate them.
6. It breaks down adhesions between fascial sheaths.
7. It separates fibrosis and breaks down adhesions that result from inflammation and trauma.
8. It helps to realign collagen fibers formed as a result of injury to produce a strong, flexible scar.

For more serious or competitive athletes, there are additional benefits of sports massage when used on a regular basis. Athletic massage accomplishes the following:

1. Encourages better performance and reduces the chance of injury.
2. Allows the athlete to reach peak performance sooner and sustain it longer.

3. Improves muscle flexibility, allowing muscles to respond more quickly and powerfully.

4. Identifies and eliminates possible trouble spots, thereby preventing injury.

5. Greatly reduces muscle stiffness due to excess acid buildup, rejuvenating muscles quicker after intense workouts or events.

6. Reduces ischemic pain and pain from spasms, splinting, and tension.

7. Assists injuries in healing quicker and stronger without loss of power due to transverse fibrosis.

8. Offers the athlete a chance to relax and recuperate more quickly.

9. Extends the overall span of the athlete's career.

Techniques of Athletic Massage

A thorough knowledge of the various massage techniques and their proper application makes the difference between an effective or ineffective sports massage therapist. Many of the techniques of athletic massage are identical with those of classical Swedish massage such as effleurage, petrissage, kneading, passive and active joint movements, percussion, vibration, and friction. One of the primary differences between Swedish massage and sports massage is that the movements are done two to three times more rapidly during pre-event sessions (the pace is slower during a post-event massage). There are some therapeutic techniques in sports massage that bear special consideration.

Compression Strokes

Compression is applied with a rhythmic pumping action to the belly of the muscle. Compression strokes cause increased amounts of blood to remain in the muscle over an extended period of time. This **hyperemia** is of value in pre-event, restorative, and rehabilitative massage.

> **hyperemia**
> is an increased amount of blood in the muscle.

Compression strokes for athletic massage use the palm of the hand to repeatedly press the muscle against the bone. The depth of pressure begins light and gradually deepens as the muscle relaxes. This procedure may be repeated three or more times along each part of the muscle, with special attention given to the body of the muscle. Large, broad muscles require several passes to cover the entire muscle.

Compression promotes increased circulation deep in the muscle at the same time that the muscle is broadened and the fibers are separated. When the compression movement is applied with short transverse motion at the deepest pressure of the compression, it also acts to stretch the muscle and separate adhesions in the muscle fascia that result from post-edemic fibrosis in the muscle fibers and fascicles.

Usually in the process of applying compressions, specific areas of the muscle are identified that contain fibrous bands, knots, or alarm points. The stroke can be changed to a cross-fiber movement to tease and separate the muscle fibers. When done correctly, this stroke mashes the

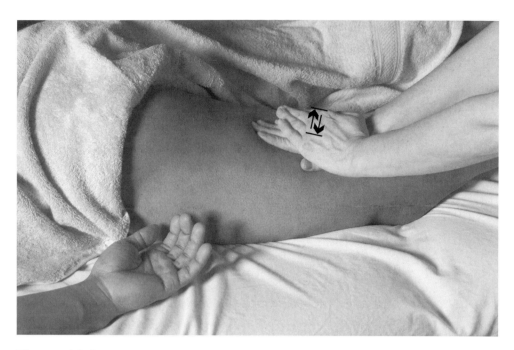

Figure 16.1

Compression strokes are applied with the palm of the hand to the belly of the muscle.

tissue and slightly stretches it, causing a broadening of the muscle and a breaking up of the binding fascia surrounding the fibers. The stroke also enhances fluid movement at the intercellular level.

The most important goal of compression is to create hyperemia in the muscle tissue. Deep compressions stretch, broaden, and separate muscle fibers and in the process release histamines (**HIS**-tah-meens) and acetylcholine (as-ee-til-**KOH**-leen). This causes the blood vessels throughout the massaged area to dilate and become more permeable to produce a lasting hyperemia (Figure 16.1).

Deep Pressure

Deep pressure is usually applied with the thumb, a braced finger, or occasionally with the elbow. The amount of pressure used varies according to the individual's pain threshold and the condition of the tissue, and the pressure should be applied with gradual increases in intensity. Deep pressure is used effectively to treat tender points that might be found in muscle, fascia, tendon, ligaments, joint capsules, or periosteum. If pressure on a point causes pain to radiate or refer to another area, that point is considered to be an active trigger point. Trigger points are found in taut bands of muscle tissue and can be active (produce and refer pain during daily activities) or latent (only producing pain when pressure is applied). Pressure is used on trigger points to deactivate them and increase function to the referred area. Left untreated, they can cause restricted and painful movement. Stress points are tender points that are usually associated with microtrauma or spasms in the muscle. They are generally located near the musculotendinous junction or attachment sites.

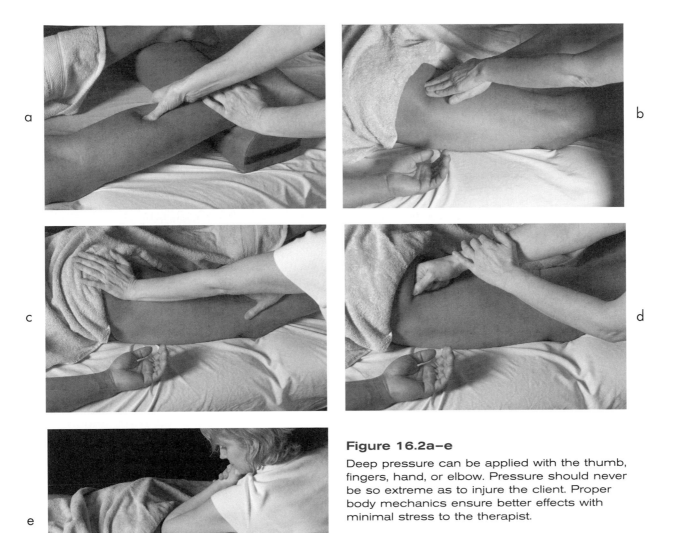

Figure 16.2a–e

Deep pressure can be applied with the thumb, fingers, hand, or elbow. Pressure should never be so extreme as to injure the client. Proper body mechanics ensure better effects with minimal stress to the therapist.

When a trigger point or stress point is located, pressure is applied directly into that point. The amount of pressure is determined by the tolerance of the athlete and the condition of the tissue. The pressure must not be so great as to cause the athlete to tense the muscles in a protective response. If the athlete were to rate the intensity of the discomfort on a scale of 1 to 10, (1 being very little discomfort and 10 being excruciating), the discomfort level should be about 5 or 6. After the therapist maintains the same amount of pressure for a short time, the intensity rating will decrease to about 2. This is an indication that the point has been deactivated, and the therapist continues with the treatment (Figure 16.2a to e).

Transverse or Cross-Fiber Friction

Transverse or cross-fiber friction is applied by rubbing across the fibers of the tendon, muscle, or ligament at a 90-degree angle to the fibers. The use of transverse friction massage for treatment of soft tissue lesions was popularized by the British osteopath Dr. James Cyriax. Cross-fiber friction effectively reduces fibrosis and encourages the formation of strong, pliable scar tissue at the site of healing injuries. Cross-fiber friction is effective at reducing the crystalline roughness that forms between tendons and their sheaths that sometimes result in painful tendonitis. Cross-fiber friction can prevent or soften adhesions in fibrous tissue.

Cross-fiber massage is used during the subacute and chronic stages of strains, sprains, and contractures or any situations where scar tissue and adhesions are present.

Cross-fiber massage is generally applied with braced fingers or the thumb and done perpendicular to the fibers. As with other types of friction, the fingers, the skin, and superficial tissues move as a unit against the deeper tissues. The pressure used in cross-fiber friction is deep enough to reach the target tissue, but stays within the pain tolerance of the athlete. The stroke must be broad enough to cover the targeted fibrotic tissues without bouncing over or plucking the fibers.

Broad cross-fiber friction can be done with the thumb, fingers, heel of the hand, knuckles or soft fist, and depending on the location, may engage more than one muscle group at a time. It is used to stretch muscles and separate fibers.

Local cross-fiber friction must be applied directly at the site of the lesion with a goal of breaking down adhesions and creating smooth fibrous tissue (see Figure 16.3).

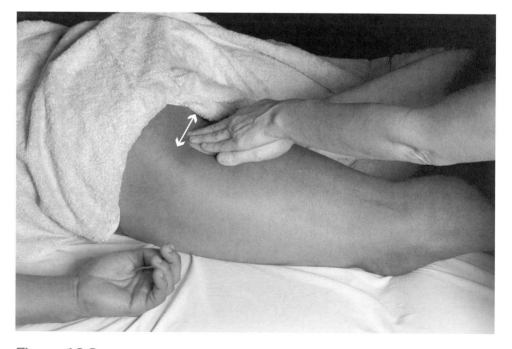

Figure 16.3

Cross-fiber or transverse friction is applied to the hamstring attachment on the ischial tuberosity. The stroke must be broad enough to cover the area and deep enough to reach the lesion.

Shaking and Jostling

A good way to relieve the intensity of deep work on the muscle is to shake or jostle the entire muscle mass or limb vigorously. This not only releases the tension that may result from the manipulations but also works to loosen fascia and improve lymph movement.

Shaking is done by grasping the body part and vigorously moving it up and down or back and forth so that the relaxed flesh flops around the bone. For example, in the supine position with the knee bent and the foot flat on the table, grasp the knee and vigorously move it laterally back and forth so that the muscles of the thigh and calf are shaken. Or, grasp the wrist with both hands. Apply a slight traction to the arm and vigorously shake the entire arm and shoulder up and down. When shaking a limb, it is important not to hyperextend any joint, especially the elbow or knee.

To jostle a muscle, place the massaging hand across the muscle belly, and then lightly grasp and vigorously move the muscle laterally across the axis.

Shaking and jostling require that the muscle be relaxed as it is moved quickly back and forth (Figure 16.4a to d).

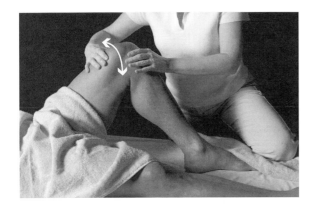

Figure 16.4a

Shaking the calf and thigh by rapidly moving the bent knee side to side.

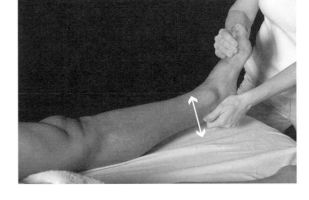

Figure 16.4b

To shake a leg, grasp the ankle as shown, apply traction, and bounce the entire leg vigorously up and down on the table. Be careful not to hyperextend the knee.

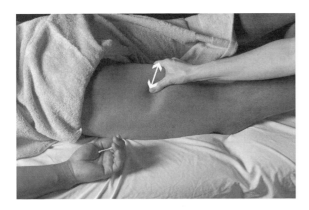

Figure 16.4c

Jostling the hamstrings. Lightly grasp the muscle and jostle it back and forth.

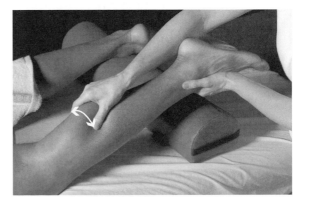

Figure 16.4d

Jostling the calf muscles.

Active Joint Movements

In the early 1950s, Dr. Herman Kabat developed a number of active movement exercises to be used in the rehabilitation of conditions such as orthopedic disabilities, spinal cord injuries, cerebral palsy, and polio. The exercises used therapist-assisted active and resisted movement in specific patterns. Dr. Kabat based the therapy on Sherington's physiological principles of reciprocal enervation, reciprocal inhibition, post-isometric relaxation, and the process of irradiation. Following Dr. Kabat's retirement, the development of the technique was continued by physical therapists Margaret Knott and Dorothy E. Voss. In 1954, this therapy system adopted the name Proprioceptive Neuromuscular Facilitation. It is better known by the acronym PNF.

Today, PNF is still one of the widest used and most effective therapy systems for the rehabilitation of neurologic and soft tissue disorders.

Active stretching movements used in athletic massage borrow from the principles of PNF. PNF stretching is based on reciprocal inhibition and post-isometric relaxation.

Another form of active joint movements that is a modification of PNF is called Muscle Energy Technique. (MET is discussed in Chapter 18.) MET helps to counteract muscle spasm, improve flexibility, and restore muscle strength. PNF stretching or MET is performed by moving a body part involving the affected muscle into an extended or stretched position to a point of pain or discomfort, then moving it back out of that position to a point where there is no discomfort. The therapist then supports the body part in this position while the client contracts the muscles for 5 to 30 seconds and then relaxes. The process is then repeated several times as the range of motion of the affected muscle or articulation increases until flexibility is restored and spasm reduced. **Caution:** The extent of these techniques is regulated by the level of pain experienced by the client. If any movement causes the client to tense due to pain, that movement is contraindicated.

APPLICATIONS FOR ATHLETIC MASSAGE

There are four basic applications for athletic massage. Each has a different goal and requires a different approach. The basic applications are

1. Pre-event massage—massage prior to an event to prepare the athlete for the exertion of all-out competition

2. Post-event massage—massage after an event to normalize the tissues and relax the athlete after competition

3. Restorative or training massage—massage during training to allow the athlete to train harder with fewer injuries

4. Rehabilitation massage—massage during rehabilitation to recover from injury more quickly with less chance of reinjury.

Pre-Event Massage

Pre-event massage, given 15 minutes to 4 hours prior to an event, prepares the body for intense activity. The massage is short (10 to 30 minutes) stimulating, and directed toward the parts of the body that will be involved in the exertion. The main goal of the pre-event massage is to increase circulation and flexibility in the areas of the body about to be used. Pre-event massage is fast paced and invigorating. Except for athletes who are extremely hyperactive, or with some adaptive sports athletes, this is not the time for relaxing movements. Pre-event massage warms and loosens the muscles, causing increased blood supply (hyperemia) in specific muscle areas. This enables the athlete to reach peak performance earlier in the event and maintain that performance longer. Increased flexibility allows the athlete more power, speed, and endurance with less possibility of injury.

Pre-event massage is not a replacement for proper warm-up before a performance, but is an adjunct to it and an aid in preparing the athlete for the all-out competition. This is not a good time for the athlete to receive his first massage because the effects of the massage may adversely effect an athlete's timing and performance. Pre-event massage is not the time to work too deeply, break down adhesions, or work on muscle spasms.

Pre-event massage uses no lubricant and is usually given through the clothing. Specific techniques are compression, light cross-fiber friction, shaking, jostling, rolling, kneading, range of motion, and stretching.

Post-Event Massage

Post-event massage is given within the first hour or two after participating in an event and can be 15 to 60 minutes in length. The goal of post-event massage is to increase circulation, clear out metabolic wastes, reduce muscle tension and spasms, and quiet the nervous system. Research shows that massage of this type promotes rapid removal of metabolic wastes and is three to four times as effective as rest in recovery from muscle fatigue. These techniques enhance the movement of blood and lymph out of the most intensely worked muscles and back toward the heart and center of the body. Lactic and pyruvic acids formed as a result of oxygen depletion are flushed from the muscles. This prevents delayed onset muscle soreness and reduces the time it takes for the body to recover from exertion.

Post-event massage is given after the athlete has had a chance to cool down from the exertion of the competition or exercise. The post-event massage should increase circulation while calming the nervous system. It is a relaxing massage that reduces the physical and mental intensity of competition.

The most effective techniques for post-event massage are light and deep effleurage, petrissage, kneading, compression, jostling, generalized friction movements, and light stretching. All movements are aimed at "stripping out" the areas of the body that have been used during the event.

Many serious athletes or teams have a massage therapist on staff to provide pre- and post-event massage. Often, sports massage therapists will be available at the site of a competition. It is common for massage areas to be set up at major athletic events such as running, cycling, swimming, and skiing competitions, as well as the Olympic and Paralympic Games.

After an exhaustive competition, the athlete cools down, replenishes fluids, and seeks out the massage area. The first step of the post-event massage is to conduct a short interview to assess the athlete's post-race condition. The therapist should be aware of signs of hypo- or hyperthermia, cramps, spasms, or muscle strain. Questions the therapist might ask of the athlete include:

- How do you feel?
- Have you had any water or fluids since the competition?
- Do you have any problems or discomfort?
- How long ago did you finish your event?
- How did you perform in the competition?
- Did you have any problems during the race?
- Are there any areas on your body that you want me to concentrate on?
- As I work on you, let me know if what I do is uncomfortable.

It is advisable to observe the athlete closely during the interview for signs of exhaustion or depression. Have the athlete sit on the table and remove his shoes during the conversational interview. Be aware of any blisters, abrasions, contusions, spasms, or strains and apply appropriate first aid or obtain the assistance of the attending medical personnel. It is a good idea to continue light conversation throughout the post-event massage.

The post-event massage concentrates on the muscle groups used during the exercise and the athlete's areas of concern. If time allows, include the rest of the body to enhance relaxation. The massage can be performed without lubricant and through the sports clothing if given on site or may include the use of some lubricant on the bare skin if private facilities are available.

The general procedure for each involved body area would include the following:

- Long effleurage strokes and kneading to flush out the area
- Light compressions to the entire area
- Jostling and traction shaking of the limb
- Range of motion and light stretching
- Repeat effleurage strokes
- Feather, nerve strokes from proximal to distal aspect of the area being massaged.

Massage During Training

Training massage—also called restorative, preventative, and maintenance massage—is the most beneficial form of massage for the athlete. It is considered a regular and valuable part of the workout and allows the athlete to train at a higher level of intensity, more consistently, with less chance of injury. Training massage increases blood and lymph circulation, which allows more efficient oxygen and nutrient supply to the cells as well as more efficient removal of metabolic waste. All these benefits make more intense and frequent workouts possible, thereby improving overall performance. The initial strokes used during regular training sessions to warm up the tissue and increase circulation provides an opportunity to find stressed areas that may require specific attention. Contractures and constricted muscle tissue containing trigger points can be released. Massage reduces minor cross-fiber adhesions resulting from microtrauma, thereby increasing muscle response and flexibility. Massage also alleviates muscle boundness (by breaking down muscle bundles) so that muscle contractions and relaxation are more efficient. This allows finer-tuned muscle response.

Another benefit of restorative massage is the breaking down of transverse adhesions that may have resulted from previous injuries. This promotes muscle power, better circulation, less chance of reinjury, increased mobility, increased flexibility, and better performance. The athlete is able to achieve maximum effort sooner, more often, and maintain it longer with fewer, if any, ill effects.

The massage process systematically involves every part of the athlete's body, concentrating on those muscle groups and body parts specifically involved in the sport and including other areas that are indirectly involved. Training massage maintains muscles in the best possible state of nutrition, flexibility, and vitality.

Restorative Massage Techniques

Techniques of restorative massage vary according to specific application. The primary techniques in this aspect of athletic massage include all the techniques of pre- and post-event massage plus deep cross-fiber friction, trigger-point therapy, active joint stretches, and neuromuscular techniques for reducing soft tissue lesions and constrictions. Effleurage and petrissage are also used, but to a lesser degree. There are a number of therapist-assisted joint movements that are very effective in this stage of massage. They include Muscle Energy Technique, strain/counterstrain, and PNF stretches. See Chapter 18 for more on these techniques.

There is no standard or set procedure for athletic massage due to the variety of sports situations to which it is applicable. However, there is a process to follow in choosing an effective treatment plan. When interviewing the client, it is important to find out the following:

- The sport or sports in which the athlete is involved
- The location and extent of present trouble areas
- The location and extent of previous injuries and surgeries
- The workout schedule and upcoming competitions
- The extent to which the athletic massage is to be incorporated in the athlete's training

By learning the client's regular sports, the practitioner can give special consideration to related muscle areas. Trouble areas can point to particular muscle groups on which to concentrate.

Previous injuries can also target trouble areas. Often an injury occurs as a result of a muscle not being flexible enough or not being able to let go. Trouble areas may also indicate fascia that is stuck or bound together. Injuries, especially when muscle spasm or tears exist, also point to synergistic, or opposing, muscles as being primary or potential problems.

Workout schedules indicate how serious a person is about a particular sport and can also reveal injury-prone weekend warriors. How much or how often the athlete wants to include massage in his training program helps the practitioner to determine the frequency and intensity of treatments. If the plan is to include only one or two sessions, the massage should be limited. However, if several regular sessions are planned, a thorough preliminary massage can be given. Work can then be done systematically on trouble areas or areas that receive continuous and intense use.

The first massage is primarily a hunt-and-search process using compression and deep stroking to seek out muscle bundles, spasms, and tender points as well as constrictions and areas of fibrosis. These bands or bundles of muscles usually feel like cords or lumpy growths that roll around or snap under the skin. Healthy, pliable muscle is smooth and evenly textured across its whole breadth and length. To the client, such trouble areas are generally painful when palpated.

Muscles often contain tender points that are either located in taut bands in the muscle body (trigger points) or where the muscle ends and joins the tendon or tendon sheath (stress points). The musculotendinous junction is where fascia and connective tissues are more prevalent. Because many muscle fibers terminate here, the area is vulnerable to strain and microtrauma. This is also where the ratio of blood vessels to tissue is less, and therefore where fatigue occurs first. Often when a muscle is headed for trouble, the first indication appears in this area (Figure 16.5).

Deep pressure on tender points gives the first clue to future problems. Early treatment of the muscles associated with the tender points can stop an injury long before it begins to affect the athlete's performance adversely. Once the trouble areas have been identified, the procedure for working on them is to deactivate the trigger point and then stretch, broaden, and strengthen the associated muscle while encouraging increased blood and lymph circulation.

Some applications of restorative massage tend to be deep and intense. Deep techniques do not mean painful techniques. All interventions must stay within the pain tolerance of the athlete. The athlete must understand that a certain amount of discomfort may be a part of a treatment and be willing to work with the therapist on deep breathing and relaxation techniques. The practitioner must not persist if in the process of working the muscle it becomes tighter. This could cause the condition to worsen or cause actual injury. The athlete and practitioner should work together for the improvement of the athlete's ability to train and condition his body.

If the restorative massage is deep and intense, it is like an intense workout and should be done on days when training is light or on days the athlete is off training. Intense restorative massage should not be given just before a competition. It is preferable to allow at least a couple of practice days between a deep massage and an event so that the athlete can adapt to changes in strength, speed, and timing.

Massage During Rehabilitation

Rehabilitation massage focuses on the restoration of tissue function following injury. The best way to treat an injury is to prevent it. Massage during training is invaluable for locating potential trouble spots and relieving them before they progress into debilitating injuries. When injury does occur, massage can be an important part of the rehabilitation program. Treatment strategy varies depending on the nature of the injury. Rehabilitation athletic massage accomplishes the following:

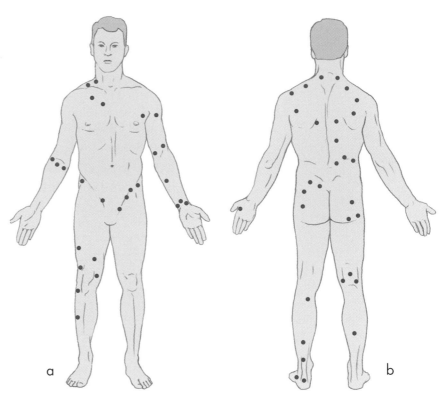

Figure 16.5

Major tender points of the body: (a) anterior and (b) posterior views.

- Shortens the time it takes for an injury to heal
- Helps reduce swelling and edema
- Assists in forming strong, pliable scar tissue
- Maintains or increases range of motion
- Eliminates splinting in associated muscle tissue
- Locates and deactivates trigger points that form as a result of the trauma
- Assists in getting the athlete back into training sooner with less chance of reinjury.

A great number of therapeutic techniques are valuable in treating injuries in any of their progressive stages of healing and/or degrees of severity. The application of proper techniques to the type of injury is important.

The massage practitioner should practice therapy at this level only after receiving proper training under the supervision of a qualified instructor who is familiar with sports injuries and the practice of therapeutic athletic massage. Before attempting rehabilitation massage, the therapist must be well trained in sound evaluation and treatment techniques. When skillfully applied, massage will reduce the healing time, with return to full function; improper application of techniques may prolong healing time and result in more severe injury.

General rules for the application of rehabilitation massage are:

- Do not massage directly on the site of an injury or trauma during the acute stage or when it is inflamed.
- Do not stretch muscle or fibrous tissue that is in the acute stage of injury.
- Never cause pain! Pain is the guide for proper application of all techniques. Less pain, more gain.
- Apply deep cross-fiber friction and stretching only after inflammation is gone and the healing process is well established.
- When in doubt—don't.

The advantages of massage therapy are numerous. Prompt application of the appropriate therapy can reduce much swelling and pain caused by an injury. Proper therapy allows the injured tissues to remain in close proximity so that healing progresses faster and with less need for the body to produce excess scar tissue. When massage is administered, the quality of healed tissue is far superior than if an injury is left to heal on its own.

Proper massage therapy improves circulation, enabling excess fluid and damaged tissue to be carried away. With improved circulation, more nutrients are brought to the rebuilding tissue so that it becomes strong and pliable and heals more quickly. Research has also shown that with massage therapy, fibrosis caused by muscle injury is reduced and the presence of transverse adhesions is almost nonexistent.

Appropriate treatment and accelerated healing of injuries mean that the athlete's downtime is cut to a minimum. With continued treatment during the rehabilitation period, there will also be fewer ill effects on performance.

Therapy may be given at the rate of once or twice a day during the time the athlete is out of training and every other day or every third day until he is back to a full training schedule. Massage for new or fresh injuries should only be given by properly trained therapists in conjunction with a physician's approval.

Athletic Injuries

It is the nature of athletes to push their abilities to their limits and beyond in order to excel at their particular sport. Because of the rigorous training and participation in competition, athletes' bodies are continuously exposed to stress, strain, fatigue, and sometimes microtrauma or more serious injury. Maximum athletic effort is physical abuse.

Most athletic injuries are either the result of trauma (contact with another athlete or in a fall) or the result of excessive and/or repeated stress to an area of the body. Injuries of the traumatic sort are often in the form of broken bones, dislocated joints, and torn ligaments. Such injuries are generally accidental and nonpreventable. Injuries of the second type are far more common and generally affect the soft tissue in the form of muscle strains, pulls and tears, or inflammation of tendons and ligaments. These are usually the result of fatigue, overtraining, poor tissue integrity, muscular weakness, imbalance, or biomechanical deviation. The majority of these injuries are preventable and treatable by massage and proper training.

Athletic injuries are categorized according to the onset and duration of the injury. Acute injuries have a sudden and definite onset and are usually of relatively short duration. Examples of acute injuries include dislocations, sprains, strains, lacerations, fractures, and contusions. Strains and sprains and their side effects respond well to massage therapy. Strains involve the tearing of muscle tissue or tendons. Sprains involve ligaments. The severity of strains and sprains is graded as follows (Figure 16.6a to c):

Grade I: Mild pain
   Severe overstretching of the fibrous tissue with little or no damage
   Full range of motion and full strength available

Grade II: Moderate to severe pain
   Swelling and possible discoloration
   Some tearing of the fibrous tissue
   Reduced range of motion and strength

Grade III: Immediate pain
   Severe or complete tissue rupture
   Extensive swelling and tissue deformity
   No strength or range of motion

Massage on acute injuries is contraindicated; however, prompt first aid greatly reduces secondary injury caused by swelling. First aid for acute soft-tissue injuries involves RICE (rest, ice, compression, elevation) for the first 24 to 48 hours to help reduce pain, swelling, and spasm. Use caution when applying ice to avoid skin burn and nerve damage. Ice massage is done directly on the skin, with the ice in constant motion for approximately 10 minutes. Another method is to put ice cubes in a resealable bag and, with a thin layer of material between the ice and skin (wrap in a light towel or place bag in a pillowcase), apply for 15 to 20 minutes. Although "frozen water" is the best method, people have also used store-bought ice packs or a bag of frozen peas—getting something cold to the area as soon as possible is the important thing! By applying ice within the first 30 minutes, the healing time is cut in half.

After one or two days of rest, the injury enters the subacute stage. The majority of swelling and inflammation has subsided, and the tissues are beginning the healing process. Contrast hydrotherapy treatments (20 minutes ice, 10 minutes heat) can be used to increase circulation to help promote healing. Each series should begin and end with cold. Massage treatments are begun to stimulate circulation to and away from the area and begin to mobilize the tissue so that as the tissue regenerates, strong, pliable, and flexible scar tissue forms. Extreme caution is used not to aggravate the injury or cause more damage to the tissues. Pain is the indicator to the athlete and

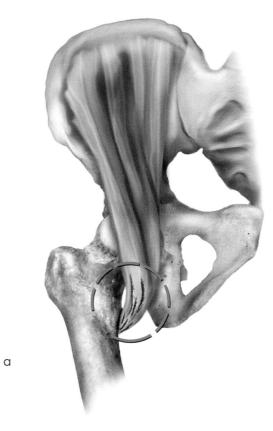

a

Figure 16.6a

Grade I: Overstretched fibrous tissue with some microtrauma.

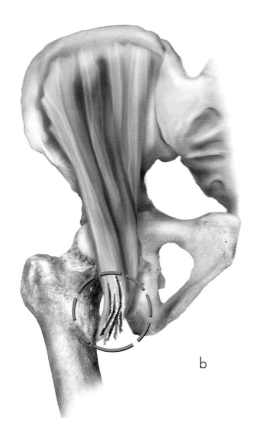

b

Figure 16.6b

Grade II: Some tearing of the fibrous tissue.

Figure 16.6c

Grade III: Severe tearing of the fibrous tissue with loss of function.

c

therapist as to the intensity of the techniques. As the tissues continue to mend and get stronger, the aggressiveness of the therapy increases until the athlete returns to full participation.

Chronic injuries have a gradual onset, tend to last for a long time, or recur often. Often they are the result of repetitive stressful activity and are sometimes labeled overuse syndrome. Repeated or extreme stresses cause microscopic lesions in the connective tissue of the tendons, muscles, the musculotendinous junction, or the tenoperiosteal junction. This in turn causes local, low-grade inflammation, selected muscle spasms (taut bands), reduced circulation to the area, pain, and dysfunction. Examples of chronic injury include chronic muscle spasm, tennis elbow, shin splints, tendonitis, fasciitis, and iliotibial band syndrome.

Though it is important to relieve the pain, identifying and eliminating the predisposing cause of the injury, if possible, is also a goal.

Soft Tissue Lesions and Injury

Skeletal muscles contain several tissues including muscle tissue, blood and other fluids, nerve tissue, and a variety of connective tissues. The structure of skeletal muscle is unique, with its arrangement of contractile fibers aligned and supported in such a way that by contracting, they exert a force on the bony levers of the skeleton, producing movement.

Muscle tissue consists of contractile fibrous tissue arranged in separate parallel bundles (fascicles), which, in turn, consist of a number of parallel muscle fibers that are held in place by an extensive and intricate connective tissue system. The connective tissue supports the muscle fibers in such a way that when the fibers contract, a force is exerted on whatever structure the muscle is attached to, causing movement.

Connective tissues form a continuous netlike framework throughout the body. Connective tissue consists largely of a fluid matrix (ground substance) and collagen fibers that support, bind, and connect the wide range of body structures. Collagen fibers provide the tensile strength in connective tissue. Depending on the consistency of the connective tissue and the varying proportions of fluid to fibers, a wide array of fibrous connective tissues are formed. Some examples are the fluid intercellular environment, the fascia of the muscles, the tendons and ligaments, and even bone.

The muscular system is a highly organized system of compartmentalized contractile fibrous tissues that work together to produce movement. The fibrous tissue is organized and supported by an intricate network of connective tissue. Connective tissue organizes muscles into functional groups, it surrounds each individual muscle, it extends inward throughout the muscle-creating muscle bundles, and eventually houses each muscle fiber. Connective tissue also creates the supporting structure for the intricate network of blood vessels and nerves. The connective tissue projects beyond the ends of the muscle to become tendons, which connect the muscles to the bones and other structures (Figure 16.7).

The layer of connective tissue that closely covers an individual muscle is the **epimysium** (ep-ih-**MIS**-ee-um). The **perimysium** (per-ih-**MIS**-

> **epimysium**
> is the layer of connective tissue that closely covers an individual muscle.

> **perimysium**
> separates the muscle into bundles of muscle fibers.

Figure 16.7
Muscles are contractile organs that are compartmentalized, organized, and supported by intricate layers of connective tissue or fascia.

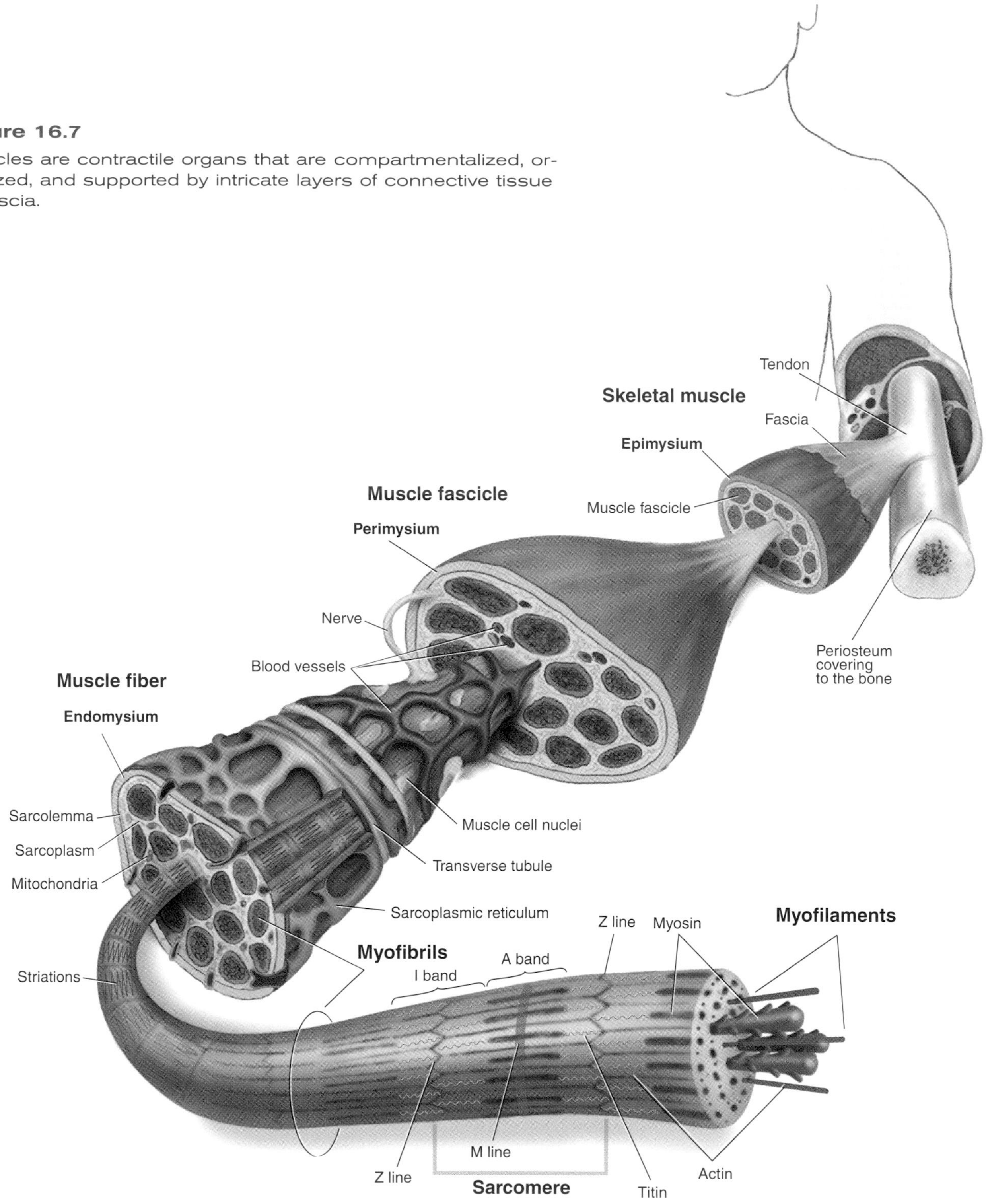

Skeletal muscle	
Tendon	
Fascia	
Epimysium	
Muscle fascicle	
Periosteum covering to the bone	

Muscle fascicle
Perimysium
Nerve
Blood vessels

Muscle fiber
Endomysium
Sarcolemma
Sarcoplasm
Mitochondria
Striations

Muscle cell nuclei
Transverse tubule
Sarcoplasmic reticulum

Myofibrils
I band
A band
Z line
Z line Myosin
M line
Sarcomere
Titin
Actin

Myofilaments

fascicle

is a bundle
of muscle fibers.

ee-um) extends inward from the epimysium and separates the muscle into bundles of muscle fibers or **fascicles** (**FAS**-ih-kls). Within the fascicle, each muscle fiber is covered by a delicate connective tissue covering called the **endomysium** (en-do-**MIS**-ee-ium). The **sarcolemma** (cell wall) of the muscle cell and the endomysium are intimately connected and act as a unit so that when the muscle fiber contracts and shortens, the connective tissue covering moves right along with it.

The connective tissue organizes the muscle fibers, connects the muscle to tendons, tendons to bones, and even bones to bone. Without this complicated system of connecting sheets, hinges, and ropes that transfer the action of the muscle fibers to the levers of the skeleton, motion and postural stability would not be possible.

Soft tissue injuries are the result of overstretching and eventual breaking of the collagen fibers in one or more layers of the connective tissue. Whether it is microtrauma in or between the muscle fibers, strained muscles, or torn ligaments, stresses to the connective tissue exceed their tensile strength resulting in the tearing of collagen fibers in the connective tissue (Figure 16.8).

The healing process in all soft tissue injuries is essentially the same. The cell damage initiates an inflammatory response. Extra fluid is infused into the area (swelling). The positive effects of swelling are to immobilize the area and supply an environment rich in leukocytes and fibroblasts so that the natural healing process of the body can start to repair the injury. The negative effect is that the swelling creates pressure in the tissue that causes further tissue damage and separates the ends of the injury and connective tissue layers, slowing healing. Inflammation and swelling are accompanied by pain.

The fluid carries an abundance of fibroblasts that within a couple of hours of the injury begin to lay down new collagen fibers to secure the injured tissue. Within two to three days, collagen formation is at its maximum. Fibroblasts generate collagen fibers that extend in random directions, forming a cobweb-like network that adheres to any structure in the vicinity. Collagen formation that reconnects the injured tissue forms scar tissue. The crisscross formation of fibers that connect to structures other than the injured tissue forms undesirable adhesions that restrict mobility and flexibility in the healed tissues.

The swelling that takes place when tissue is injured also creates space between the various layers of fascia. Wherever swelling has separated tissues, collagen fibers form to adhere the separated tissue. The more extensive the swelling, the more extensive the formation of fibrosis and adhesions. Also, the more severe the injury and the greater the separation in the injured tissue, the more extensive the formation of scar tissue. As long-term swelling is reduced, the fibrosis left

endomysium
is the delicate connective tissue covering of muscle fibers.

endurance
The act, quality, or power of withstanding hardship or stress.

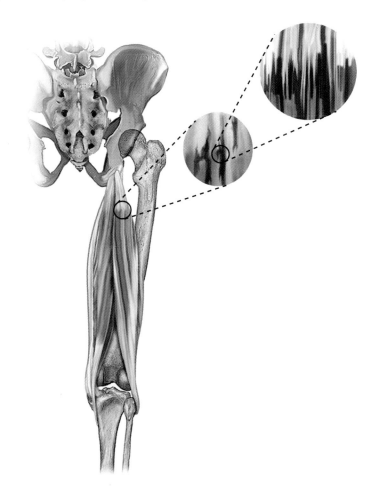

Figure 16.8

Soft tissue injuries occur when the tissue is pulled and stretched to the point that the integrity of the collagen fibers is broken.

behind sticks or glues the adjoining layers of fascia together. This type of gluing may also be the result of stressed and confined muscle movement over a long period of time. The resulting fibrosis reduces mobility and flexibility, leaving a reduction of power and a greater chance of reinjury. Both of these conditions can be greatly reduced with proper first aid and athletic massage therapy.

Proper first aid greatly reduces swelling, and the accompanying secondary trauma. With reduced swelling, the space between the ends of the injured tissue and between associated connective tissue layers is minimized. This minimizes the formation of scar tissue, fibrosis, and adhesions.

As the tissue heals, proper therapy, including massage, encourages new fibers to form along appropriate lines of stress. Properly applied transverse friction massage helps to organize and align collagen fibers to produce strong, pliable tissue at the same time as it breaks down unwanted interfiber cross-links and adhesions.

CONTRAINDICATIONS

The athlete's physician (employed by the organization or school) takes case histories and is responsible for preseason evaluations and for advising the athlete on health care and care of injuries. The physician treats illnesses and injuries and is responsible for rehabilitation of the athlete. The massage practitioner or trainer works under the direction of the physician and follows her guidelines when massage is to be a part of treatment or rehabilitation of injuries.

The physician or practitioner avoids doing anything that might make her liable or subject to malpractice. Negligence is defined as imprudent action or failure to act properly or failure to take reasonable precautions. Athletes understand that there are always some risks involved and that a physician or therapist is not held liable for poor judgment on the part of the athlete. Athletic massage is contraindicated in any abnormal condition, acute injury, illness, or disease except as advised by the athlete's physician.

There are times when an amateur or school athlete will request the services of the massage practitioner. The same contraindications for massage apply for this client as for the professional. The client must take responsibility for his own health and provide a physician's report if deemed necessary. Any heart condition, anemia, diabetes, thyroid disorders, liver and lung conditions, cancer, skin disease, varicose veins, hypertension, internal injuries, wounds, or like conditions are contraindications for massage. In these cases, massage would only be done by an experienced massage therapist who has continued her education, by the recommendation of the client's physician, and at the request of the client.

GENERAL PROBLEM AREAS AND SUGGESTED MASSAGE

The following are common areas of potential stress that may be addressed during restorative massage.

The Foot and Ankle

The heels take a lot of shock in sports such as jogging and running, and muscles can become painful to pressure (Figure 16.9).

Massage: To apply general massage to the foot, have the athlete lie facedown with feet over the edge of the table. You may sit on a stool if you are more comfortable. Use your finger or thumb to apply deep friction to sore spots. Apply cross-fiber friction for about 10 counts, pause, then repeat the movement. Flex and rotate the foot.

Achilles' Tendon

The Achilles' tendon, located just above the heel, is a sheathed tendon that may become swollen and painful if the ankle has been strained or if the tendon has been pulled at its attachment to the heel. Stress points may have formed at the attachment to the calf muscle.

Massage: At the musculotendinous junction, use your thumbs to apply 10 or more direct pressure movements, followed by cross-fiber friction. Repeat direct pressure to the tendon, followed by compression with your thumb. Search the calf muscle for related fibrosis or knots. Caution: It is contraindicated to do deep strokes along a fibrous tendon like the Achilles' tendon because it tends to aggravate abnormal conditions such as pulls and tears. Since the Achilles' is a sheathed tendon, it is necessary to stretch the tendon before applying cross-fiber friction. To do this, with the athlete lying prone, dorsal flex the ankle. With one thumb, move the tendon to the side and with a braced finger of the other hand apply transverse friction massage to the site of tendonitis (Figure 16.10).

Metatarsal Cramp or Fatigue

An athlete often suffers muscle cramps, tightening, and spasms of the muscles in the foot.

Massage: Hold the foot steady as you use the tip of your thumb to apply pressure to the stress point near the big toe. Follow pressure with deep cross-fiber friction for 10 to 20 counts, then release and repeat the movement. Move your thumb to the stress point near the little toe, and repeat the same movements. Check for stress points near the heel. Apply deep strokes from toes to heel, and gently stretch the plantar tendon.

Ankle Strains and Twists

The feet and ankles play an important part in sports and, due to the varied and stressful movements, are prime targets for injury and fatigue.

Massage: Use your thumb and forefinger to apply pressure and cross-fiber friction to the stress points near the ankle bone. Continue for 20 counts. Release and repeat. This must be done gently, as the area may be painful. Apply friction to the instep, working gently

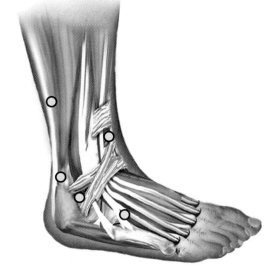

Figure 16.9

Common stress points of the foot and ankle.

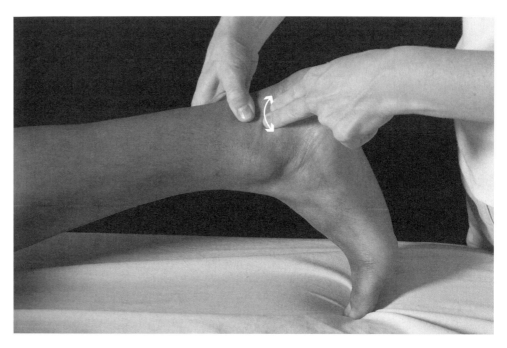

Figure 16.10

To apply transverse friction to a lesion on a sheathed tendon, like the Achilles', the tendon must be stretched while friction is applied. The foot is dorsal flexed. The tendon is displaced to one side with the thumb of one hand. Transverse friction is applied with a braced finger directly to the site of the lesion.

and from the toes to the heel. Move to the stress point of the outer ankle, and apply direct pressure for 10 counts. Release and repeat the movement. Shake and rotate the foot, then gently stretch it in every direction. Finish the massage with friction.

The Thigh, Calf, and Knee

Sports such as skiing, skating, ice hockey, surfing, horseback riding, and cycling all require quick reflexes and muscle power. Though the neck, shoulders, and back are under stress in these sports, the muscles of the lower back and hips also undergo stress and strain. Often, there is pain in the knee area and thigh after a day of heavy exertion.

Massage: Use the tips of your fingers to apply direct pressure to the stress points of the knee, and then follow with cross-fiber friction. Repeat the sequence several times. Use your fingertips to apply circular friction over the knee. Use your fist to finish with circular friction movements. Locate the stress areas in the thighs above the knee and in the groin and inguinal fold. With your thumb, apply pressure for 10 counts; release and repeat the movement several times. Apply cross-fiber friction for 10 counts. Apply compressions to the entire thigh. Finish the massage by applying deep strokes from knee to hip, shaking, jostling, and rolling the thigh (Figure 16.11).

Golf Knee

In golf, the twisting movements of the torso cause the knee to rotate until the ligaments are sometimes strained. Golf appears to be a mild enough game, but injuries to the knees (and back) do occur.

Massage: Locate the stress points. Use the middle finger or thumb to apply direct pressure. Hold for 20 counts. Release and repeat the movement. Apply cross-fiber friction for 20 counts; release and repeat the movement. Apply friction around the patella. Movements should be gentle.

Calf

Tennis and similar games place stress on the muscles of the calves and ankles, often causing spasms.

Massage: Have the athlete lie facedown. Bend the knee and flex the ankle several times. Locate the stress points at the outside of the knee joint. Use your thumbs to apply direct pressure, holding for 10 counts. Release and repeat the movement. Follow with cross-fiber friction on the stress points. Repeat the direct pressure and friction on the lower stress points of the ankle. Use the palm of your hand to apply deep compression all over the calf muscles. Apply cross-fiber friction along fibrous bands in the muscle. Apply deep strokes from heel to knee, followed with shaking and jostling of the muscle and effleurage.

Runner's Cramp

Runners will often suffer muscle cramps, spasm, muscle tightening, and calf pull. Ice may be applied to the spasmed area. Have the athlete tighten and relax the antagonist muscle to the one in spasm several times while slightly stretching the spasmed muscles between contractions (reciprocal innervation).

Massage: To massage the leg, have the athlete lie facedown on the table. After the spasm subsides, bend and flex the knee several times. Flex the ankle, and rotate it several times. Locate the stress points below the knee joint, then with your thumb, apply pressure for 10 counts, release, and repeat the movements. Find the stress point on the ankle, and repeat the same movements. Apply steady, firm compression movements to the calf. Compress stress points for 10 counts, release, and follow with cross-fiber friction. Repeat the compression. Apply several deep strokes from heel to knee. Shake and jostle the calf muscle from knee to ankle and apply effleurage to the area.

Strain to Hamstrings

Sports requiring sustained leg tension for some time can lead to strain. Examples of such sports are dance and distance running. Generally, the strain will be in the back mid-thigh extending to the back of the knee.

Massage: Use your thumb to locate the stress point behind the knee and in the gluteal crease. Apply direct pressure for 10 counts. Release and repeat. Apply cross-fiber friction for 10 counts. Release and repeat. Slightly flex the knee while supporting the ankle. Use the palm of your

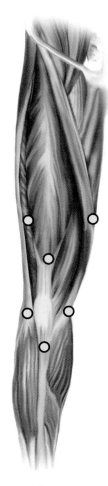

Figure 16.11
Common stress points around the knee.

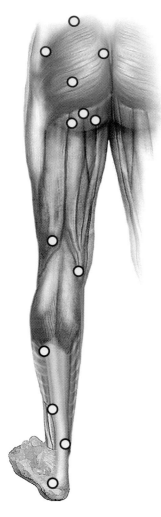

hand to apply compression over the entire back of the thigh from the buttock to the knee. Release and repeat. Finish the massage with deep strokes along the hamstring from knee to hip for 10 counts (Figure 16.12).

Hip, Leg, Buttock, and Groin

Sports such as golf cause strain to the back because of the twisting and swinging motions.

In the hip area, there are four main stress points with which you need to be concerned: the side of the hip, the leg, the buttock, and the groin area.

Massage: Have the athlete lie facedown on the table. Use the point of your thumb to apply direct pressure all over the buttock area. Locate tight stress areas. Apply pressure for 10 counts, release, and repeat the movement several times. Controlled use of the elbow is very effective in this area. Apply cross-fiber friction for 20 counts. Release and repeat the movement. Use the thumb to apply direct pressure to the lateral side of the leg to 10 counts. Release and repeat. Apply direct pressure to the lateral side of the midcalf. Find the pressure point in the buttock and along the iliac crest. Apply deep direct pressure for 10 counts; release and repeat the movement. Apply cross-fiber friction for 10 counts to each affected area; release and repeat the movement. Repeat the cross-fiber friction for 10 counts; release and repeat the movement. Apply direct pressure again using the thumb or elbow. Apply for 10 counts; release and repeat the movement. Repeat the cross-fiber friction, and finish with deep shaking and vibration movements.

Figure 16.12

Common stress points of the posterior leg and buttock.

The Elbow and Arm

The muscles in the arm and shoulder may be weakened by overuse or strain from an activity such as tennis. Muscles can become stiff and sore. Generally, the extensor muscles of the forearm will be affected. In the acute state, this condition is characterized by inflammation, swelling, and intense pain near the lateral epicondyle of the elbow.

Massage: Using the heel of your hand, apply compression to the wrist for 10 counts. From the wrist, work up to the elbow, the shoulder, and then back down to the wrist so that the entire arm is covered. Find the pressure point at the side of the elbow, and with your thumb, apply direct pressure for about 10 counts. Release and repeat the pressure three or more times. Using cross-fiber friction, move to the next pressure point. Follow along the length of the muscle, repeating the cross-fiber friction where the muscle fibers seem stuck together. Follow this with several more compressions along the muscle. Apply deep stroking movements along the muscle from insertion to origin, and follow these with shaking and jostling movements. Repeat the same procedure to other stress points, and finish with general compression on the entire arm, gentle passive-joint movements, stretching, and soothing effleurage. Instruct the athlete to rest the arm, and repeat the treatment daily until all symptoms are gone (Figure 16.13).

The Wrist

The ligament, tendons, and muscles of the wrist can be affected by tension caused by grasping and tensing for long periods of time. Examples are grasping the handlebars of a bicycle and lifting weights.

Massage: Find the pressure point. Use your fingertips to apply direct pressure to the stress point, holding for 10 counts. Release and then repeat the movements several times. Apply cross-fiber friction for 10 counts; release and repeat. Use your thumb to apply cross-fiber friction all around the wrist and back again. Do this for about 15 to 20 counts; release and repeat the movement. Follow with a series of compressions using the heel of your hand. Apply compression up the forearm from wrist to elbow going all around the arm. Repeat these movements several times. Finish the massage by applying direct pressure to the stress points for 10 to 20 counts; release and repeat the movement (Figure 16.14).

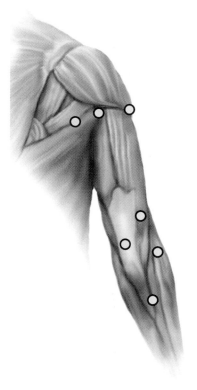

Figure 16.13

Common stress points of the elbow and arm.

Back, Shoulder, and Neck

The back and shoulder muscles are often strained during weightlifting, bowling, golf, and other sports. Shoulder joint injuries are due to such sports as baseball, bowling, basketball, and other sports requiring exertion of the arm and shoulder. These usually result in injury to the rotator cuff or associated muscles.

Massage: Have the athlete lie facedown on the table. Use the thumb to apply deep pressure and cross-fiber friction at high stress areas for 10 counts. Release and repeat the movement. Do this sequence about four times. Apply cross-fiber friction to the side of the neck and downward on the shoulder. Apply for 10 counts; release and repeat until the area has been covered. Find the stress points on the shoulder blade. Apply direct pressure for 10 counts; release and repeat the action. Apply cross-fiber friction for 10 counts; release and repeat the movement. Do this sequence several times. Find the stress points around the shoulder blade and repeat the direct pressure for 10 counts. Release and repeat the cross-fiber movements for 10 counts. Finish the massage with compression done with the palm (Figure 16.15).

Midback and Lower Back

Massage: Have the athlete lie on the table facedown. Find the stress points in the muscular bands along each side of the spine. With your thumb, apply direct pressure for 10 counts. Release and repeat the movement all the way down the back. Do the sequence

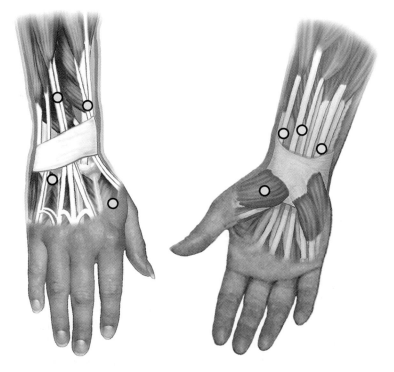

Figure 16.14

Common stress points of the wrist.

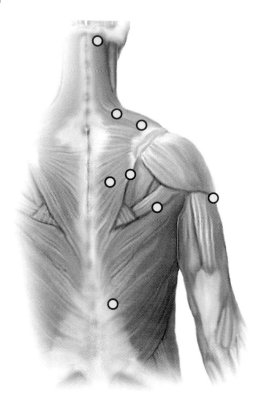

Figure 16.15

Common stress points of the back and shoulder.

down the back several times. Work with the client's breathing. Apply pressure on the exhale and release on the inhale. Apply cross-fiber friction with your thumb for 10 counts. Release and repeat the movement moving an inch or so down the back. Use the palm of your hand to apply several compressions on the muscle. Use your thumb to apply cross-fiber friction on the outside of the muscle. Return to cross-fiber friction with your thumbs for 10 counts. Release and repeat the movement. Do this sequence several times. Apply deep strokes with the thumbs from the top of the shoulders down to the tailbone, and then shake and vibrate the muscles back up to the shoulders. Apply compressions to the buttock with the heel of your hand, and finish by flushing out the area with effleurage.

Racquetball Shoulder

This is somewhat like tennis elbow but can be more severe. It affects the trapezius and deltoid muscles.

Massage: Begin with direct pressure on the stress points, holding for 10 counts. Apply friction over the back, including the neck, for about 20 counts. Use compression movement on the shoulders. Release and repeat the movements. Massage the entire back from the waist upward over the shoulders. Massage over the deltoid muscle. Find the pressure points of the shoulders and apply deep compression for 10 counts and release. Continue with cross-fiber friction for 10 counts and release, and then finish with compression, using deep stroking to stretch the fibers. Shake the involved areas to release tension. Apply repeated pressure to the stress points once more, and then apply effleurage to the entire area.

Triceps Strain

This is a condition usually occurring when the muscle is overused and stressed.

Massage: Find the stress point. Use your thumb or fingertip to apply direct pressure for 10 counts. Release and repeat the movements. Apply cross-fiber friction for 10 counts. Release and repeat the movements. Do this sequence (gently) several times. Apply deep strokes from elbow to shoulder; then shake and flush out the area.

The Groin

The groin is more likely to be pulled in sports such as horseback riding, gymnastics, and soccer. This is a painful condition caused by overstretching of the gracilis and adductor muscle located high on the inner thigh.

Massage: Have the athlete lie on his side with the affected leg on the bottom. The knee of the top leg is bent, and the bottom leg remains fairly straight. Stand behind the athlete and apply compressions to the inner thigh with the palm of the hand. Use your thumb to apply pressure and cross-fiber friction for 20 counts. Release and repeat the movement. This area will be quite tender, so it is necessary to be gentle. Find the spasm area and apply compression with your fingertips. Release and repeat the movement.

The Chest and Abdomen

During some sports, especially weightlifting, the pectorals and the intercostal muscles may be strained. There may be spasm, soreness, and tenderness (Figure 16.16).

Massage: The athlete should lie on his back with the body relaxed. Apply circular compressions using the palm of your hand to the pectoral muscles, moving from the breastbone to collarbone across the chest and shoulders. Avoid doing movements over or near the nipples even on men because this is a sensitive area. Follow compression movements with effleurage. Apply light percussion (hacking movements) with the little finger sides of your hand over the pectoral muscles. Finish with a few light strokes over the entire chest area.

The Abdomen

The rectus abdominis is often affected by sports that involve bending and twisting movements. Tension, soreness, and spasm may develop in the area around the navel. Keep in mind that the abdominal region of the body is sensitive to pressure. The athlete should lie on his back with knees slightly raised and feet flat on the table. Raising the knees helps to relax the abdominal area. Use gentle movements and direct pressure downward (never upward) from the waistline toward the pubic bone.

GENERAL PROCEDURE FOR PRE- OR POST-EVENT MASSAGE

In this chapter, we have covered the techniques and types of sports massage. Training and rehabilitation massage will generally be done in the training facility or your clinic and may incorporate several types of massage modalities (Swedish, sports, lymphatic, shiatsu, etc.). In this setting, you will become familiar with the client and the client's needs during a series of visits. This will allow you preparation time to create a plan of action for the next visit using the techniques you have learned.

However, at a sporting event where pre- and post-event massage is given, it is wise to have a general routine prepared that you can then adapt to the sport and any injuries or complications an athlete has incurred. As you use these routines more, you will begin to find a pattern that is comfortable for you. With event experience, you will get a feel for what techniques are best for the athlete and when certain ones are not

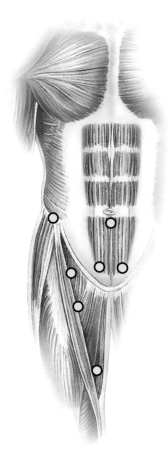

Figure 16.16
Common stress points of the groin and abdomen.

beneficial. Body support cushions® may also be used and are extremely comfortable for the athlete who has just run 26 miles or biked 100 miles!

The following is a general event sports massage routine that may be used if you joined a state team or was accepted as a team member to provide massage at a national or international event (such as qualifying events, Olympics/Paralympics, or World Games). The sidebars give you ideas for stretches as well as sports-specific common problems.

As you escort the athlete to your table, introduce yourself and conduct an interview. Following are sample questions and why they are important; this will give you an idea of the athlete's overall attitude, frame of mind, level of concentration, and focus. A triage person at the registration table may ask these questions also.

Pre-Event

- When and what is your event?

  Determines speed, amount of time available for your session; enables you to be sports specific to the athlete's needs.

- How did your training go? Are you feeling prepared?

  Determines their frame of mind—whether the athlete is disappointed, ready, anxious, nervous, calm, focused, eager, or the like.

- Did you incorporate massage during your training?

  If yes and on a regular basis—once a week, twice a month—the athlete can tell you what works for him, the pressure and techniques he is used to, and so on. If no, you know not to do deep or trigger-point work that could affect his performance.

- Do you have any chronic or acute injuries?

  Makes you aware of sensitive areas and any specific work or treatments the athlete has received.

- What do you want me to focus on?

  Remember, the person on the table is the one living in his body—he may want you to focus on legs if he is running, or upper body if he is swimming . . . or relaxing if he is anxious. Listening is a key component when working with athletes.

- Let me know if my pressure is too deep or light or if something hurts.

  Initiates good communication and rapport.

Post-Event

- How long has it been since you finished your event?

  Gives you an idea whether the athlete has allowed himself time to cool down (physically and mentally).

- Have you had something to eat or drink?

  Lets you know whether the athlete has replenished his body with nutrients and fluids.

- Have you cooled down, stretched, walked around?

  It is important to do this before massage; it allows the recovery process to begin.

- How do you feel about your performance?

  Determines the athlete's state of mind—disappointment, excitement, determination to continue to the next level, ideas on what he needs to improve on, and so on.

- Did you have any problems (falls, cramping, injuries) during the event? If so, have you been to first aid/medical? How are you feeling now?

  Helps you focus on problem areas immediately, or determine whether the athlete needs to be referred to a medical professional.

- Where do you need work done; where would you like me to focus?

  Allows you to meet the athlete's needs in order to recover more quickly or address a weak or injured area, or complement his cooldown/recovery/relaxation process.

- Let me know when my pressure is too deep or light or if something hurts.

  Communication and rapport.

Remember that pre-event should be done at a faster pace (with some exceptions) than post-event.

Have the athlete lie on the table (either supine or prone is fine to start). Make sure to use a bolster under the knees when supine to reduce strain on the low back, and under the ankles when prone (or have the feet hanging off the edge of the table) to reduce cramping in the calves. You may help him remove his shoes (if post-event, look for blisters he may not know about).

Prone—Back/Upper Body

- Begin with gentle rocking, starting with the back, then going down each leg. Use this time to assess the body, noting any tense or sensitive areas.

- Begin with compressions on the gluteals, move up the erectors to the trapezius, rhomboids, and scapulas; continue the rocking motion.

- On the next pass, apply circular friction to this same area using the heel of your hand or fingertips.

- Apply direct pressure to stress points, paying attention to the athlete's response.

SCAPULA RELEASE

Bring the arm above the head, apply traction for 2 to 3 seconds. Return the arm to the side of the body, then place the hand on the low back (check for any shoulder injuries first, then comfort level of this position). Place your bottom hand under the shoulder, top hand on the scapular with fingers wrapped around the medial board of the scapula, and apply a gentle traction (see Figure 16.17a to c).

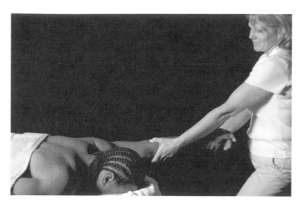

Figure 16.17a

Bring the arm above the head, apply traction for 2 to 3 seconds.

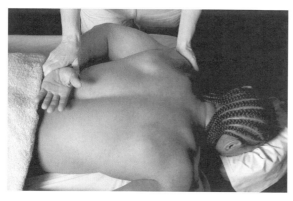

Figure 16.17b

Return the arm to the side of the body, then place the hand on the low back. Check for any shoulder injuries first, then the comfort level of this position.

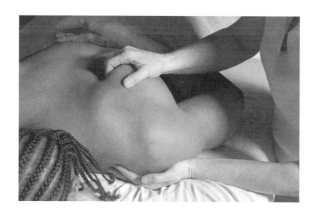

Figure 16.17c

Place your bottom hand under the shoulder, top hand on the scapula with fingers wrapped around the medial board of the scapula, and apply a gentle traction.

- Apply circular friction with the thumbs from the base of the neck to the occiput, then gently squeeze the neck.
- After compressions into the belly of the upper traps, a general kneading can be done.
- Apply compressions to the triceps.
- Let the arm hang off the side of the table. Grab it around the biceps/triceps with both hands and jostle. Return the arm to the table (see sidebar for stretch).
- Light tapotement can be done for pre-event.

Repeat the routine on the other side of the body.

Prone—Lower Body

- Bend the knee to 90 degrees, grasp the ankle with both hands, and lift the leg slightly off the table; gently shake the leg. Extend the leg, returning the foot to the bolster.
- Apply compressions on the gluteals and hamstrings (2 to 3 passes).
- Jostle then petrissage the hamstring.

- Spread hamstring muscles (see the accompanying sidebar and Figure 16.18a and b for a description).

- Apply compressions on the gastrocnemius.

- Grasp and lift the gastrocnemius with gentle shaking.

- Bend the knee to 90 degrees; use a wringing motion on the gastrocnemius from the knee to the Achilles'.

- Lift and shake the leg (as in Step 1).

- Quadriceps stretch: Heel toward buttocks to athlete's tolerance. Hold for 2 to 3 seconds, release, and repeat several times.

- External and internal hip rotation: With one hand on the buttocks, use the other hand on the ankle to rotate the leg externally, then internally for gluteal and piriformis stretch.

- With the knee still at 90 degrees, rotate the ankle clockwise and counterclockwise, then dorsiflex the ankle to stretch the gastrocnemius. Return the leg to extension.

- Foot (optional at events): Using fist, knuckles, or thumbs, apply compressions to the sole of the foot, then circular friction. You may end with tapotement (be aware of blisters or injury, especially post-event).

- Repeat on the other leg.

Before asking the athlete to turn over, do some gentle rocking of the whole body to bring it together.

SPREADING THE HAMSTRING

With fists together on the hamstring, apply pressure then slowly bring the fists apart, spreading the fibers apart (Figure 16.18a and b).

Supine–Lower Body

Quadriceps

- Standing at the end of the table, cup both ankles/heels in your hands and apply traction for a few seconds. Release and rock the legs. Repeat traction and rocking again.

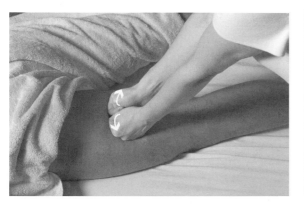
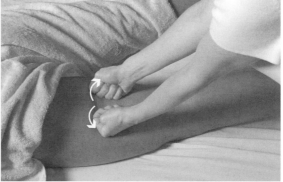

Figure 16.18a and b

Spreading the hamstrings: With fists together on the hamstring, apply pressure, then slowly bring the fists apart, spreading the fibers.

QUADRICEPS STRETCH

Have the athlete lie on his side, keeping the spine straight. The lower leg should be bent at the knee and hip (knee to chest). The upper leg (parallel to the table at all times) should be bent at the knee with the upper hand holding it at the ankle (a towel may be wrapped around the ankle if he cannot grab it). The hamstring should first engage to extend the leg, then the athlete (or therapist, if assisting) will pull on the ankle to get a little more stretch in the quadriceps. Hold for 2 seconds, release to starting position, and repeat five or more times. The body should be in alignment at all times, not rolling back when the quad is in full stretch. The stretch should be felt at the top of the quadriceps (see Figure 16.19a and b).

- Apply compressions to the upper leg, proximal to distal, covering all quadricep muscles.
- Jostle the quadriceps.
- Place outside hand under the leg (on hamstring) and top hand on the quadricep. Lift and drop the leg, like bouncing a basketball.
- Apply spreading technique as done on the hamstring.
- Jostle.
- Bend the knee to 90 degrees, flex at the hip to 90 degrees; take the knee to the chest and do range of motion for the hip. Extend the leg back to the table.

Knee and Lower Leg

- With opposing thumbs, effleurage around the patella OR use cross-fiber friction on patella tendon/ligament above and below patella.
- Apply compressions on the tibialis anterior and peroneus muscles.
- With thumbs, apply circular friction to the tibialis anterior.
- Flex the foot to stretch the gastrocnemius.
- Traction the leg again.
- Repeat on the other leg.

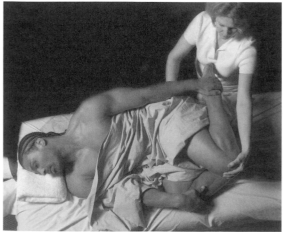 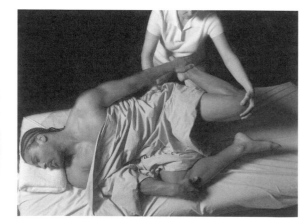

Figure 16.19a and b

Quadriceps stretch.

Upper Body

Chest and Arms

- Hold the hand and laterally raise the arm to the side of the table (shoulder height). With flexed elbow, shake the arm. Return it to the table.

- Apply compressions to the pectoralis, deltoids, biceps, and forearm.

- Petrissage the deltoids, biceps, and forearm.

- Use the tips of fingers to apply friction to the palm of the hand and around the wrists.

- Apply long effleurage strokes up the arm.

- Do range of motion for the shoulder.

- End by shaking the arm.

Shoulders, Neck, and Head

- Stand or sit at the head of the table and knead the upper trapezius muscles of the shoulders and up the neck.

- Do gentle stretching of the neck (flex right and left, lift chin to chest).

- With your fingertips, apply circular friction to the scalp.

- To end, place your hands on the shoulders and apply pressure (pressing the shoulders down toward the feet).

- You may end with nerve strokes or gentle rocking.

Abdominal Massage (Optional)

- Have the athlete bend his knees, keeping his feet flat on the table.

- Begin with kneading movement over the entire abdominal region, graduating from gentle to stronger movements.

- Apply circular effleurage clockwise over the abdomen.

QUESTIONS FOR DISCUSSION AND REVIEW

1. What is athletic/sports massage?

2. Define adaptive sports massage.

3. In addition to a thorough understanding of human anatomy and physiology, which four major body systems and their functions must the therapist know?

4. What is the overload principle?

5. What are negative effects of exercise?

6. What techniques are commonly used in athletic massage?

7. What is the primary goal of compression?

8. In athletic massage, what does the term *hyperemia* refer to?

9. In athletic massage, how is deep pressure used?

10. Who popularized the use of transverse friction massage for treating soft tissue lesions?

11. What is the objective of using cross-fiber friction in athletic massage?

12. What are the four basic applications for athletic massage?

13. What is the goal of each athletic massage application?

14. When is massage considered to be the most beneficial to the athlete?

15. What are stress points, and where are they generally located?

16. Why must the therapist be sure to apply proper techniques at all times?

17. What is the best way to treat an athletic injury?

18. What are some beneficial advantages of rehabilitation massage?

19. How does massage therapy affect the healing time of injuries?

20. Who is qualified to give athletic massage to new or fresh injuries?

21. What is RICE?

22. Differentiate between acute and chronic injuries.

23. What massage techniques should be used at the site of acute muscle injuries?

24. Differentiate between a strain and a sprain.

25. When is athletic massage contraindicated?

Massage in Medicine

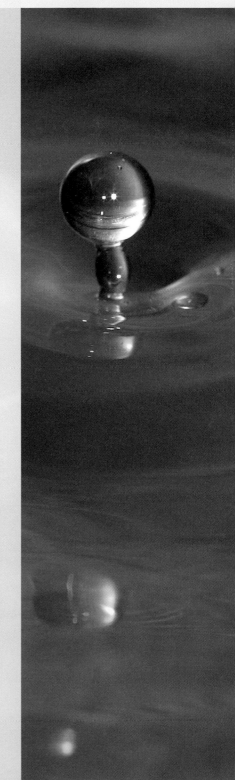

LEARNING OBJECTIVES

After you have mastered this chapter, you will be able to:

1. Explain the historical significance massage has played in medicine.
2. Explain how massage re-emerged in the United States as alternative medicine.
3. Differentiate among alternative, complementary, and integrative medicine.
4. Explain the role of massage in integrative medicine.
5. Describe the role of the patient in integrative medicine.
6. Define CAM.
7. Explain how massage may fit into a hospital setting.
8. Define medical massage.
9. Demonstrate billing insurance for massage.

MASSAGE IN MEDICINE THROUGHOUT HISTORY

Many massage techniques were developed and used as part of healing or medical practice. The earliest medical literature from Persia, Egypt, Japan, and China all make reference to various treatments that include the use of massage techniques, though the actual term *massage* did not appear in medical literature until the end of the nineteenth century. There is evidence that the Greeks in the times of Hippocrates and Asclepiades employed massage-like treatments for medical purposes. Exercise, diet, bathing, and massage were an important aspect of Roman culture to preserve health. The fall of the Roman Empire ushered in the Dark Ages (AD 470–1500), a time when few Western medical or historical books were written and much recorded history was lost. As the Roman Empire declined, the Arabic Empire flourished. In Persia, physicians such as Rhazes and Avicenna authored important texts on medical practices that included references to the use of exercise and rubbing for the treatment of disease and preservation of health.

In the West, by the sixteenth century, medical practitioners again began using mechanotherapy. French physician Ambrose Pare (1517–1590)

677

wrote about the positive effects of friction treatments in the healing process. In 1569, Mercurialis of Italy published *De Arte Gymnastica,* which included the benefits of manual therapies when integrated into other treatments. The sixteenth, seventeenth, and eighteenth centuries saw literature from English, French, Italian, and German authors describing the use of massage-like treatments, exercises, and other physical treatments for the purpose of maintaining health and treating disease.

References to massage techniques are found in medical literature from the United States and Europe dating from the 1700s to the present day. Techniques were referred to as rubbing, frictions, gymnastics, medical movements, and medical rubbing.

Per Henrik Ling developed a system of movements he called medical gymnastics and, in 1813, opened the Royal Swedish Central Institute of Gymnastics, where he taught the Ling System until his death in 1839. The popularity of what was to become known as the Movement Cure or the Swedish Movements spread throughout Europe. In 1858, Dr. Charles Fayette Taylor traveled to England to learn the Cure and returned to New York to practice and teach the technique. At the same time, his brother, George Henry Taylor, attended the Sotherberg Institute in Stockholm and completed a full training in the Movement Cure before returning to New York to join his brother Charles. Though their combined practice lasted only about a year, they both continued to practice, write about, and teach the Cure until their deaths in 1899.

In 1902, Douglas Graham, M.D., of Boston published *Manual Therapies, A Treatise on Massage,* which clearly described the effects of massage and helped massage gain more credibility in the medical profession.

James Mennell (1880–1957) published *Physical Treatment by Movement, Manipulation and Massage* in 1917. He was a medical officer and lecturer of massage in England and was very influential in the early development of physical therapy.

Mary McMillan received her training and early experience in England. She moved to the United States to become the director of massage and medical gymnastics at Children's Hospital in Portland, Maine, and later took a position at Walter Reed Hospital. She was an instructor for reconstruction aides in physiotherapy during World War I and became Director of Physiotherapy at the Harvard Medical School from 1921 to 1925, where she wrote the definitive text *Massage and Therapeutic Exercise.*

Massage for treating orthopedic conditions continued to expand in the United States until about 1945. Massage as physiotherapy was used extensively in reconstruction and rehabilitation of those wounded in World War I and World War II. Massage was also a common prescription for victims of the polio epidemic during the 1940s and 1950s.

The use of massage in physiotherapy declined between 1940 and 1950 due to the fact that it was strenuous, it was time-consuming, and it required extensive training. Physical therapy began relying more on exercise and the use of a variety of machines, medicines, and mechanical modalities for treatment. The use of massage in the medical field in the United States was nearly nonexistent after the early 1950s.

Even though the use of massage in medicine declined, exercise and massage continued its long relationship for the maintenance and promotion of physical health. Swedish massage, which included Swedish movements, hydrotherapy, and sometimes colon irrigation and diathermy, remained popular with natural health enthusiasts. Swedish massage practitioners could find employment in health clubs or spas, sanatoriums, YMCAs, and resorts.

Manual therapies and massage-like procedures have been considered part of medical practice since ancient times. Massage practices of physical manipulations and applications have also flourished in nonconventional healing practices and folk medicine. After falling into obscurity in the 1950s, massage began to re-emerge during the human potential movement of the 1960s and 1970s. The re-emergence of massage in the United States happened outside of **allopathic medicine.** Classic Swedish massage was joined by reflexology, shiatsu, acupressure, and other alternative practices. More therapeutic modalities began to emerge, each carrying the name of the person who devised it, such as Riechian Therapy, Rolfing, Alexander Technique, Feldenkrais, and Trager, among others. Cross-fiber techniques of James Cyriax and trigger-point therapies described by Simons and Travell gained acceptance and popularity. English osteopaths Stanley Lief and Boris Chaitow developed Neuromuscular Technique (NMT), which has been popularized in the United States by Judith Walker and Paul St. John. John Upledger developed Craniosacral Therapy. In the 1980s, massage gained popularity among athletes due to its effects of reducing the stress of intense workouts, enhancing performance, and its effectiveness in promoting the healing of soft tissue injuries. Many techniques found to be effective when addressing soft tissue conditions in athletes also were effective for hypertonic or dysfunctional conditions in the general population.

Massage had turned a corner from being simply relaxing and feeling good to being therapeutic and directed toward improving an individual's physical condition. All these modalities were developed outside Western medical practices and were considered alternative practices. More and more people began to regularly seek out the services of these alternative practitioners to help maintain and improve their health. Massage and massage-like practices were accompanied by a wide array of health and healing practices that were considered as alternative medicine.

> **allopathic medicine**
> treatment of disease or injury with the use of medications and surgery.

ALTERNATIVE AND COMPLEMENTARY MEDICINE

The popularity of massage and other alternative practice steadily increased from the 1960s through the 1990s. A survey conducted by David Eisenberg in 1990 showed that Americans were using alternative and complementary therapies at the rate of $13.7 billion annually, with massage being the third most used modality, behind chiropractic and relaxation techniques. To put this figure in perspective, the out-of-pocket expenditure for hospitalization in the United States the same time was estimated to be $12.8 billion.

alternative medicine

is a term that implies using services other than those usually accepted from allopathic physicians.

complementary medicine

is the term that took the place of "alternative medicine" and implies that the alternative practices can work along with more conventional medicine for the benefit of clients.

The term **alternative medicine** implied that people were seeking services of alternative health practitioners instead of going to allopathic physicians. In fact, many were using the services of conventional doctors and alternative practitioners for the same physical conditions. Many times, this was done without clients informing their medical doctors that they were visiting alternative practitioners at the same time. In the 1980s, the term **complementary medicine** emerged and began to gain popularity implying that the alternative practices could work along with more conventional medicine for the benefit of the client. A change in terminology was accompanied with a change in attitude. Some alternative practices, massage among them, were becoming more socially acceptable and more accepted in the medical community.

The establishment of the National Center of Complementary and Alternative Medicine (NCCAM) as a part of the National Institutes of Health (NIH) generated increased research in CAM therapies (http://nccam. nih.gov). Senate bill 2440 established the NCCAM in the fall of 1998. On July 13, 2000, President Clinton, by executive order, appointed members and the chair for the White House Commission on CAM policy to develop administrative and legislative recommendations to increase benefits and protect the public by providing consistent and credible research. Results of clinical studies were published in the *Journal of the American Medical Association* and other prestigious scientific and medical journals.

Research continues at hospitals and academic institutions across the United States. Due to reported findings, more medical doctors are supporting the use of various CAM therapies along with prescribed medical care. More doctors are using CAM therapies for their own health maintenance. Nearly half of U.S. medical schools are offering some education on CAM.

Complementary and alternative medicine (CAM) encompasses a number of healing practices, philosophies, and therapies that conventional Western medicine does not include, study, accept, or generally offer.

COMPLEMENTARY AND ALTERNATIVE MEDICINE DEFINED

The Panel on Definition and Description, CAM Research Methodology Conference, Office of Alternative Medicine, National Institutes of Health, Bethesda, Maryland, April 1995, defined complementary and alternative medicine as a broad domain of healing resources that encompasses all health systems, modalities, and practices and their accompanying theories and beliefs, other than those intrinsic to the politically dominant health system of a particular society or culture in a given historical period. CAM includes all such practices and ideas self-defined by their users as preventing or treating illness or promoting health and well-being. Boundaries within CAM and between the CAM domain and the domain of the dominant system are not always sharp or fixed.

Alternative versus Complementary versus Holistic versus Integrative Medicine

Complementary and alternative medicine encompasses many therapies that have developed outside of the Western medical model and are not necessarily based on surgical or biochemical theories. The term *CAM* is well recognized, partially due to the creation

BOX 17.1 CAM MODALITIES

There is a wide variety of health or healing practices that are included in CAM. Here is a partial list:

Acupuncture	Hydrotherapy
Alexander technique	Imagery
Aromatherapy	Light therapy
Ayurveda	Massage
Biofeedback	Meditation
Chelation therapy	Music therapy
Chinese herbal medicine	Naturopathy
Chiropractic	Neurolinguistic programming
Color therapy	Nutrition counseling
Diet therapy	Pet therapy
Folk medicine	Prayer and spiritual healing
Glandular therapy	Reiki
Guided imagery	Shiatsu
Herbal medicine	Sound therapy
Homeopathy	Visualization
Humor therapy	Yoga

in 1998 of the National Center of Complementary and Alternative Medicine at the National Institutes of Health. Other terminology is often used interchangeably, such as holistic medicine, body-mind therapies, or integrated medicine, although each of these has special considerations.

Holistic means to look at the whole picture. When applied to health, holistic takes into account the whole person rather than just the symptoms. All the things affecting the health of the individual—including spiritual, physical, mental, emotional, social, and environmental—are considered. Holistic treatment may include medical intervention combined with music in a conducive setting while the patient would also receive massage, acupuncture, Reiki, or hypnosis and participate in a support group. Holistic approaches also emphasize wellness, healthy lifestyle, and active participation by the person in her healing process where diet, imagery, positive thinking, meditation, and motivational tools are commonly used.

Mind-body medicine considers the power of the mind or thought processes and their effect on the physical. Techniques include positive attitude, hypnosis, guided imagery, as well as meditation, relaxation techniques, tai chi, and yoga. Mind-body response is supported by studies in

BOX 17.2 COMPLEMENTARY OR ALTERNATIVE?

In 2002, the Medical Subject Headings Section staff of the National Library of Medicine classified alternative medicine under the term *complementary therapies*. This is defined as therapeutic practices that are not currently considered an integral part of conventional allopathic medical practice. Therapies are termed as *complementary* when used in addition to conventional treatments and as *alternative* when used instead of conventional treatment.

Integrative medicine

combines complementary and alternative medicine with allopathic medicine.

---

psychoneuroimmunology and is the source of healing from within, spontaneous healing, and the placebo effect.

Integrative medicine combines complementary and alternative medicine with allopathic medicine. In an integrated model, a health care team, including doctors, massage therapists, acupuncturists, nutritionists, other selected health providers, and the patient meet together and cooperate to create a plan to best benefit the health maintenance of the patient. Integrative medicine effectively combines high tech and high touch to provide the best overall support for the patient. Recognizing that mind, body, spirit, emotion, and environment all play a part in healing the whole person, where no one system has all the answers, many resources can be combined to support health on many levels.

According to Andrew Weil, alternative insinuates instead of; complementary indicates a nice add-on, fluff; integration is a true coming together and cross acceptance of the medical models. It is the meeting of the minds, worlds, and philosophies. In keeping with Dr. Weil's model, he is training physicians in the practice and implementation of integrative medicine, but the physician is still the director and decides what course to take, whereas in a true integrative model, the patient is the director. Innately, patients know what they need. If they are interested in their health, they can make choices when given the appropriate information.

In 1993, David Eisenberg published a study in the *New England Journal of Medicine*[1] that surveyed people across the United States in 1990 that revealed startling use of unconventional therapies and CAM modalities for chronic or serious health problems. Thirty-four percent of the respondents reported using at least one unconventional therapy the previous year. The survey showed that 83 percent of those visiting alternative practitioners for serious medical conditions also visited allopathic doctors in the same year for the same condition; however, 72 percent of those did not tell their conventional doctor that they had sought out or used alternative therapies.

---

[1] D. M. Eisenberg, R. C. Kessler, C. Foster, N. E. Norwalk, D. R. Calkins, T. L. Delbanco, "Unconventional Medicine in the United States: Prevalence, Costs and Patterns of Use," *New England Journal of Medicine* 328 (4):246–253, 1993.

Another study by Eisenberg in 1997[2] indicated that 40 percent of all Americans and over 50 percent of individuals between the ages of 30 and 55 used some form of alternative therapy. Indeed, in 1997, there were an estimated 629 million visits to alternative practitioners, compared with 386 million visits to primary care physicians. Both surveys indicated that an overwhelming majority of individuals seeing alternative practitioners were also seeing allopathic physicians. The study also showed that in 1997, Americans spent more than $27 billion on alternative therapies, which exceeded the out-of-pocket spending for all U.S. hospitalizations.

The surveys show that the American public continues to use and support the use of alternative therapies. Patients are choosing to use CAM with their pocketbooks.

CHIROPRACTIC AND MASSAGE

A large number of massage therapists work in chiropractors' offices. The relationships between the chiropractic and massage practices vary between offices. Often, the massage therapist is an independent contractor who simply rents a space in the chiropractor's office. The massage therapist may be responsible for scheduling his own appointments and may work entirely independent from the chiropractor. On the other hand, the office receptionist may handle all scheduling and billing for services. Occasionally, the chiropractor may refer one or more of his patients for massage when soft tissue conditions need to be addressed. The chiropractor may suggest that the patient receive a short massage before the adjustment because it helps her relax and prepares the tissues so that the chiropractor's manipulations are easier and more effective. Some patients prefer a massage after being adjusted by the chiropractor. They feel the effects of the combined treatment far exceed the effects of either treatment given by itself. The chiropractor may also diagnose a soft tissue condition and refer the patient to the massage therapist for a number of therapy sessions.

Massage therapy and chiropractic together can address structural alignment issues and the soft tissue conditions that so often accompany them. The massage therapist spends the time to work with the soft tissue to increase circulation, reduce spasms, deactivate trigger points, and increase range of motion. The chiropractor is then easily able to adjust the spine and other joints to improve the overall structure and function of the client.

[2]D. M. Eisenberg, R. B. Davis, S. L. Etner, S. Appel, S. Wilke, M. Van Rompey, R. C. Kessler, "Trends in Alternative Medicine Prevalence and Costs 1990-1997: Results of a Follow Up National Survey," *Journal of the American Medical Association 280,* 1569–1575, 1998.

INTEGRATIVE MEDICINE

Integrative medicine combines conventional allopathic medicine with appropriate complementary and alternative medicine (CAM) modalities to provide the highest benefit to the client. Integrative medicine programs focus on assisting patients in the creation of customized wellness plans for optimal health that are as responsive to patient's initial concerns as they are to patient's changing health needs, taking into consideration all aspects of well-being. They include recommendations from a wide range of appropriate therapeutic interventions from both conventional and complementary/alternative practices, such as conventional medications and diagnostic medical screenings and examinations, herbal supplements, Oriental medicine and acupuncture, physical therapy, nutritional therapy, movement, and exercise assessments. These plans may include suggestions among the diversity of stress reduction and mind-body interventions such as biofeedback, massage, art and music therapy, yoga, and meditation. Above all, these plans are founded in mutual trust and respect between patient and practitioner, with the understanding that each individual has a significant, innate capacity for healing that can be supported and enhanced.

By combining modalities to reduce symptoms, by enhancing the ability to control pain and anxiety, and by better managing stress and improving quality of life, integrative medicine is particularly successful at assisting patients who have chronic medical conditions. Patients with chronic health problems, ranging from arthritis to headaches to life-threatening illnesses such as heart disease and cancer, combine traditional medical care with integrative methods to ensure that their physical as well as emotional well-being are addressed. A close collaboration among the physician, integrative medicine team, and the patient enables choosing treatments and services that are thoroughly integrated into the patient's overall medical care.

Integrative medicine is a health care program that is principled in science and tradition where the patient is treated as a whole person and respected as an individual. The patient in an integrative medicine program is encouraged to participate fully in health care choices in order to attain optimal health. Patients are listened to and treated with respectful consideration as a partner in the development of their health plan. They are given recommendations founded in Western/conventional medicine combined with appropriate lifestyle recommendations such as diet and exercise, as well as appropriate complementary and alternative treatment options such as herbal medicine, acupuncture, massage, biofeedback, yoga, and stress reduction techniques. A care plan is tailored to fit each patient's needs in order to honor at patient's personal healing process. The patient is also given the help needed to sort through the myriad complexities within complementary, alternative, and conventional health options to customize a health plan that is right for that individual.

Many health centers and hospital complexes around the United States have opened centers of integrative medicine. These centers offer a variety of services mostly directed to offering alternative or complementary health services in conjunction with mainstream Western allopathic medical practices. Practitioners from a wide variety of CAM modalities are available to provide their services. Each practitioner is part of the health team integrating services to support and enhance the health and well-being of the patient. Many of the integrative health services provide wellness services to hospital staff and outpatient services to people in the community. Many also provide services for hospital inpatients in certain circumstances and under supervision of the medical staff.

Because integrative clinics are connected to hospitals, the CAM modalities used at those clinics are gaining acceptance and recognition by parts of the medical community and the community at large. Integrative medicine programs see themselves as agents of change, dedicated to the transformation of health care from a disease-oriented, physician- and technology-centered model into a wellness, patient-centered orientation that understands and empowers the integration of body, mind, spirit, and community in health care.

As the medical community gains a better understanding of the level of interventions available from different types of massage and other CAM therapies, patients will benefit by integrating CAM and conventional medical practices with their physician's referral, recommendation, or at least, knowledge and cooperation. Reports from patients of positive outcomes about the use of CAM modalities are part of what changes the attitudes and opinions of the medical community. Educating the medical community and the community at large is an ongoing function of the integrative clinic, the practitioners who practice there, and the participants who benefit from the services.

Massage is often the first choice, or at least on the top of the list, for patients using integrative medicine. Massage may be the therapy that is directed toward the remedy of a specific condition, or massage therapy may be an adjunct therapy to complement a therapy regime. Massage therapy is one of the most effective CAM modalities for relieving stress and managing pain that is associated with so many pathological conditions. Massage is the most popular and requested CAM modality. It is the most familiar. Massage therapy is the mainstay of many CAM and integrative clinics.

Just as there are numerous complementary and alternative practices in integrative medicine, there are also many different styles of massage and touch therapies used in integrative medicine clinics according to the circumstances and needs of the patient/client. Some of the variations of massage therapy found in integrative clinics include Swedish, neuromuscular therapy, trigger point methods, craniosacral, Rolfing®, manual lymph drainage technique, infant massage, pre- and postnatal massage, and energy modalities including Reiki, therapeutic touch, and shiatsu.

Classic Western or Swedish massage is very popular when the client is seeking respite from the rigors of more stressful conventional medical treatments. Circumstances may prompt special considerations, such as cancer treatment, AIDS, prenatal care, pre-op preparation, postsurgical recovery, or following a traumatic accident. Massage increases relaxation, promotes well-being, and reduces anxiety in patients undergoing more invasive therapies. Massage is about touch and human contact. It is a key to wellness.

Lymph drainage therapy is offered in many integrative clinics to assist patients who experience lymphedema following the surgical removal of lymph nodes or other congestive conditions.

Massage services may also be requested that are specific to the client's condition. This may be the request of the patient, the suggestion of the integrative team coordinator, or a prescription from the client's physician. Specific massage may be orthopedic massage to reduce pain and increase range of motion and function to a particular body area, or scar tissue massage to reduce the detrimental effects of excessive scar formation. If there is any consideration of submitting billing to insurance, a prescription from the client's physician is required. (More on insurance billing can be found on page 695.)

The experience of working in an integrative clinic helps the therapist become more aware and knowledgeable about other therapies. A massage therapist who is knowledgeable about other CAM therapies is able to suggest other CAM modalities or refer clients to other therapists who may be able to support the client in her healing journey. Massage becomes a doorway to help open clients to using other CAM therapies.

Working in an integrated system, especially a hospital-related program, the massage therapist will be required to follow set guidelines and protocols. Protocols will be established for each CAM service offered. Protocols and procedures delineate the standard of care to the patient; define relationships and communication between practitioners, staff, and administration; reflect professional standards; and ensure that all practices are within the policies of the hospital and other legal entities. The Joint Commission on Accreditation of Healthcare Organizations routinely reviews hospital operational policy and practices providing accreditation for their continued operation. During these surveys, protocols, policies, and procedures must be clearly stated and meet professional standards before the hospital or the program is accredited.

If an integrative clinic is a hospital department or massage therapists are employed by the hospital, therapists may need to meet certain competencies in order for the hospital to maintain its accreditation. Those competencies may be evaluated through written tests, hands-on demonstrations of competence, verbal exams, or a combination of the three. If a massage therapist is working in a particular department, such as the birthing center, and is doing postpartum massage, she will be required to show that he has knowledge of positioning the patient, understands precautions about working with new mothers, and is knowledgeable about epidurals or C-sections. There may be competency exams for each massage modality.

Record Keeping

Clear and accurate documentation is required when working in an integrative setting. When working in an integrative clinic, especially in a hospital setting, a massage therapist must follow hospital regulations regarding patient safety, record confidentiality, and patient information. Patient records provide communication from patient to provider and from provider to provider. Records must be accurate, stating what you saw and what you did. Accurate records become the communication tool between various modalities and the means by which the coordinator follows the patient's progress and counsels with the patient regarding health care decisions.

Documentation of massage services is included in the patient's chart. Clear, concise language describes the services provided. Documentation of massage includes the assessment, type of massage given, effects of the treatment, any physical observations, and follow-up recommendations. Most hospitals use a central charting system where all health providers, doctors, nurses, physical therapists, and CAM practitioners document in the same chart. The SOAP system of documentation is commonly used in the medical community and is well suited to CAM practices. However, many settings use a descriptive explanation of services. The practitioner should learn and follow the documentation procedure the facility uses.

HOSPITAL-BASED MASSAGE

Hospital-based massage takes place in a hospital environment. The therapist may be employed by the hospital, may be an independent contractor, or even may be a volunteer or work through an associated hospital program, such as an associated integrative clinic. Sometimes the therapist will be associated with the physical therapy department. Therapist services may be available to hospital staff, patients, or patients' families. Benefits of massage to staff include decreased staff turnover, increased productivity, improved morale, decreased sick time, decreased worker compensation claims, and improved quality of patient care. Benefits of providing massage to patients include improved sleep, reduced need for pain medication, earlier discharge, and more satisfaction regarding patient care.

Providing massage services to patients requires a recommendation, referral, or prescription by the patient's doctor. Even without a prescription, the physician must provide a recommendation or release for the massage. A prescription is required before any third-party (insurance coverage) payment can be pursued. If the therapist is working as an employee of the hospital and has a prescription to provide massage, insurance reimbursement may be available through the hospital's patient billing

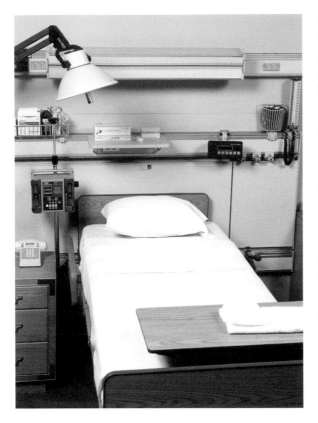

Figure 17.1

For patients staying in the hospital, massage from a caring massage therapist can reduce anxiety, improve sleep, and improve the overall sense of well-being.

services. Usually the patient requests the massage. Services are generally provided on a cash basis, whereby the patient pays the therapist directly. Services are usually performed with the patient in her hospital bed. The therapist may encounter a wide variety of medical conditions. Careful consideration must be given to medical equipment. The massage therapist must have a clear understanding of related pathologies and indications and contraindications of each of his clients when working in a hospital environment.

Hospitals can seem impersonal and intimidating (Figure 17.1). Receiving a massage from a caring massage therapist helps to relieve the feeling of being institutionalized and improves the patient's overall sense of well-being. Studies have found that massage reduces anxiety, improves sleep, and reduces requests for pain medication.

Some areas in the hospital where massage is performed include prenatal, postnatal, pre-op, and cancer treatment areas. Massage before surgery helps reduce a patient's anxiety. It also seems to reduce time spent in recovery.

Massage services have become a common addition to birthing centers. Massage helps promote relaxation during the birthing process. It also helps reduce the back pain often associated with labor. Acupressure can help stimulate contractions and ease the process.

Massage during cancer treatment provides a service that feels good when most treatment feels bad. Given before invasive treatments such as radiation or surgery, massage can help reduce anxiety. Massage has also been found to reduce pain. After surgery and the initial healing, massage can help reduce scar tissue, relieve edema, and help the client regain a better sense of self.

Massage is valuable after trauma, such as auto accidents, to help people reintegrate bodies that many times have gone through radical changes.

Often the massage services provided are modifications of classical Swedish massage to help soothe and reduce stress. There are usually special considerations and precautions because of the population receiving the massage services. It is essential that the massage therapist be knowledgeable of the pathologies present, be aware of the indications and contraindications for massage, and follow the recommendations of the attending physician.

We are a touch-deprived culture, especially in the hospital. In an environment where most procedures tend to be invasive, there is not much touch that is sensitive to the person. By providing services like massage and therapeutic touch in the hospital, we can begin to bring compassionate touch back into health care.

MASSAGE AS A THERAPEUTIC AID IN NURSING PRACTICE

Massage is one of the most beneficial services for patients during convalescence. Exercise and massage are often prescribed as a means of restoring the patient's fitness and sense of well-being. Swedish massage movements are most frequently used by nurses. The basic movements (manipulations) are effleurage, petrissage, friction, and joint movements.

In nursing, general massage consisting of basic movements or manipulations to increase the psychological and physiological well-being of the patient may be recommended. There are also specialized treatments in which the nurse is called on to deal with some abnormal condition affecting the patient's body systems. In the case of specialized massage, the patient's physician may assign therapy procedures to a physical therapist who is trained to work with nurses and physicians. Exercise, massage, electrotherapy, hydrotherapy, and related techniques may be used in the treatment of specific diseases and injuries. For example, a knee or hip replacement may require special care, such as a heat or ice treatment, before massage.

Massage is valuable in the treatment of injuries to soft tissues and joints and is prescribed in a wide range of conditions. Massage is used in some cases to treat nervous fatigue, insomnia, headache, tension, stress, and other disorders.

The nurse or health care practitioner should have a thorough understanding of anatomy, physiology, and pathology in order to determine the effects of various massage manipulations on the functions of the body's organs and systems. It is important to know when the patient will benefit from massage and when there are contraindications.

Nurses and other health care professionals are expected to practice the same code of ethics as other massage practitioners. They must have the same concern for the patient's comfort, privacy, and self-esteem. The main difference between nurses and massage practitioners is that nurses deal with patients who have a health problem or injury that requires hospital and physician care. The massage practitioner may also work under the supervision of a physician but may be employed in a private practice, a health facility, or a sports complex. The massage practitioner usually works in an environment where massage is part of a client's regimen for keeping fit and healthy rather than as an aid to recovery from disease or injury.

In nursing and health care, massage is used as part of the physiological and psychological rehabilitation process. When a person becomes ill or is injured, it is common to feel a sense of apprehension, insecurity, and anxiety, which often leads to restlessness and insomnia. A good massage will increase the patient's comfort, induce relaxation, and help to relieve anxiety. When a patient is confined to bed for a period of convalescence, muscles lose their tone, joints become stiff, and skin develops sensitivity. Unless a patient is turned or is able to move, bedsores may develop. Massage helps to prevent these problems.

In addition to increasing the patient's comfort, massage aids healing by increasing the number of white and red blood cells and by improving circulation, which in turn nourishes the tissues. Massage, when done correctly, improves the action of the lymphatic system. It also helps to promote blood supply to the brain and nerves so that the patient feels more in control of her faculties. Massage is used as an aid to preventing constipation by improving the peristaltic action of the small intestines and colon. There are numerous ways in which massage has been found to benefit patients of all ages. Many doctors recommend it as an aid to a speedier recovery.

Contraindications for Massage in Nursing and Health Care

Unlike the practitioner who deals with healthy clients, the nurse or massage therapist in a health care setting often works with people who are ill, injured, or recovering. The stage of the person's illness or injury will often determine the extent that massage might be given beneficially, or whether it should be given at all. It is important to be sure that massage is approved by the patient's physician.

Massage brings more fluid, blood, nutrients, and oxygen to affected areas of the body, but there are times when massage must not be given to or near an affected part. The patient's physician will note deterioration of muscles or skin that could benefit from massage and will also be aware of contraindications for massage. The nurse or therapist does not apply massage in cases of illness or injury without the supervision or permission of the patient's physician.

The following is a general review of contraindications:

- Bleeding (internal or external)
- Skin problems such as rashes, growths, lesions
- Newly formed scar tissue, scabs, wounds, and burns
- Infections, swollen areas, pain, inflammation, heat in the area
- Nausea, vomiting, and fever
- Edema: Excessive lymph fluid often causes swelling in feet and legs, particularly in elderly people. Sometimes the physician will recommend gentle effleurage or lymph drainage therapy in the direction of the lymphatic flow to help relieve this condition.
- Varicose veins: Veins in the legs become dilated and lengthen due to increased blood pressure. In mild cases, massage may be done on nearby areas but not directly on the affected part.
- Inflamed joints such as arthritis and bursitis: Massage is not done on the area when it is painful and inflamed.
- Cancer: When any symptom of cancer is detected or if any condition is suspected to be cancerous, massage is avoided on or near the area.

The following are warning signs that are associated with cancer and are contraindications for massage. Clients who show any of these signs should be referred to a doctor:

- Any sore that has not healed normally
- A mole, skin tag, or wart that is changing in color or size
- Lumps underneath the arms or in the breasts
- Persistent hoarseness, coughing, or sore throat
- Abnormal functioning of any internal organ, such as changes in the bladder or bowels
- Discharge or bleeding from any part of the body
- Persistent indigestion or difficulty in swallowing

MASSAGE AS MEDICINE

Currently, massage and manual therapies are experiencing a resurgence in popularity within the medical profession. As research continues to verify the benefits of massage and patients continue to profess its value and request referrals from their doctors for massage, more doctors are writing prescriptions for massage (Box 17.3). Some of these physician-prescribed massages take place in hospitals and integrative or medical centers; however, most of the time, medically prescribed massages occur in the office or studio of independent massage therapists. A massage to address a condition diagnosed by a physician can be considered a medical massage (Box 17.4).

Medical massage is sometimes defined as medically prescribed massage performed with the intention of improving pathologies diagnosed by a physician. Medical massage is generally practiced on patients to bring about a medical goal for health improvement. Medical massage is part of the medical treatment. The role of the massage therapist of medical

BOX 17.3   A CASE OF NECK PAIN

A prospective client comes for a massage for relief of headaches, neck and shoulder pain, and pain and tingling in her arm that has been intermittent but persistent since an automobile accident she was in several months ago. Before proceeding with any massage treatments, the therapist refers the client to her physician for a full examination and an accurate diagnosis. The client can also request a prescription from the physician for massage and provide for release of medical information so that the massage therapist may contact the physician. In so doing, the massage therapist protects the client and himself by making sure that there is an accurate diagnosis and that there are no hidden medical conditions. Having a prescription for massage also opens the possibility of obtaining insurance coverage for the massage services. This may increase the likelihood of more extensive and consistent massage services to achieve lasting relief to the client.

BOX 17.4 CONDITIONS THAT BENEFIT FROM MEDICAL MASSAGE

Medical massage can be an effective treatment for a number of conditions, especially when stress or musculoskeletal issues are involved. Some diagnosed conditions that are referred for medical massage include:

Anxiety	Neck pain
Athletic injuries	Osteoarthritis
Back pain	Postinjury rehabilitation
Carpal tunnel syndrome	Repetitive strain injuries
Edema	Sciatica
Emotional stress	Sprain/strain
Fibromyalgia/fibrositis	Temporomandibular joint dysfunction
Headaches	Tendonitis and other tendon injuries
Insomnia	Thoracic outlet syndrome
Migraines	Whiplash
Myofascial pain	

massage is to apply techniques that positively and directly affect the diagnosed condition. The therapist must be familiar with the pathologies involved and with therapeutic modalities to positively address the conditions. The therapist may use a variety or combination of modalities or procedures during the treatment, such as Swedish massage, neuromuscular therapy, craniosacral therapy, myofascial release, lymphatic drainage, massage for cancer patients, orthopedic massage, trigger-point therapy, soft tissue mobilization, acupressure, and so on, depending on the condition and the skills of the therapist. Medical massage is specifically directed to resolve conditions that have been diagnosed and prescribed by a physician and will focus treatment on the areas of the body related to the diagnosis and prescription.

Medical massage is directed toward a diagnosed medical condition or at least is given with the consideration of a medical condition being present. The massage may be directed toward a soft tissue condition to improve function, relieve tension, increase range of motion, and/or relieve associated pain. Massage may also be prescribed to help manage stress and anxiety related to pathologies or medical conditions that are otherwise unaffected by the massage.

Medical massage sessions follow a therapeutic procedure. The prospective client comes to the session with some condition or injury and seeks a massage to remedy or improve the medical condition. A physician or chiropractor has previously diagnosed the condition, and the client has a prescription or recommendation for massage. A concise health and client history will help to better understand the client's conditions and concerns. A thorough assessment at the beginning of the first session further determines the tissues involved. The therapist must have an acute awareness of indications and contraindications for the diagnosed conditions. Techniques are chosen, a care plan is created, and the treatments commence. The therapist will continually assess the tissues and responses of the client as they provide appropriate techniques to address the condition. Massage services are directed toward the affected condition according to the doctor's diagnosis. Sessions of medical massage are usually shorter and more frequent. Full-body massages are generally not warranted. When the condition subsides or improves to a level where there is no further improvement, the goal for the treatments is accomplished and further treatments are discontinued.

INSURANCE REIMBURSEMENT FOR MASSAGE

Massage therapists in many parts of the United States are experiencing the advantages and frustrations of obtaining reimbursement from insurance companies for the work they do on massage clients who have been injured and referred to them from a doctor or chiropractor. The decision to accept insurance cases into your practice requires some consideration of the pros and cons of working with the clientele and their insurance companies.

Working with the clients can be very rewarding as they find relief from their injuries with the soft tissue interventions of medical massage. With the doctor's recommendation and prescription, the regular massages are therapy that would otherwise be unavailable to the client.

The therapist, however, must be willing to provide services to the client and prepare the necessary paperwork to bill the insurance company, then patiently wait or battle for reimbursement while the insurance company processes the claim. Usually reimbursement payments are fairly prompt; however, the insurance company may request more information or review a claim. Sometimes the waiting continues for months or even years after which the therapist's fees for service may be reduced or even denied. Knowledge of proper billing practices reduces the frustration of resubmitting claims and increases the promptness and probability of being paid by the insurance companies. Proper billing requires close attention to detail when preparing claims, clear communication with the company agent, and accurate record keeping while documenting client progress and billing information.

There are a wide variety of types of insurance providers. Most do not reimburse massage therapists for the services provided. HMOs and PPOs will not cover the services of a massage therapist unless the therapist is listed as a provider in the group. Even then, massage services are usually only available to the subscriber at a reduced rate. Government health insurance such as Medicare and Medicaid do not cover massage services. Most major medical insurance policies do not cover massage therapy at this time. As massage becomes more recognized as a cost-effective alternative, this may change.

The types of insurance cases that are more likely to cover massage therapy are state Worker's Compensation, auto insurance, and some personal injury (PI) cases. In Washington state, legislation was passed in 1996 requiring insurance companies to reimburse licensed massage therapists for services performed on patients when prescribed by a doctor. The state of Florida also has some legislation that requires insurance providers to reimburse massage therapists for some types of services.

When you, as a therapist, decide to accept insurance cases, it is a good idea to start slow, learn the ropes, and become comfortable with the process. Begin with one or two insurance claims. Learn the intricacies of correctly filling out and submitting the necessary paperwork and communicating with insurance agents. Proper filing of insurance claims requires considerable time. If your business decides to accept several insurance clients, consider contracting with a billing service to file claims, thereby leaving more time for you to see clients.

Filing a Claim

The process in which insurance billing is done is fairly standardized. Following a procedure when working with insurance cases and billing insurance companies, even though it is a rather involved process, will actually simplify the process and increase the chance of prompt payment from the insurance company. Organization, clear documentation, perseverance, patience, attention to detail, and promptness are required to successfully reap the benefits of insurance reimbursement.

In order for a claim for massage therapy to be considered by an insurance company, the massage treatments must be considered to be medically necessary. Medical necessity can only be determined by a doctor, chiropractor, or possibly a physical therapist and is documented via a letter of referral and/or a prescription. A referral to a massage therapist must include a statement of medical necessity and a prescription that includes a diagnosis of the condition, an order for services to be preformed, the frequency of treatments and how long the treatments will continue until the patient is re-evaluated by the doctor. The billing to the insurance company must reflect massage services as they appear on the prescription.

If during the intake assessment the massage therapist recognizes conditions related to the client's injury beyond those indicated on the doctor's prescription, the therapist may request that the doctor rewrite the prescription to include the additional conditions so that they may be included in the insurance claim. The client can return to the doctor and ask that the related condition be added to the diagnosis, or the therapist can call and inform the doctor of his observations, and ask whether the physician would consider amending the prescription. Otherwise, even if the therapist addresses the additional conditions during the therapy session, he may only bill the insurance company for the work done on the conditions listed on the prescription.

When making the first appointment with a new client, determine whether it is an insurance case. If it is, have the client bring the necessary information to the first appointment, or better yet, get the necessary preliminary information over the phone in order to obtain verification from the insurance carrier before the client arrives for the first appointment. Always obtain verbal verification from the insurance company before providing any services to the client.

Verification or Authorization

Before beginning any massage on a new insurance client, obtain verification over the telephone from the insurance adjuster that the massage services are covered on the client's policy. You should have the following information before calling for verification: client name, name of policyholder if different from the client, insurance company name, adjuster's name and phone number, insurance ID number (Social Security Number), claim number, and date of incident/injury. You must also have a prescription and preferably a referral letter from a physician or chiropractor. The prescription should include a diagnosis and a treatment plan to include the number, frequency, and duration of the massage treatments to be given.

Obtain verification of the following: Does the client have coverage for your services as a massage therapist? What **current procedural terminology (CPT) codes** are covered? Is there a limit on coverage either in number and frequency of treatments or monetary limit of benefits? What is left under the limit? Is there a deductible? How much and what portion has been met? When does the deductible renew? What percentage of fees does insurance reimburse? Is there **co-pay**? What is it? If it is a worker's compensation claim, get an authorization to proceed.

Worker's compensation requires authorization before services are rendered. Any services provided before authorization is obtained do not have to be reimbursed by the insurance carrier. Rules for worker's compensation vary from state to state. Before accepting any claims, call the Worker's Compensation Division of the Department of Employment in your state for information and ask for a fee-for-service manual. Worker's Compensation is generally provided from an insurance company designated by the client's employer at the time of the injury. By the time the client comes to you, she should have a prescription from the physician, the name of the claims agent or case manager, the agent's phone number, and a claim number. The prescription must include the diagnosis, the prescribed treatment, the frequency of treatments, the duration of treatment, and the physician's license number and signature. The prescription must prescribe "massage therapy" or include specific CPT codes that are within the massage therapist's scope of practice.

When communicating with an adjuster or insurance claims agent, be sure to document the conversation. Record the date and time (to the

current procedural terminology (CPT) codes

were developed and are maintained by the American Medical Association that categorize and quantify medical services and provide a common language and a base for communication between physicians, therapists, patients, and insurance companies.

co-pay

is the portion of the fee for service that the patient is responsible for at the time of service.

BOX 17.5 CLIENT INFORMATION REQUIRED FOR INSURANCE VERIFICATION

The following information is required to obtain verification or authorization from the insurance carrier that your services are covered by the client's policy. Do not expect to be paid for any services provided to the client before obtaining verification. Even getting verification does not guarantee payment for all the services you may submit for reimbursement. You will need the following information from the client to contact the insurance company for verification:

- A prescription or a doctor's referral that contains:

  Physician's name and license number

  Diagnosis (ICD-9 code)

  Prescribed treatment (CPT codes)*

- Insurance information

  Name of the insured person

  Name of the insurance company

  Adjuster's name and phone number

  Name of policyholder if different than name of insured

  Policy number

  Claim number

  Date of injury

While you are speaking to the adjuster, verify what will be covered by insurance.

- Will insurance cover the services of a massage therapist?

- Verify that the CPT codes for the prescribed treatment will be reimbursed?

- What is the amount of time allowed per treatment per diagnosis?

- What is the duration of treatments or number of sessions allowed?

- Ask about the deductible:

  How much is the deductible?

  Has the deductible been met?

  When does it renew?

- Ask about co-pay:

  Is there a per visit co-pay?

  How much is it?

- Ask about percentage of coverage information.

  Remember that verification does not guarantee payment.

*ICD-9 and CPT codes are described on page 704.

minute), the name of the person or persons with whom you are speaking, and exactly what was said. If an agent transfers you to another party, get the name and the direct phone number of the person you are being transferred to in case you get cut off in the transaction.

Always obtain a verbal verification of a client's insurance coverage over the telephone before performing any services on that client. Follow up the telephone authorization or verification with a confirmation letter restating what was verified during the telephone conversation and fax or mail it to the insurance carrier, requesting a written confirmation of coverage.

Documentation for an Insurance Claim Client

During an initial interview, the client with an insurance claim will complete several forms and a preliminary assessment. At the initial interview, the client completes and signs a Medical Information Release Form and an Agreement for Payment Form. The Intake Form and the doctor's prescription will have sufficient information to contact the insurance adjuster for verification of coverage. The Medical Information Release Form is required by law and allows you to share information regarding the client's health (related to the injury) with the insurance company, other

BOX 17.6 DOCUMENTATION FOR INSURANCE CLIENTS

During the initial visit, the client will be requested to fill out several documents, including:

- Client Intake Form: Design this form so that the information it contains will transfer to the HCFA 1500 form.

- Medical History Form: May be part of the Intake Form or a separate document.

- Medical Information Release Form (Figure 17.2): This is required to share confidential information with insurance companies, physicians, or attorneys.

- Agreement for Payment Form (Figure 17.3): This states that the client is responsible for any fees not covered by insurance.

- Assignment of Benefits Form (Figure 17.4): This instructs the insurance carrier to pay you, the therapist, directly for services billed.

- Informed Consent Form

- Initial Assessment Form: This will contain current findings related to the physician's diagnosis.

The preliminary visit of an insurance client will require extra time to fill out required documents and to perform an initial assessment. The insurance company may or may not reimburse for the extra time required for the initial assessment.

Medical Information Release Form

Client's Name _____

Address _____

I hereby authorize _____ to release to any physician, insurance company, or attorney directly involved in my case any medical records or other information necessary for the purpose of administration, evaluation, or payment of debt related to my illness/injury sustained on (date) __/__/____.

This authorization remains valid from the date it is signed until revoked by me, in writing to both this provider and the insurance company.

Signed _____ Date _____

Figure 17.2

Medical information release form.

Agreement for Payment Form

I understand that I am responsible for all fees charged for professional services rendered. All fees are due at the time of service unless other arrangement are made in advance. If insurance is billed for services, I understand that I am responsible for any charges not covered including co-payments, unpaid percentage of coverage, and deductibles. In the event of insurance nonpayment or denial, I also understand that I am responsible for all fees and will make whatever arrangements possible to make full payment.

I understand that your time is valuable and that 12 hours' notice is required for cancellations and I will be charged for missed appointments without giving proper notice.

Client's Name _____

Address _____ City _____ State ____ ZIP _____

Client Signature _____ Date _____

Figure 17.3

Agreement for payment form.

health practitioners related to the case, or lawyers or the courts involved with the case. Do not release any patient information without the patient's authorization, and then provide only necessary information and only to those professionals involved or related to the case. The Agreement for Payment Form establishes the client's responsibility for any payment of fees for services that is not paid by the insurance company or in a court settlement. The client should also sign an Assignment of

---

Assignment of Benefits

I hereby direct my insurance provider _____ to assign and make direct payment to _____, my health care provider, all monies for medical claims submitted by them on my behalf for medically necessary treatment.

Client's Name _____

Address _____ Policy Number _____

Client Signature _____ Date _____

Figure 17.4

Assignment of benefits form.

Benefits form, a copy of which will be sent to the insurance company with the first claim so that the carrier will send the claim benefits directly to the therapist for the services he performs. Another copy is kept in the client's file so that when sending in future claims, and the client is not available to sign forms, the proper blank can be filled in with "Signature on file."

Another important form when dealing with insurance companies is a receipt for services. The receipt should include all information necessary for the insurance company, the client, and the therapist regarding the session. The receipt should include the following information:

Date of service

Client's name

Charges for service

Payments and adjustments

Previous and current balance

ICD-9 (diagnosis) and CPT (procedural) codes

Therapist's name, address, phone number, and provider number, if there is one

Client's next appointment

During the initial evaluation, carefully document any conditions relevant to the client's injury or complaint. The physician's prescription will designate specific areas of the body to apply selected procedures. Palpate the tissues in the designated area(s) and note the condition of the specific muscles on the preliminary assessment form. Indicate tension, trigger points, hypertonicity or hypotonicity, inflammation, swelling, or any other condition. Following the session, note changes to these conditions.

When performing medical massage or filing for insurance payment, every massage or therapy session must be clearly documented. Usually, this documentation is kept only in the client's files and is not included when filing a claim unless requested by the insurance company. A narrative SOAP note style of documentation is preferred.

You may be required to submit documentation to insurance companies or, if the case goes to court, to attorneys, so it is imperative to keep clear, concise client records.

When performing massage for medical purposes, whether at the request of a physician or from the prescription, or when expecting reimbursement from insurance, it is essential to keep accurate documentation of each and every therapy session. Documentation includes forms completed during the intake procedure, individual session notes, and a receipt for services. Progress or session notes document each session and help the therapist and the client follow the course and progress of the treatment. Documentation is required for communicating with others involved such as medical personnel, insurance companies, and even lawyers or the courts. Clear session notes provide documentation that the session happened. They also show proof of progress, which is vitally important to insurance companies as they review and determine to continue payment of benefits.

Insurance companies pay only for services that are deemed medically necessary. The insurer determines medical necessity by reading documentation presented by the service providers. The client's medical history, especially related to the current injury or condition, the referral and prescription from the doctor, your initial assessment, and your progress notes are essential documents with which the insurer determines whether or not to reimburse for your massage therapy services.

Most of the documentation remains in the client files, except the receipt for services, a copy of which is given to the client and a copy is kept in a file for bookkeeping. Copies of the client's medical history, initial assessment, physician's referral and/or prescription, session notes, and the assignment of benefits form will accompany the **HCFA 1500 form** as attachments with the initial claim that is sent to the insurance company. Remember to keep copies of everything that is sent to the carrier. Follow-up submissions of claims for the same incident may only require the HCFA 1500 form, unless the insurance company requests session/SOAP/progress notes and a copy of the prescription with each claim submission. Ask the claims adjuster during the initial verification to determine the particular company policy regarding what documentation accompanies submitted claims.

Insurance companies usually prefer progress notes to be in a story form following a SOAP format. The use of abbreviations is discouraged. If abbreviations are used, include a key with every report. Session notes should be typed or written very clearly and be easy to read and understand.

The initial SOAP documentation includes the name of the client, name of the physician, name of the therapist, the date of service, location, and type of visit (initial or the number in the series) in the header

HCFA 1500 form

is a standardized form created by the Health Care Financing Administration to be used by service providers when billing insurance for medical expenses.

of the document. The **S** (subjective) portion contains the client's experience of the condition, including complaints and symptoms, when and how it started, what makes it better or worse, what has been done about it and the results, and the client's impression or response to the treatment. The **O** (objective) portion contains the therapist's observations of visual and palpatory findings as well as results of any exams and tests. Remember, when billing insurance, all objective and subjective findings must directly correspond to the diagnosis on the physician's prescription. The **A** (assessment) portion of the report contains the physician's findings or diagnosis as well as the functional outcome of the massage session. The **P** (plan) portion contains the treatment plan as directed by the physician, including the type, duration, and expected outcome or results.

SOAP documentation for follow-up sessions is somewhat more brief. The header contains the same information as the initial session document. The S portion contains the client's updated, current experience of her condition, including reactions or responses to the previous massage session. The O portion contains the therapist's visual and palpatory findings as well as the results of any exams or assessments. The A portion reports any functional outcome the therapist observes or the client reports as a result of the session. The P portion describes the procedure used and any suggested exercises.

HCFA 1500 Form

Insurance companies have adopted a standardized form for billing purposes. The form HCFA 1500 was created by the Health Care Financing Administration and is now used throughout the insurance industry, eliminating the confusion of different forms for every company. The Center for Medicare and Medicaid Services (CMS) uses an identical form and refers to it as form CMS 1500 for billing of Medicaid and Medicare part B services. The forms HCFA 1500 and CMS 1500 are identical and interchangeable.

The HCFA 1500 form was designed to be read by optical character recognition (OCR) software, which is the reason that it is printed with specialized red ink. The form ideally should be filled out using a typewriter or a computer using black ink. Handwritten forms cannot be read by computer and may result in a delay of payment. If the form is handwritten, use black ink and very legible handwriting. If using a computer, make sure the printer is aligned properly so that all entries are clearly readable. Use all uppercase (capital) letters and an easily read (Courier or Arial, 10 or 12 point) font. Do not copy, staple, paper clip, tape, or fold the form. There are a few software companies that have developed programs to assist in the preparation of the HCFA 1500 forms using client information from client intake and history documents.

Design your intake form so that it contains all the necessary information to transfer to the HCFA 1500 form.

> **ICD-9 codes** are a system of decimal numbers that correspond to medical conditions diagnosed by doctors. ICD-9 is an acronym for International Classification of Disease, 9th Revision, and is published annually by the U.S. Health Services and Health Care Financing Administration.

The HCFA form also requires the use of procedural codes that refer to the services provided (CPT codes), diagnostic codes that refer to the doctor's diagnosis (ICD-9 codes) and place of service codes indicating where service is provided.

ICD-9 codes are published by the U.S. Health Services and Health Care Financing Administration and specifically relate to the condition of the client as diagnosed by a physician. ICD-9 is an acronym for International Classification of Disease, 9th Revision, Clinical Modification. The system was first created by the World Health Organization (WHO) and has been modified in the United States. Every health condition has an assigned decimal number that is used on insurance forms to aid in the uniform reporting of ailments. A medical diagnosis and corresponding ICD-9 codes can only be provided by the doctor. It is preferred that the doctor or the physician's office includes the ICD-9 codes on the prescription. If you receive a prescription without an ICD-9 or CPT codes, call the physician's office and ask for the codes. Usually the doctor's office will be very cooperative about supplying the proper codes. Remember, as a massage therapist, it is outside your scope of practice to diagnose or provide ICD-9 codes. However, it is the therapist's responsibility to enter the correct ICD-9 code for the client's condition on the HCFA 1500 forms.

Current procedural terminology codes were developed by the American Medical Association to accurately categorize and quantify medical services. The codes provide a common language and a base for communication between physicians, therapists, patients, and insurance companies. CPT codes also list the allowable fees for each listed procedure. It is necessary to verify with the insurance adjuster as to what codes are currently being recognized and reimbursed. Worker's compensation claims also require the use of CPT codes; however, worker's compensation may only update codes covered in their fee schedules every several years, so contact the office in your state to obtain the most recent fee schedule.

CPT codes are arranged according to medical specialty, where specified levels of medical training or certification are required to use particular codes. Massage therapy falls into the category of physical medicine. You must have proper training for the codes you bill for even to the extent that you could explain the technique and reasons for using it in a court of law. Use only these codes you are trained or certified to use within your scope of practice. As of the latest revision of this text (2005), the following CPT codes are most commonly suggested to be used by massage therapists. Always verify with the insurance carrier as to which codes will be considered for reimbursement.

97010	Application of a modality to one or more areas; for example, hot or cold packs.
97124	Therapeutic procedure, one or more areas, each 15 minutes; massage, including effleurage, petrissage, and/or tapotement (stroking, compression, percussion)

97139   Therapeutic procedure, one or more areas, each 15 minutes; unlisted therapeutic procedure (specify)

Note: Consider reporting such procedures as shiatsu, Reiki, Qi Gong, etc. with this code. You will be required to submit a written description of the procedure and justification for its use.

97140   Manual therapy techniques (e.g., mobilization/manipulation, manual lymphatic drainage, manual traction); one or more regions, each 15 minutes

Note: This code replaces 97250 (deleted in 1999). Use this code for all therapeutic work. See 97124 for standard massage.

Codes change often. Because of the widening acceptance of massage and other complementary health practices, new codes are being considered to better describe the various therapies. Stay informed of changes in the CPT codes. CPT codes are revised yearly with a new CPT manual published annually. Manuals are sold at most major book sellers or can be obtained through the American Medical Association or on their Web site, www.ama-assn.org. Rather than purchase the code books, the therapist may determine the proper codes to use from the physician's office or the insurance carrier. Contact each claims adjuster when beginning a new case to verify what codes to use. Insurance may or may not pay for the evaluation done during the preliminary client visit. If the insurance company wants evaluations and will pay for them, ask the adjuster what code to use to cover this service.

Insurance usually will only pay for one hour of "physical medicine" per date of service and for a maximum of four, 15-minute procedures. Many carriers only allow two units or procedures on a specified area of the body. Each CPT procedure delineates a 15-minute increment, so four increments or units would constitute one hour. When listing the procedures on HCFA 1500, put one unit on each line. It is the therapist's responsibility to know that the codes he uses are proper and within his scope of practice.

State worker's compensation determines the reimbursement scale for every procedure listed in the CPT codes that is covered by worker's compensation. It is necessary to get authorization for every worker's compensation claim. When calling for worker's compensation authorization, call the insurance adjuster of the company carrying the policy, NOT the state worker's compensation office. After authorization is received, the therapist agrees to accept the payment schedule from worker's compensation insurance and not charge the client anything above what is paid by the insurance company. The therapist may request a claim's guide or a fee for service manual from the state worker's compensation office that should include what procedures are covered and the fee allowed for each procedure.

Place of service codes on the HCFA 1500 form go in box 24b. Codes that massage therapists might use are these:

11	office
12	home
21	inpatient hospital
22	outpatient hospital
34	hospice
61	inpatient rehabilitation facility
62	outpatient rehabilitation facility

Complete the HCFA form including services provided specific to the diagnosed conditions and the individual and total cost of those services. Be sure to include your tax I.D. number—either your Social Security number or your Employer Identification number—the address where services were provided, and your business or billing address; then sign and date the document.

Send the completed HCFA 1500 form along with the required supporting attachments to the insurance adjuster. If it is an initial filing, include a copy of the prescription, initial assessment, typed session progress notes, and the assignment of benefits form. Insurance companies will only pay for medical care that is considered medically necessary. The company makes the determination of medical necessity according to the documentation, including physician's referral and prescription, the initial visit/history documents, and the individual session progress notes. It is important for these documents to be complete and clear. The insurance carrier may or may not require progress notes from each session to be included with subsequent claim submissions. Remember, your treatment and documentation must coincide with the physician's prescription and diagnosis of the patient's complaints to be considered by the insurance company for reimbursement. Be prompt when submitting claims. File the first claim as soon as possible after the client's initial visit. It is preferred not to include more that two or three visits on a single form. Smaller claims seem to be paid more quickly. Always retain a copy of everything that is sent to the adjuster.

Insurance companies are supposed to respond to claims within 30 days from when they were submitted. If you do not receive any notification in six weeks (include time for mail delivery), contact the adjuster to inquire as to the status of the claim. Document the inquiry. If it is a phone call, document the date and time (down to the minute), the person with whom you spoke, what was said, and the tone in which it was said. The agent may say that the claim is under review or that they need more documentation. If denial or reduction of fees is part of the conversation, be sure to document any and all reasons. Be as diplomatic as possible when working with insurance adjusters. It is better to have them as an ally rather than an adversary. If diplomacy fails, persistence and assertiveness may be required to move the process. If the insurance company continuously delays action or payment on a claim, you might inform the client and have her or her attorney contact the company. Another avenue of recourse is to contact your state insurance commissioner to file your concerns. If all else fails and the claim is denied or fees reduced, contact the client, inform her of the decision, and remind her that according to your signed agreement, she is now responsible for the balance due.

SUMMARY

Many of the techniques now referred to as massage were developed as health-promoting remedies or part of a medical treatment in the earliest development of these practices. The earliest medical literature from Persia, Egypt, Japan, and China all make reference to various treatments that include the use of massage-like techniques, though the actual term *massage* did not appear in medical literature until the end of the nineteenth century. Massage-like practices continued to be a part of healing and remedial practices in many cultures around the world throughout history. In Western cultures, references to massage techniques are found in medical literature from 1700 on to the present day. In the early 1800s, Per Henrik Ling developed a system of movements he called medical gymnastics, which was to become popular throughout Europe as the Movement Cure or the Swedish Movements and eventually spread to the United States. The brothers George Henry and Charles Fayette Taylor traveled to Europe and studied the Cure at different schools and then returned to New York in 1859 to practice, teach, and write about the Movement Cure until their deaths in 1899.

During the first half of the twentieth century, massage continued to gain within the medical field in the form of physiotherapy. It was practiced in hospitals and rehabilitation sanatoriums as a part of the rehabilitation of wounded soldiers returning from World War I and World War II. Physiotherapy was also used for recovering victims of the poliovirus. By the 1950s, the use of massage in physiotherapy declined due to the fact that it was strenuous, time-consuming, and required extensive training. Physical therapy began relying more on exercise and the use of a variety of machines, medicines, and mechanical modalities for treatment. The use of massage in the medical field in the United States was nearly nonexistent after the early 1950s.

Swedish massage maintained a relationship in the natural health field and was practiced in health clubs or spas, sanatoriums, YMCAs, and resorts. Massage began to re-emerge during the human potential movement of the 1960s and 1970s outside of allopathic medicine. Classic Swedish massage was joined by reflexology, shiatsu, acupressure, and other alternative practices. In the 1980s, massage gained popularity among athletes due to its effects of reducing the stress of intense workouts and its effectiveness in promoting the healing of soft tissue injuries. Many of the techniques found to be effective when addressing soft tissue conditions in athletes also were effective for hypertonic, painful, or dysfunctional conditions in the general population. Clients were seeking the services of massage practitioners to remedy their aches and pains as an alternative to seeking medical treatment. Massage became classified as an alternative medicine along with other practices such as acupuncture, nutritional therapy, herbal therapy, and other practices that are not considered an integral part of conventional allopathic medical practice. A study by David Eisenberg in 1991 indicated that an astonishing number of people were seeking out the services of alternative practitioners. The study showed that there were more visits to alternative practitioners than to doctors and expenditures to alternative practitioners exceeded the out-of-pocket money paid to hospitals. The study also showed that clients visiting alternative practitioners were also seeing their medical doctors for the same condition although most were not telling their doctors that they were seeing the alternative practitioners. In the 1980s, the term *complementary medicine* gained popularity, implying that the services of the alternative practitioner would complement those of allopathic medicine rather than be an alternative to it. The National Center of Complementary and Alternative Medicine (NCCAM) was established in 1998 as a part of the National Institutes of Health to develop administrative and legislative recommendations to increase benefits and protect the public by providing consistent and credible research. Research into the effects of massage and other complementary pratices continues at hospitals, academic institutions, and in private clinics across the United States. Due to reported findings, more medical doctors are supporting the use of various CAM therapies along with prescribed medical care.

Integrative medicine combines complementary and alternative practices with allopathic medicine to create a care plan that is tailored to fit each patient's needs in order to honor each patient's personal healing process. It includes recommendations from a wide range of appropriate therapeutic interventions from both conventional and complementary/alternative practices to provide the highest benefit to the client. A patient may meet with an integrative team consisting of her medical doctor and a wide variety of alternative practitioners to develop a care plan to best serve her individual needs.

Integrative medicine is particularly successful at assisting patients who have chronic medical conditions by combining modalities to reduce symptoms, to enhance the ability to control pain and anxiety, and to better manage stress and improve quality of life. A close collaboration between the physician, integrative medicine team, and the patient enables a choice of treatments and services that are thoroughly integrated into the patient's overall medical care.

Integrative medical clinics are often associated with a hospital and offer a variety of alternative and complementary services to hospital patients and staff. A massage therapist working in a hospital-related program will be required to follow set guidelines and protocols that delineate the standard of care to the patient; define relationships and communication between practitioners, staff, and administration; reflect professional standards; and ensure that all practices are within the policies of the hospital and other legal entities. Accurate documentation that follows hospital protocols is essential in that it is the communication tool between providers and the means by which the coordinator follows the patient's progress and counsels with the patient regarding health care decisions.

Massage in the twenty-first century is re-emerging as an integral part of an individual's health practice. Whether it is to manage stress or pain on a regular basis or as part of an integrated treatment plan for dealing with cancer or other illness, massage and bodywork are becoming a common choice for individuals seeking better health. As research continues to verify the benefits of massage and patients continue to profess its value and request referrals from their doctors for massage, more doctors and patients are making massage a part of their medical treatment. Massage that is prescribed by a physician or chiropractor to address a diagnosed condition can be considered a medical massage and is part of a medical treatment. The therapist may use a variety of techniques with the intention of directly and positively addressing the diagnosed condition. Medical massage is especially effective for musculoskeletal and stress-related conditions.

A client seeking medical massage has seen a physician and has a prescription for massage. That prescription should contain a diagnosis, an order for massage therapy services to be performed, the frequency of treatments, and how long the treatments will continue until the patient is re-evaluated by the doctor. The massage session should follow a therapeutic procedure with a thorough assessment, treatment plan, massage, and evaluation. Massage services are directed toward the affected condition according to the doctor's diagnosis. Sessions of medical massage are usually shorter and more frequent. When the condition subsides or improves to a level where there is no further improvement, the goal for the treatments is accomplished and further treatments are discontinued.

Because medical massage is done according to a doctor's prescription, certain types of insurance reimbursement may be available. There are pros and cons to working with a clientele and their insurance companies that the therapist must consider before accepting insurance cases. Working with the clients can be very rewarding; however, insurance billing requires extra paperwork, and sometimes dealing with the insurance companies can be time-consuming and frustrating. Whereas most major medical policies, HMOs, PPOs, and government insurance such as Medicare and Medicaid do not cover the services of a massage therapist, personal injury from auto insurance and Worker's Compensation claims are more likely to pay for massage therapy when prescribed by a doctor or chiropractor. Filing an insurance claim is a fairly standardized yet rather complicated process. Successful reimbursement requires close attention to detail when preparing claims, clear communication with the company agent, and accurate record keeping while documenting client progress and billing information. Medical necessity must be established. The client must have a prescription that contains a diagnosis including ICD-9 codes and an order for massage including CPT codes. The billing to the insurance company must reflect massage services as they appear on the prescription. Different insurance companies require different documentation when filing a claim; however, almost all companies use the standardized HCFA 1500 form accompanied by other documentation. It is necessary to contact the claims agent for the case to verify that services will be covered and what documentation is required. Patience and persistence are necessary when depending on insurance companies to pay for services provided to clients. It may take months or even years to be reimbursed, or in some cases, the claim may be reduced or denied, in which case it is imperative that the client understands she is responsible for payment for any services not reimbursed by insurance.

Historically, massage is closely associated with medical practices when working with musculoskeletal conditions and physical rehabilitation. In the mid-twentieth century in the United States, massage fell out of favor in the medical community only to re-emerge as a most popular form of complementary and alternative therapy. In the latter half of the twentieth century and into the twenty-first century, continuing research, better training, and patient demand are restoring massage therapy as a viable and valuable component of the health care system.

QUESTIONS FOR DISCUSSION AND REVIEW

1. What did Charles Fayette Taylor and George Henry Taylor have in common?

2. Define CAM.

3. Differentiate between alternative medicine and complementary medicine.

4. What is integrative medicine?

5. What is the role of massage in integrative medicine?

6. What are some considerations for hospital-based massage?

7. What are seven early warning signs for cancer?

8. Define medical massage.

9. Why should a massage therapist obtain verification before providing massage services for a client seeking insurance reimbursement?

10. What is an HCFA 1500 form?

11. What are ICD-9 codes?

12. What are CPT codes?

13. What documents should be included in an initial insurance claim?

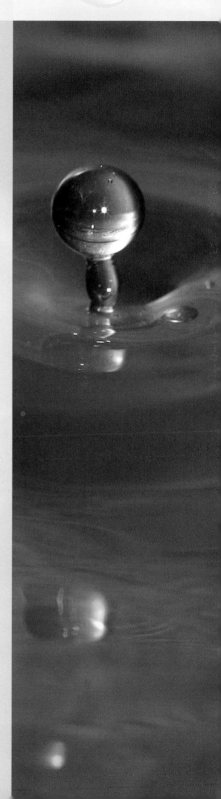

Other Therapeutic Modalities

LEARNING OBJECTIVES

After you have mastered this chapter, you will be able to:

1. Explain the benefits of prenatal massage.

2. Explain contraindications for prenatal massage.

3. Explain the benefits of lymph massage.

4. Describe the basic functions of the lymphatic system.

5. Explain the purpose of structural integration.

6. Define a trigger point and describe its location.

7. Describe how to treat trigger points.

8. Describe techniques used in neuromuscular therapy.

9. Describe the techniques used in muscle energy technique.

10. Define passive positioning and the bodywork styles that incorporate passive positioning.

11. Explain the basic philosophy of acupressure and acupuncture.

12. Describe shiatsu as related to pressure points of the body.

13. Define reflexology.

INTRODUCTION

In recent years, there has been a resurgence of interest in various massage therapies that relate to the maintenance of physical, mental, and emotional health. Many of these techniques are related to or are descendants of Swedish massage in that they encourage relaxation, increase the movement of body fluids, and soothe the nervous system. Others have origins in the far Eastern philosophies of Japan and China. Some touch techniques are referred to as bodywork.

It is not within the scope of this book to cover in detail every therapy style. However, serious students or practitioners are encouraged to continue their training by exploring various styles and sharpening their skills to better serve their clientele. Continuing education through advanced programs at schools or in workshops is necessary to stay current regarding new developments and techniques available to the massage professional. There is a wealth of reference material listed in this book's bibliography. The brief discussions in this chapter will acquaint the practitioner with the basic concepts of a variety of techniques. At the end of the chapter is a partial list of other popular somatic therapies the serious student will want to explore.

PRENATAL MASSAGE

During pregnancy, a woman's body experiences many changes to accommodate for the gestation and delivery of a baby. The changes are both physical and hormonal. Physical changes include an enlarging abdomen and breasts and weight gain. Strain is increased on the lower back, hips, and lower extremities from bearing the shifting and increasing weight. Hormonal changes soften some connective and ligament tissue in preparation for delivery and may play a part in the emotional swings some expectant mothers experience.

In normal, healthy pregnancies, massage has proved to be beneficial to both mother and unborn child. Properly applied massage can aid relaxation, benefit circulation, and soothe nerves. Prenatal massage is applied like any regular massage except for the following considerations.

Positioning: The client may take any of several positions depending on which is more comfortable. Early in the pregnancy, before the abdomen starts to protrude, the prone and supine position may be used as in any regular massage. When the fetus has grown enough to "show," special considerations to provide comfort to the mother and safety to the fetus must be made. If the client takes a supine position, arrange pillows under her back to support her in a semireclining position. Also place a pillow or a small bolster (6 or 8 inches) under the bend of her knees to take the strain off her lower back and abdominal muscles (see Figure 18.1).

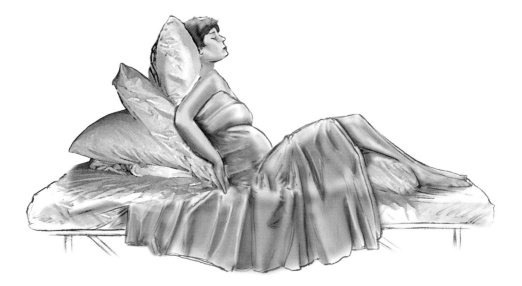

Figure 18.1

A supported reclining position is comfortable and safe during the later stages of pregnancy.

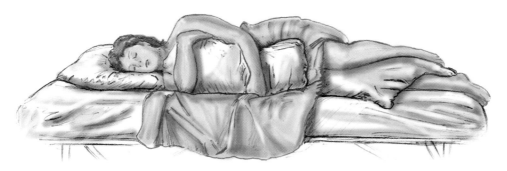

Figure 18.2

The side-lying position is a comfortable position to be used throughout pregnancy.

During the second half of the pregnancy, use the supine position with great caution because in this position the weight of the fetus may press on the descending aorta and impede the flow of blood to the placenta.

The mother may prefer lying on her side, especially during the final months of pregnancy. Use plenty of pillows to comfortably support the head, womb, and between the knees (Figure 18.2). Ask the client to indicate if at any time during the treatment she becomes uncomfortable.

During the first two to three months of pregnancy, the prone position may be used. However, as the abdomen becomes larger, pillows placed underneath the client's head, chest, pelvis, and legs will add to her comfort. During the second and third trimester, a preg-pillow can be used for a safe and comfortable prone position. A preg-pillow is a cushion, 6 to 8 inches thick, with space cut out for the enlarged abdomen and breasts. There are commercially available cushions and bolsters specifically designed for prenatal massage that safely and comfortably support the mother in side-lying and prone positions (Figure 18.3).

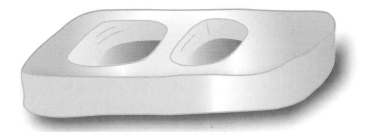

Figure 18.3

A preg-pillow is a special supporting cushion with cutouts for the womb and breasts that can be used to allow even a full-term mother to lie safely and comfortably in the prone position.

Body Areas Subject to Discomfort

Areas of the body that appreciate special attention during pregnancy are the neck, upper and lower back, hips, legs, and feet. The upper back and neck often feel strained because of the head-forward position that is common during pregnancy. Tension in this area can lead to tension headaches. The neck is most easily accessed with the client in a supine or side-lying position.

The lower back experiences extra strain, especially in the later stages of pregnancy due to the extra weight of the protruding abdomen and the hormonal changes that soften the ligaments in preparation for delivery. Massage to the lower back can be applied in the side-lying position, or if a preg-pillow is used, in the prone position. Lateral and abdominal muscles are also under strain from carrying the extra weight and from stretching to accommodate the growing fetus. Effleurage and light petrissage are soothing and will help relieve the tension in the muscles. Massage directly on the abdomen is contraindicated during pregnancy.

The added weight and reduced activity that accompany pregnancy often result in fatigue and minor swelling in the legs and feet. Regular, gentle massage of the feet and legs helps to reduce the fatigue and swelling. If edema is minimal, it is acceptable to massage (effleurage) the legs and arms. If the edema is serious, massage should not be done, and the client should be referred to her physician.

Be present to assist the client onto the table and into a comfortable position. A step stool is helpful for the client to easily get onto and off the table. Have lots of bolsters and pillows on hand to provide comfortable positioning. A bathroom should be easily accessible because the growing fetus tends to press on the mother's bladder prompting frequent and urgent urination. Plan on a relatively short massage. Most pregnant women will not remain comfortable lying down for more than 45 or 50 minutes. Women often comment on how pleasant and soothing they find massage to be during pregnancy because of its calming and reassuring effects.

Contraindications for Prenatal Massage

There are some special considerations when performing massage on a pregnant woman. Before beginning a prenatal massage, it is important to ask the expectant mother whether there is any reason why massage would not be advisable. Massage is contraindicated if the woman is experiencing morning sickness, nausea, or diarrhea, or has any vaginal discharge or bleeding. High blood pressure, excessive swelling in the arms or legs, abdominal pain, or a decrease in fetal movement are contraindications for massage and warning signs for immediate referral to a physician. High blood pressure and excess edema are contraindications and should be referred to a physician. Pre-eclampsia, a type of toxemia, is a condition sometimes occurring in the latter half of pregnancy and is characterized by high blood pressure, edema (swelling of hands, feet, and face), and sodium retention. Indications of this condition include excessive weight gain or protein in the urine. The expectant mother may suffer headaches and dizziness and, in serious cases, convulsions. When toxemia is suspected, the expectant mother should see her physician without delay.

Varicose veins are often a problem during pregnancy due to the effects of progesterone on the blood vessels and to the increased pressure on the main blood vessels that return blood from the legs. Light effleurage can be done around, but not on, affected areas.

If there are any other health concerns, obtain permission and possibly a recommendation from the woman's primary health care provider before providing massage services. During pregnancy, do not give massages when contraindications are present. Problems can occur during pregnancy, and the expectant mother should be under her physician's care regarding diet, exercise, and massage. However, many physicians recommend massage for its therapeutic effects.

Massage During Labor

A physician may recommend light effleurage on the patient's abdomen and upper legs as a means of obtaining relief between contractions. Lower back pains can also be relieved by the application of firm continuous counterpressure. During a contraction, counterpressure can be applied to both sides of the spine in the area of the sacrum.

Massage Following Birth

Often a mother will request massage throughout her pregnancy and after the child is born. Massage helps to relieve neck, shoulder, and lower back discomfort and is an aid in the relief of tension. When combined with proper exercise and diet, massage will be of value in regaining normal weight and firming slack muscles.

LYMPH MASSAGE

Lymph or lymphatic massage is a descendant of Swedish massage. Dr. Emil Vodder, Ph.D, of Copenhagen, Denmark, pioneered the practice of manual lymph drainage massage in the 1930s, although because he was not a physician, the therapeutic value of his techniques was not really recognized until the 1960s. He is credited with having discovered the benefits of lymphatic massage and for the development of massage techniques widely used today. Dr. Vodder's method of manual lymph drainage massage uses light, rhythmical, spiral-like movements to accelerate the movement of lymphatic fluids in the body.

In 1967, a German physician, Johannes Asdonk, conducted a scientific study of over 20,000 patients and published a report on the effects, indications, and contraindications for lymph drainage massage. Now, in many parts of Europe, lymph drainage massage is recommended by doctors for the management of lymphedema. More recently, Dr. Bruno Chikly of France has developed methods to recognize the rhythm and flow of both superficial and deep lymph movement and techniques to map lymph flow to better assist its movement with lymph drainage therapy.

Before beginning the study of lymph massage, the practitioner or student must have a thorough knowledge of anatomy, particularly of the lymphatic system. Lymph drainage massage requires careful training procedures. Vodder's manual lymph drainage massage and Chikly's lymph drainage therapy are taught in the United States, Canada, and Europe. Students and therapists interested in practicing these techniques are urged to enroll in training under the guidance of qualified instructors.

The following overview will be helpful to understanding the basic functions of the lymphatic system and the principles of the lymph massage.

The Lymphatic System

The lymphatic system is a system of vessels and nodes supplementary to the blood-vascular system and provides another pathway for fluids of the circulatory system to return to the heart. In contrast to blood circulation, which is a closed loop, lymph circulation is one-way, beginning when interstitial fluid enters the closed-end lymph capillary and ending when lymph re-enters the venous blood flow in the subclavian vein at the junction of the internal jugular vein in an area called the **angulus venosus**, just before the blood returns to the heart. The lymphatic system consists of lymph, lymph vessels, and lymph nodes. Lymph vessels include initial lymphatics or lymph capillaries, precollectors, collectors, and lymph ducts or trunks.

> **angulus venosus**
>
> is the juncture of the jugular and subclavian veins.

Lymph Vessels

The walls of lymph capillaries are composed of a single layer of flat, endothelial cells. The outer surface of these cells have fine anchoring filaments that connect the capillaries to the surrounding tissue (Figure 18.4). Movement of the tissue or fluid pressure in the connective tissue pull on the filaments, thereby opening the space between the cells of the capillary walls and allowing the tissue fluid to enter the lymphatic capillary. These anchoring filaments play an important part in lymph drainage massage in that the gentle movements of the massage tug on the filaments, encouraging fluid into the lymph system. The spaces created between the cells in the walls of the lymphatic capillaries act as tiny valves that allow fluid from the interstitial spaces to enter the capillaries. Once inside the capillaries, the fluid is considered lymph. Lymph is carried from the capillaries into slightly larger pre-collectors containing bicuspid valves that prevent backflow and direct the lymph into even larger collector vessels. Collectors are the main transporting vessels that carry the lymph toward the lymph nodes, then on to the larger trunks or ducts. The walls of the collector vessels are several cells thick and contain smooth muscle that helps propel lymph through the system. Smooth muscle in the lymph collector vessels is under the control of the autonomic nervous system and is most active when activated by the parasympathetic impulses. Trunks or ducts are the largest lymph vessels that carry lymph to the deep veins at the base of the neck where the lymph is reunited with the blood just before it re-enters the heart.

Specialized lymph vessels in the walls of the small intestine called lacteals carry away fat that is absorbed in the digestive tract. The milky fluid that collects in the lacteals is called **chyle.**

Lymph

Lymph is interstitial fluid that is absorbed into the lymphatic system. Interstitial fluid is derived from blood plasma and continuously bathes the cells and connective tissues. Tissues receive nourishment and building materials from this interstitial fluid and also release waste products and toxins into the fluid. Without it, tissues would soon dry out and degenerate. Between 80 and 98 percent of this fluid, containing dissolved gases, waste products of metabolism, and water, is reabsorbed into the blood vessels. Between 2 and 20 percent

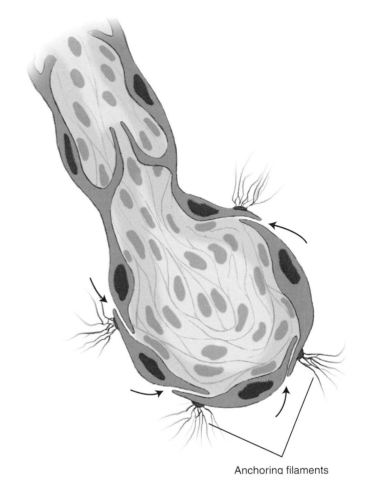

Anchoring filaments

Figure 18.4

Initial lymph capillary with anchoring filaments.

of the fluid is absorbed into the lymphatic system to become lymph.

Lymph is comprised of approximately 96 percent water and may contain proteins, fats, hormones, enzymes, lymphocytes, phagocytes, tissue debris, cell parts, bacteria, viruses, or other toxins, including cancerous tissue. The reabsorption spaces in lymphatics are four to five times larger than those in the venous capillaries. This allows the lymphatic capillaries to absorb larger proteins, antigens, and other waste elements that are too large or toxic to be absorbed into the venous system. Contaminants that may be harmful if left to circulate freely through the vascular system are carried in the lymph by way of the afferent (inward) lymph vessels and deposited in the lymph nodes. Here, antigens, damaged cells, and toxins are acted on, broken down, or devoured by the lymphocytes. They are turned into harmless substances and passed out of the lymph nodes through efferent (outward) vessels. Eventually, they pass through the lymph ducts and back into the blood system to be eliminated through the liver, kidneys, lungs, or digestive system.

Lymph generally flows toward the heart. Superficial lymph flow in a generally healthy, nonobstructed system is toward the nearest lymph nodes responsible for draining the area. Lymph flows from lymphatic capillaries to pre-collectors and then to larger collectors that carry the fluid

chyle
is a cloudy liquid, consisting mostly of fats, that passes from the small intestines, through the lacteals, and into the lymph system.

toward the lymph nodes. Lymph travels from the lymph nodes into deeper collecting vessels toward the thoracic duct from the lower extremities and toward the venous re-entry site at the base of the neck from the upper extremities. Lymph from the right side of the head and neck, the right upper extremity, and the right side of the torso above the belt line flows into the right lymphatic duct before re-entering the venous blood system near the junction of the right subclavian vein and right jugular vein (Figure 18.5). Lymph from the lower extremities flows toward the inguinal lymph nodes and then toward and into the cisterna chyli at the base of the thoracic duct. It is joined by chyle from the lacteals. Lymph from the left side of the head and neck and the left upper extremities flows toward and into the left thoracic duct before it re-enters the venous blood flow at the left subclavian vein near the junction of the left jugular vein.

Lymph flow may become inhibited for many reasons, including lack of physical activity, stress, fatigue, or emotional trauma. Surgeries may remove lymph nodes or create scar tissue that obstructs lymph flow.

Lymph circulation is vital to life: When it slows down, waste products can accumulate and stagnate. The tissue often becomes puffy and shows signs of edema. The movement of lymph is maintained by the ac-

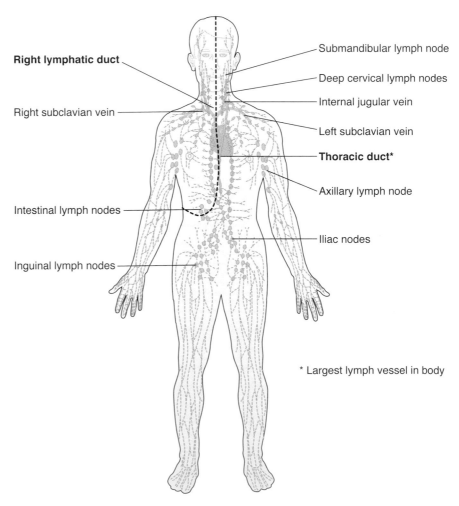

Figure 18.5

Areas of the body drained by the right lymphatic duct and the thoracic duct.

tions of the smooth muscles in the larger lymph vessels, by normal respiration, and by muscular movements of the body in general.

Lymph Nodes

Lymph nodes are small masses of lymphoid tissue. They vary in size and shape but are usually less than 1 inch (2.5 cm) in length. They are often beadlike or bean-shaped compact structures that lie in groups along the course of lymphatic vessels. There are an estimated 400 to 1,000 lymph nodes in the body. Superficial lymph nodes are located in areas of the body where it folds, except the wrists. Major areas of nodes that drain the flow of superficial lymph are the sides of the neck, the axillary area, and the inguinal crease. Nearly half the lymph nodes in the body are located deep in the abdomen, and they collect lymph from intestines and other organs of the body. When inflamed and swollen, lymph nodes can be felt beneath the skin.

Functions of the lymph nodes include the following:

- The filtration of toxins and other elements from the lymph

- The breakdown or destruction of harmful substances by the action of lymphocytes and phagocytes

- Concentration of lymph by reabsorbing fluid back into the venous system

- Production of monocytes and lymphocytes

Lymph nodes are usually distributed in groups. Regional lymph nodes include the following:

- Submaxillary nodes are located beneath the mandible.

- Preauricular nodes are located in front of the ear.

- Postauricular nodes are located behind the ear in the region of the mastoid process.

- Occipital nodes are located at the base of the skull.

- Superficial cervical nodes are located at the side of and over the sternocleidomastoid muscle.

- Deep cervical nodes are located along the carotid artery and internal jugular vein.

- Axillary nodes are located in the armpit. Constituting the main group of the upper extremity, axillary nodes receive lymph from vessels that drain the wall of the thorax, mammary glands, upper wall of the abdomen, and the arm.

- Supratrochlear nodes are located in the elbows.

- Inguinal nodes, located in the groin and constituting the most important group of the lower extremity, receive lymph from the leg, external genitalia, and lower abdominal wall.

- Popliteal nodes are located behind the knee.

- Abdominal and pelvic cavities also contain numerous lymph nodes.

Lymph nodes are part of the lymphoid system and the immune system. The immune system produces lymphocytes and other cells in response to the presence of inflammation, antigens, bacteria, viruses, and other cellular debris in the body. Lymphocytes are active in the immune responses of the body and play a major role in the healing of wounds and fighting infections. The primary lymphoid organs are the bone marrow and the thymus gland where the majority of the lymphocytes are produced. B-lymphocytes are produced and mature in the bone marrow. Lymphocytes produced in the bone marrow that migrate and mature in the thymus are termed T-lymphocytes. When an antigen enters the body, B-lymphocytes produce antibodies that counteract the antigen and produce an immune response that protects the body from future exposures. When an antigen enters the body, T-lymphocytes activate and destroy the foreign invader.

Secondary lymphoid organs include the spleen, tonsils, adenoids, appendix, and the lymph nodes. Lymphocytes reside in the secondary lymphoid organs in high concentrations, ready to actively counter any problematic substances they encounter. Lymphocytes also penetrate all tissues and are abundant in blood, mucous membranes, connective tissue, skin, and all body organs except the central nervous system. (For more information of the lymph system, refer to Chapter 5, page 219.)

Influence of Massage on Body Fluids

It is important to understand the influence of massage on circulation of fluids in the human body. Both the lymphatic and venous circulation are accelerated by massage movements. Lymph massage activates the movement of lymph into and through the lymph system. Lymph massage stimulates the activity of the lymph nodes, increases the production of lymphocytes, and improves body metabolism. It helps drain stagnant interstitial fluids, toxins, and proteins from the interstitial fluid, helping to rid the body of toxins and waste materials. Lymph massage stimulates the immune system by bringing more antigens in closer contact with lymphocytes in the lymph nodes. The slow rhythmic pace of lymph massage is very relaxing and stimulates the parasympathetic nervous system, which in turn is helpful in relieving stress, depression, and some types of insomnia.

Lymph massage promotes balance of the body's internal chemistry, purifies and regenerates tissues, helps to normalize the functions of organs, and enhances the function of the immune system.

Contraindications for Lymph Massage

Contraindications for lymph massage are generally the same as for general Swedish massage. If there is any question about a condition, refer the client to a doctor and work under the guidance or supervision of a physician or other qualified health practitioner.

Contraindications for lymph massage include the following:

- Acute infections and fever
- Inflammation (heat, redness, swelling, pain)

- Cardiac problems; congestive heart failure, uncontrolled high blood pressure, cardiac insufficiency

- Venous obstructions (phlebitis, thrombosis)

- Bleeding, hemorrhage, or weeping sores

- Malignant illness; cancer when the tumor is still present; lymphomas. Lymph massage has proven beneficial as a postsurgical treatment to manage secondary lymphedema resulting from the surgical removal of regional lymph nodes. This should only be done by experienced therapists trained in lymph drainage massage, under the supervision of a physician, and with the informed consent of the client after having signed a release form.

- Edemas of unknown origin: Avoid work on edemas caused by kidney, heart, or liver dysfunction. Always consult the client's physician if there is any doubt.

Techniques of Lymph Massage

The techniques of lymph massage are gentle, rhythmic, slow, and somewhat circular movements that encourage the flow of lymph into and through the lymphatic capillaries and toward the lymph nodes that drain the area being massaged. Light circular movements create a wavelike action that encourages the movement of lymph through the lymph vessels.

The practitioner's hand lightly contacts the client's skin and gently and slowly moves the skin over the subdermal layers. The pressure is between 1 and 8 ounces per square inch (1 to 8 oz./in^2). The more delicate the tissues, or severe the edema, the lighter the pressure. The maneuvers are somewhat circular or elliptical with the hand in contact with the skin and slightly more pressure applied in the direction of lymph flow. The rhythm is slow with five to ten repetitions per minute depending on the natural, personal rhythm of the client. The movement is repeated in the same area several times before moving to an adjacent area. With some practice and awareness, the practitioner is able to attune to the rhythm of the lymph movement.

The target of lymph massage is the superficial lymphatic capillaries located just a few millimeters below the skin surface in the dermis. It is estimated that superficial lymph circulation accounts for approximately 70 percent of the lymph in the body. The hand pressure against the skin is very light. If the practitioner is feeling any of the deeper structures or tissues, the pressure is probably too heavy. The pressure is just enough to feel the fluid nature of the subdermal tissue. The pressure is lightest on the delicate tissues of the face. It will be only slightly more on the thicker tissues of the arms or legs. Pressure may be a little more where lymph nodes are located in the axial and inguinal areas.

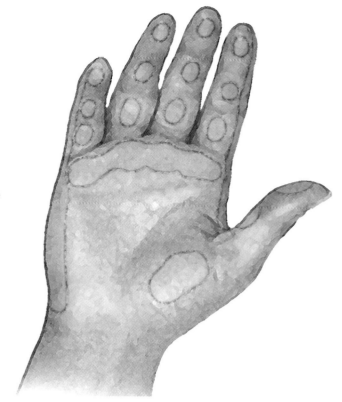

Figure 18.6

The soft pads on the palm of the hand make contact during lymph massage.

Touch and Pressure

The touch is very light, using the soft pads of the fingers, thumb, and palm of the hand (Figure 18.6). Just enough pressure is used to encourage fluid into the delicate lymph capillaries. Too much pressure would tend to collapse the lymphatics and increase the volume of fluids filtrating from the blood capillaries, which would be directly counterproductive to the intention of lymph massage. The very light circular movements of lymph massage are gentle, rhythmic, and in harmony with the natural body rhythms of the client.

Rhythm

The rhythm is slow. Move according to your client's natural rhythm. Each pulsation of the circular movement is between 4 and 10 seconds. Quietly tune into and enhance the unique wave of fluid movement.

Frequency

The movement is repeated in the same area five to seven times, sometimes more, sometimes less before moving to the next, adjacent area. There is a discernable softening or warming of the tissues as the fluid begins to move.

Successful lymph drainage massage depends on the expertise and sensitivity of the practitioner. He must consider the effects to be achieved by various movements. For example, body fluids can be displaced intravascularly (within vessels) or extravascularly (in the interstitial spaces). This displacement of fluid is achieved by manual strokes.

Sequence of Movements

The sequence of movements generally begins and ends at the site of the collecting lymph nodes draining the area being massaged or at the re-entry site where lymph rejoins the venous blood at the angulus venosus. Lymph massage on the neck and head begins and ends inferior and superior to the clavicles near the sternal notch. Lymph massage on the extremities begins and ends at the site of the lymph nodes in the axilla or inguinal crease respectively. The lymph massage sequence begins proximally to clear out the lymph channels and works distally and then again from distal to proximal, finishing by once again helping to clear the area of the lymph nodes.

Movements are first directed toward the regional lymph nodes and then progress away from the nodes while directing the movements to encourage lymph flow toward the nodes. On the arms, the movements begin in the axillary area and progress down the arm to the hand. The slow rhythmic movements encourage lymph flow toward the medial aspect of the arm and toward the lymph nodes in the axillary area. Likewise, on the legs, the movements begin in the inguinal crease to clear the inguinal nodes and progress down the leg to the foot. Movements direct the lymph flow toward the inguinal area. After massaging all the way to the foot, the therapist works back up the leg, finishing by once again clearing the inguinal nodes. On the back of the thigh, movements are directed toward the inguinal area on the medial aspect of the thigh or around the lateral aspect to the front leg and then on toward the inguinal nodes. On the back of the lower leg, movements are directed toward the popliteal space behind the knee, location of some minor nodes. Superficial lymph flow on the torso is generally directed toward the closest concentration of lymph nodes. Above the belt line, approximately at the level of the umbilicus, lymph flow is toward the axillary nodes of the same side of the body. Below the belt line, lymph moves inferiorly toward the inguinal nodes on the same side of the body (see Figure 18.7a and b).

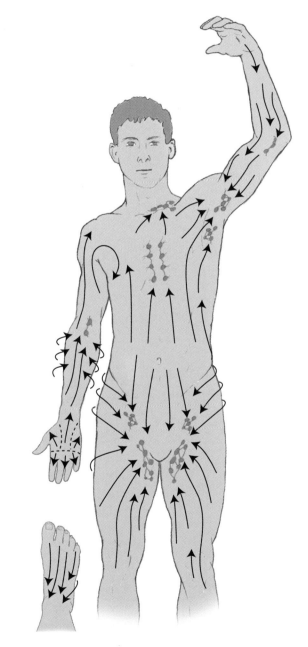

Figure18.7a

Direction of superficial lymph flow on the anterior of the body.

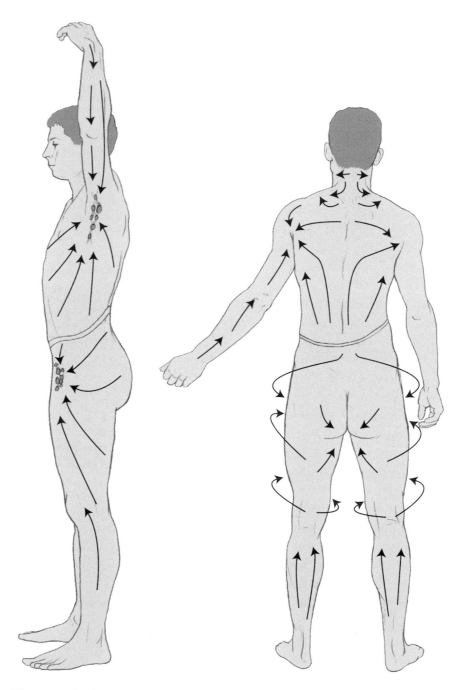

Figure 18.7b

Direction of lymph flow on the lateral and posterior aspects of the body.

Before attempting lymph massage, the practitioner should be thoroughly familiar with the functions of the lymphatic system. Lymph massage is done to enhance, but not force, the movement of lymph through the lymphatic system. The procedure begins at the junction of the right thoracic lymph ducts and the subclavian vein adjacent to the junction of the jugular veins, and just behind the clavicle near its articulation to the sternum. This is where the lymph system dumps into the venous blood.

PROCEDURE FOR A LYMPH MASSAGE

The following procedure should be done only under the supervision of a qualified instructor.

1. Neck: There is a high concentration of lymph nodes in the neck to protect the organism from infectious invasion through the mouth, nose, eyes, and ears. It is a valuable practice to methodically encourage lymph movement through and out of this area. Lymph massage begins where lymph circulation ends, at the base of the neck, just superior to the clavicles, close to their sternal attachment. The client is positioned supine on the massage table, and the practitioner is preferably seated above the client's head (Figure 18.8a). The pads of all four fingers are used to contact the area just superior to the medial clavicle on both sides of the neck. Small, light, circular or elliptical movements encourage lymph movement toward the angulus venosus, which is the junction of the subclavian and the jugular veins. The movements are slow, approximately six to ten rotations per minute, and repeated several times in the same spot. Move slightly superior and posterior (Figure 18.8b) and continue the soft, circular movements with the soft pads of the fingers, directing the flow toward the base of the neck. After five to ten repetitions or revolutions, move your finger up to the next adjacent area (Figure 18.8c) and continue the slow, gentle wavelike movements, directing the lymph flow down the neck. Methodically proceed to massage the entire lateral aspect of the neck from the anterior border of the sternocleidomastoid muscle to the lateral aspect of the spenius capitis or the trapezius and from the base of the neck to the base of the ear and the occiput at the top of the neck (Figure 18.8d).

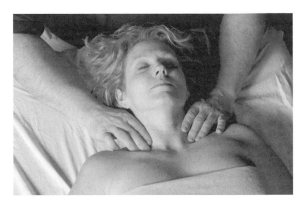

Figure 18.8a

Begin the lymph massage with the therapist's fingers just superior to the medial clavical near the angulus venosus.

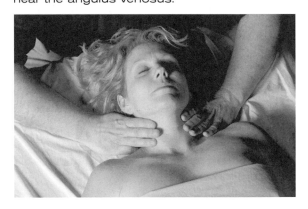

Figure 18.8b

Move the hands superior and continue the slow movements of lymph massage.

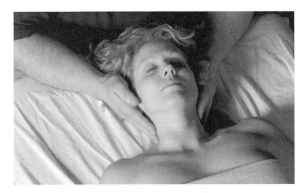

Figure 18.8c

Continue with the lymph massage movements directing the lymph flow downward while working up the neck.

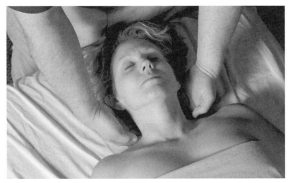

Figure 18.8d

Turn the hands over to massage the posterior aspect of the side of the neck from the bottom to the top.

Finish with superficial effleurage in a downward direction on the entire side of the head and neck.

2. **Pectoral and axillary area:** Superficial lymph from the central, upper chest flows toward the clavicles and the angulus venosus. Light circular strokes along the sternal and subclavicular borders are therefore directed toward the angulus venosus. Massage can continue just inferior of the clavicle all the way to the axillary fold, directing the flow toward the angulus venosus.

Lymph from the axillary lymph nodes flows into deeper collector vessels and toward the midclavicular region and the angulus venosus. Initial massage to the axillary lymph nodes can begin bilaterally by gently placing the fingers deep into the axillary fold and directing the movements in a midclavicular direction (Figure 18.9a and b). Access to the axillary nodes can be increased by abducting and laterally rotating the client's arm (Figure 18.10a to c). Continue the gentle, circular, wavelike movements in different aspects of the axillary area that can be easily accessed from this position. Remember, slow movements repeated several times in the same area. Continue to direct the lymph deep toward the midclavicular direction. Complete this area of massage by again clearing the subclavicular and supraclavicular areas near the lymphatic trunks and the angulus venosus.

The preceding massage maneuvers are performed with the practitioner seated above the client's head. The following movements are done with the practitioner standing on the same side of the client as is being massaged.

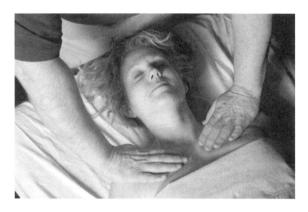

Figure 18.9a

Lymph flow is directed toward the angulus venosus from the subclavicular areas.

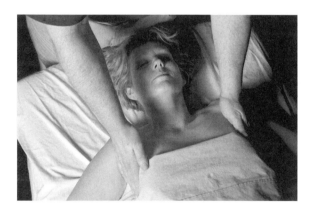

Figure 18.9b

Lymph in the axilla is directed toward the midclavicular area.

The Upper Quadrant

3. **Axillary area (continued):** Superficial lymph from the upper quadrant generally flows to the axillary nodes on the same side of the body. (An exception is when axillary nodes have been surgically removed or otherwise damaged, lymph may adopt other pathways into neighboring quadrants.)

Continue massage directed at the axillary area from a standing position at the client's side. Gently place the soft pads of the fingers onto areas of the axilla that were not addressed previously. Apply slow, rhythmic, circular, wavelike movements directed deeper into the axilla. Approach the area from different directions until the entire area has been covered (Figure 18.11a to c).

4. **Upper quadrant of the torso:** Superficial lymph from pectoral area, breast, and upper torso flows toward the lymph nodes in the axillary

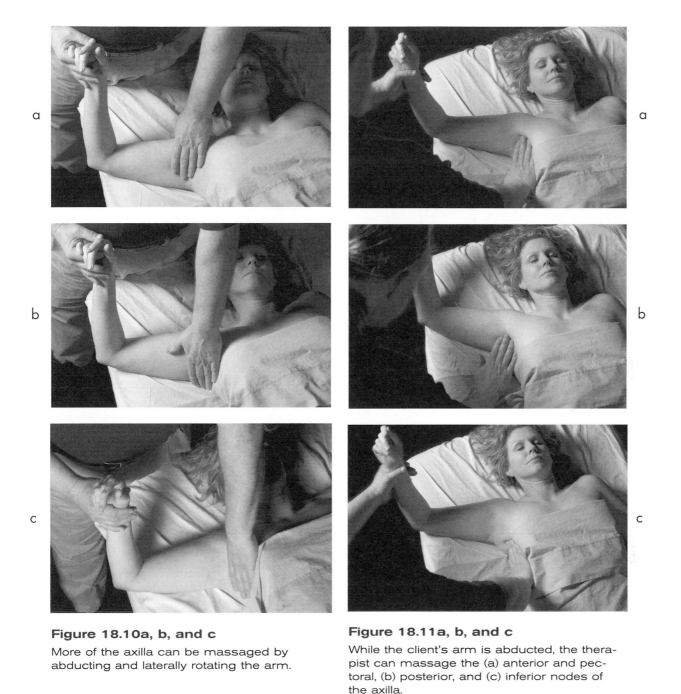

Figure 18.10a, b, and c

More of the axilla can be massaged by abducting and laterally rotating the arm.

Figure 18.11a, b, and c

While the client's arm is abducted, the therapist can massage the (a) anterior and pectoral, (b) posterior, and (c) inferior nodes of the axilla.

area of the same side. Lymph massage in this area begins proximal to the axillary fold (Figure 18.12a and b). Movements can be applied with the entire hand, or even both hands when appropriate (Figure 18.12c and d). Place the hand close to the axilla with as much of the hand making contact as possible. Apply gentle, circular, wavelike movements directed toward the axillary nodes. Repeat the slow, rhythmic movements five to ten times in the same place and then move the hands to an adjacent area just distal and repeat the movements. Apply movements over the lateral and anterior rib cage. You may want to work in sections. Begin just inferior of the axilla and

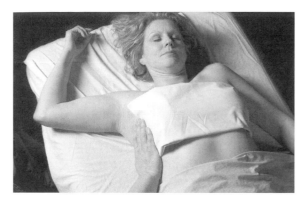

Figure 18.12a

Lymph massage on the lateral torso begins near the axilla.

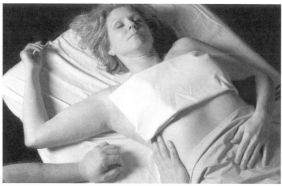

Figure 18.12b

Lymph massage continues down the side directing lymph toward the axilla. Two hands may be used.

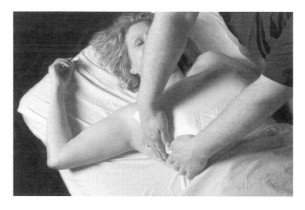

Figure 18.12c

The therapist may stand on the opposite side of the table while applying lymph massage to the torso.

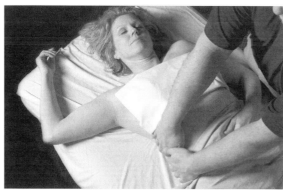

Figure 18.12d

Continue working down the side of the torso while directing lymph flow toward the axilla.

apply movements with the intention of moving lymph toward the axilla while working in increments to the bottom of the rib cage, then repeat the movements moving closer to the axilla. Massage the pectoral area in the same way, beginning close to the axilla, moving incrementally away to cover the pectoral area and then back to the axilla, all the time directing lymph flow toward the axillary nodes. On male clients, begin near the axilla and apply movements first below the nipple line and then above the nipple line (Figure 18.13a and b). On female clients, apply movements above and below, but avoid massage of the breast tissue (Figure 18.14a and b). Although lymph massage of the breast is a benefit in some circumstances, instruction on this methodology is beyond the scope of this text. The serious student will seek advanced training in lymph therapy to offer this highly beneficial service. Breast massage is also illegal in some jurisdictions.

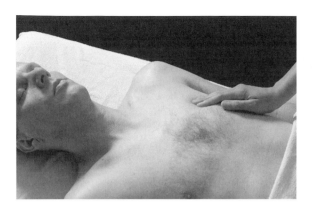

Figure 18.13a

Lymph is directed from the pectoral region to the axilla.

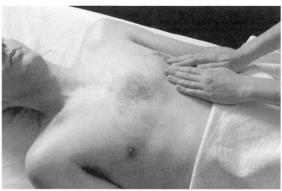

Figure 18.13b

Two hands can be used in some areas.

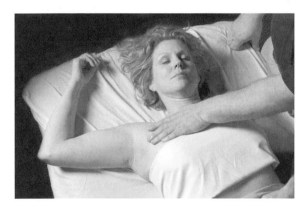

Figure 18.14a

Proper draping is used on female clients. Apply lymph massage on the upper pectoral area.

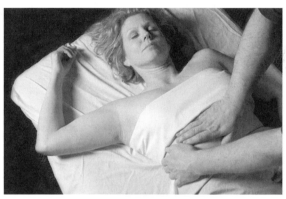

Figure 18.14b

Apply massage below the breast. Avoid the breast tissue.

Massage of the upper quadrant may continue by repeating the lymph massage to the axillary nodes or by proceeding to the arm.

5. Arm: Lymph from the arm flows to and through the axillary nodes. To gain access to the axillary nodes, abduct and laterally rotate the arm to expose the axilla and underside of the arm and support it in this position. Begin lymph massage of the arm in the axillary fold, directing the lymph flow toward the angulus venosus. Using the soft pads of the fingers of both hands, apply the gentle rhythmic movements of lymph massage to the posterior, medial, and anterior aspects of the axilla (Figure 18.15a to c). Spend a minute or more

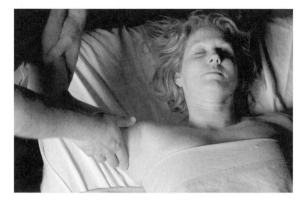

Figure 18.15a

Lymph massage of the arm begins at the axilla.

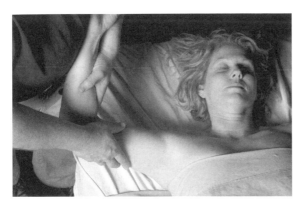

Figure 18.15b

Massage continues down the brachial aspect of the arm, directing the flow towards the axilla.

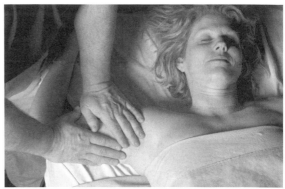

Figure 18.15c

One or two hands can be used on the inner arm.

in each position. Thoroughly cover the entire axillary space. Continue movements down the brachial aspect of the arm from axilla to the elbow and then from the elbow to the axilla. Replace the arm to the client's side on the table.

Continue lymph massage of the arm by placing one or both hands near the shoulder, over the deltoid muscle and apply the gentle, slow, circular, wavelike movements of lymph massage with the entire palmar and finger pad surface of the hands (Figure 18.16a). After five to ten revolutions, or about a minute, move the hands down the arm to an adjacent area and continue the movement (Figure 18.16b). Continue moving down the arm in increments to include the forearm, hands, and fingers, all the time directing the lymph flow up the arm toward the axilla (Figure 18.16b to e). Briefly repeat the movements from the fingers to the shoulder. Spend extra time in any areas that seem to be congested, again clearing proximal vessels to allow move-

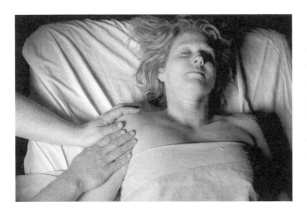

Figure 18.16a

Arm massage continues on the shoulder with one or two hands.

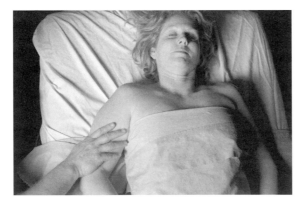

Figure 18.16b

Lymph massage continues down the arm with the intention of directing lymph toward the axillary nodes.

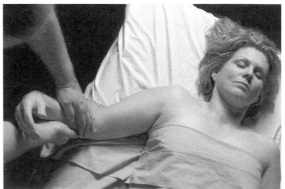

Figure 18.16c

On the lower arm, lymph flows up and around to the soft side of the arm and on up to the axillary nodes.

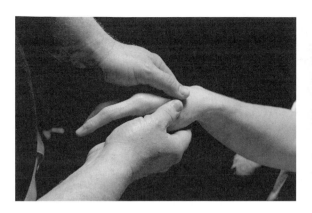

Figure 18.16d

Massage the back of the hand and the palm with light pressure with the thumb and fingers.

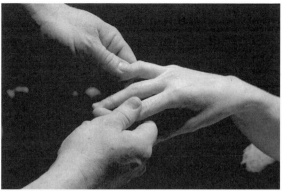

Figure 18.16e

Apply light circular pressure to each finger and the thumb.

ment from the area. Signal the end of the arm massage with very light effleurage from the hand to the shoulder.

This procedure illustrates the process in lymph massage of beginning at the site of the central lymph nodes, then working from proximal to distal and then back to proximal again. This regime can be applied to any area of the body.

Conclude lymph massage of both upper quadrants by moving to the head of the table and again applying massage to the axillary nodes, along the inferior and superior aspects of the clavicles, and finally at the base of the neck near the angulus venosus.

6. Lower quadrant: Superficial lymph from the lower quadrant generally flows toward lymph nodes just inferior to the inguinal ligament and then into deeper iliac nodes and to the cisterna chyli at the inferior end of the thoracic duct, deep in the abdominal cavity. The upper boundary of the lower quadrants of the body is roughly defined by a belt line about the level of the umbilicus. Superficial lymph from the lower abdomen flows inferiorly toward the inguinal nodes on the same side of the abdomen. Superficial lymph from the hips, gluteals, and lower back tend to flow more laterally toward the front of the body and the inguinal nodes. Lymph from the lower extremity flows up the leg toward the inguinal crease. Lymph from the lateral aspect of the thigh tends to flow around toward the front of the leg and on to the inguinal nodes (see Figure 18.17).

Lymph massage of the lower quadrant begins in the area of the inguinal lymph nodes. The inguinal lymph nodes are located in an area that is quite vulnerable, touchy and even ticklish, with the lower nodes located very near the genital area. Discuss the

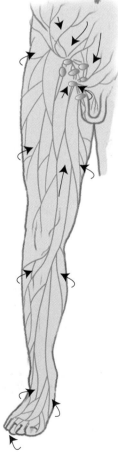

Figure 18.17

Major lymph nodes and superficial lymph flow of the lower quadrant.

lymph massage of the inguinal area with your client before the session and obtain informed consent to work in this area. As you begin massage in this area, alert the client and explain your hand placement and movement. Be extremely discreet and gentle with your hand placement. Use excellent draping skills.

7. Anterior Legs: Massage of the leg and lower quadrant begins at the site of the inguinal lymph nodes, which are located along a line just inferior to the inguinal ligament. Begin the massage of the anterior leg by slightly flexing, laterally rotating and abducting the hip. Support the flexed knee with either your body or a pillow (Figure 18.18a). First contact the lateral, more superior area, just below the inguinal ligament with the soft pads of your fingers and begin to apply gentle, slow, rhythmic movements, encouraging the movement of lymph into the deeper vessels. Repeat the wavelike movements ten to twenty times and then reposition your fingers medially and inferiorly until the lower hand borders on the gracilis muscle, then continue the movements (Figure 18.18b).

With the leg in the same position, lymph massage can easily be applied to the medial aspect of the thigh from the inguinal crease to the knee. Begin with hand positions proximal to the inguinal nodes, applying five to ten slow repetitions and move incrementally toward the knee (using two hands if so desired) until the medial thigh has been massaged (Figure 18.18c). At this point, light effleurage

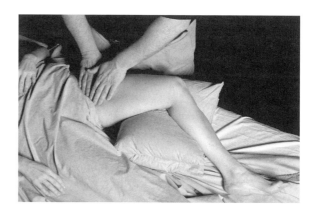

Figure 18.18a

Lymph massage begins at the site of the inguinal lymph nodes. Flexing and abducting the thigh slightly provides easy access to the inguinal nodes.

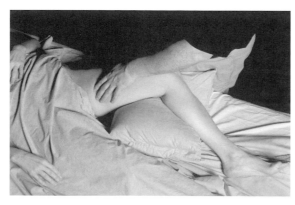

Figure 18.18b

Lymph massage progresses down the medial aspect of the leg.

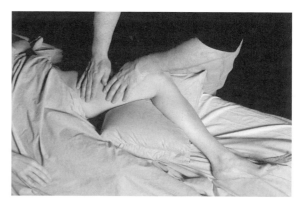

Figure 18.18c

Two hands can be used to cover a larger area of the leg.

could be applied from the knee to the hip, or for a more thorough treatment, the lymph massage steps can be reversed. Beginning at the medial aspect of the knee, apply the lymph massage movements, working up the leg and finishing on the inguinal nodes. These return movements can be of a shorter duration.

To continue lymph massage of the anterior leg, straighten the leg so that it is resting on the massage table (Figure 18.19a). Begin with hand positions on the upper thigh near the ilium. Two hands can be used on much of the legs to cover a larger area in less time. Apply the gentle, slow, circular, wavelike movements of lymph massage with the entire palmar and finger pad surface of both hands. After five to ten revolutions, or about a minute, move the hands down the leg to an adjacent area and continue the movement (Figure 18.19b). Continue moving down the leg in increments to include the foot (Figure 18.19c to e), all the time directing the flow

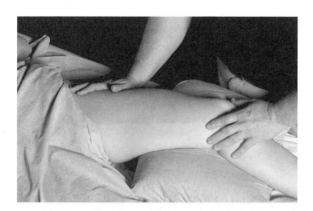

Figure 18.19a

Lymph massage on the upper lateral thigh is directed toward the inguinal nodes.

1

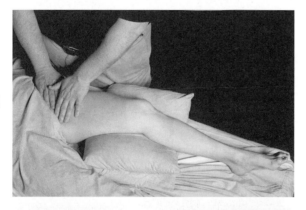

2

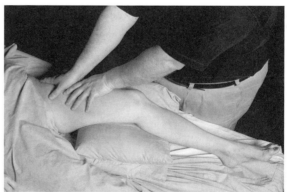

3

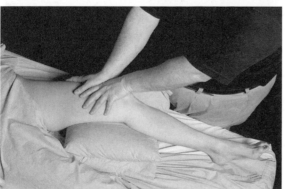

Figure 18.19b, 1, 2, and 3

Two hands can be used on larger areas of the thigh. Begin near the inguinal nodes and progress down the leg, directing the movements toward the inguinal nodes.

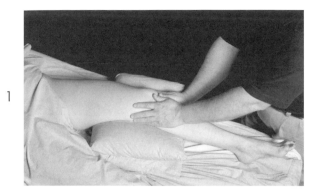

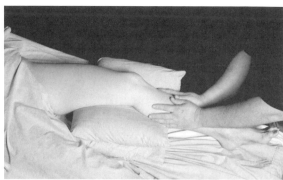

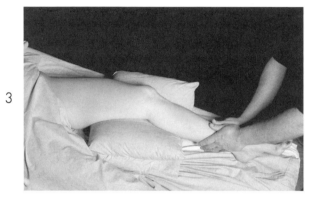

Figure 18.19c, 1, 2, and 3
Continue massage down the lower leg, directing lymph flow up the leg.

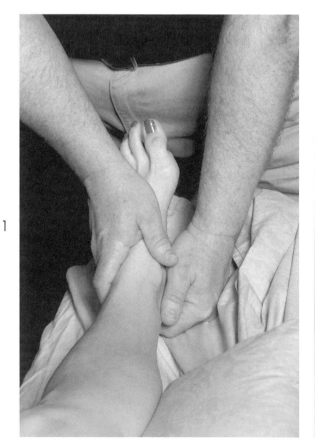

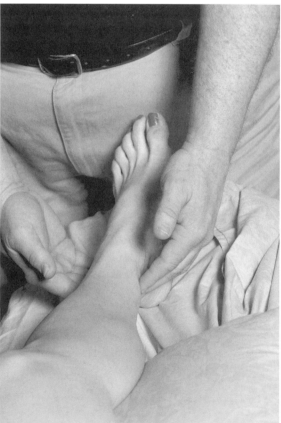

Figure 18.19d, 1 and 2
Beginning with the ankle, apply lymph massage to the foot.

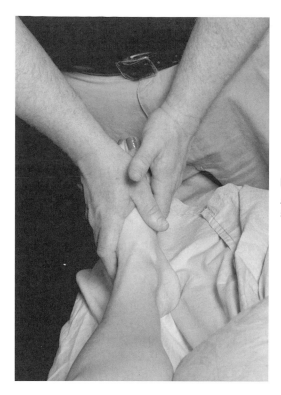

Figure 18.19e
Apply lymph massage movements to the top while supporting the bottom of the foot.

up the leg towards the inguinal nodes. When the entire leg has been massaged, continue from the foot and work back up the leg using the same slow, gentle technique with a shorter duration and finish at the inguinal nodes. Signal the end of the leg massage with a few light effleurage strokes.

8. Lower abdomen: Lymph massage on the areas of the lower quadrant superior to the inguinal nodes directs the flow inferiorly toward the nodes. After the inguinal nodes have been massaged, massage continues just superior of the inguinal ligament and medial to the ASIS. Use the pads of the fingers of one or both hands to gently apply movements directed toward the inguinal nodes for five to ten repetitions. Reposition the hands just superior on the abdomen and repeat the rotations. Continue new hand placements until the abdomen below the umbilicus has been massaged.

9. Posterior legs: The client assumes a prone position on the table. Superficial lymph in the posterior aspect of the lower quadrant still flows toward the inguinal nodes (Figure 18.20). In the upper portion of the quadrant, including the lower back, hips, and most of the gluteal muscles, lymph tends to flow laterally around to the anterior of the body and on to the inguinal nodes. Therefore, lymph massage on these areas has the intention of enhancing the flow in this direction.

Lymph flow on the posterior thigh divides with lymph from the medial aspect moving directly toward the inguinal nodes while lymph from the lateral aspect finds its way around to the anterior thigh and on toward the inguinal nodes. This creates

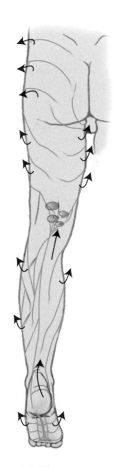

Figure 18.20
Superficial lymph flow on the posterior lower quadrant on the body.

what is termed a **watershed** somewhere near the center of the posterior thigh where the lymph flow splits. Lymph massage movements on the posterior thigh must take this into consideration.

Lymph massage on the lateral aspect of the posterior leg begins in the neighborhood of the greater trochanter. Movements are made with the intention of enhancing lymph flow toward the front of the body. Movements may progress either up over the gluteal area or down along the lateral aspect of the leg to the knee.

Lymph massage on the medial half of the posterior thigh begins at the gluteal crease near the ischial tuberosity and directs the lymph flow anteriorly toward the inguinal nodes. Massage on the medial portion progresses down toward the knee and then back up the medial thigh, always directing lymph flow toward the inguinal nodes.

On the posterior aspect of the lower leg, superficial lymph flows toward lymph nodes located in the popliteal space behind the knee. Lymph from these nodes often bypasses the inguinal nodes and flows into deeper nodes in the pelvic cavity. Massage on the lower leg begins by addressing these popliteal nodes. Bend the knee slightly and apply gentle lymph massage movements with the soft pads of the fingers to the soft area just superior to the crease in the back of the knee. Apply ten to twenty repetitions to this area and then move down to the back of the knee and continue with ten to twenty more repetitions. Lower the foot to the table and proceed with lymph massage movements, working down the back of the leg to the heel.

After applying lymph massage on the entire back of the leg, from the hip to the heel, begin at the heel and apply the movements, in an abbreviated form, but still slowly, back up the leg to the hip. Complete the leg massage with light effleurage movements.

10. Upper posterior quadrant: Superficial lymph of the back generally flows toward the closest lymph nodes. Above the umbilical belt line, which is approximately at the level of the first lumbar vertebrae, lymph flows toward the axilla on the same side of the body. Below the belt line, lymph flows around to the anterior of the body toward the inguinal lymph nodes. Lymph massage on the back of the body therefore is directed to enhance lymph movement toward these areas.

Lymph massage on the upper back begins near the axilla, directing movements toward the axillary nodes. Movements proceed medially to the spine and inferiorly to cover the posterior and lateral aspects of the rib cage.

While the client is in the prone position, lymph massage can also be applied to the posterior aspects of the shoulder and the upper arm. Movements in these areas are also directed toward the axillary lymph nodes.

Conclude the lymph massage by asking the client and then assisting her to turn over to a supine position. Once again, clear the axillary lymph nodes, the infra- and supraclavicular spaces, and the area of the angulus venosus. Finish with a gentle, relaxing neck and shoulder massage.

Lymph massage is very soothing and relaxing. Allow your client to relax and assimilate the effects of the massage for a few moments and then assist her to first roll onto her side and then sit up on the side of the table. Allow the client to sit on the table for a moment to reorient and make sure that any dizziness has passed. Discuss any homework and possibly demonstrate self-massage techniques or exercises the client might use on her own. Assist the client off the table, toward the dressing area.

CRANIOSACRAL THERAPY

Craniosacral therapy has been developed largely by Dr. John Upledger, D.O. In 1970, while assisting in surgery to remove plaque from the spinal cord of a patient, Dr. Upledger observed a rhythmic movement of the cord that was independent of the patient's heartbeat or respiration. The phenomenon intrigued him, as he could not find an explanation for it from colleagues or in textbooks. He did learn of the work of fellow osteopath Dr. William Sutherland, who since early in the twentieth century had contended that the bones of the cranium were structured to allow movement and, in the 1930s, developed a system of cranial osteopathy. The common belief of the scientific and medical community was that the sutures of the skull held the cranial bones in a solid, immovable structure. Dr. Upledger surmised, however, that if there was indeed movement of the cranial bones, there would be a feasible explanation for the rhythmic movement he had observed in the spinal cord during surgery.

While serving as a clinical researcher and professor of biomechanics at Michigan State University from 1975 to 1983, Dr. Upledger had the opportunity to lead a research team made up of anatomists, bioengineers, physiologists and biophysicists to explore the existence of cranial bone motion. The research confirmed Dr. Sutherland's theory and provided a better understanding of the actual mechanisms creating the movement—that is, the craniosacral system—which led Dr. Upledger into the development of craniosacral therapy. In 1985, Dr. Upledger established the Upledger Institute in Palm Beach Gardens, Florida, as a facility to do further research, train practitioners, and provide a state-of-the-art treatment center for craniosacral therapy. Since then, more than 60,000 practitioners have been trained in craniosacral therapy, including osteopaths, medical doctors, chiropractors, psychologists, dentists, physical therapists, acupuncturists, and massage therapists.

> **craniosacral therapy**
> is a gentle, hands-on method of evaluating and enhancing the functioning of the craniosacral system.

The Crainiosacral System

Craniosacral therapy is a gentle, hands-on method of evaluating and enhancing the functioning of a physiological body system called the craniosacral system. The craniosacral system is a semiclosed hydraulic system comprised of the meninges, the cerebrospinal fluid that surrounds and protects the brain and spinal cord, the physiological structures that control fluid input and outflow, and related bones. The meninges is made up of three layers. The pia mater is the inner layer, closely associated with the brain and spinal cord tissue that is highly vascularized, providing nutrients to nervous tissue. The middle layer, the arachnoid membrane, is a thin layer separated from the pia mater and dura mater by a fluid-filled space, allowing relatively independent motion between the three layers as the spine turns, bends, and twists. The outer layer of the meninges, the dura mater, is made of a tough, rather inelastic connective tissue that surrounds the central nervous system, contains the cerebrospinal fluid, and therefore encloses the hydraulic craniosacral system. The dura mater is closely associated with the cranial bones of the skull, the sacrum, and the fascia surrounding the spinal column so that the craniosacral rhythm is palpable on many parts on the body.

During craniosacral therapy, trained practitioners use a light touch, equivalent to a nickel's weight, to feel the rhythmic motion theoretically created by the movement of the cerebrospinal fluid within the craniosacral system. Practitioners check the rate, amplitude, symmetry, and quality of this wavelike motion in places where the craniosacral membrane barrier attaches to bones such as the skull, sacrum, and tailbone. The craniosacral rhythmic motion is most readily palpated on the cranial bones of the head, but because of the close association of the dura mater with the body's fascial system, with practice, the craniosacral rhythm can be perceived almost anywhere on the body. The craniosacral system normally moves through a flexion and extension phase at a rate of six to twelve cycles per minute. On the cranium, flexion is palpated as a transverse widening and a front-to-back shortening of the skull. Conversely, extension is sensed as a transverse narrowing and a front-to-back lengthening of the cranium. Craniosacral motion is transmitted throughout the fascia of the body with flexion noted as a gentle external rotation and widening on the body, an extension palpated as an internal rotation and a very slight narrowing of the body. The cranial motion is most easily perceived at the ankles, thighs, pelvis, thorax, and head.

With practice, the pulse of the craniosacral motion is easily differentiated from the cardiovascular pulse and respiration. Craniosacral motion is palpated and monitored by lightly touching the client with as much of the surface of the hand as possible and noting the extent and quality of the motion. It is necessary for the client and therapist to be in a relaxed and quiet space. With the client lying quietly and faceup on a massage table, the therapist sits at the head of the table and lightly places his hands so that the thumbs are near the temple and the palms and fingers lightly contact the back of the head. With eyes closed, the therapist allows his hands to meld with the client's head yet maintains the lightest pressure possible to maintain contact. The therapist becomes aware of the proprioceptive information of his arms. Soon the slight narrowing and lengthening followed by pause and then a widening and shortening of the cranium is sensed.

Craniosacral therapy treatment techniques are noninvasive, usually indirect, approaches intended to resolve restrictive barriers and restore symmetrical, smooth craniosacral motion. When an abnormal motion or restrictive barrier to motion is palpated, indirect technique would attempt to release the restriction by encouraging movement away from the restriction and toward ease. When monitoring the motion, the practitioner quietly follows the movement. To apply indirect technique, the practitioner will follow the movement in the direction that it moves most freely. At the furthest extent of the movement, the practitioner simply becomes immovable, holding against the cyclic return as the craniosacral movement continues through its cycle. As the motion progresses through another cycle, it moves further into its direction of ease, at which time the practitioner simply takes up the slack and again becomes immovable, holding the tissue in the furthest extent of its cycle. This is repeated through several cycles until there is no further movement into the direction of ease or until the craniosacral system becomes quiet and still. This is referred to as a *still point*. The stillness may continue for a matter of seconds to several minutes. After a still point has been induced, the practitioner releases the hold and returns to monitoring the motion. As the still point subsides, craniosacral motion will resume, usually in a more symmetrical manner with less or no restriction.

A restriction in one part of the craniosacral system can affect the entire system, so treatment may involve working at a point distant from an overt symptom. Any restrictions or blockages are treated with light-touch adjustments.

Craniosacral therapy is effective for a wide range of physiological conditions associated with pain and dysfunction and is used as a preventive health practice because of its ability to improve the function of the central nervous system and bolster the body's resistance to disease.

Students interested in learning craniosacral therapy can contact the Upledger Institute to locate seminars in their area on the Web site, www.upledger.com.

DEEP TISSUE MASSAGE

The term **deep tissue massage** refers to various regimens or massage styles that are directed toward the deeper tissue structures of the muscle and fascia. Some of the techniques focus just on the physiological release of tension or bonds in the tissues, whereas others use bodywork in conjunction with or as a means of psychological release. In most deep tissue massage techniques, the aim is to affect the various layers of fascia that support muscle tissues and loosen bonds between the layers of connective tissues. Some deep tissue massage techniques are named after the person who developed or specialized them, such as Rolfing after Ida Rolf; Trager after Milton Trager; Hellerwork after Joseph Heller; and Feldenkrais after Moshe Feldenkrais. The following are brief explanations of some of these techniques.

> **deep tissue massage**
>
> refers to various regimens or massage styles that are directed toward the deeper tissue structures of the muscle and fascia.

Structural Integration

As the name implies, structural integration attempts to bring the physical structure of the body into alignment around a central axis. This is done by manipulating the fascia of the structural muscles. After structural integration sessions, both physical and psychological balance are often experienced by the client.

Throughout life, traumas, both physical and emotional, may cause a reduction of movement that results in a shortening or binding together of the connective tissue surrounding muscles. Restriction may affect fibers, bundles, and whole muscles. This condition can also come about as a result of habitual postures while sitting, walking, and standing. Poor posture can be learned by imitating parents, from environmental factors, or as a reaction to some forms of punishment and emotionally charged situations. Structural integration can be beneficial when given by a practitioner who knows the methods and understands how to achieve the desired results.

Rolfing

Rolfing®, a brand of structural integration, is a deep connective tissue massage originated by Dr. Ida Rolf, a biochemist. Dr. Rolf discovered that in a normal, healthy body, the spine and body segments are correctly aligned, allowing the organs to function properly. However, during childhood and in early adult formative years, poor posture habits are often formed, throwing the body off center or out of its normal, healthy alignment. This in turn causes structural problems. Incorrect body alignment can also cause tension in muscles and connective tissues that may interfere with normal functioning of internal organs. Dr. Rolf originated a series of treatments called Rolfing to bring the body into proper structural alignment.

The goal of Rolfing treatments is to reshape the body's physical posture and to realign the muscular and connective tissue. The benefits of Rolfing also include increased suppleness of the muscles, improved appearance, and a renewed sense of well-being.

Rolfing techniques involve the use of heavy pressure applied carefully to the client's body with the fingers, a knuckle, a fist, or sometimes an elbow. Rolfing is usually done in a series of 10 treatments of one-hour duration each. During this time, the practitioner (Rolfer) works on various portions of the body.

Contraindications for Rolfing are the same as for any other type of massage. When in doubt about the use of this type of treatment, the client's physician should be consulted. The practitioner who wishes to pursue Rolfing techniques should study under the supervision of a qualified instructor.

NEUROPHYSIOLOGICAL THERAPIES

Several therapy systems are emerging that are directed toward neurophysiological processes that affect the musculoskeletal system. These systems recognize the importance of neurological feedback between the nervous system and the musculoskeletal system in maintaining proper tone and function. Alterations or disturbances in the neuromuscular relationship often result in dysfunction and pain. Neurophysiological therapies utilize methods of assessing tissues and delivering soft tissue manipulative techniques to normalize the tissues and reprogram the neurological loop to reduce pain and improve function. These neurophysiological therapies include trigger-point therapy, neuromuscular therapy, and passive positioning therapies.

TRIGGER-POINT THERAPY

Musculoskeletal dysfunctions that may include restrictions in joint mobility, myofascial pain, and constricted muscles commonly involve contractile tissues that house myofascial trigger points. In most cases, deactivating the trigger points reduces pain and improves musculoskeletal function.

Trigger points are hyperirritable nodules associated with dysfunctional contractile tissue that illicit a pain response when digital pressure is applied. There are several different classifications of trigger points depending on where they are located and whether or not they refer pain when palpated. Trigger points are classified by Travell and Simons (*Myofascial Pain and Dysfunction, Second Edition,* 1998) according to their response to pressure and their location.

An *active myofascial trigger point* is a hypersensitive spot associated with a palpable nodule located in a taut band of muscle that prevents full lengthening of the muscle and refers pain or other definable sensations to referral areas when digitally compressed.

A *latent myofascial trigger point* is tender when compressed but does not refer pain to other areas. Latent trigger points may become active trigger points with continued stresses.

A *central trigger point* is an active or latent trigger point that is located near the center of the muscle body and is closely associated with the motor endplate that activates the muscle.

An *attachment trigger point* is located at the musculotendinous junction or at the osseous attachment of the muscle and is caused by the continuous tension of the taut band caused by a central trigger point. Attachment trigger points are often inactivated when the central trigger point is inactivated.

A *primary or key trigger point* in one muscle may activate a *satellite trigger point* in another muscle. By deactivating the key trigger point, the satellite trigger point will also inactivate.

A *satellite trigger point* forms as a direct result of the dysfunction of the primary myofascial trigger point. The satellite trigger point may appear in the pain referral area or in the antagonist or synergist muscles to the muscle housing the primary trigger point. Many times, deactivating the primary trigger point will inactivate the satellite trigger points.

An *associate trigger point* is located in another muscle and forms concurrently and due to the same overload or abuse that is the source of the primary trigger point. Deactivating the primary trigger usually does not inactivate an associate trigger point.

trigger point
is a hyperirritable nodule associated with dysfunctional contractile tissuc that illicits a pain response when digital pressure is applied.

Trigger points may also be located in the skin, scars, ligaments, joint capsules, and fascia. Nearly 70 percent of common trigger points are located at the site of known acupuncture points.

A trigger point is commonly palpated as a nodule in a taut band in muscle tissue. When pressure is applied, sensations of pain, tingling, numbness, or some other sensation may radiate from the point to another area of the body that is usually not associated by nerve or dermatomal segment. If this happens, it is defined as an active trigger point. The pattern of referred pain is generally characteristic of a specific point. Active trigger-point referral areas are very predictable and have been mapped by Travell and Simons in *Myofascial Pain and Dysfunction,* Vol. 1&2. A client may be experiencing pain in an area of the body that can be directly correlated to referral areas of a specific trigger point. Deactivating that trigger point often relieves the related pain.

When a suspicious nodule or point is palpated and only local pain is experienced with no referred sensation, it is considered to be a latent trigger point. Latent trigger points may or may not radiate pain around the point. Latent trigger points may become active under conditions of continued or exaggerated stress. Active trigger points can also become latent trigger points if aggravating circumstances are reduced.

Trigger points may become active due to many factors, including acute or extended overload, trauma, joint dysfunction, arthritic conditions, visceral disease, and emotional stress. The presence of trigger points is often associated with the report of poorly localized pain, aching, or even numbness in muscles, joints, or subcutaneous tissues. This pain and discomfort may be distant from the trigger point but in the common referral area of the trigger point. This is differentiated from numbness or prickling pain often associated with nerve entrapment.

Trigger points, whether latent or active, result in dysfunction. Muscles containing trigger points will be prevented from reaching their full stretch length and will be restricted in strength and endurance. Muscles containing trigger points tend to fatigue more quickly and are more likely to be painful when stressed.

Trigger points are associated with dysfunctional neurological reflex circuits. A **physiopathological reflex arc** is a self-perpetuating neurological phenomenon that not only affects the muscle where the trigger point is located but also will have referred effects in tissues supplied by associated nerves of both the peripheral and autonomic nervous system. In other words, a trigger point is more than a tender nodule. A trigger point is an indication of physiological dysfunction. The trigger point may be reflexively related to any of the following:

- Contracture in the muscle
- Increased muscle tonus
- Constriction and hypersensitivity in the skin in local or referred areas

physio-pathological reflex arc

is a self-perpetuating dysfunctional neurological circuit.

- Increased pressure in the joints associated with the muscle
- Decreased activity in visceral organs associated through depressed autonomic nerve activity
- Constriction in local circulation resulting from hypertonus and constriction in the muscle
- Vasoconstriction in referred areas from effects in the autonomic nervous system
- Development of satellite and associated trigger points due to compensating from the effects of the primary trigger point

Research and practice indicates that deactivating the trigger point reflexively improves the function of the associated referred phenomena. When an active trigger point is successfully quieted, the referred pain and dysfunction will decrease.

A central myofascial trigger point is centrally housed in a palpable taut band of myofibrils in the belly of the muscle at the site of the motor endplate of the associated nerve. According to Travell and Simons, dysfunction at the motor endplate sets the conditions for continued contraction of the section of the muscle fiber close to the endplate, forming the nodule. Contraction of the sarcomeres in the area of the endplate causes tension throughout the muscle fibers, resulting in the palpable taut band. Continuous tension of the taut band on the connective tissue attachment sites sets up conditions to produce attachment trigger points at the musculotendinous or tenoperiosteal junction of the muscle. Releasing the central trigger point usually results in release or reduction of the attachment trigger points. Locating and deactivating trigger points are valuable for reducing pain and improving function in the location of the trigger point and in the referral areas.

Trigger points usually become active either after a clearly identifiable event or movement or as the result of prolonged and repetitive activity. To effectively treat trigger points, it is necessary to deactivate the point and change or eliminate the activity that activated it.

In the case of an acute, single-incident onset, the client will be able to describe the activity that initiated the pain. It may have been an accident, a fall, or injury such as a fracture, sprain, or trauma to the tissue. After the initial healing of the tissues, the deactivation of the related trigger points should be fairly straightforward. Because the trigger points were a result of a single incident, the chance of their reoccurrence is quite small.

Trigger points that have a gradual onset are often the result of chronic overload to a muscle, and it may be more difficult to identify the cause. If the activity or conditions that initiated the trigger point are not identified and altered, treatment of the symptoms will only provide temporary relief. Gradual onset trigger points may result from poor postural habits, improper ergonomic positions at work, emotional issues, visceral conditions, or other hidden causes. The client is encouraged to pay close

attention to situations that aggravate or intensify the pain to try to identify and modify any perpetuating activities. Without eliminating or altering the perpetuating factors creating the trigger point activity, any
attempt to inactivate the trigger point will be short-lived and rather futile.

Palpating for Trigger Points

Palpation skills are essential when working with trigger points and
trigger-point release techniques. Through palpation, the therapist recognizes variations in tissue texture and can differentiate between normal
soft tissue; constricted, hypertonic tissue; fibrotic tissue; taut bands in
muscle; and the congested, hyperirritable nodules associated with myofascial trigger points (Figure 18.21a). Palpatory skills also come into
play when monitoring the tender points during and after position release or trigger-point pressure treatment.

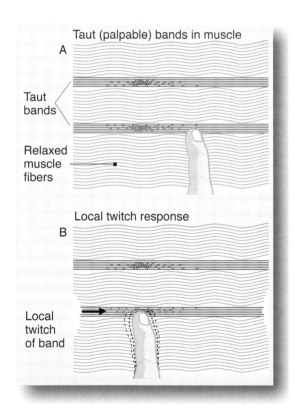

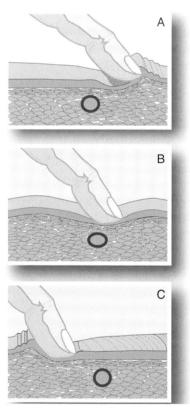

Figure 18.21a

Taut bands, myofascial trigger points, and a local
twitch response seen in a longitudinal view of
the muscle. (a) Palpation of a taut band (straight
lines) among normally slack, relaxed muscle
fibers (wavy lines). The density of stippling corresponds to the degree of tenderness of the taut
band pressure. The trigger point is the most tender spot in the band. (b) Rolling the band quickly
under the fingertip (snapping palpation) at the
trigger point often produces a local twitch response that is most clearly seen toward the end
of the muscle, close to its attachment.

Figure 18.21b

Flat palpation of a taut band and its trigger point. Flat
palpation is used for muscles that are accessible
from only one direction, such as infraspinatus. (a)
The skin is pushed to one side to begin the palpation. (b) A fingertip is slid across the muscle fibers to
feel the cordlike texture of the taut band rolling beneath it. (c) The skin is pushed to the other side at
the completion of the snapping palpation.

When assessment findings indicate a limitation in range of motion, constricted movement, or myofascial pain in a referral area, trigger-point activity can be verified by palpating the suspect muscle tissue. Palpation is done with the fingertips or thumb. **Flat palpation** is done either in line with or perpendicularly across the fibers of the muscle tissue (Figure 18.21b). Enough pressure is applied to engage and feel the muscle tissue through the skin and either glide along or across the fibers. The skin and subcutaneous tissue are moved over the fibrous muscle tissue to detect ropey, fibrous, or flaccid conditions beneath. A hypersensitive nodule may be encountered when gliding along parallel to the muscle fibers.

Pincer palpation can be employed in areas where the muscle tissue can be picked up between the thumb and fingers of the same hand (e.g., sternocleidomastoid muscle). The belly of the muscle is rolled between the thumb and fingers in search of taut bands, fibrotic tissue, or sensitive nodules (Figure 18.21c).

Palpation is done with the suspect muscle in a slightly elongated position. In this position, the muscle fibers are not stretched, but any taut bands will be more easily identified. The taut band is located by palpating across the muscle. A palpable band will be apparent to the sensitive fingers. When a taut band is identified, the therapist explores the length of it to locate a nodule or hypersensitive spot, which identifies the trigger point. If the client reports pain, discomfort, or other sensations referred to another area when the point is compressed, it is confirmed as an active trigger point. The area of referred pain may be a recognized reproduction of the client's symptomatic pain. If a hypersensitive nodule is found that does not produce a referral pattern upon mild compression (deeper compression may produce a referral pattern), it is considered a latent trigger point. Central trigger points are generally palpated near the middle of the taut band. There may also be trigger points near the ends of the taut band or at the attachment of the muscle to the bone. Attachment trigger points form as a result of continuous tension due to the

flat palpation
is done with the fingertips or thumb either in line with or perpendicularly across the fibers of the muscle tissue.

pincer palpation
is employed in areas where the muscle tissue can be picked up between the thumb and fingers of the same hand (e.g., sternocleidomastoid muscle) where the belly of the muscle is rolled between the thumb and fingers.

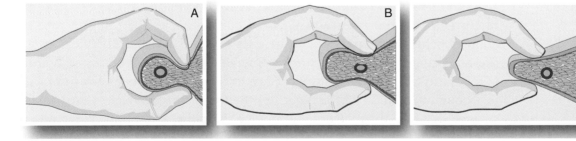

Figure 18.21c

Pincer palpation of a taut band at a trigger point. Pincer palpation is used for muscles that can be picked up between the digits, such as the sternocleidomastoid, pectoralis major, and latissimus dorsi. (a) The muscle fibers surrounded by the thumb and fingers are shown in a pincer grip. (b) The hardness of a taut band is felt clearly as it is rolled between the digits. The change in the angle of the distal phalanges produces a rocky motion that improves discrimination of the fine detail. (c) The edge of the taut band is sharply defined as it escapes from between the fingertips, often with a local twitch response.

contraction of the fibers in the taut band associated with the central trigger point. These attachment trigger points often disappear when the central trigger point is deactivated. Active trigger points become a priority for inactivating, but latent trigger points and attachment trigger points should still be addressed during the treatment.

Deactivating Trigger Points

According to Travell and Simons, there are several ways to address and deactivate trigger points and by so doing reduce myofascial pain and increase the neuromusculoskeletal function of the client. Though several of these modalities are outside the scope of practice of massage therapy, other very effective treatment modalities are well within the scope of soft tissue manipulation. Following is a list of possible modalities that are divided as in or out of the scope of a massage therapist.

Injection of an agent into the trigger point. Common agents including procaine, lidocaine, or a saline solution are injected into the trigger point with a syringe. This practice falls outside the scope of practice of the massage therapist.

Dry needling or acupuncture into the trigger point is done with an acupuncture needle. This practice falls outside the scope of practice of the massage therapist.

Spray-and-stretch techniques use a vapocoolant spray applied over the trigger point and associated muscle, followed by stretching the involved muscle. Cool-and-stretch techniques use ice applied with a stroking movement over the trigger point and muscle, followed by stretching the involved muscle.

Travell and Simons found spray-and-stretch techniques to be some of the most effective at relieving trigger-point activity (p. 128, Vol. 1). Unfortunately, the products used to spray as a vapocoolant either contain fluorocarbons, in the case of Fluori-Methane, or are unavailable or are too volatile for safe use, as in the case of ethyl chloride. Ice has been used as a substitute but with somewhat less effective results.

The coolant is applied in parallel lines over the muscle in the direction toward the referral area. The coolant is applied at the rate of about 4 centimeters per second in parallel lines that barely overlap. As the coolant is applied, the underlying muscle is passively stretched to take up any slack. A maximum of two to three passes over each area will be enough to cool the surface but not the underlying muscle. Cooling the surface acts as a distraction, suppresses the pain, and allows for a relaxation and gentle stretching of the affected muscle fibers. (For more detailed discussion, refer to *Myofascial Pain and Dysfunction*, Vols. 1 and 2.)

Ischemic compression with gentle stretching, **position release**, and **muscle energy technique** are three therapeutic modalities available to the massage therapist to reduce trigger-point activity and restore muscle and fascia to a more normal, pain-free, functional length. These three methods can be combined to very effectively address and release trigger points.

ischemic compression
involves digital pressure directly into a trigger point.

position release
is a method of passively moving the body or body part toward the body's preference and away from pain, seeking the tissue's preferred position. Movements are toward ease and away from bind, away from any restrictive barrier and toward comfort.

muscle energy technique
(MET), or PNF stretching, uses neurophysiological muscle reflexes to improve functional mobility of the joints.

Trigger-Point Pressure Release

Pressure point release or ischemic compression involves digital pressure directly into the trigger point. Ischemic compression was popularized by Bonnie Prudden and is used extensively in the practice of Myotherapy. The idea is that pressure on a point causes hypoxia or a lack of oxygen, therefore the name "ischemic." Deep pressure is usually applied with the thumb, or sometimes with the elbow, to a specific point, either a trigger point or an acupressure point.

The pressure must be deep enough and held long enough to deactivate the trigger point. Too much pressure will cause the client to react by tightening muscles in a protective response that defeats the purpose of the treatment. Pressure on a trigger point will cause pain. The deeper the pressure, the more intense the pain. The amount of pressure must be regulated to stay within the tolerance of the individual client. In other words, on a pain scale from 1 to 10, where 0 is no pain and 10 is excruciating, the target level is 5 or 6. Pressure is increased until the client begins to elicit a pain reaction. As the pressure is maintained, the pain intensity usually decreases. As this happens, the pressure can be increased to maintain the level of intensity. When the point has been inactivated, the pain level will reduce to an intensity rating of 1 or 2.

Paul St. John, in St. John Method Neuromuscular Therapy, suggests applying enough pressure to a hypersensitive nodule to cause mild discomfort for 8 to 12 seconds, during which time the discomfort should diminish.

Travell and Simons suggest applying digital pressure to a trigger point until a restrictive barrier is approached. The pressure is enough to cause a noticeable discomfort, but not pain. The pressure is maintained until the therapist notices a release of tension in the tissues, at which time the pressure is released and repeated at a somewhat deeper pressure, again deep enough to engage the restrictive barrier.

Dr. Leon Chaitow suggests applying enough pressure to the trigger point to either elicit a response of 5 to 7 on the pain scale or enough to produce referred pain symptoms and holding the pressure for about 5 seconds, letting off for 2 to 3 seconds and then repeating the process for up to 2 minutes or until the referred pain diminishes.

Position Release to Inactivate Trigger Points

Position release techniques are very effective to inactivate trigger points and release the taut bands that house them. (Read more about position release techniques on pages 761–768). Both central trigger points and attachment trigger points respond well to position release and can effectively be used as monitor points to find a preferred position. A working knowledge of muscle action and attachments is crucial to effectively use position release techniques when addressing trigger points. When a trigger point is identified, knowing what muscle it is in, the orientation of the muscle fibers, and the action of the muscle all play an important role in successfully positioning the muscle and deactivating the trigger point.

Finding the release position will involve passively moving the joint in the same direction that the involved muscle would if it were to contract. This will, in effect, move the ends of the taut band toward the trigger point. The precise position may include dynamic movement in all planes (flexion or extension, adduction or abduction, side bending, and internal or external rotation). Usually the preferred position is in the midrange of the muscle's range of motion.

The indicator for the correct position is a change in the trigger point. Trigger points can be palpated as nodules that are hypersensitive. They are especially sensitive when digital pressure is applied to them. When a position for release is achieved, the sensitivity in the associated trigger point will diminish by 70 to 100 percent, and the palpable nodule softens and often disappears.

Beside monitoring palpable changes in the trigger point, feedback from the client is essential when finding the preferred position. Chaitow suggests using a pain scale where an amount of pressure is applied to the trigger point and the client is instructed to rate that amount of discomfort as a 10 on the scale. The therapist maintains the same amount of pressure on the point and begins moving the joint in positions to approximate the ends of the muscle's fibers while asking the client to rate the discomfort at the palpated point. When the client reports a discomfort level of 3, 2, or less, and the palpable point has diminished, that is a good indication that a preferred position has been found.

After the preferred position is achieved, Jones and Chaitow suggest holding the position for 60 to 90 seconds and then very slowly and passively returning the joint to a neutral position, rechecking the trigger point, and looking for other associated points.

It is the author's experience after years of practice that after the preferred position is achieved, a slight compression into the joint from the approximate muscle attachments should be incorporated. The compression is only enough to engage the nerve receptors in the joint, approximately 5 to 7 pounds of pressure. It is theorized that feedback from these receptors as well as the proprioceptors of the muscle activate, reorganize, and normalize after the muscle fibers are shortened and stress is removed.

While the position is held, the therapist is encouraged to continue monitoring the trigger-point area with a light touch to note any changes. Common palpable signs are what feels like an unraveling at the point, and very often a pulse is noted, an indication that circulation is flowing back into the area. When a pulse is felt, it is only necessary to hold the position for about another 10 seconds for maximum benefit. Gently release the compression and passively and very slowly, without any help from the client, return the body part to a neutral resting position. Again, it is important to release the position slowly and slowly return the joint to a neutral position. Recheck the alarm point and other related points such as synergist and antagonist muscles.

Restoring the Muscle to Its Resting Length

Regardless of the technique used, after the trigger point is inactivated, it is very important that the muscle that housed the trigger point be restored to a normal resting length. If the muscle is not restored to its normal resting length, its function will be reduced, and the chance that the trigger points will return is increased. Gentle stretching may be used to restore the muscle to its functional length; however, there is a chance of retraumatizing the tissue. A preferred technique would be muscle energy technique using the antagonist. Read more about MET on pages 752–758. When applying MET using the antagonist, the joint the muscle acts upon is moved so that the muscle is lengthened until it approaches its resistive barrier. The practitioner supports the joint or limb in that position and instructs the client to inhale as she continues the movement with about a 20 percent effort. The practitioner matches the client's effort, thereby allowing no movement for about 7 to 10 seconds, at which time the client is instructed to relax and exhale. As the client exhales, the joint is moved, and the muscle is lengthened to its new resistive barrier. This process is repeated until there is no increase in muscle length.

Combining Techniques to Inactivate Trigger Points

Trigger points are effectively inactivated by combining these various techniques.

1. A trigger point is identified through assessment and palpation.

2. Trigger-point pressure release is applied for 8 to 10 seconds, let off for 3 to 5 seconds, and repeated several times.

3. Pressure is applied to the point to elicit a pain response from the client. The client is asked to rate the pain as a 10, and position release is applied, positioning the joint so that the ends of the taut band move into closer approximation until the pain sensation has reduced to a 2 or less. The position is held for 60 to 90 seconds, then slowly returned to a neutral position.

4. Muscle energy technique using the antagonist is employed to help restore the muscle to its normal resting length.

NEUROMUSCULAR THERAPY

Neuromuscular therapy (NMT) was originally developed in the 1930s by Stanley Leif in England. Dr. Stanley Leif was born in Latvia, one of the Baltic States, and was raised in South Africa. He received training as a chiropractor and naturopath in the United States before World War I. He established a healing resort in England and there, along with his cousin Boris Chaitow, developed the system of soft tissue manipulation called neuromuscular therapy. Dr. Leon Chaitow, D.O., Boris Chaitow's nephew, has carried on with the scientific development of neuromuscular techniques. He continues to research, lecture, teach, and write, including more than 50 books on NMT and related subjects. A recent collaboration between Chaitow and Judith Walker-Delany of the United States produced *Clinical Applications of Neuromuscular Techniques* Volumes 1 and 2. These two texts contain comprehensive descriptions of neuromuscular techniques from both the United States and Europe to address every area of the human body. In the United States, Paul St. John has popularized and advanced a method of neuromuscular therapy that is taught through a series of seminars.

The body continuously endures stresses from trauma, improper body mechanics, poor posture, as well as tensions of a psychological or emotional nature. Regardless of the nature of the stress—be it mechanical, postural, or emotional—the adaptive tendencies of the body will attempt to compensate for the stress by producing neuromuscular changes. Many of the changes result in reduced mobility, pain, fatigue, and depression. Neuromuscular dysfunctions become apparent in the soft tissues of the musculoskeletal system as contractures, hypersensitive areas, and tissue restriction. Neuromuscular dysfunction is self-perpetuating. When an area of the body is restricted from pain or mobility impairments, other areas of the body compensate, resulting in further physiological dysfunction.

NMT identifies soft tissue abnormalities and at the same time manipulates the soft tissue to normalize its function. In so doing, the perpetuating cycle is broken, much of the referred pathologic activity is reversed, and overall function is improved.

NMT depends on anatomical knowledge and palpatory skills to assess the tissue condition and treat neuromuscular lesions. Careful and systematic examination of the muscle and associated soft tissue identifies abnormal signs, including:

- Postural and biomechanical deviation
- Congestion in the tissues
- Contracted tissue or taut, fibrous bands
- Nodules or lumps
- Trigger points
- Restrictions between the skin and underlying tissues
- Variations in temperature (warmer or cooler than surrounding tissues)
- Swelling or edema
- General tenderness

Neuromuscular lesions are always hypersensitive to pressure and often associated with trigger points. NMT recognizes the importance of trigger points and their relation to local and referred dysfunction and pain. Beside trigger points, NMT also takes into account other natural and physiologic laws that account for hypersensitive or painful areas on the body. For example, acupuncture points and neurolymphatic reflexes not associated with trigger points are often tender. Tenderness usually means some degree of dysfunction in the associated tissues or organs.

General NMT treatment often stimulates the reflex improvement of the associated or referred function.

NMT treatment involves assessment and soft tissue manipulation. Postural assessment is important to determine any postural distortion. Postural distortion indicates an imbalance in the tone of structural muscles and is an indicator of chronic stress patterns. Palpating the tissues with initial light strokes and progressively deeper strokes reveals areas of tension, contracted tissue, and hypersensitivity.

Treatment manipulations are similar to the gliding and pressure techniques used to palpate and assess the tissue. Many NMT treatment techniques are incorporated from other modalities. They include but are not limited to:

- Gliding: The primary technique of NMT generally uses the thumb to move across, along, and through the tissues. Gliding strokes are applied to the tissue in one direction at a time using varying amounts of pressure. Light pressure assesses the superficial tissues and stimulates circulation of lymph and blood. Deeper stroking assesses deeper structures and stretches the fascia, releasing fibrotic adhesions.

- **Ischemic compression:** When painful spots and trigger points are located, pressure is held directly on these points. The depth of the pressure is determined by the tolerance of the client. The pressure should be deep enough to elicit a mild amount of discomfort in the client. Pressure that is too deep causes the client to tense up and is counterproductive. Pressure that is too light is usually ineffective. Duration of the pressure, according to St. John, is from 8 to 12 seconds and is repeated.

ischemic compression
involves digital pressure directly into a trigger point.

- **Skin rolling:** When there is tightness between the skin and the underlying tissues, the skin is picked up and rolled between the thumb and fingers of both hands in several directions across the area. This tends to loosen the superficial fascia and improve nerve and fluid circulation to the underlying structures.

skin rolling
is a variation of kneading in which only the skin and subcutaneous tissue is picked up between the thumbs and fingers and rolled.

- **Stretching:** After hypersensitive spots have been quieted and trigger points inactivated, the involved muscle and connective tissue must be stretched to achieve their normal resting length. This is accomplished with passive and active stretching. Slow, sustained passive stretching is encouraged to regain and maintain length of the connective and muscle tissues. Active stretching is valuable in overcoming contractures and neuromuscular programming that restricts mobility. Active stretching, also known as muscle energy technique (MET), is discussed in the following section.

stretching
is passive and active stretching of muscle and connective tissue to achieve normal resting length.

To maintain improvements achieved with NMT, the stresses that precipitated the soft tissue dysfunctions must be addressed and, if possible, eliminated. It is also helpful to monitor the areas of dysfunction with follow-up NMT sessions and incorporate a program of regular exercise to improve strength, endurance, posture, and stamina.

MUSCLE ENERGY TECHNIQUE

Muscle energy technique (MET) is a soft tissue mobilization technique that was developed in the osteopathic profession. Elements of MET have been documented and described for many years using different terminology. Kabat, Knott, and Voss developed techniques in the 1940s and 1950s called *proprioceptive neuromuscular facilitation* that used many of the same physiological mechanisms. Dr. T. J. Ruddy developed a technique he called *resistive duction* in which the therapist resisted multiple, rapid, small muscle contractions of the client meant to increase blood flow and strengthen muscles. It is Fred Mitchell Sr., D.O., F.A.A.O., who is given credit for the development of modern muscle energy technique. He developed the techniques in the 1940s and 1950s and published his work in the yearbook of the American Academy of Osteopathy in 1958.

MET is a valuable tool when addressing soft tissue conditions that involve tense or shortened muscles. Muscle spasms are effectively quieted. Joint mobility can be improved and lengthened, or weak antagonistic muscles can be toned. MET can be applied in several different ways, depending on the condition of the tissue and the intended response. It may be used to increase joint mobility where constricted contractile tissue restricts movement, to release hypertonic muscles, and to reduce fibrosis in chronically shortened muscles.

MET involves the active participation of the client, who is instructed to contract isolated muscles against a counterforce provided by the therapist. MET uses active muscle contraction followed by relaxation and subsequent passive stretching to reduce constrictions in the muscle and increase range of motion of the related joints. Muscle energy technique utilizes neurophysiological muscle reflexes to improve functional mobility of the joints. By employing active joint movements, muscle activity that restricts movement is inhibited, allowing for better mobility.

There are two basic inhibitory reflexes produced during MET manipulations:

postisometric relaxation

means that following an isometric contraction, there is a period of relaxation during which muscle impulses are inhibited.

reciprocal inhibition

occurs when a muscle acting on a joint contracts and the opposing muscle is reflexively inhibited.

- **Postisometric relaxation:** Following an isometric contraction, there is a brief period of relaxation during which impulses to the muscle are inhibited.

- **Reciprocal inhibition:** When a muscle acting on a joint is contracted, the muscle responsible for the opposite action on that joint is inhibited.

MET involves the contraction of a muscle by the client against the resistance provided by a therapist. The direction of the contraction and the position of the muscle and the limb previous to the contraction are determined by the condition and movement restrictions of the joint and target muscle or muscle groups. Range of motion and palpation assessment techniques are used to determine the nature of the restriction and the direction of maximum limitation. Depending on the intended outcome of the treatment, the force applied by the therapist may be equal to that of the client, allowing no movement; be less than that of the client, allowing movement in the range of motion; or may overcome the force of the client. Various outcomes include relaxing and lengthening hypertonic muscles, stimulating and strengthening weakened muscles, and lengthening chronically shortened fibrotic muscles.

Muscle energy techniques have many variations, depending on the condition of the target tissue, the condition of the client, and the intended outcome of the treatment. Some variations include the following:

- The starting position
- The direction of the client's effort
- The amount of effort applied by the client
- The length of the effort
- Whether the therapist's force matches, overcomes, or is less than the client's force
- How the breath is incorporated
- Whether there is a passive, active, or no stretch after the contraction
- Whether or not to stretch through the barrier after a contraction
- Whether or not to repeat the sequence
- Whether to use MET with other techniques

MET Applications for Hypertonic Muscles

Hypertonic muscles are usually shortened, many times containing trigger points and taut bands of muscle tissue and are often involved in joint constriction. They may or may not be painful and may be the site of an acute or chronic injury. These conditions are determined during the assessment procedures.

There are three main variations of muscle energy technique that are effective in lengthening tense and shortened muscles:

- Contract relax or agonist contract
- Antagonist contract
- Contract-relax-contract the opposite

Contract Relax or Agonist Contract

The most common MET procedure used to relax constricted and hypertonic muscle involves contracting and then relaxing and lengthening the target muscle. The **contract-relax technique** incorporates the *postisometric relaxation* theory that as soon as an isometric muscle contraction releases, the muscle is inhibited and relaxes.

To perform the contract-relax or agonist-contract technique (Figure 18.22a to d):

1. Position the limb so that the target muscle is in a lengthened but comfortable position. This can be done by moving the limb until the resistive barrier is engaged or to the point of resistance and then backing off slightly. (In the performance of MET, the resistive

> **contract-relax technique**
>
> incorporates postisometric relaxation theory that as soon as an isometric muscle contraction releases, the muscle relaxes.

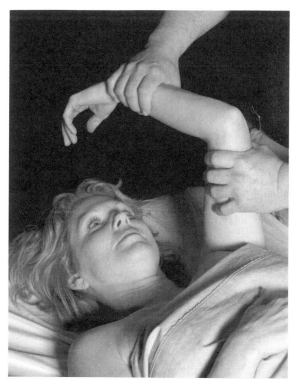

Figure 18.22a

To perform contrast-relax or agonist-contract MET on the triceps, move the arm until the muscle approaches its resistive barrier and support it while the client contracts the muscle.

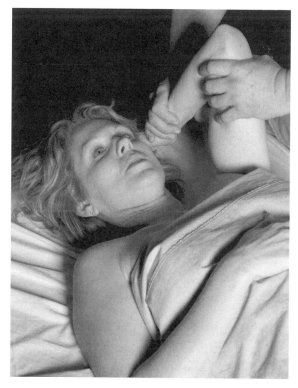

Figure 18.22b

After 7 to 10 seconds, the client relaxes and takes a breath, and as she exhales, the therapist moves the arm to a new barrier and repeats the procedure.

barrier in a joint movement is when the first resistance is met when moving a limb or joint through its normal range of motion. This resistive barrier is usually encountered before the physiological limit of the possible joint movement. The resistive barrier is the beginning of the soft tissue constriction to the joint's flexibility.)

2. Support the limb in that position securely, ask the client to inhale, and have the client contract the target muscle isometrically against the resistance for 5 to 10 seconds. It is not necessary for the client to perform a maximal contraction. A contraction of 20 percent is adequate for this procedure. The contraction should not cause acute pain. If the contraction is painful, try the antagonist-contraction procedure discussed next.

3. After about 7 to 10 seconds, ask the client to exhale and slowly relax the contraction.

4. Ask the client to again inhale and exhale, and as she exhales, move the limb until a new resistive barrier is felt. The range of motion should increase slightly.

5. Repeat steps 1–4 two to five times or until there is no more increase of ROM when moving to a new barrier.

Alternatives may include increasing the client's effort to up to 50 percent, and/or increasing the time of the contraction up to 20 seconds.

Antagonist Contraction

If muscle tissues are in a subacute stage of healing or if there is any pain when the target muscle contracts, the preferred MET technique would involve the antagonist. Antagonist contraction takes advantage of a physiological process known as **reciprocal inhibition**. When a muscle acting on a joint contracts, the muscle that causes the opposite action is reflexively inhibited. Remember, if the procedure causes pain, STOP. To perform the antagonist-contract technique (Figure 18.23a and b):

> **reciprocal inhibition**
>
> occurs when a muscle acting on a joint contracts and the opposing muscle is reflexively inhibited.

1. Position the limb so that the target muscle is in a lengthened but comfortable position. This can be done by moving the limb either to the middle of the range of motion or until the resistive barrier is approached, then back off several degrees.

2. Support the limb securely in that position and instruct the client to attempt to continue the movement with only a 20 percent effort. Resist the movement for a couple of seconds and then allow the movement to continue slowly. The contraction should not cause acute pain. If there is acute pain on both contract-relax and antagonist-contract techniques, pathologies may be present that contraindicate MET.

3. After 7 to 10 seconds, instruct the client to exhale and relax (hold the limb in the same position).

4. Ask the client to inhale and exhale again, and as she exhales, passively move the limb to its new barrier and again back off several degrees.

5. Repeat steps 2–4 two or three times or until there is no more improvement in the lengthening muscle and therefore no more increase in ROM before the barrier is encountered.

The amount of effort can be increased up to about 50 percent, and the length of the contractions may be increased to as much as 20 seconds.

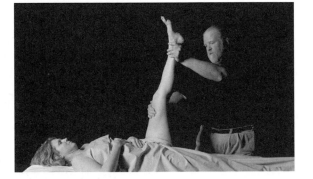

Figure 18.23a

To perform antagonist-contract MET on the hamstrings, flex the hip with the leg extended until the restrictive barrier is felt and then back off a few degrees. Hold the leg in that position and instruct the client to continue the movement.

Figure 18.23b

After 7 to 10 seconds, instruct the client to relax the contraction and inhale, and as she exhales, move the leg to a new resistive barrier. Back off from the barrier, support the leg, and repeat the procedure.

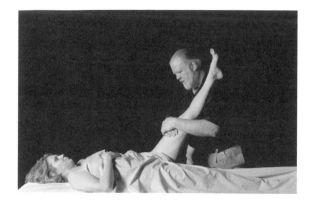

Figure 18.24a

To perform contract-relax, contract the opposite for the hamstrings, flex the hip with the leg extended until the resistive barrier is approached and support the leg in that position. Hold the leg in that position, then have the client inhale and contract the target muscle for 7 to 10 seconds.

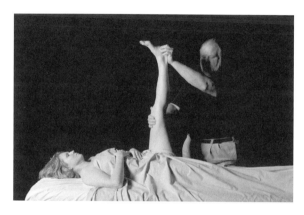

Figure 18.24b

After 7 to 10 seconds, instruct the client to relax, exhale, then inhale again and actively contract the quadriceps to move the leg further toward the barrier.

Contract-Relax-Contract the Opposite

This technique, sometimes called contract-relax-antagonist-contract (CRAC), essentially combines the two previous techniques. To perform Contract-relax-contract the opposite technique (see Figure 18.24a to d).

1. Position the limb so that the target muscle is in a lengthened but comfortable position. This can be done by moving the limb until the resistive barrier is engaged or to the point of resistance or pain and then backing off slightly.

2. Support the limb in that position securely and have the client inhale and contract the target muscle isometrically against the resistance for 5 to 10 seconds.

3. Instruct the client to exhale and relax the muscle and then contract the muscle opposite the tight muscle (the antagonist). In so doing, the client actively moves the limb in the direction of the intended stretch. The therapist may or may not assist in the final stretch.

4. After a short rest, repeat the procedure.

Pulsed Contractions of the Antagonist

During the 1940s and 1950s, Dr. T. J. Ruddy, D.O., developed a system of rapidly pulsed contractions against a resistance he called "rapid rhythmic resistive duction technique." A more simplistic, modern term is *pulsed muscle energy technique*. Many times when joint constriction involves a hypertonic muscle, often con-

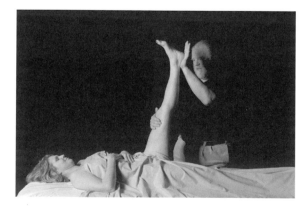

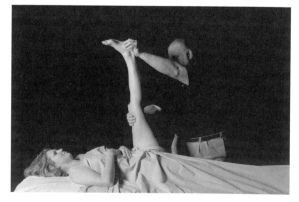

Figure 18.24c, d

Hold the leg in the newly achieved position and repeat the procedure two to five times or until there is no more increase in range of movement.

taining trigger points, the antagonist is found to be hypotonic and inhibited. Pulsed MET is directed at the inhibited muscle to facilitate proprioceptive re-education, increase circulation, stimulate the weakened muscle, and further inhibit the opposing hypertonic muscle (RI). According to Ruddy, the technique produces more oxygenation and better lymph and venous flow to the muscle. To practice PMET:

1. Move the limb so that the hypertonic tissue is lengthened to its resistive barrier and support the body part in that position.

2. Ask the client to begin a series of rapid, minute contractions toward the barrier (contracting the antagonist). The contractions are small and at a rate of about two per second. The effort is small and, in Ruddy's words, creates "no wobble or bounce."

3. Continue for about twenty contractions, rest for 10 seconds, and then repeat.

PMET is a valuable adjunct therapy to use after the constricted, hypertonic muscles have been treated directly by methods such as stretching. After the hypertonic muscles have been lengthened, stimulating and facilitating the hypotonic or weakened antagonists will improve the overall function of the joint.

A number of factors determine the effectiveness of MET. It is essential to identify the contractile tissue involved in the movement limitation and direct the resistance to the contraction directly toward or away from those restrictions. Generally, pathological changes to structures of the joint other than contractile tissues will not respond to MET. The success of MET is dependent on the skill of the therapist in the following:

- Assessing the muscles involved
- Determining the direction of maximum limitation
- Determining when the joint movement is approaching its limitation
- Choosing a postisometric relaxation or reciprocal inhibition technique
- Instructing the client in the direction, duration, and intensity of the contraction

Muscle energy techniques are contraindicated for acute soft tissue injuries, such as muscle strains, for at least the first 72 hours after the injury is sustained. During the acute period, the preferred treatment is designated by the acronym RICE—rest, ice, compression, and elevation.

After the initial acute period is a subacute period when appropriate therapeutic interventions will accelerate the healing process, reduce scarring and adhesions, and apply therapeutic stresses to return the tissues to optimum function. Appropriate therapeutic interventions apply gentle stresses and cause no pain to the injured area. Muscle energy techniques using the antagonist along with other appropriate techniques such as position release techniques and cross-fiber massage are invaluable when rehabilitating soft tissue injuries.

A naturally occurring neuromuscular process known as *splinting* causes muscle fibers closely associated to the injured fibers to shorten in order to protect the injured area. This splinting and the associated hypertonic tissue often persist beyond the time the injured tissue heals. MET is a method that will encourage those tissues to return to their normal resting length.

MET for Improving Strength

There are two other variations of MET that are valuable for toning weak muscles or reducing fibrosis in the muscle fascia.

During the course of treatment, it may be beneficial to stimulate a hypotonic muscle, tone a weakened muscle, or re-educate an injured or habitually misused muscle. There are many reasons why a muscle or muscle group may be underutilized, resulting in postural distortion or joint dysfunction. A form of MET that employs an isokenetic contraction helps awaken, stimulate, and tonify the muscle.

To improve tone or strengthen a weakened muscle, the client is instructed to move the limb through the full available range of motion as the therapist provides resistance directed against the target muscle. For maximum effect, movement through the full range of motion should take about 3 to 4 seconds. During the first repetition, the client uses approximately 20 percent effort. On subsequent repetitions, the resistance is increased until maximum resistance is achieved. The resistance is continuous during concentric and eccentric contractions. The resistance from the therapist is continuous during the entire movement. When a muscle is identified to be hypotonic, deficient, or in a weakened state, the procedure is as follows:

1. The therapist moves the target muscle and related joint passively through its range of motion to demonstrate to the client intended movement.

2. The therapist instructs the client to move the joint through the described range of motion using about a 20 percent effort as the therapist resists the movement with a gentle resistance throughout the full range of the movement. (*Note:* The therapist's hands should be placed to isolate the target muscle during the entire range of motion. For instance, for movements of the shoulder, one of the therapist's hands should contact the distal portion of the humerus near the elbow to resist the movement while the other hand supports the client's hand during the movement or supports the shoulder to isolate the movement.)

3. The client is instructed to repeat the movement several times. Each time, the therapist increases the resistance until maximum resistance is achieved or the muscle begins to fatigue.

Rapid gains in strength are experienced with this type of exercise. The use of this technique may be limited, depending on the strength of the therapist relative to the strength of the target muscle. The therapist may not be able to provide enough resistance for large muscles or muscle groups such as the hip flexors. The therapist must be aware of positioning and body mechanics to avoid injury to self or to the client.

MET for Reducing Fibrosis

Fibrosis in the muscle fascia may be the result of trauma, inflammation, strain, or aging. Fibrosis causes contractures and loss of mobility. Constriction in contractile tissues may be due to fascial sheaths gluing together with collagenous cross-hatching. Neuromuscular therapy gliding techniques and myofascial release stretching are helpful in these conditions, as are MET isolytic techniques. A MET manipulation that may be effective in reducing fibrosis involves a resistance that overpowers a muscle contraction. As the client contracts the target muscle, the therapist provides a resistance greater than the force of the contraction and forces the muscle to lengthen (Figure 18.25a to c).

To perform isolytic MET:

1. The therapist positions the associated body part so the target muscle is in a mild stretch, near its resistive barrier.

2. The therapist supports the joint in that position and instructs the client to inhale and gradually contract the muscle to a near maximum effort.

3. When at a maximum effort, the client is instructed to exhale and maintain the contraction as the therapist overpowers the contraction and moves the joint further toward (but not beyond) the physiologic barrier.

4. The client is instructed to relax as the therapist releases the stretch.

5. Repeat steps 1–4, two or three times.

Isolytic MET may cause mild discomfort or burning, but it should not cause acute pain. When using this technique, a maximum contraction is most effective, but the client must be instructed to contract the muscle to the extent that is within the comfort level. The therapist must not use ballistic movements against the contractions. The resistance must be steady and forceful enough to overcome the client effort.

Extreme caution must be used by the therapist to avoid further injury to the muscle tissue.

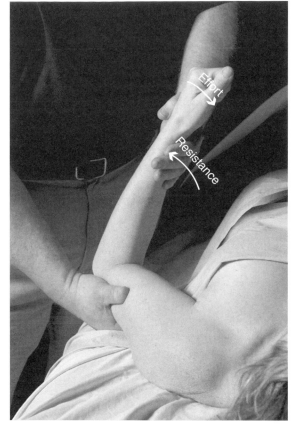

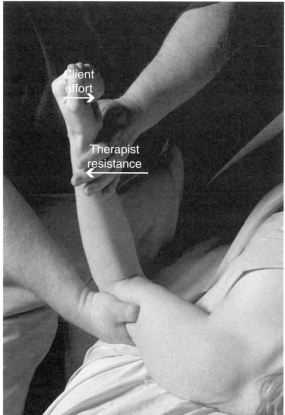

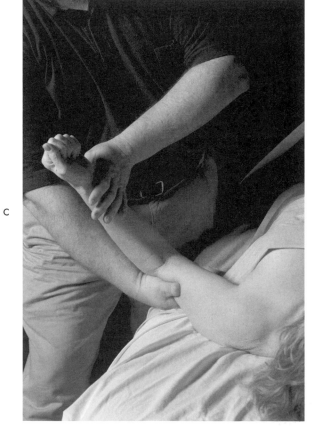

Figure 18.25a, b, and c

To help reduce fibrotic conditions of the sub-scapularis muscle, as the client contracts the muscle, the therapist gently overpowers the contraction to lengthen the muscle.

PASSIVE POSITIONING TECHNIQUES

Passive positioning techniques are perhaps the gentlest of soft tissue manipulations when addressing mobility restrictions due to pain and soft tissue dysfunction. As the name implies, passive positioning involves the gentle, passive movement of a joint into a position of maximum comfort, holding it there for an appropriate time and then very slowly returning it to its normal resting position.

Three bodywork systems that incorporate this technique are strain-counterstrain, orthobionomy, and structural muscular balancing. Although each system utilizes passive positioning, each determines the appropriate position for maximum release in a different manner and will be discussed individually.

Strain-Counterstrain

The strain-counterstrain (tender point) technique was developed by Lawrence Jones, D.C. Dr. Jones happened upon the basis of the technique by accident when a patient came into his office in a great deal of pain. At the time, Dr. Jones was very busy and was not able to treat the patient immediately. He instructed his assistant to take the person into the next room, tell him to lie on the table, and make him as comfortable as possible. The assistant did as instructed. The patient lay down, and using various cushions and pillows, the assistant positioned the patient's body so that he was virtually out of pain and then left him there until the doctor was able to see him. When the doctor finally came in, he carefully removed the pillows and gently positioned the client flat on the table and asked where the pain was. It was then that the patient realized the pain had disappeared.

Dr. Jones was able to produce similar results with other patients by positioning and supporting them in pain-free comfortable positions. Through his own research, he developed the technique he calls strain-counterstrain.

Dr. Jones postulated that impaired joint mobility is often due to protective proprioceptive reflexes that fire when the muscle is shorter than its resting length. In other words, as the body attempts to move through its normal range of motion, a premature myotatic reflex (stretch reflex) causes the muscle to contract, thereby limiting movement. Often, the contraction is accompanied by spasm and pain. Jones theorizes that this pathologic reflex may have been initiated when the joint was in a stretched position and a panic reaction to return to a normal position caused the muscles opposite the stretched muscles to spasm. For example, a woman bends over for a short time. When she attempts to stand up, there is a sharp pain and she is not able to stand up without pain. There is a position, however, somewhere between the bent-over position and an erect position that is pain free. An overcontraction of the antagonist of the stretched muscle resists any attempt to return to a normal position.

Jones feels that a quick stretch of the shortened antagonist muscle caused the spindle cells to report to the central nervous system (CNS) that the muscle was being strained. A physiopathologic reflex circuit is created that maintains the antagonist muscle in a hypertonic state. This phenomenon can also result from muscle splinting following trauma. Once the reflex has been initiated, the body has no way to reset it.

Jones found that by positioning the joint in a position of comfort, which was usually close to the position where the spasm occurred, the pain ceases. By holding that position, which is usually a more exaggerated angle than the painful posture, then very slowly and passively returning to a normal position, the muscle shortening and the pain and spasm are eliminated.

Jones also noted that most joint problems have associated tender spots. When movement of a joint is restricted, pressure on the associated myofascial tender point will be painful. As the joint is moved into the position of maximum comfort, the pain in the tender point will diminish. By monitoring the sensitivity of the associated tender points while positioning the joint, the ideal angle for maximum benefit can be determined. When the client indicates that the pain in the point is reduced and there is a noticeable "letting go" in the palpated tissues, the pain or discomfort in the joint is also reduced and the client is in a comfortable position. Hold that position about a minute and a half (90 seconds), and then slowly return the body to a neutral position. The pain and restriction are often eliminated, and the pain in the associated tender spot has disappeared.

Orthobionomy

Orthobionomy was developed by an English osteopath named Arthur Lincoln Pauls. After reading of the work of Dr. Lawrence Jones, Dr. Pauls began to develop a healing system based on the body's self-correcting reflexes. Ortho means to correct or to straighten. Bionomy is the study of life processes. Dr. Pauls defines the term **orthobionomy** as the correct application of the natural laws of life.

Dr. Pauls feels that disease and injury are often the result of the body's inappropriate response or reaction to some stimulus or situation. The inappropriate reaction is a misinterpretation or a misunderstanding brought on by fear or habit. Orthobionomy works to restore the body's natural understanding by safely and slowly moving the body into and through those places where fear or habit is holding it in patterns that block vital energy, restrict movement, or cause pain.

Techniques include both methods that use physical contact and those that address energy systems of the body (*chi,* aura, etheric energy). The hands-on manipulations used in orthobionomy are passive positioning methods that relax tense ligaments and muscles by moving them into their position of greatest comfort and gently supporting them there. Techniques combine contact of trigger points with passive movement of the joint to produce the release of pain and tension in the

> **orthobionomy**
> is a healing system based on the body's self-correcting reflexes.

related muscles. There are movements to release every joint of the body that increase circulation and relaxation throughout the body. The client experiences movement through a wider range of motion with less pain and tension.

Because of the gentle, caring, and loving way orthobionomy is done, the release of muscular tension is often accompanied by mental and emotional release. As areas of the body begin to unwind, especially in areas where there has been trauma (physical or emotional), the stored body memories will also release. The release of physical and emotional restrictions along with the restoration of circulation and energy flow provides an environment in which the self-healing powers of the person can function.

Structural/Muscular Balancing

Structural/muscular balancing integrates techniques from several body-work systems including those of Drs. Lawrence Jones and Arthur Pauls. Dr. Ray Lichtman incorporated the passive positioning techniques of Pauls and Jones with precision muscle testing into a system he called positional release. Mark Beck and Marcia Hart further adapted the techniques of positional release to include tools to identify and balance the body-mind or psychophysical aspects that are intimately related to physical dysfunction.

Structural/muscular balancing (SMB) is a method of:

- Gently moving the body away from pain and toward more comfort
- Improving neuromuscular communication in the body
- Rebalancing the energy flow in the muscles
- Releasing tension which limits body range of motion (From *Structural Muscular Balancing,* Hart, 1992)

SMB provides an extremely gentle, noninvasive method of working with a client's unique self-knowledge to locate and release constricted tissues that cause pain and rigidness. SMB uses a variety of techniques to address the physical, neuromuscular, energetic, and psychoemotional aspects of an individual's dysfunctional patterns. The main physical techniques used in SMB include precision muscle testing, passive positioning, directional massage, and deep pressure. The aim of SMB is to release tension in the structural muscles and reset the neuromuscular reflexes that perpetuate tension, spasms, and the associated pain.

Precision Muscle Testing

Precision muscle testing is a type of specialized kinesiology that is used to evaluate energetic imbalances in the body and determine exactly what remedies will work best for the individual at that particular time. Whenever there is a dysfunction in a muscle, organ, tissue, or mental or emotional process, it will cause an energetic imbalance that can be revealed through muscle testing even before it becomes symptomatic.

Precision muscle testing evolved from the original work of Dr. George Goodhart, D.C., a Michigan chiropractor, who since the 1960s has guided research in the development of a system called applied kinesiology for detecting imbalances in the body. The system was simplified and popularized by Dr. John Thie, D.C., with the publication of *Touch for Health* and the development of Touch for Health seminars. Specialized muscle testing has been adapted to several alternative health practices as a way to determine physical or emotional imbalances and the effects of corrective measures or stresses on the systems of the mind or body. Precision muscle testing as it is used in SMB was refined by the work of Gordon Stokes and Daniel Whiteside of Three in One Concepts, Burbank, California.

In SMB, precision muscle testing is used to indicate the following:

- Where imbalances or lesions are in the body
- What parts of the body will be worked on
- What techniques will be used on each part
- Priorities as to what needs to be done in what order
- Relationships between two or more dysfunctional patterns

Precision muscle testing is the information-gathering tool that directly accesses the body's wisdom and self-knowledge. Through muscle testing, the body reveals where tension or imbalances exist and what corrective techniques it prefers.

Positional Release

Position release addresses muscle tissue that is tense, hypertonic, over-contracted, or in spasm. Muscles in a hypertonic state generally are ischemic, contain trigger points, have a high level of nerve activity, and may be painful. The presence of tight muscles in one area of the body usually is an indication of muscle imbalance in other areas as well. This is especially true with structural muscles of the pelvis and trunk.

The tense muscle is attempting in vain to bring its ends closer together. The tension may be the result of a protective reflex, muscle splinting, or strain. Tension is often self-perpetuating. The static tension of tight muscles restricts the flow of blood and fluids in those tissues. Tension causes increased metabolic activity, requiring more nutrients and producing more metabolic wastes. This ischemia and congestion impede the function of the muscle and may cause pain. Pain causes spasm, muscle splinting, and protective posturing, which further perpetuate the dysfunction.

Neuromuscular activity is increased. Proprioceptive feedback maintains the local tension and facilitates imbalances in the immediate area and in other related areas of the body. A viscious cycle of tension-pain-dysfunction builds on itself to a point that activity becomes restricted or stopped.

Positional release breaks the tension cycle by gently allowing the body to achieve the exaggerated positions it has been attempting without straining or initiating protective reflexes.

Contracted tissues are gently moved into their direction of contraction (preferred position). The body part is slowly and passively positioned so that the ends of the hypercontracted muscle tissue are brought closer together. When the right position for release is achieved, a slight compression into the joint is applied. The proprioceptive information created during the positioning resets the pathophysiologic reflex circuits that have held the joint and associated tissues in a state of tension. After holding the position for 30 to 90 seconds, the body part is slowly and passively returned to its normal position. Muscle tension is reduced, and associated trigger points are inactivated.

Directional Massage

Directional massage uses a short "hook and stretch" or J stroke on a specified body area or muscle. As the name implies, the stroke is done in one direction either up, down, or across the muscle. The area of the body and the direction of the stroke are determined with precision muscle testing. Tension and pain in the tissue are reduced, and energy flow is improved.

Deep Pressure

Occasionally, deep pressure is applied to specific hypersensitive spots. Deep pressure as it is used in SMB is similar to the ischemic compression used in trigger-point techniques. Deep pressure is used when passive positioning to release the affected tissues is not possible or does not completely inactivate the points.

INCORPORATING POSITIONAL RELEASE TECHNIQUES IN THE MASSAGE PRACTICE

Position release techniques can easily be incorporated into a massage practice. Whenever tight, constricted tissue is encountered, position release techniques can be employed to gently release the constriction and restore the tissues to an improved functioning state.

Position release is a very noninvasive system of soft tissue manipulation that originated in osteopathic practices. It is a gentle technique that affects the deepest neuromuscular mechanisms to relieve pain and dysfunction and restore normal function. The benefits of position release are increased local circulation and a neurological resetting of the proprioceptive mechanisms that had maintained the dysfunctional state. Position release affects the neuromuscular mechanisms and the proprioceptive system by passively relieving the shortened, constricted tissue, allowing circulation into the area to nourish the tissues and flush out toxins. The feedback at the annulo spiral ends of the spindle cells has a chance to reset to a more normal state, and the gamma feedback to the Golgi tendon organs is reduced. Position release is less effective on tissues with chronic fibrosis than on areas of hypertonicity and spasm.

Applying Position Release Techniques

There are several different methodologies for practicing position release, but they all involve the passive positioning of the body or a body part in such a way as to reduce the tone in restricted contractile tissue. Position release is done by passively moving the body or body part toward the body's preference and away from pain, seeking the tissue's preferred position. Movements are toward ease and away from bind, away from any restrictive barrier and toward comfort. Positioning is done slowly in such a way as to not cause any increase in pain. Positions are held for a period of time, usually 60 to 90 seconds. After the correct position for release is achieved and held for an appropriate period of time, it is essential that as the position is released, the body part is passively and slowly returned to a neutral position.

When a painful or dysfunctional area has been identified, one method to find the position for release would involve simply and passively moving the body part or joint associated with the painful condition into its preferred position. To find the preferred position, first flex and extend the joint. Choose the direction that is away from pain and toward comfort. Next, abduct and adduct the joint, again choosing the direction away from discomfort and toward comfort. Finally, rotate the joint first clockwise, then counterclockwise. Once again, choose the direction toward the most comfort. Now, combine the three movements that were toward comfort. For instance, flex, adduct, and rotate the joint clockwise into the middle of the range of movement until a resistive barrier is encountered. The position should be very comfortable. After the body part is in position, add a slight compression into the joint and hold the position for 30 to 90 seconds. After holding the position for about a minute, release the position and slowly and passively return the limb to a neutral position. Reassess the area for improvement and continue the massage or apply position release to another area.

Joint and neuromuscular dysfunctions usually have one or more associated hyperactive myofascial tender points that respond favorably to position release techniques and therefore are effective monitors for finding the correct position for release. These hypersensitive points may be trigger points in the target muscle, or occasionally the points may be located in the antagonist or a synergist to the target muscle. Position release techniques create an environment where the hypersensitive points deactivate and the dysfunctional tissues are restored.

Releasing Muscles with Trigger Points

Positional release has been found to be very effective in relieving constricted muscles with central trigger points in taut bands of muscle. Trigger points in myofascial tissue are excellent monitors when performing position release. Identifying the muscles that contain trigger points and knowing the actions those muscles perform help determine the preferred direction in which to move the body part to achieve the correct position for release. The body is positioned to bring the attachments of the affected muscle into closer proximity, passively mimicking the action of the muscle. Monitoring the myofascial tender point while fine-tuning the position ensures the most appropriate position for release.

In his books *Position Release Techniques* and *Clinical Applications of Neuromuscular Techniques,* Dr. Leon Chaitow incorporates a pain scale to elicit feedback from the client to help find the preferred position. Contact is made on an identified tender point or trigger point, and an amount of pressure is applied to the point of manageable discomfort. The client is instructed to gauge the discomfort as a 10 on the pain scale. The therapist maintains the same pressure and begins to passively move the body part into its preferred position, usually bringing the attachments of the muscle closer together. The client is asked to report the discomfort level at the contact point as the therapist continues to adjust the body toward the muscle's preferred position. When the discomfort at the point is reduced to a response of 3, 2, or less, this is the indication that affected tissue is in a position of ease. The practitioner holds the limb in this position and applies a slight compression into the joint the target muscle acts upon. The position is held for 60 to 90 seconds, and then slowly and passively the limb is returned to its neutral position. The practitioner reassesses the area for improvement and continues the massage or applies position release to another area (see Figure 18.26a to c).

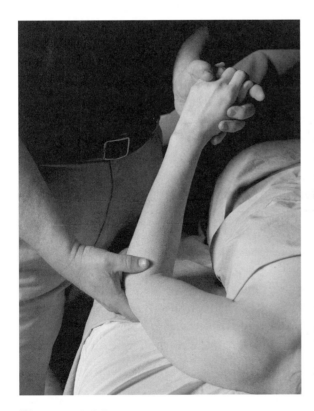

Figure 18.26a

Apply position release to the forearm extensors by first locating the trigger point in the muscle belly near the elbow.

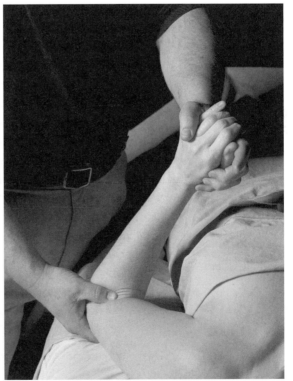

Figure 18.26b

Press on the trigger point to elicit a pain response from the client and position the arm by passively flexing the elbow, extending the wrist, and rotating the forearm in one direction, then the other. Experiment with different positions until the pain response at the point greatly diminishes or disappears.

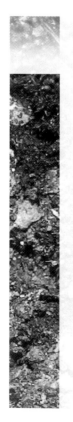

Figure 18.26c

Hold this position and compress gently into the wrist and elbow for 60 to 90 seconds, then release the compression and passively return the forearm to the table.

BOX 18.1 POSITION RELEASE PROTOCOL

1. Contact the alarm point in muscle tissue. It is felt as a nodule and will be tender to the touch. Apply pressure to the contact point to elicit a pain response.

2. Passively articulate the joint to bring the end points of the target muscle closer together (mimic the action of the muscle). It may be necessary to use all components of movement to find the preferred position of the muscle (flexion/extension, adduction/abduction, and rotation). The tenderness in the point will subside or the point may disappear as the correct position is achieved.

3. When the preferred position is achieved, maintain that position and gently and lightly compress into the joint that the muscle is acting upon. Continue to lightly monitor the alarm point. Often, a release and a gentle pulse may be felt at the point.

4. Hold the position for 30 to 90 seconds, or until a pulse is felt at the point plus another 10 seconds.

5. Gently release the compression and passively and slowly, without any help from the client, return the body part to a neutral resting position.

6. Recheck the alarm point and other related points such as synergist and antagonist muscles. For instance, on the neck, after releasing one side, it is a good idea to release the other side at the same level.

ENERGETIC MANIPULATION

Throughout the philosophies of Eastern countries is the premise that there is a force, or vibration, common to all living matter. It is believed that the smooth flow of this force is the predeterminator of good health.

When this flow is out of balance in the body, the person experiences physical illness and a sense of uneasiness. Techniques have been developed that detect imbalances in the flow of the force in the body and affect it in such a way as to bring it back into balance, or homeostasis.

Some techniques based on these theories are acupuncture (a traditional medical procedure rather than a massage technique), acupressure, shiatsu, polarity, Reiki, and reflexology. The following is a brief explanation of some of these techniques.

Acupuncture

Acupuncture is said to have originated in China more than 5,000 years ago. It is recognized around the world today as a remedial and medical technique. Throughout history, more people have been treated with acupuncture than all other therapies combined. Acupuncture is not a massage technique, but the basic philosophy underlies to some degree many of the energetic massage techniques. Touch is an integral part of acupuncture treatment. Acupuncture is a traditional Chinese medical practice whereby the skin is punctured with very thin needles at specific points for therapeutic purposes. Acupuncture must be done only by highly trained practitioners.

It is not within the scope of this book to cover the philosophy that supports such therapies as acupuncture and shiatsu, but the following information will help the beginning practitioner or student gain a better understanding of the therapies that originated in the ancient cultures of China and Japan.

Eastern Thought

Religious philosophies of the Far East speak of *Tao* or "the way" and refer to the law of the universe or "that which is all there is." The belief is that *tao* was split into two parts, and those two parts became opposed and dynamically in motion, thus creating the energy that sustains the whole. These two parts are represented by *yin* and *yang*.

Yin and *Yang*

The *yin* and *yang* theory demonstrates the natural process of continuous change where nothing is of itself but is seen as aspects of the whole or as two opposite, yet complementary, aspects of existence. Therefore, *yin* and *yang* are seen as opposites of the same phenomenon and exist only in

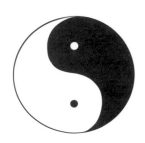

Figure 18.27

Yin yang symbol depicting balance and change.

relation to one another (Figure 18.27). The following list of words shows *yin* and *yang* contrasts:

Aspects of Yin and Yang

YIN	YANG
dark or night	light or day
low	high
cold	hot
inside	outside
contracting	expanding
passive	active
deficient	excessive

Yin and Yang on the Body

YIN	YANG
front of the body	back of the body
inner body	outer body
lower body	upper body
underactive	overactive
coldness	hotness
weak	forceful

Although *yin* and *yang* are diametrically opposed, one has no meaning without the other. There is continuous and constant vying as one creates and transforms into the other while at the same time holding the other in check. It is said that when *yin* and *yang* are in balance, there is harmony and well-being. The outcome of long-term disharmony is disease. If *yang* is too strong or excessive, *yin* will appear to be too weak. If *yang* is weak, *yin* will be overbearing. If the imbalance becomes too severe, *yin* and *yang* will separate, and the result is death of the organism. Breathing, digestion, metabolic rest and activity, and even the seasons are examples of this interaction. This relationship is considered to be the source of all change and movement.

Chi or Bioforce

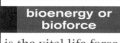

bioenergy or bioforce

is the vital life force in all living matter.

In the constant interplay of *yin* and *yang*, a subtle vibratory substance or a force or energy existing in all life forms is created. Many philosophers recognize this force as the vital force of growth and change. *Chi* (China) and *ki* (Japan) are two of the words used to describe this concept, while **bioenergy** and **bioforce** are terms in current usage that reflect similar ideas. There is no one word in English that adequately translates the *yin* and *yang* concept of *chi* (*ki*).

In discussing *chi* as it relates to health, it is much clearer to speak in terms of function. *Chi* in the body comes from three major sources: heredity from parents, the food we eat, and the air we breathe. These three sources combine and permeate our beings. According to ancient philosophy, *chi* (or *ki*) manifests itself as five interrelated aspects of en-

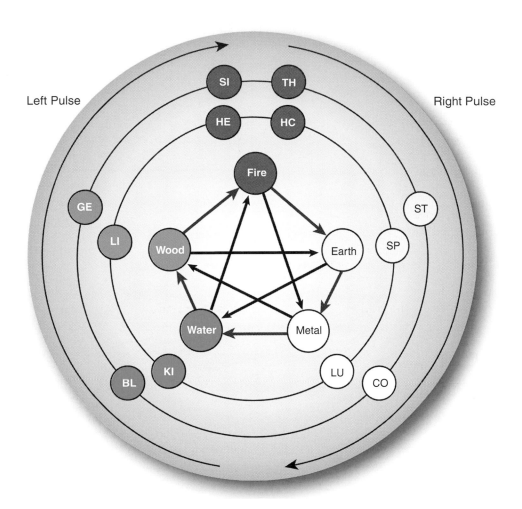

Figure 18.28

The relationships of the five elements to each other and their related organs are depicted in this diagram. The arrows in the center that look like a star depict the *ko* or control cycle: Wood controls earth by covering it or holding it in place with roots. Earth controls water by damming it or containing it. Water controls fire by dousing or extinguishing it. Fire controls metal by melting it. Metal controls wood by cutting it. The next arrows that form a pentagon depict the *shen* or creative cycle: Water engenders wood. Wood fuels fire. Fire creates earth (ashes). Earth engenders metal. Metal engenders water. The two rings indicate the solid (*yin*) and hollow (*yang*) organs that are associated with the elements. The outer arrowed circle indicates the location of the pulse points that are used for diagnosis.

ergy, which are the five elements. These are fire, earth, metal, water, and wood. Everything is created from one or more of these elements. Humans are said to be combinations of all five (Figure 18.28).

Meridian *chi* refers to the energy that circulates in a network of meridians, channels, and collaterals in the body. Channels and meridians are like rivers of *chi* (energy) that course along the extremities into the body and through related organs. There are 12 bilateral meridians, or channels, that are associated with organs, and 8 extra meridians that have regulatory effect. The extra meridians or collaterals flow from meridian to meridian and allow for regulation and harmonization of *chi*.

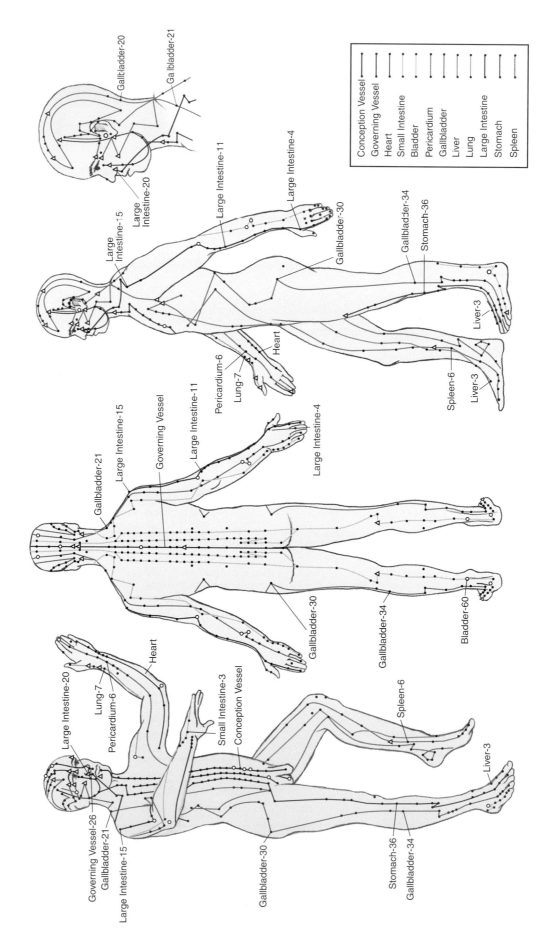

Figure 18.29

The 12 organ meridians are located bilaterally on the body.

Along these meridians are small areas of high conductivity called acupoints (acupuncture points), where *chi* can be affected by a number of modalities such as pressure, heat, electricity, needles, and touch. There are 365 acupoints located on the meridians where the *chi* (or *ki*) flow can most easily be influenced. A number of extra acupoints are not located on a specific meridian. It is at these points that the acupuncturist will insert needles or the therapist will apply pressure.

Meridians have been mapped on the body very specifically in terms of location and direction of energy flow. The practitioner who is seriously interested in pursuing the mastery of the subject must learn the location of each meridian, the direction of *chi* flow within the meridian, and the commonly used meridian points (Figure 18.29).

ORGAN MERIDIANS—*YIN* AND *YANG*

ORGAN MERIDIAN	*YIN* OR *YANG*	ELEMENT	LOCATION
Lung	Yin	Metal	Chest to end of thumb
Large intestine	Yang	Metal	Index finger to face
Stomach	Yang	Earth	Face to front of body to end of second toe
Spleen	Yin	Earth	Middle side of large toe to inside of leg to chest
Heart	Yin	Fire	Chest to inside of arm to end of little finger
Small intestine	Yang	Fire	Small finger to back of arm to side of face
Bladder	Yang	Water	Medial side of eye, over head, and down back and back of leg to little toe
Kidney	Yin	Water	Bottom of foot and along inside of leg to upper chest
Pericardium	Yin	Fire	Chest to end of middle finger
Triple heater	Yang	Fire	End of ring finger back to side of head
Gallbladder	Yang	Wood	Side of head and body and alongside leg to fourth toe
Liver	Yin	Wood	Big toe and along inside of leg to chest
Governing vessel	Yang		Tip of tailbone, up midline of back, and over the heart to upper lip
Conception vessel	Yin		Perineum and up front of midline to bottom lip and chin

The 8 meridians that have a regulatory effect are:

Conception vessel	Governing vessel
Regulatory channel of *yin*	Regulatory channel of *yang*
Connecting channel of *yin*	Connecting channel of *yang*
Belt channel	Vital or penetrating channel

Achieving the balance of *yin* and *yang* is the aim of most energy therapists. Imbalance in the body is recognized by a number of signs and symptoms. Various therapists have differing means of recognizing imbalances and offering techniques for affecting and regulating energy flow so that a more healthful condition might be achieved.

Acupressure

Acupressure refers to any of a number of treatment systems that incorporate various manipulations of acupoints. The basic philosophy comes from the traditional Chinese. Most Eastern societies incorporate some touch pressure in their traditional touch remedies. A number of acupressure techniques have been developed in Western societies.

Acupressure is often used to facilitate better circulation of blood and *chi* to an affected area and to relieve pain. Techniques usually include touching, pressing, or rubbing one or more points, depending on what is to be achieved. Acupressure as well as many of the health practices of Oriental origin are used in conjunction with diet, exercise, and meditation. The goal is to balance the physical and psychological aspects of a person's being into a holistic (wholesome) way of life.

Shiatsu

shiatsu
is similar to acupuncture but uses finger pressure instead of needles.

The Japanese word **shiatsu** (composed of *shi* [finger], and *atsu* [pressure]), means pressure of the fingers or digits. In a sense, it is like acupuncture without the use of needles. The purpose of shiatsu is to increase circulation and restore energy balances in the body. It is also an aid in soothing the nervous system and is said to be particularly effective in relieving headache, fatigue, insomnia, nervous tension, sore and stiff muscles, and such disorders as constipation and high blood pressure.

Like acupuncture, shiatsu recognizes strategic points (called *tsubo*) or energy pathways situated on the meridians that do not correspond entirely to the Chinese method. Instead of using needles, the shiatsu expert uses the ball of the thumb to apply pressure. The treatment can be given to the entire body to restore complete harmony or according to specific needs. By applying pressure to the points, the natural recuperative powers of the body are generated, toxins are dispersed, muscles are relaxed, circulation of blood and lymph are improved, energy is released or balanced, and the entire body is revitalized.

To be effective, the practitioner must build strength and dexterity of the fingers, thumb, and entire hand. Pressure is applied with only the tips of the fingers pointing straight into the point. One finger with another finger placed over it as a brace is used. The palm of the hand is sometimes used to apply pressure over a larger area. Three fingers held together may be used generally for the face, abdomen, and adjacent areas. The thumbs are used most often in shiatsu. Only the ball of the thumb is used to press straight down (no rubbing motions) on the pressure points. Pressure is exerted perpendicularly to the surface of the skin with the pads of the fingers or thumb, for 2 to 5 seconds or more, depending on the area being treated.

Pressure Points

To become better acquainted with pressure points, study Figure 18.30 and Figure 18.31, then note the basic benefits attributed to pressure points on specific areas of the body. The practitioner who wishes to become proficient in the art and science of shiatsu must study the philosophy and techniques under the direction of a skilled teacher. Shiatsu is not exceptionally difficult to learn, but it is an art that cannot be learned correctly by hit-or-miss methods or experimentation. Certain contraindications, as with other massage techniques, must be observed.

Shiatsu need not be applied in the order listed next. Judge the area to be treated, and then determine the duration of pressure and procedure to follow for maximum benefit to the individual.

Anterior View of Pressure Points

The following list refers to points indicated on Figure 18.30, reading clockwise from the head.

1. Frontal crown of the head, forehead, temple, and mastoid process. Use the thumbs on pressure points to relieve headache and tension.

2. Sides and front of the neck. Use the thumbs to press first the right and then the left carotid artery. Pressure here relieves stiff neck and fatigue.

3. Intercostal area. Gentle pressure with thumbs encourages relaxation.

4. Upper arm, cubital fossa forearm, elbow joint. People who use their arms a lot enjoy relief from fatigue when this technique is used. Apply pressure to points using the thumbs.

5. Descending colon and sigmoid flexure. Use the palms of the hands and the fingertips on pressure points. Pressure here relaxes tension and improves metabolism.

6. Outside of thigh and outside of lower leg. Use the fingers on the pressure points to relieve fatigue and sore muscles.

7. Toes, metatarsus, and ankle. Use the thumbs to press the toes several times each. Repeat on the metatarsus and ankle. This relieves fatigue, tension, and soreness.

8. Knee joint, front, and inside of the thigh. Use the thumbs to work down the front and inside of the thigh. Apply pressure above and below the kneecap. Relieves strained muscles and prevents soreness.

9. Palm of the hand. Use the thumbs on the pressure points to relieve strained muscles, stiffness, and soreness.

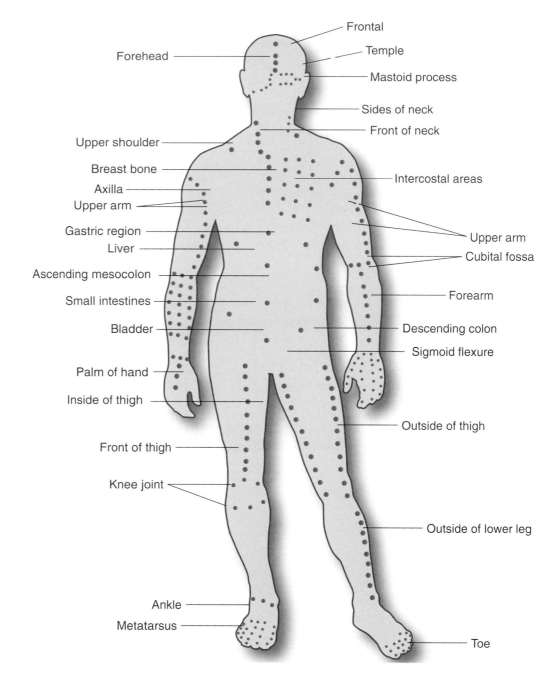

Figure 18.30

Anterior view of pressure points.

Labels on figure: Frontal, Forehead, Temple, Mastoid process, Sides of neck, Front of neck, Upper shoulder, Breast bone, Axilla, Upper arm, Intercostal areas, Gastric region, Liver, Upper arm, Cubital fossa, Ascending mesocolon, Small intestines, Forearm, Bladder, Descending colon, Sigmoid flexure, Palm of hand, Inside of thigh, Outside of thigh, Front of thigh, Knee joint, Outside of lower leg, Ankle, Metatarsus, Toe

10. **Bladder, small intestines, ascending colon.** Use fingertips to apply pressure to the points, and use the palm of the hand to apply pressure to the abdomen. This stimulates the flow of blood to the area and relieves constipation.

11. **Gastric region and liver.** Use the tips of the fingers to apply pressure. This relaxes nerves and promotes good digestion.

12. **Inside upper arm and axilla.** Use the thumbs on the pressure points to relieve strain and soreness.

13. **Breastbone.** Use the fingertips to apply pressure. This stimulates the endocrine gland.

14. **Shoulder.** Use the fingertips on pressure points to relieve soreness, strain, and fatigue of muscles.

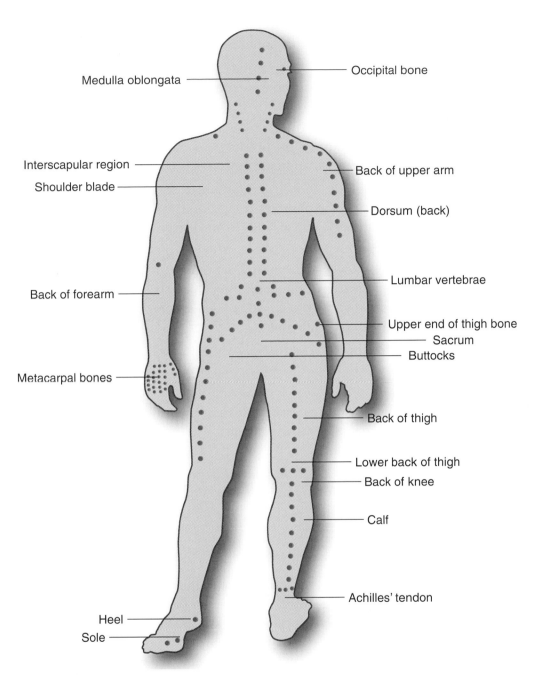

Figure 18.31

Posterior view of pressure points.

Posterior view labels:
- Medulla oblongata
- Occipital bone
- Interscapular region
- Back of upper arm
- Shoulder blade
- Dorsum (back)
- Lumbar vertebrae
- Back of forearm
- Upper end of thigh bone
- Sacrum
- Buttocks
- Metacarpal bones
- Back of thigh
- Lower back of thigh
- Back of knee
- Calf
- Achilles' tendon
- Heel
- Sole

Posterior View of Pressure Points

The following list refers to points indicated on Figure 18.31, reading clockwise from the head.

1. **Occipital.** Use the thumbs on the pressure points to help regulate blood pressure and relieve fatigue, insomnia, and headache.

2. **Back of upper arm.** Use the thumbs on the pressure points to relieve fatigue, soreness, and stiffness.

3. **Dorsum (back).** Use thumbs on pressure points to increase circulation, relieve tension, relax muscles, and soothe anxieties.

4. **Lumbar vertebrae and upper end of thigh bone.** Use thumbs on the pressure points to stimulate circulation to the area, relieve fatigue, and impart a sense of well-being.

5. Buttocks and sacrum. Use thumbs on the pressure points to relieve aching lower back, fatigue, and feelings of anxiety.

6. Back of thigh, lower back of thigh, and back of knee. Use the tips of the fingers on pressure points to relieve soreness, fatigue, and strain in muscles.

7. Calf and Achilles' tendon. Use the fingers to pinch the calves, and use the thumbs to press the points from calf to ankle. This relieves soreness, strain, and fatigue in muscles.

8. Heel and sole of the foot. Use the thumbs on the pressure points of the instep and the plantar arch (sole). Pressure here relieves strain and soreness, relaxes nerves, and strengthens muscles of the foot.

9. Metacarpal bones, hand, and fingers. Press the tips of all the fingers on the surfaces of the hand. Move pressure until all fingers have been treated. This technique adds strength and flexibility and improves general well-being.

10. Back of forearm. Use the thumbs on the pressure points from wrist to elbow to relieve muscles that are fatigued, strained, and sore.

11. Shoulder blade and interscapular region. Use the thumbs on the pressure points to improve circulation to the area, soothe nerves, and relieve anxieties.

12. Medulla oblongata. Use the fingertips on the pressure points to relieve fatigue, restore energy, soothe headaches, and promote alertness.

Reflexology

> **reflexology**
>
> stimulates particular points on the surface of the body, which in turn affects other areas or organs of the body.

Reflexology is the art and science of stimulating the body's own healing forces by locating and stimulating certain points on the body that affect organs or functions in distant parts of the body. A form of compression massage, reflexology is based on the principles that reflex points in the hands and feet are related to every organ in the body. By applying pressure to a reflex point, the practitioner can effect certain beneficial changes. For example, when reflex massage is given on the big toe, it is said to relieve headache and tension. Various parts of the hands and feet are linked with specific glands, organs, and muscles. Activating these links through reflex massage can relieve tension, improve the blood supply to certain regions of the body, and help to normalize body functions (Figure 18.32).

In recent years, public interest in reflexology has been aroused. Some people are skeptical whether this form of massage is beneficial, whereas others credit the method with remarkable success.

Practitioners do not claim reflexology to be a major cure-all. They encourage those who are interested to be sure to master the techniques well before attempting to use them.

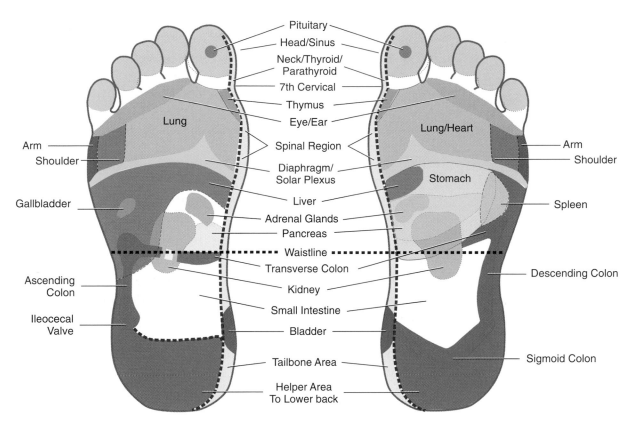

Figure 18.32
Foot reflexology chart indicates points on the foot that reflexively correspond to other areas of the body.

STRESS THERAPY AND RELAXATION MASSAGE

Stress is a condition that affects both the body and the mind. Originally it was caused by certain physical reactions in humans and animals that served as lifesaving signals to enable the organism to react quickly when danger threatened. This became known as the "flight or fight" response. Today, we face different kinds of stress situations, but the body still reacts in somewhat the same manner. To prepare the body to flee or to confront a problem, the sympathetic nervous system increases blood pressure and elevates the pulse rate. Hormones (adrenaline and noradrenalin) are released, and energy reserves are mobilized.

In cases of extreme fright or certain forms of nervous tension, a person may perspire profusely. The skin may become affected by the contraction of the erector pilorum muscles around a hair follicle. This condition, resembling a profusion of small bumps with erect hairs, is referred to as gooseflesh.

A certain amount of stress is normal and desirable, but there is a difference between positive and negative stress. Stress is an involuntary response. Whether it is positive or negative, the body deals with it in the same way. Positive stress expels excess energy, stimulates motivation, and is advantageous, whereas negative stress can cause adverse responses. For example, when under stress, the body's metabolism changes, and, if prolonged, body systems begin to react. A person may develop internal problems such as ulcers or skin problems such as psoriasis, hives, and problem blemishes. The great danger of stress is that when it becomes a chronic condition rather than an occasional reaction, it can eventually lead to serious health problems. Continued anxiety, tension, or hypertension can lead to allergies, arthritis, indigestion, constipation, high blood pressure, heart disease, insomnia, and many other conditions.

Stress-related illnesses account for most of the reasons for nonproductivity on the job as well as for problems that affect people personally and socially. When a person is suffering from negative stress, incidents that are normally accepted as minor or inconvenient are blown out of proportion as to their actual seriousness. Often the affected person will react by exhibiting excessive anger and frustration. Stress tends to deplete the body's supply of vitamins and minerals; therefore, people under stress should pay attention to their dietary habits. When under stress, there is a tendency to eat too fast and to eat meals lacking essential nutrients. Sometimes stress stimulates a craving for food or causes a feeling of fullness without satisfaction. Also it is not uncommon for the stressed individual to lose her appetite.

A sense of hopelessness is often associated with stress. When depression sets in, a person may turn to drugs or alcohol or both, hoping to find relief. However, alcohol and drugs only compound the problem. The most effective way to deal with stress when it becomes unmanageable is to seek counseling and treatment. It is important to identify causes and look for a solution. For example, when stress is work related, making a list of daily, weekly, and monthly activities may be helpful in pinpointing stress-producing activities that can be rescheduled or eliminated.

Individuals respond differently to the same stressful situations. For example, major life changes, a new job, illness, or financial setback may be devastating to one person, whereas another will be able to handle such events with less distress. Those individuals who have stressful life experiences should make an effort to balance their lives with some type of enjoyable recreation such as a hobby or special interest. A good balance of work and relaxation helps to combat stress.

Doctors often recommend massage for the relief of tension, anxiety, worry, and anger—all causes of stress. Many practitioners create a restful environment with relaxing background music for clients who are experiencing stress and for those who want to prevent stress-related illnesses. The goal is to induce complete mental and physical relaxation. When working with clients who are highly stressed, the practitioner should be aware of the effects of pressure, rhythm, and duration of each movement as well as the client's response. In some cases, the client may experience deep relaxation that is somewhat like a hypnotic state.

A great deal can be determined during the consultation, so the client should be encouraged to express her feelings. Also, the practitioner will want to know how long the beneficial effects of the massage lasted; clients often experience renewed energy and relief from stress for several days or longer.

When giving relaxation massage, the practitioner's hands are much better than any machine. In stress therapy and relaxation massage, human contact is most important. The massage practitioner is not expected to serve as the client's personal psychologist or counselor, but he should have an instinct for what is right for the client and an understanding of human feelings in order to apply a therapeutic healing touch.

CHAIR MASSAGE

Chair massage (Figure 18.33) is a growing, highly visible branch of professional massage. In airports, shopping malls, convention centers, supermarkets, street corners, dentists' offices, the workplace, and other venues, chair massage practitioners are introducing thousands of people, who ordinarily might not consider receiving table massage, to the benefits of skilled touch.

History

The origins of chair massage can be traced to the earliest history of bodywork. Centuries-old Japanese block prints illustrate bathers, newly emerged from the tub, receiving massage while seated on a low stool. Indeed, many styles of East Asian table or floor massage traditionally perform a portion of each session (often at the beginning or end) with the client sitting up rather than lying down. In the modern bodywork tradition, modalities such as Rolfing, Feldenkrais, and Alexander techniques regularly work with clients in a seated position.

However, as a discrete segment of the contemporary profession, this style of bodywork was popularized by David Palmer, a former massage school owner. Palmer began experimenting with massaging seated clients in 1982 as a way of making it easier for his students to introduce their services to potential clients. In 1986, he developed the first specialized chair for seated massage and began training practitioners at other bodywork schools throughout the country.

Today, massage chairs are available from more than a dozen different manufacturers. Most bodywork schools include some form of chair massage in their core curriculum. Seated massage is widely available around the world and is considered an integral part of the massage profession.

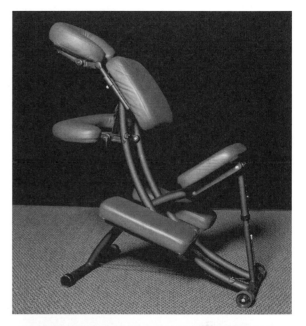

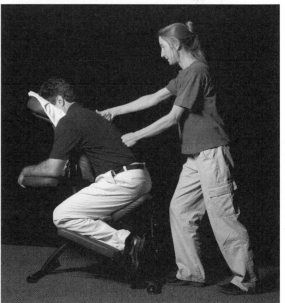

Figure 18.33

Seated massage uses a massage chair or face rest that attaches to the top of a desk.

Advantages of Chair Massage

Chair massage has made skilled touch physically, psychologically, and financially accessible to the general public. Because the client does not disrobe and no lubricants or lotions are used, a practitioner with a portable massage chair is no longer restricted to working in a private room behind closed doors. Chair massage has been performed on planes and trains, in gyms and beauty salons, at the beach and state fairs, in RV parks and flea markets, on movie sets, and in professional ballparks. The variety of locations is limited only by the imagination of the practitioner.

This accessibility creates a psychological safety net for potential clients who are still burdened with "massage parlor" associations.

For those who have a personal history of negative touch experiences, chair massage is a way to reintroduce positive touch into their lives. Shelters for battered women and programs assisting victims of physical, sexual, and emotional abuse or other forms of post-traumatic stress disorders often include chair massage among their services. Chair massage can be helpful in reconnecting clients with emotions that need to be processed for successful recovery.

Finally, because a typical chair massage session lasts only 5 to 20 minutes, not only is it well-suited to the fast pace of urban living, but it also makes a massage significantly more affordable. Whereas relatively few people will choose to spend $45 a week on a table massage, $5 to $15 a week is more manageable. The low cost of chair massage makes it the easiest way to experience massage for the first time and, on an ongoing basis, to integrate regular massage into a healthy lifestyle.

The Process

Because chair massage is done mostly through the clothing without lubrication and tends to be high-volume (larger numbers of clients in a day than table massage), certain adjustments are necessary.

Gliding or effleurage movements are generally not possible through clothing. Without these "resting" strokes, kneading movements tend to quickly tire the hands. Consequently, superficial or deep touch, combined with friction, percussive techniques, and perhaps some simple stretches are more commonly employed. Virtually all the acupressure techniques of East Asian massage, traditionally done through clothing or a towel, are ideally suited for this style of bodywork.

The head, neck, shoulders, arms, back, and hips of a client seated in a massage chair are most readily accessible to the practitioner. However, in one newer method of chair massage—a lower leg and foot massage—the client is seated in a traditional chair or turned around backward in a massage chair.

The determining factors in the creation of your own chair massage routine are the length of the massage and the special needs of the target market. For example, if you provide services to a large number of people in a short time span, each session will necessarily be shorter. If your clients are wheelchair bound, the lower back may not be as accessible as in other clients, and that factor will dictate the kind of massage you can perform.

There are also a few special hygiene considerations. Because the chair is not draped with a sheet, particular care must be exercised in cleaning the vinyl surfaces that come in contact with clients' skin. The face cradle and armrest (and knee rest and chest pad if the client is in shorts or without a shirt) should be sanitized with an antimicrobial wipe or spray solution after each use. Likewise, without a sink nearby, practitioners should be prepared to sanitize their hands using a similar procedure.

In addition, face cradle covers should always be used and changed with each client. Because the face cradle is typically tilted, try to pick covers that will not slide off the vinyl. Although cloth covers work well, if you are massaging 20 or more clients a day, laundering may become a major expense. A less labor-intensive choice is a set of disposable caps with elastic bands around the edges (worn by nurses and food service workers). They are available from medical supply stores or massage chair manufacturers at a very low price.

As with table massage, every client needs to be screened before sitting in a massage chair. Although chair massage can be utilized as part of an overall remedial treatment plan, by far its most common uses are to provide relaxation, reduce stress, and promote health. An abbreviated version of your standard table screening will probably suffice, with strong adherence to the rule "When in doubt, don't." Because time pressures often do not permit extended assessment, a conservative approach to screening is more appropriate for chair massage.

There is one special screening consideration: Because the client is seated rather than prone, she may experience a sudden drop in blood pressure, possibly leading to symptoms of fainting. This rarely occurs when a client is lying on a table because gravity keeps blood (and thus oxygen) moving to the head. The most common reasons seated clients might faint or experience symptoms of fainting is because they missed a meal and their blood sugar is low, or because they have a history of fainting. If they have missed a meal, a quick snack—a muffin or a glass of juice—will make them feel more comfortable. If they have a history of fainting, ask them to let you know immediately if they feel any lightheadedness, nausea, sudden sweating, or clamminess. In addition, be alert during the massage for fidgeting, particularly if you see the client lift her head away from the face cradle. Stop the massage and ask her if she feels all right. If not, immediately position her so that she can place her head between her knees or is lying prone. Though not a common experience, the potential for fainting does exist, and a wise practitioner is prepared to handle it.

The Role of Chair Massage in a Bodywork Practice

Because the best way to learn massage is by doing massage, the versatility of chair massage makes it ideal for students and new practitioners. It is much easier to learn than table massage, and students can begin their practice massages sooner. Because chair massage is so user-friendly, more people are willing to offer their bodies for practice. If you are setting out on a massage career, chair massage is one of the best ways to introduce clients to your touch and market your table practice.

A regular chair massage clientele also provides good balance to a table practice by helping to prevent the "cabin fever" syndrome that occurs when practitioners begin to tire of the same four walls 40 hours a week. Seated massage also allows bodyworkers to interact with their community in a broader, more spontaneous way, which some practitioners find helps to keep their practices, and their lives, fresh and exciting.

A growing number of practitioners now make chair massage their exclusive bodywork practice. Some prefer it for the same reason the general public does: the perceived safety and control that come with not having to deal with modesty issues behind closed doors. Others see chair massage as the best way to accomplish the goal of introducing new markets to professional touch. It is a valuable addition to every bodyworker's toolbox.

OTHER SOMATIC THERAPIES

Somatic therapies include many different applications of techniques that affect the well-being of the individual. Most of these therapies are hands-on techniques; however, they may focus on various aspects of the body/mind. Many of these therapies may be classified according to their intent or the aspect of our being to which they are directed. Some therapies are directed at the energetic aspect, others at movement, and others at physiologic tissue manipulation.

Listed here are some of the somatic therapies that are popular today. They are organized according to the broad classifications of energy, movement, or manipulative therapies. Using this type of classification is somewhat difficult because several of the therapies fit into more than one classification—for example, shiatsu is a manipulative technique that affects the energy systems of the body.

Energy Techniques

> *Do-in*
> Five-Element Shiatsu
> *Jin Shin Do*
> *Jin Shin Jyutsu*
> Polarity Therapy
> Reiki
> Therapeutic Touch
> Touch for Health
> *QiGong*

Movement Techniques

> Alexander Technique
> Aston Patterning

Feldenkrais
Tai Chi Chuan
Yoga

Manipulative Techniques

Anmo
Ayurvedic Massage
Bindegewebsmassage or Connective Tissue Massage
Esalen Massage
Lomi Lomi
Myofascial Release
Pfrimmer Deep Muscle Therapy
Rolfing/Structural Integration/Hellerwork
Soft Tissue Release
SOMA Neuromuscular Integration
Thai Massage
Trager Method
Tui Na
Watsu
Zero Balancing

Other Related Therapies Not Classified Above

Applied Kinesiology
Aromatherapy

QUESTIONS FOR DISCUSSION AND REVIEW

1. How does prenatal massage benefit the expectant mother?

2. What are the major benefits of lymph massage?

3. What are lymphocytes?

4. What is lymph?

5. What is deep tissue massage?

6. What is the purpose of structural integration?

7. What is the basis for neurophysiological massage therapies?

8. What is a trigger point?

9. Where are myofascial trigger points located?

10. What techniques deactivate trigger points?

11. Who developed the system known as neuromuscular therapy?

12. What are the abnormal tissue signs that indicate neuromuscular lesions?

13. What are the primary treatment techniques used in neuromuscular therapy?

14. Name the two inhibitory reflexes utilized in muscle energy technique.

15. What are the three primary active joint movements used in MET?

16. What are passive positioning techniques?

17. What are three important considerations when using passive positioning techniques?

18. Who developed the technique known as strain-counterstrain?

19. How is the preferred position determined in strain-counterstrain?

20. What are the primary tools used in structural/muscular balancing?

21. What is precision muscle testing?

22. Where is acupuncture said to have originated?

23. In Eastern thought, there are two parts that contrast or exist as opposites of the same phenomenon. What are these two parts called?

24. What are the three main techniques used in acupressure?

25. What is the meaning of the Japanese word shiatsu?

26. Why do doctors often recommend massage to people who are suffering from stressful life experiences?

27. What is the main purpose of reflexology?

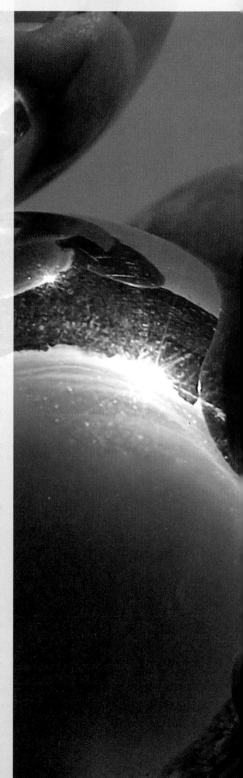

Business Practices

LEARNING OBJECTIVES

After you have mastered this chapter, you will be able to:

1. Explain the relationship between attitude, self-image, and business success.

2. List the major expenses related to starting a massage business.

3. Explain the difference between a partnership, a corporation, and a sole proprietorship.

4. Explain the advantages and disadvantages of operating your own business.

5. List the various permits and licenses required to operate a massage business and where to obtain them.

6. List the types of insurance a massage business owner should carry to protect the business.

7. Describe a physical layout for a beginning business operation.

8. Explain the importance of business location to the success of a personal service business.

9. Explain why careful planning is important before opening a business.

10. Explain the application of rules of professionalism to business practice.

11. Explain why keeping accurate records is necessary in a successful business.

12. List the major ingredients of a basic bookkeeping system.

13. Explain the importance of marketing to business success.

14. Define target market.

15. Make a checklist of factors to consider before opening a business.

INTRODUCTION

One of the greatest rewards of being a massage professional is seeing the relaxed smile on a client's face after a good massage. Of course, another objective of becoming a massage therapist is to produce an income. Most people who decide to become massage practitioners do so because they want to help people feel better. Many people have an ideological notion of how easy it would be to take a few massage classes then go out and start making money giving massages. As the emphasis on wellness and physical fitness continues to grow, there will be more business opportunities for ethical and well-trained massage practitioners. However, because there are not a large number of massage positions available, many massage practitioners opt for self-employment. It is wonderful to have the independence of operating your own business, but it is also your responsibility to make sure that your business thrives and supports you in the manner you wish. As a self-employed massage businessperson, you are owner, organizer, manager, bookkeeper, sales staff, and advertising executive as well as maintenance person and janitor. To be successful—to attain a desired level of practice and comfort—the self-employed person must develop some sense of business practice.

The practitioner who wishes to gain valuable experience may look for employment in a health club, at a resort hotel or spa, on a cruise ship, in conjunction with a medical facility, or as a freelance professional. An ambitious practitioner may choose to open her own business or occupy space within an established salon, clinic, or studio. Regardless of the environment in which the practitioner works, it is important to know something about business procedures. This includes keeping records, understanding laws and regulations, being familiar with insurance requirements, and much more. The practitioner who understands business procedures is more likely to succeed because she will be more aware of the importance of good customer relations, more involved in the overall operation of the business, and more profit conscious. This chapter is directed toward basic business skills that will provide the basis for a successful massage practice.

ATTITUDE/SELF-IMAGE/PUBLIC IMAGE

As a massage therapist, you are not only a health care practitioner, you are also a businessperson. To be a successful businessperson, a positive self-image is essential. A positive self-image means that you feel good about who you are and what you are doing. A good self-image is a positive attitude reflected in the enthusiasm and quality exhibited in your work and other activities. There is a sense of excitement about what you are doing. Often, this is accompanied by a desire to be involved and to learn more. A positive attitude and an inner knowledge that "I will attain my goals" is a major advantage in being successful.

A good self-image and a positive attitude are the foundations for creating a good public image. Your public image is the way you are perceived through your appearance, the way you do business, and how you interact with your clients and associates. Your public image relates to your reputation and the degree of professionalism with which you operate. Success is dependent on a good reputation, a good public image, and a high degree of professionalism.

BUSINESS PLANNING

Business planning starts when a business is first conceived and continues throughout the life of the business. Planning is the first step in setting the stage for the development of the business. Planning involves clarifying your purpose, stating a mission, setting goals, and determining priorities.

A **mission statement** is a short general statement of the main focus of the business. Developing a mission statement requires careful consideration. The mission statement expresses the intent of the business and can be used on promotional material as a reflection of the business's public image.

A **purpose** is a theme that is derived from your dreams and ideals. You may have several purposes for doing business. Clarifying those purposes allows you to direct your energies toward those purposes.

Some examples of a purpose might be:

To provide a pleasant, environmentally friendly working environment

To make a positive difference for my clientele

To prosper and enjoy

Goals are specific, attainable, measurable things or accomplishments that you decide on and make a commitment to achieve. The business goals you set support your mission and reinforce your purpose. Setting goals clarifies your intentions and directs your creative energy toward realizing your dreams, toward success.

Goals may be short term or long term. You can have lifelong goals, 5-year goals, 1-year goals, 6-month goals, goals for next week, goals for tomorrow, or goals for today. Although it is helpful to include a deadline with a goal, it is not necessary. Keep your goals personalized and in the present tense. Make your goals realistic and attainable, but do not hesitate to think big. The more specific your goals are, the better.

The following are some examples of goals:

- I will see 20 clients per week.
- I will attend the next national convention.
- I will spend at least three evenings a week at home with my family.
- I will increase my income by 20 percent this year.

mission statement
is a short, general statement of the main focus of the business.

purpose
is the business theme that is derived from the owner's dreams and ideals.

goals
are specific, attainable, measurable accomplishments that you set and make a commitment to achieve.

Develop a Strategic Plan

It is helpful to write your goals. Refer to them often to see how you are progressing. Setting goals is only a clarification of where you are heading. Once you set goals, it takes planning and commitment to realize them. Some goals are simple: "I will maintain my client files daily." Others are more complicated and have many subgoals contained within them. "I will increase my income by 20 percent this year." To accomplish the larger goal, it helps to break it into doable chunks, examine them, and develop a course of action.

List the benefits of attaining the goal. Brainstorm possible steps needed to reach the goal. Note potential obstacles or conflicts and solutions to those problems. Then develop a step-by-step plan of how to reach the goal. Include in the plan resources and timetables of what actions to take. After the plan is formulated, *do it!!*

BEGINNING IN BUSINESS

As a business owner and manager, you must have knowledge of your field, good business sense, a sense of diplomacy, and clear business goals. In addition, you must keep accurate records and understand all business procedures involved in your kind of business. You can hire tax consultants and bookkeepers to do some of the more extensive work, but it is you, the owner, who is responsible for the success of the business.

Most people who succeed in the personal service business gain experience by learning while working for someone else. They learn efficiency of management, motivating employees, promoting good customer relations, and numerous other business procedures. After a practitioner has gained experience and knowledge, she may decide to start a business or look for an established business to buy or manage.

If you are beginning a new business, there are several things you must consider. What type of a business operation will it be? How will you finance the costs of equipment and other start-up costs before you can begin to generate income? Other considerations in starting a business are choosing a location, acquiring permits and licenses, and selecting adequate insurance coverage.

Determining Whether to Be Self-Employed or Employed

There are many opportunities and capacities in which a massage practitioner can work. However, the majority require the practitioner to be self-employed. Unless you live in an area where there are established massage establishments, spas, or medical facilities that employ massage therapists or you work for a concessionaire in a resort area or on a cruise ship, the chances are you will have to create a place to practice.

One of the first steps in planning how you are going to practice is to consider what kind of massage business operation you want to work in or to have. Regardless of the situation you choose, there will be both advantages and disadvantages. The following will explore some possible practice alternatives for the massage practitioner.

If the option is available, you may choose to work in an established massage practice or business. In an established business, the novice practitioner has the opportunity to gain valuable experience without the time and financial commitment of running a business. When working for someone else, you may be paid by the hour or on a commission basis, in which case you would be paid a portion of the fees collected for the massages you perform.

Besides gaining valuable experience, advantages include having facilities, supplies, scheduling, and reception services provided; receiving a steady paycheck with taxes withheld; and receiving any employee benefits that may be included.

Some disadvantages are that you receive only a small portion of the money and working on someone else's time schedule.

Deciding to work for someone else means that you will probably have to seek out an employer. A number of possible employment situations include the following:

Alcohol or abuse treatment centers

Athletic clubs

Athletic teams

Beauty salons

Chiropractic clinics

Cruise ships

Dance companies or schools

Hospitals

Hotels or resorts

Physical therapy or medical clinics

Ski resorts

Spas

Sports medicine clinics

What Kind of Massage Operation Do You Want?

The majority of massage practitioners are self-employed. There are many opportunities for qualified and industrious practitioners to be successful entrepreneurs. The following is a list of possible self-employment situations. Add to this list other situations that you can think of. Make a list of pros and cons (advantages and disadvantages) for each situation.

Independent Contractor

Working as an independent contractor may be very similar to being employed by someone else except that as an independent contractor, you determine your own work schedule, provide your own supplies, get paid a flat fee, and are responsible for your own taxes (including self-employment tax). Many times as an independent contractor, you simply rent a space and operate your business within another business. An example might be providing massage services in a spa or full-service beauty salon. You might also be hired as an independent contractor to provide massage services for an organization such as a dance company, sports team, or corporation.

Working Out of Your Home

Operating a massage business out of your own home may be an economical alternative to having a separate office if you have a suitable space in your home that you can dedicate to your massage business. It is important to have an easily accessible bathroom, a clear entryway, and a waiting area. Not only is a massage business in your home economical, there are certain tax advantages in operating a home business. Check with your accountant for full details.

There are also disadvantages. There may be zoning restrictions. Having people coming into your home restricts your privacy. You must keep your home/office clean and sanitary. You must also maintain a quiet, professional atmosphere. This setup generally does not work well if there are children or if the household has a lot of traffic through it.

Outcalls Only

Some massage practices are set up as portable offices. With a portable table and/or massage chair, the practitioner goes wherever the client is. The overhead of such an operation is minimal. The convenience to the client is high, but for the practitioner, it is low. The workspace is whatever the client has available. The practitioner must carry her equipment in, set it up, then tear it down and carry it out at the end of each appointment. When doing only a few appointments a day or a week, this may be an ideal setup, but going to several appointments everyday may get exhausting.

Safety may also be a factor. Carrying a portable table into awkward locations may result in strain and injury. Going into unknown situations alone may result in a threatening encounter. Practitioners who do outcalls should have a system to protect themselves from the potential risk. When doing outcalls in a questionable situation, ensure your safety by making a telephone call to a colleague when you arrive at the appointment, giving the name and address of the party and the approximate time you will be finished, and then another call to let your colleague know that you have finished and are leaving. Your phone calls will dissuade the client from any wrongdoing.

Working Out of a Separate/Private Office

A popular option among massage therapists is to rent a small private office. Depending on the size of the business, the office may be just one room or a complex of rooms where several practitioners work as employees or partners. For a one-person operation, it is helpful to have at least two rooms, one a therapy room and the other an entry/waiting area.

Renting a Space in a Larger Office Complex

Another popular option for a therapist is to rent a space in conjunction with another, complementary business operation, such as any of the following:

- A full-service beauty salon
- A chiropractor's office
- An athletic gym
- A sports clinic

- A hospital
- An alternative health clinic
- A doctors' complex
- A spa

These arrangements have many advantages in that the massage business has ready access to clientele as well as receptionist and waiting room facilities.

There are a number of possible alternatives when working out of or renting from another business regarding how the rent is paid and what is included. They range from renting/leasing raw space (you bear all costs of modifications, maintenance, support services, and supplies) to a turnkey situation (landlord prepares the space, supplies all the needs, and all you have to do is tell him what you want and come in and go to work). The amount of rent depends on what is included. In some cases, the rent is a flat amount; in other cases, it is a percentage of your sales. (In most situations, this author does not recommend this kind of agreement.)

It is essential that whatever the terms of the agreement, they be put in writing in the form of a lease agreement that is signed by both parties.

Co-op an Office with Other Therapists

Often massage therapists rent a facility together, sharing the expenses of rent, utilities, and a receptionist/bookkeeper. This option is a way to provide an attractive facility for a number of practitioners, yet keep the overhead affordable. It also provides flexibility in scheduling so that practitioners can work hours that suit them and clients have the option of receiving services at their convenience.

These are only a few of the many options available to the enterprising massage entrepreneur. Every option has its advantages and disadvantages. For each of the options given here, make a list of pros and cons. Think of other possible options for a massage practice. What would be the ideal massage practice you would like to work in?

TYPES OF BUSINESS OPERATIONS

A business may be organized as a sole proprietorship, a partnership, or a corporation. Each has advantages and disadvantages.

As a **sole proprietor,** you are an individual owner and carry all expenses, obligations, liabilities, and assets. You would receive all profits from your business and be responsible for all losses. Business obligations and debts are the owner's personal responsibility. Legally as a sole proprietor, you and the business are one and the same in the eyes of the law. If the business gets too far into debt, or in legal trouble, you as an individual are liable. There is the potential for numerous tax advantages, but you must comply with all tax responsibilities, including self-employment

> **sole proprietor**
> is an individual business owner responsible for all expenses, obligations, liabilities, and assets.

taxes. Many people prefer being a sole proprietor if they can handle the financial and personal responsibilities involved.

Most massage therapists are self-employed and are sole proprietors. Being self-employed means being your own boss and setting your own schedule. It also means that you are responsible for the success or failure of your business. Being self-employed requires you to be self-motivated and disciplined. You are solely responsible for not only working with clients but also all promotional and operational activities.

A **partnership** may be the answer if you know someone who wants to invest and who is qualified to share the responsibility. The combined ability and experience of two people can make a business easier to operate. Although a partnership can relieve a sole proprietor of the pressures of doing everything herself, there are some drawbacks. A partnership is a relationship wrought with all the bonuses and misunderstandings of any interpersonal association.

> **partnership**
>
> is a business setup in which two or more partners share responsibility and benefits of running the business.

One key to a good working partnership is a clear partnership agreement. Though it is not a legal requirement, a written partnership agreement will clarify the rights and responsibilities of each partner and strengthen the relationship. A partnership agreement should include the business goals, what each partner will contribute (money, material, and time), how the profits will be divided, and how the business will continue should one partner want out.

Legally, in a partnership, each partner carries the same responsibilities as a sole proprietor in the case of debt and liability. There are also certain tax regulations specific to partnerships. An accountant and a lawyer may be helpful if you are considering setting up a partnership.

> **corporation**
>
> is a business setup subject to state regulation and taxation. A charter must be obtained from the state in which the corporation operates.

A **corporation** has advantages and disadvantages. It is subject to regulation and taxation by the state, and a charter must be obtained from the state in which the business operates. Management of the corporation is in the hands of a board of directors who determine policies and make decisions in accordance with the charter. Stockholders share in profits but are not legally responsible for the actions of the corporation. Stockholders and corporate owners are not directly liable for lawsuits and debts against the corporation. However, as a professional, the corporation will not shield you from the liability of actions of gross negligence that result in a malpractice suit. If you are considering incorporating, consult with knowledgeable authorities to determine whether it is worth the time, money, and effort it will take.

> **limited liability companies**
>
> are a form of legal entity, something between a partnership and a corporation.

Limited Liability Companies (LLCs) are a form of legal entity that are something between a partnership and a corporation. LLCs offer many of the benefits of a corporation with much less paperwork and other complications. Most states require an LLC to have at least two owners or members and to file an IRS Form 1065. The owners in an LLC are a separate entity from the business and are shielded from some of the personal liability of the business. Profits and losses from the business are divided among the owners and recorded on their individual income tax returns.

START-UP COSTS AND NEEDS

The start-up costs for beginning a business include all the expenses incurred before any revenues are collected. Those costs vary according to the size and complexity of the operation. Start-up costs are out-of-pocket expenses that must be considered during the planning stage and recovered before a profit is realized.

The two main reasons small businesses fail are undercapitalization and poor management. Most massage practitioners are self-employed. They work out of their home, a small office space, a space shared with another practitioner, or in conjunction with another health care provider (doctor, chiropractor, etc.). Regardless of where you locate your practice, there will be certain expenses in setting up your practice.

Start-up expenses may include:

- Rent or lease: May include first and last month's rent and a cleaning/damage deposit
- Utilities: Hook-up charges and deposits for electric, gas, telephone; telephone answering service
- Equipment and supplies: Table, bolsters, therapy equipment, linens, massage oils, and so on
- Furniture: Desks, chairs, supply cabinets, music system, file cabinet, lighting, and so on
- Decorating supplies: Paint, curtains, plants, and so on
- Office supplies: Calculator, printer, computer, pens, staple gun, writing paper, filing supplies, appointment and receipt books, and so on
- Advertising expense: Ads and announcements, and so on
- Printing expense: Business cards, stationery, information forms, brochures, and so on
- Insurance and license costs
- Initial operating expense: Opening business checking account with enough capital to cover miscellaneous expenses until the business is up and running

When planning a business operation, it is important to establish good credit and banking relations. Many businesspeople rely on getting business loans when necessary in order to have sufficient working capital. It usually takes time to build clientele, so money must be available to take care of necessary expenses. Always know where your money is being spent and operate with sufficient cash flow. A major cause of small business failure is the owner's inexperience in judging overhead expenses and having inadequate capital to carry the business through slow periods. As income and profits grow, the budget may be increased for expansion of facilities, advertising, and other areas of growth.

BUSINESS LOCATION

One of the most important decisions you may make concerning the success or failure of your business is where it is going to be located. Depending on how you structure the business, possible locations will vary. Massage businesses may be operated out of the practitioner's home, in a rented space in another business, or out of a freestanding office.

There are many factors to consider when renting or leasing a space for a massage business. The building in which a personal service business is located should be in good condition and in a fairly prosperous location. Choose a site that will accommodate your business needs, be pleasing to your clients, fit your image, and is properly zoned and within your budget. It must be easy to locate, with the address clearly visible from the street. It should be easily accessible and relatively quiet. An ideal space would have one or more massage rooms, a reception/waiting area, an office, and bathroom facilities with a shower. The first impression your clients will have of you is the one they get when they walk into your place of business, so ask yourself, "Does this facility represent the quality with which I want to be associated?"

If a business is large enough to support a consistent advertising program, it may be located in an out-of-the-way, prestigious location. However, a smaller, less affluent business should be located near other active places of business in order to attract the attention of potential clients. Being near public transportation and having adequate parking facilities are important considerations.

After you have determined your space requirements, have a clear price range in mind and an idea of the kind of location you want, and check the resources in your area. Realtors and the chamber of commerce may be good leads. If you want to work within another business, check out the local business directory or the yellow pages for businesses of the type you want to associate with.

Before signing a rental agreement or lease, make certain that the space fits your needs. If remodeling is necessary or if the building must be "brought up to code," the costs may be overwhelming. Some questions you may want to ask are: Does the massage area have individual heating and air-conditioning controls, and is it well ventilated? Will the massage rooms be quiet? Is the lighting appropriate, and are there sufficient outlets? Is there sufficient storage? How are the maintenance and utilities handled? Who is responsible for what and how much can I expect to pay? If you plan to lease a location or business, be sure that you insert into the lease agreement any options for removing or replacing fixtures, making repairs, changing specific structures, or installing equipment, plumbing, and electrical work.

When you are satisfied with the location, it is important to get the lease agreement in writing. Do not necessarily sign the first lease the landlord puts in front of you. Read the lease carefully to make sure all provisions are clearly explained. If you have any questions, it is a good idea to consult a lawyer.

Many therapists choose to work independently out of their homes. This is an inexpensive alternative but may require a special use permit because of local zoning regulations. When working out of your home, it is imperative that the portion of the home that is used for an office is kept clean and neat. A clean bathroom, preferably with a shower, should be available for your clients. There are certain tax deductions that can be claimed for having an office in the home (check with your tax accountant).

BUYING AN ESTABLISHED BUSINESS

You may have an opportunity to buy an established business, in which case you must weigh the advantages or disadvantages. Be sure the business has a good reputation, that it is worth the price being asked, and that it has an established clientele. It is a good idea to question customers as well as other business owners in the vicinity regarding the reputation of the business. Of course, you will want to know why the present owner is selling. It will not be to your advantage to buy a business that is being sold because it is failing. Generally, the owner is moving, retiring, or changing occupations.

It is important to consult a lawyer who can handle all legal aspects of the transaction to the satisfaction of everyone involved. A written purchase and sale agreement will be needed. You will also need a complete inventory of all fixtures, equipment, supplies, and materials as well as the value of each article that is to be part of the agreement. To avoid future misunderstandings, it is advisable to take photographs of furnishings and equipment. This will help to ensure that you receive the exact items listed. It is also necessary to examine all records to understand the assets and liabilities of the business you are buying. An investigation should be made to determine any outstanding debts or obligations that may be held against the business.

LICENSES AND PERMITS

There are local, state, and federal regulations that must be considered when beginning, locating, or relocating a business. It is to the advantage of the business owner to be aware of and comply with all regulations in the process of organizing the business rather than to be surprised after the fact and have to pay heavy penalties or restructure or relocate the business. Following is a partial list of permits and licenses that may be required and who to contact to determine how to comply.

Fictitious name statement (DBA): Required if the business name is different from the owner's name. A fictitious name statement, also called DBA (Doing Business As), is filed with the county to ensure that no other business uses the same name when doing business. *Contact:* County clerk's office.

Business license: May be required to operate a business in the city. *Contact:* City government, business licensing department.

Massage license: May be a city, county, or state requirement to perform massage services for a fee. *Contact:* County/city licensing bureau or the state agency in charge of occupational licensing.

Sales tax permit: Required if you sell products or if services are taxed. Provides information and materials to collect and file sales tax. *Contact:* State department of revenue.

Planning and zoning permits: Required to ensure that the operation and location of the business is in compliance with local zoning requirements. This may especially affect those who operate a business out of their home. *Contact:* County or city planning and zoning board.

Building safety permit: May be required to obtain a business or professional license. May be issued after the place of business has been inspected and found to comply with building and fire codes and be free of conditions that may pose a hazard to you or your clients. *Contact:* Local fire department.

Employers identification number (EIN): This is the federal tax identification number issued to businesses and is used on all tax-related forms. An EIN is required of partnerships and businesses that hire employees. *Contact:* Internal Revenue Service.

Provider's number: This is an identification number issued to licensed health care providers. It is used and required when submitting claims to and receiving payment from medical insurance companies for services rendered. Massage practitioners in most states are not eligible to hold a provider's number but do receive third-party payments (insurance payments) by contracting with, billing through, or being an employee of a licensed provider (doctor, chiropractor, physical therapist, etc.).

PROTECTING YOUR BUSINESS

You will need to have adequate insurance against fire, theft, and liability. To determine the specific types and amounts of coverage to cover your business and yourself, consult with one or more insurance agents. If you work out of your home, review your homeowner's policy concerning the liability of operating a business out of your home. If you lease an office, check the lease to determine which liability responsibilities are yours and which are the landlord's.

Following is a list of some types of insurance you may want to obtain.

Liability insurance covers costs of injuries and litigation resulting from injuries sustained on your property. This is usually a part of a homeowner's policy but may not cover business-related occurrences. Check your policy.

Professional liability insurance protects the therapist from lawsuits filed by a client because of injury or loss that results from alleged negligence or substandard performance of a professional skill. Professional liability insurance can be purchased reasonably through some professional organizations such as the American Massage Therapy Association and the Associated Bodywork and Massage Professionals.

Automobile insurance full coverage provides medical and liability insurance to the driver and any passengers, and covers the vehicle and its contents regardless of who is at fault.

Fire and theft insurance covers fixtures, furniture, equipment, products, and supplies. If you rent or lease an office, the landlord may carry this insurance. Make sure it is adequate. *Renter's insurance* is available through most major insurance companies for a relatively small premium that will cover the loss of furniture and equipment in the case of theft, vandalism, fire, or other natural disasters. If you have an office in the home, be sure your homeowner's policy is adequate to cover your office.

Medical/health insurance helps cover the cost of medical bills, especially hospitalization, serious injury, or illness.

Disability insurance protects the individual from loss of income because she is unable to work due to long-term illness or injury.

Worker's compensation insurance is required if you have employees. It covers the medical costs for employees if they are injured on the job.

PLANNING THE PHYSICAL LAYOUT OF A BUSINESS

The layout of a business takes careful planning in order to achieve efficiency and economy of operation. After the building or space within a building has been decided, the interior must be designed. An efficient salon, studio, or clinic offering massage should have the following:

1. Air-conditioning and heating systems that will provide warmth and comfort to your clients

2. Appropriate plumbing for showers and restrooms

3. Adequate and appropriate lighting for the entire operation, including indirect lighting in the massage rooms

4. A private massage room with adequate space for a massage table, maneuvering space around the table, a supply cabinet, possibly a dressing area, and, if consultations will take place in the room, a desk with two chairs.

5. Proper equipment and adequate space for its use

6. Accessibility to all areas

7. Furniture that is appropriate, attractive, durable, and in keeping with the dignity of the business

8. An attractive and comfortable private consultation area

9. An attractive and comfortable reception area

10. An area suitable to carry out business practices such as client files, correspondence, telephone, and appointments.

Clients form either a positive or negative first impression of a business operation by the appearance of the office facility. The decor and appointments need not cost a fortune, but should give the impression that the business and the people employed there are highly professional. Your office can be one of your best promotional tools if the client is favorably impressed. Design the office so that it is comfortable, uncluttered, and professional.

Massage Business Floor Plans

When planning a massage business, all facilities must be considered. A business may be located within another business such as a hairdressing and skin care salon, athletic club, or chiropractic office. The reception area, storage, restrooms, and other facilities might be shared between the office, club, or salon.

Floor plan A shows adequate space for a larger business with room for several practitioners (Figure 19.1). The basic floor plan B (Figure 19.2) and the functional floor plan C (Figure 19.3) show only essential furnishings of a massage room. This is often the ideal plan for the beginning practitioner and to maintain a low operational cost.

Figure 19.1

Floor plan A—ideal space, 28′ x 50′.

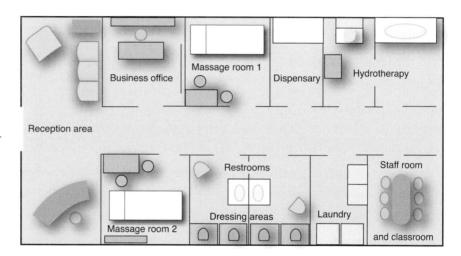

Figure 19.2

Floor plan B—basic space, 10′ x 12′.

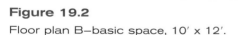
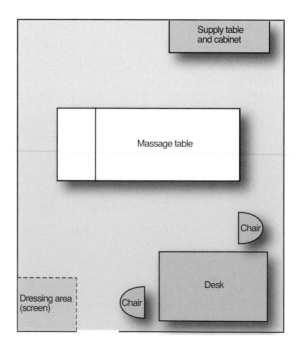

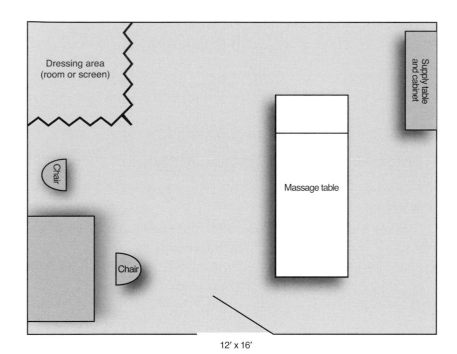

Figure 19.3
Floor plan C—functional space, 12′ x 16′.

OFFICE MANAGEMENT

Establishing business practices and office procedures may be the farthest thing from a massage practitioner's mind or desires. Most people who become massage therapists do so for the personal contact and the chance to enhance their intuitive and creative abilities through healing touch. Generally, they have a limited background at best about office management or bookkeeping and may consider it an unsavory or even incomprehensible task.

BUSINESS ETHICS FOR THE MASSAGE PRACTITIONER

A massage practitioner must always practice according to a professional code of ethics. Ethics are standards of acceptable and professional behavior by which a person or business conducts business. Chapter 3 discusses ethics. Good ethics provide guidelines for professional conduct. The following guidelines reflect ethical behavior for the massage practitioner:

1. Always present a professional appearance.
2. Maintain a sense of dignity and professionalism in your work.
3. Project a pleasant, optimistic personality.
4. Treat each client with courtesy.
5. Maintain good health habits.
6. Keep surroundings neat, clean, and attractive.
7. Follow a systematic plan and organize your work properly.

8. Space appointments so that sufficient time is allowed.

9. Keep clients' records and conversations confidential.

10. Keep accurate records of all treatments.

11. Keep an active card file and mailing list of regular and prospective clients.

12. Use professional business cards and stationery.

13. Make periodic mailings of services that are offered.

14. Be sure that all advertising represents your business in the most professional manner.

15. Let physicians and other professional people know about your work and how you may be of valuable assistance to them.

16. Make every effort to eliminate negative concepts of your business by speaking before groups and educating the public about your work.

17. Join professional organizations that strive to upgrade, improve, and set high standards for your business.

18. Continue to promote your own personal and professional growth.

19. Work to eliminate any activities that cast unfavorable light on your business and profession.

20. Be responsible in keeping your word and meeting your obligations.

21. Obey all laws and legal requirements regulating the practice of massage and your business operation.

22. Charge a fair price for services rendered.

23. Continue to build a good reputation by your own work and conduct.

24. Recommend massage treatments only as the client requires and desires them.

25. Be loyal to your employers, associates, and clients.

26. Keep your professional and private lives separate by not discussing your personal problems with your clients.

SETTING YOUR FEES

As a businessperson offering a personal service, your income is dependent on the fees you charge for your services. In determining your fee structure, there are several factors to consider. There are various strategies you may use to set your fees.

You are a professional massage therapist selling a valuable service. Set a fee that compensates you fairly and reflects your credibility. Consider the market and your competition. A little research will tell you what services are offered by other practitioners in the area and what they charge for those services. Set your fees in accordance with others in your area.

If you offer a unique service in high demand, your fee may be higher. If you are just beginning and want to attract more of the market, you may set a lower fee or offer special introductory rates.

If you are self-employed and massage is your sole source of income, you must consider all the costs of operating your business and determine how many sessions you must do at what rate in order to earn a living. If you are working for someone else, you may work for an hourly wage or for a percentage for each massage you perform. You must determine what you are willing to receive for each massage you perform. The percentage you receive may depend on who furnishes the equipment, supplies, and services such as telephone, receptionist, advertising, and the like.

YOUR BUSINESS TELEPHONE

The business telephone is a powerful advertising tool. It is your contact with potential and steady clients. Anyone placing or receiving calls must know and use proper telephone techniques and courtesies. Your telephone number will accompany your business ads in telephone directories or newspapers and will be printed on your business cards. Therefore, the person answering your telephone should know how to do the following:

- Give accurate information and encourage a potential client to make an appointment.
- Make or change appointments for clients when necessary.
- Take messages accurately.
- Return all calls promptly.
- Place orders for supplies and other items when needed.
- Handle any complaints tactfully.
- Remind clients of appointments or needed services.
- Build goodwill and new business.
- Screen calls.

In addition to the foregoing, your business telephone serves as a security instrument in calling for help in case of emergency. For the protection of your employees and clients, the following phone numbers should be displayed near your business telephone:

- Nearest fire station
- Nearest ambulance service and hospital emergency service
- Police, local and state
- Taxi service
- Companies that provide needed services such as telephone, utilities, and the like
- Names and telephone numbers of owners, managers, custodians, and employees

- Names, addresses, and telephone numbers of all clients, which are kept in a private file but available in case of emergency

If you work out of your home and use your personal telephone for business purposes, there are a few special considerations. Business telephone expenses are tax deductible. If you use your home telephone for business purposes, the portion of your home telephone bill that is business related (i.e., long-distance business phone calls) is tax deductible if you maintain a telephone log book with the date, destination, and purpose for the call. (The base charges for your personal home phone are not deductible.) If you use your home phone number on your business cards and other advertising, it is considered a business phone and is subject to higher business telephone rates. If your phone is a business telephone (you pay business rates), the entire bill is tax deductible.

BASICS OF BOOKKEEPING

A good recordkeeping system is essential to the success of a business. You will need to keep client records as well as records of income from both services and sales of products. Receipts, canceled checks, and invoices should be kept in appropriate files for tax purposes. Even though businesses hire accountants, it is still important for the self-employed practitioner, business manager, or owner to understand the basics of the system. It is more difficult to manage a business if you do not understand the principles of sound business administration and management. It is a plus for an inexperienced person to have some training in business administration before opening a business.

Without a proper bookkeeping system and accurate records, the owner or manager of a business would not be able to determine the progress of the business, especially the cost of doing business in relation to income. Business records are necessary to meet the requirements of local, state, and federal laws pertaining to taxes and employees. The manager of the business should see that records are kept properly for social security and taxes (state, local, federal taxes). If employees are involved, the manager should also be aware of recording payroll, wage and hour laws, worker's compensation, and any other laws or regulations that apply to hiring (or firing) employees.

A bookkeeping system should only be as complicated as the business requires. For a self-employed individual, a simple system that records income and disbursements is sufficient. Once a good system is set up and kept current, it reduces the year-end tax preparation drudgery and offers an accurate accounting of the business's financial position. Consulting an accountant is helpful when setting up a bookkeeping system and advisable when preparing taxes. A good accountant knows the changing tax laws and can often find many deductions you may otherwise miss.

Accounting packages have been designed specifically for the massage therapist. They may be advertised in one of the massage industry's journals or magazines. Make sure they are updated and meet your needs.

A Word or Two about Using Computers

If you have a computer and are somewhat comfortable using it, the right software can make the process of bookkeeping much easier. There are several programs that enable the user to easily enter information and create a number of reports. In programs like Quicken® and Quickbooks®, by entering the information from your checkbook register (or writing your checks by way of the computer), you can generate a wide variety of reports and graphs. When recording checks, you enter the payee and the category of the expenditure. Another feature allows you to break down your deposits into various income categories. With a couple of key strokes you can create cash flow charts, income statements, accounts payable, accounts receivable, balance sheets, and a number of other reports.

Other computer accounting programs allow even more functions, such as writing invoices and inventory control. There is a growing number of computer software packages that have been designed specifically for the massage business to manage client files, including appointments, SOAP notes, insurance, and financial files. Most of these programs, however, do not include business accounting. Obtain the computer software that will do what you need it to do. Make sure that the software and hardware are reliable, and *always* back up your work.

If you do not have a computer and are not familiar with how to operate one, this is probably not the best time to start. You have enough on your hands getting your new business off the ground and most likely do not have a lot of capital in the bank to invest in the hardware and software that are required.

There are several ingredients to a workable bookkeeping system. The following are some of the basics.

Business Checking Account

A business checking account enables you to separate personal and business expenses. Open a separate account under the name of the business. Deposit all business income into the account. This will provide a record of your earnings. Use it whenever making cash disbursements. Pay all business bills by check, which will provide a record of your expenditures. Write checks out of the business account to pay yourself. Then cash those checks or deposit them into your personal account in order to pay personal bills. This is called "personal draw" or "owner's expense." Do not use the business account to pay personal or nonbusiness expenses.

When a check is written, be sure to clearly record in the check register the check number, the date the check was written, to whom the check was written, what the check was written for (the category or type of expense), and the amount of the check. All this information must be recorded in the disbursement journal. If any of it is missing, it makes bookkeeping more difficult. An updated checkbook ledger is a good way to register disbursements and income. More complete ledgers are necessary to track a business's financial standing.

Petty Cash Account

petty cash fund
is maintained to pay small disbursements for incidentals.

A **petty cash fund** can be maintained to pay small disbursements for incidentals. Receipts should be kept for each transaction, which should be properly recorded in the ledger. Occasionally, a check should be written from the business checking account to bring the petty cash fund back to a desired level.

Bank Statements and Reconciliations

Each month, the bank will send a bank statement listing the deposits you have made for the month, the checks that have been processed through your account, any bank charges or interest payments, and the balance left in the account. All these figures should be compared with your records to make sure neither you nor the bank has made any mistakes and that you agree on the balance in your account. On the back of most bank statements is a worksheet that can be used to reconcile your account. Be prompt in reconciling the statement with your checkbook. Note any errors, omissions, or miscalculations. Correct your mistakes and notify the bank immediately of any problems. Keep all bank statements, reconciliations, and canceled checks in your files a minimum of ~~three~~ seven years as proof of expenditures.

Credit Cards

You might consider acquiring a credit card to use solely for business purposes. Credit cards are wonderful if you are going to do any business traveling. You can use them to reserve and pay for hotels, plane tickets, or restaurant tabs. They are convenient, and all expenditures are listed on the credit card billing, which simplifies your bookkeeping. You must, however, still retain cash reciepts for your tax records.

Just as checking accounts have a variety of charges and benefits, credit cards have different cost and amenities. They vary in the annual fee, the interest charged on the balance in the account, and the grace period allowed after a purchase is made before interest is charged on the balance. Your credit line may also vary, from $1,000 to $100,000 or above. Some credit cards have added benefits such as free travel insurance, discounts on car rentals, or no-fee traveler checks. Several credit card companies offer a rewards program in which each dollar spent earns points toward airline travel, hotel stays, merchandise, or even cash back. By shopping around a little, you may be able to save in the long run. Regardless of the credit card you decide on, if you pay off the balance promptly every month and keep the balance at zero, you will avoid paying exorbitant finance and interest charges.

Income Records

There are two basic steps to recording business income. The first step takes place when the income is first received and an invoice or sales slip is filled out. The second step is when the invoices are totaled, summarized, and recorded in an income ledger.

Writing out an invoice or a cash receipt every time money is taken in is a convenient way to keep track of how much money has been brought in and specifically for what. Invoices should be written in duplicate. The original goes to the client for his records, and the copy goes into the cash box or daily records. At the end of the day or week or whatever recording period you choose, the invoices are tallied and recorded on the income ledger.

For a business that does only massage, a simple invoice that indicates how much the massage service costs is sufficient. If the business offers a variety of services and products, the invoice may be more complex. In states that have a sales tax, the invoice should have space for nontaxable services (or items), taxed items (retail sales), amount of sales tax, and the total. If you offer credit, it is a federal law that the terms of credit and finance charges are clearly disclosed on the invoice.

The invoice should include the following:

- Your business name
- The date
- The client's name (and address)
- A description of services given
- Amount charged for services
- A description of goods sold
- Amount charged for the goods sold
- Amount of sales tax
- The total
- A space to indicate the date paid

If you extend credit, you must include on the invoice your credit terms and finance charge. Keep a copy of the invoice for your records and give a copy to the client.

The income ledger is a summary of all cash receipts or invoices. The information from sales invoices is tallied and posted on the income ledger. It is one of the most important business documents you have. It shows you where your money is coming from and when it is or is not flowing. It is a primary source for preparing cash flow summaries, sales tax reports, and income taxes. It is also helpful when planning advertising, expenditures, and vacations.

How frequently the information is posted into the income ledger depends on the volume of business. The information you need to note on a ledger sheet depends on the nature of your massage business. If all your income is strictly from doing massage in your studio, the income ledger could be very simple. If your business sells any products or offers a variety of services, your income ledger will be more sophisticated to reflect the different sources of incoming funds.

If your sales volume is quite large, daily posting may be appropriate. However, in most individual massage practices, weekly posting is sufficient.

A word to the wise: Don't let the paperwork pile up! Be prompt and do the book work regularly. It really becomes a headache when you get behind. Each time you tally up your receipts to deposit your incoming funds in the bank, record your totals onto your income ledger, and your book work is done.

The income ledger should have a sufficient number of columns to list the classifications and sources of money coming into your business. Provide a column for income from massage services. If your business provides a variety of massage services that you want to track, you may want to include a column for each of those services. Examples might be outcalls, seated massage, hydrotherapy, or tanning booths. If your business sells massage-related products, include a column for retail or taxable sales and another column for sales tax. The sales tax column greatly simplifies filing quarterly sales tax documents. If you have any nontaxed income such as wholesale, out-of-state sales, or freight, include another column for nontaxed income. The last column on the ledger should record your total sales.

The sample ledger in Figure 19.4a has columns for the date, massage income, gift certificate income, nontaxed retail, taxable income, and sales tax. There is also a column for other income with a space for description of the income source. This might include freight, reimbursement for travel, or royalties. Finally, there is a column for the total. The amount in the total column should equal the sum of the other columns and be the amount that is recorded on the bank deposit slip.

Regardless of how often you post information into your books, keep the months separate and run monthly totals. This will become important information when planning specials, advertising, expenditures, and vacations. You can record monthly totals on a summary sheet like the one in Figure 19.4b in order to better track your business activity. It also simplifies quarterly and year-end taxes.

File all your sales invoices and keep them for a minimum of three years. Every month, bundle all the invoices together for that month and store them in a file. They are documents that support your records and tax returns, and you may need them if you ever get audited.

Disbursement Record

The disbursement ledger is your record of all the expenditures the business pays out, including bills, loan payments, and the money you pay yourself (personal draws). Some of these expenditures are tax deductible, and some are not. A huge advantage of being self-employed is that much of what you do or buy can be considered business related and is therefore tax deductible. Obtain and keep receipts for all expenditures and record them in the disbursement ledger. The function of the disbursement ledger is to separate and classify business expenditures both for tax purposes and so that you can easily identify where your money is going. You are thereby able to plan and budget better.

Daily Income Ledger for Month of _____ 20_____

Date	Massage Income	Gift Certificates	Other Income	Nontaxable Retail	Taxable Retail	Sales Tax	Total Income
Total							
YTD							

Figure 19.4a

Sample income ledger.

Yearly Summary Income Ledger for 20_____

Month	Massage Income	Gift Certificates	Other Income	Nontaxable Retail	Taxable Retail	Sales Tax	Total Income
January							
February							
March							
1st Quarter							
April							
May							
June							
2nd Quarter							
July							
August							
September							
3rd Quarter							
October							
November							
December							
4th Quarter							
Yearly Total							

Figure 19.4b

Sample yearly income summary ledger.

Nearly all the information that goes into the disbursement ledger comes from the checkbook register or credit card statement. If for some reason there are any cash outlays or payments made with money orders, those should be posted in the disbursement ledger as soon as possible. Try to make ALL business expenditures from the checkbook or credit card. Even though information on the disbursement ledger comes from the checkbook, it is still necessary to maintain both. The information that each document furnishes is different and important. The checkbook allows you to keep a running balance of your account. It also provides a space for marking off canceled checks and posting deposits. The disbursement ledger includes expenditures paid by cash or money order and categorizes expenditures so that you can easily see how much you have spent on what.

Ideally every entry on the disbursement ledger can be validated by a receipt. When you pay your bills, pay them by check, put the check number on the receipt from the billing, and file that receipt. It is a good idea to bundle the receipts together each month, put them in an envelope, label it with the month and year, and keep it in a file. Keep all receipts a minimum of three years in case you are audited.

The disbursement ledger (Figure 19.5) is divided into several columns. The first four columns contain the date of the expenditure, the check number (or if the payment was made with cash or money order), the payee, and the amount of the check or payment. The rest of the columns represent the category of the expenditure. There are literally dozens of possible categories. Following later is a list of 36 categories that are common in a massage practice. It is not practical to have a separate column for every category. The example disbursement ledger in this chapter has nine columns, most of which actually have two categories. One column is a catch-all "misc." column.

Most disbursements are tax deductible; however, some paid-outs such as loan payments and owner's expenses are not. Be sure to allow a separate column for nondeductible expenses. The last column is for the "owner's draw" or the money that you pay to yourself. At the bottom of the ledger is a space to total the figures in each column. The total of the category columns should equal the total of the "check amount" column. If it does not, recheck all your figures and find your mistake.

It is a good idea to total all the columns of the disbursement ledger every month and record those totals on a summary sheet. This is a good way to keep track of your expenses and adjust your expenditures.

Note: If you use a computer, a variety of software companies have accounting programs that include checking, income, and disbursement functions.

List of Business Expenses

Business expenses are partially or totally deductible from the business income when determining the profit or loss of the business. These categories can be used when writing checks and on the disbursement ledger.

The following are possible expenses:

- Accounting expense
- Advertising
- Automobile expense

  Fuel

  Maintenance

  Payments

  License fees

Expenditure From _____ 20___ **To** _____ 20___

Date	Check No.	Payee Description	Check Amount	Advertise Insurance	Inventory Education	Cleaning Labor	Tax, Lic. Dues	Postage Supplies	Rent Repair	Utilities Tele	Misc	Owner's Draw
		Total Line A										
		Total Line B										
		GRAND TOTALS										

Figure 19.5

Sample disbursement ledger.

- Bad debts
- Bank fees
- Cleaning and janitorial
- Contract labor
- Convention costs
- Cost of products to be sold
- Depreciation
- Donations to charity
- Dues to business and professional associations
- Education expense

    Seminars, professional journals, books, and the like

- Entertainment
- Equipment expense
- Furnishings and fixtures
- Insurance premiums

    Auto, liability, malpractice, fire, theft

- Interest paid on loans
- License and permit fees
- Office supplies
- Payroll, wages, and withholdings
- Postage, freight, and shipping
- Professional, legal, or consulting fees
- Refunds for services or products
- Rent
- Repair and maintenance
- Supplies
- Taxes

    Sales, property, state, federal

- Telephone
- Travel, business related
- Utilities

An expenditure that is not considered an expense is the owner's expense or salary paid to yourself.

Business-Related Receipts

Keep all receipts for every purchase or expenditure related in any way to the business. After recording transactions, file the receipts. Each month, create a new file so that the receipts are separated to reflect and support the entries in the monthly disbursement ledger. For tax reasons, keep all receipts for a minimum of three years.

Accounts Receivable

If you extend credit and bill your clients, you will have to keep an ongoing record of each transaction. This does complicate the bookkeeping process considerably. To keep it simple, require cash payments at the time of service for everything except gift certificates, advance payments, insurance billings, and credit card payments (i.e., Visa and Mastercard). *Accounts receivable* is a record of moneys owed to you by other persons or businesses. Record each charge and payment, including the date of the transaction and current balance.

Accounts Payable

If you buy supplies or services on credit, keep a file for each account or business that extends you credit. *Accounts payable* records the moneys you owe other persons or businesses. File statements and purchase orders so that you have an accurate record when it is time to pay the bills. Trades and barters should be recorded on a separate record.

Assets and Depreciation Records

Items and equipment purchased to be used in your business for an extended period of time (more than a year) are considered business assets. Supplies and inventory are not considered assets. Maintain a current record of business assets that includes an item description, date of purchase, and purchase price. Add new items when purchased and remove items when they are sold or retired from use.

Depending on the purchase price of a durable item and the business's financial situation, you may choose to declare it, for tax purposes, as a one-time business expense or depreciate its cost over a number of years. Methods and schedules for depreciating different items vary according to the length of the useful life of the item. It is not within the scope of this book to discuss depreciation methods. Consult with your accountant or refer to *The Tax Guide for Small Business*, published by the IRS, for detailed instructions. Maintain a depreciation record for all depreciable assets.

Keep a file on all major items and equipment, including purchase records, instruction manuals, service records, warranties, and guarantees.

Inventory

A good inventory system helps to ensure that you will not run out of supplies or be overstocked on items that do not move well. Supplies to be used are classified as consumption supplies, and those to be sold are classified as retail supplies. You may need to keep records of sales tax on supplies sold.

If you sell products as part of your business, you are required to take an inventory at the end of the year to determine cost-of-goods-sold for the year. The cost-of-goods-sold is a business expense. The inventory you still have on hand at the end of the year is considered an asset and will not be considered as cost-of-goods-sold until the time it is sold.

In order to determine cost-of-goods-sold:

	Determine cost of inventory as of January 1 of the tax year
+	Inventory purchased during the year
=	Total inventory available for sale
−	Cost of inventory as of December 31 of the tax year
=	Cost-of-goods-sold for the year

Mileage Log

All business-related travel should be recorded for tax purposes. Expenses for operating a vehicle for business are deductible from taxable income. This does not include travel from home to the place of business. There are two ways of determining this deduction: the standard mileage allowance or actual automobile expense.

When an automobile is used in the course of the business, keep a mileage log and record all business travel. For each trip, record the destination, beginning and ending odometer readings, total miles traveled, and purpose of the trip. According to 2003 tax laws, a deduction of 37¢ a mile could be taken for business-related automobile use. (This figure may vary. Check with an accountant or the IRS for the current rate.)

If you deduct the actual auto expense, keep an itemized record of all expenses (fuel, service, insurance, license fees, parking, and depreciation records of actual purchase price). The auto expense is prorated between business use and personal use. For example, if you drove the vehicle 12,000 miles in a year and 4,000 miles was business related, you would deduct 33.3 percent of the total auto expenses from the business income.

Updated Client Files

The client file is the mechanism practitioners use to record pertinent client information and document the work they have done with clients. The information a practitioner keeps in the client files varies as much as the massage routines of different practitioners. Updated client files help the practitioner render prompt and efficient service and ensure access to current information regarding the client. Information that is often found in a client file includes intake information (Figure 19.6a), a treatment plan, informed consent, session documentation, and a record of payment (Figure 19.6b). Intake information includes name, address, phone, and medical information and history. A treatment plan provides a kind of a blueprint for the sessions that is updated periodically. Each session is documented with the type of service given, the date given, the products used, and the results obtained. A payment record lists the amount charged and received for each item and service. Keeping accurate and updated records is a tedious but essential part of a professional operation.

Appointment Book

The appointment book is possibly the most important document for organizing a successful and prosperous business. It is an important tool in time management. A well-kept appointment book ensures that appointments are not missed and are scheduled so that you can be prompt and

Massage Clinic
Client Information Form

Name_____   Birth Date _____

Address _____   Telephone _____

_____   Business Phone _____

City/State/Zip _____   Social Security # _____

Occupation _____   Other Activities_____

General Health Condition_____   Blood Pressure _____

Have you had any serious or chronic illness, operations, chronic virus infections, or trau-

matic accidents? _____

Are you in recovery for addictions or abuse?_____

Are you under a doctor's, chiropractor's, or other health practitioner's care? _____

If so, for what condition(s)? _____

Are you on any medication?_____ If so, what? _____

Do I have permission to contact your doctor/therapist?_____

Names of doctors, chiropractors, or health practitioners:

Name_____   Name _____

Address _____   Address _____

Telephone _____   Telephone _____

Why did you come for our services? (relaxation, pain, therapy, etc.)_____

_____

What results would you like to achieve with our work? _____

Have you had any massage therapy before?_____If so, by whom? _____

How did you find out about our services? _____

Were you referred to this office?_____By whom? _____

In case of emergency notify: Name_____Phone_____

I have completed this information form to the best of my knowledge. I understand the
massage services are designed to be a health aid and are in no way to take the place of
a doctor's care when it is indicated. Information exchanged during any massage session
is educational in nature and is intended to help me become more familiar and conscious
of my own health status and is to be used at my own discretion.

Our time together is precious, and I agree to cancel 24 hours in advance. Unless there
is an emergency, if I miss an appointment, I agree to pay the full appointment fee.

Date_____ Signature _____

Figure 19.6a

Sample intake form.

Client Name _____ Date 1st Session _____

Address _____ City_____ St_____ ZIP_____

Phone (h)_____ (w)_____ Insurance _____

Date	Service	Products	Tax	Charges	Credits	Balance	Comments

REFERRAL RECORD

Client Referred By _____ Date _____

New Clients Referred by This Client

Name	Date 1st Session	Acknowledged

Figure 19.6b

Sample payment record.

on time. There is nothing more embarrassing than to have two people show up for a massage at the same time. Keep your appointment book handy and always up-to-date. If you carry an appointment book with you, it can become a portable file to record mileage, important phone numbers, business expenses, as well as appointments. It is still advisable to maintain a client appointment book at your office. Be sure to transfer information from your portable appointment book to your office book to avoid double bookings.

The appointment book should have enough space to record each client's appointment time, name, phone number (address and directions if it is an outcall), and possibly the amount you receive from each client.

Some clients will book the same time on a regular basis. These regular customers are the mainstay of many businesses because they can be counted on for a certain amount of regular income.

Bookkeeping Tips

Record keeping is an essential part of maintaining a successful business. Once a filing and bookkeeping system is established, be persistent by continually updating the files. Here are a few tips that will simplify the task:

- Keep all records current.
- Review client files before each session and document each session promptly after the session.
- When writing checks, record the amount and expenditure category in the check register.
- Keep and file all business-related receipts.
- Update income and disbursement ledgers regularly.
- Reconcile bank statements promptly.
- Keep all tax-related records:

Receipts	(at least 3 years)
Ledgers, canceled checks, and so on	(at least 3 years)
Tax returns	(at least 10 years)
Real estate and business contracts	(indefinitely)

Preparation of Federal and State Taxes

If you have a net annual income of more that $600, you must file federal income tax forms. If you are a self-employed massage therapist, you will be required to include a Schedule C (Sole Proprietorship Business or Profession Profit or Loss Form) and a Schedule SE (Social Security Self-Employment Tax Form) along with your federal income tax. If you had any subcontractors to whom you paid more than $600 during the year, you must also file 1099s and the accompanying 1096 forms. Taxes are filed each year before the April 15 deadline. If you are self-employed, you may expect to pay estimated state and federal taxes quarterly. The estimated tax is approximately one fourth of the previous year's income tax, and payments are due by the 15th of April, June, September, and January respectively.

If you have been diligent in keeping your books, tax preparation is much simpler. Most of the information you need for tax forms comes right off your income and disbursement ledgers and summaries. Your disbursement ledger will list the amount and description of most of your business expenses. The exceptions will be bad debts, automobile expenses, and business use of the home (if you work out of your home).

There are innumerable tax laws (including new ones almost every year), and unless you have a natural disposition toward preparing taxes, it is usually a good idea to seek the help of a tax preparation professional. A competent tax preparer is well worth the expense and can usually save you money by pointing out deductions you would otherwise miss and by making sure that all the proper forms are prepared correctly, thereby saving you mistakes and possible penalties. Even if you do use a tax preparer, however, you are ultimately responsible for your taxes. Being familiar with tax requirements will affect your bookkeeping, your business profits, and your relationship with your tax accountant. Besides, it may result in tax savings your tax preparer fails to recommend. A good publication that provides up-to-date tax information is the *Tax Guide for Small Business,* prepared by the Internal Revenue Service and available at your local IRS office.

MARKETING

Marketing is all the business activity done to promote and increase your business. Some marketing activities include advertising, promotion, public relations, referrals, and client retention. Marketing is an educational process of getting yourself and what you do known. It is the enticement that encourages an individual to seek your services. Marketing is an ongoing activity in your business. The goal of marketing is to create and maintain a thriving practice. When developing marketing materials and practices in the field of massage, be certain that they reflect the image you want to portray.

Assess Marketing Needs

Your particular marketing needs are determined by several factors, including the amount of time or money you can afford, your target market, and the size of your practice. If you are starting out in your practice, you may not have a large clientele and therefore have a lot of time and not a lot of money. More time can be spent on making contacts, giving presentations, writing articles, and making personal appearances. Concentrate on activities that are low-cost but may be more time-consuming. Actively educate the public as to what you do and how it will benefit them.

If you have a fairly busy practice already, time may be limited, but you have a larger advertising budget. You may concentrate more on client retention, developing referrals, direct mail, and targeted advertising to announce special services.

There are many marketing techniques to choose from that can be selected and designed to best suit your personal marketing needs.

Analyze Target Markets

Massage is a service that tends to appeal to specific segments of the population. Target groups are various segments of the population that have similar characteristics. Your target market consists of those target groups that you prefer to attract to your services. Selecting a target market enables you to modify your advertising and promotional activities to appeal to the specific group.

The parameters of target groups are innumerable. They may be very broad (i.e., women or athletes or the elderly or professional people). They can be specific (i.e., low birth weight infants, female runners, accountants, or abuse survivors). Several attributes that depict groups are age, gender, income, occupation, interests, and location.

There are at least two ways to determine your particular target market. One is to consider what type of clientele you want to attract. When you have made your choices, contact clubs and organizations in your area that cater to individuals from that group. Offer to be a speaker or do a demonstration. Create brochures highlighting benefits of massage for the specific conditions common to that group. Place ads and articles in magazines and newsletters. Make personal contact with individuals and participate in activities common to your target market.

Another way to determine your target market is to assess your client files to determine who is presently using your services and what they have in common. Then design promotional activities that reach that segment of the population.

It is wise to have more than one or even several target markets. The number depends on your preference, your expertise, and the size of your practice.

Business Promotion

The objective of promotion is to become known, to be visible to those in the community that may seek your service. It is also to create the desire in potential clients to use your services. Promotional activities, especially in a service industry such as massage, are largely educational in nature. They let your target population know who you are, what you do, and how your services will benefit them.

Common methods of business promotion include public speaking and appearances, articles in newspapers and professional magazines, and booths at health fairs and other public functions. These provide excellent opportunities to educate prospective client groups. An excellent promotional tool to familiarize the public with the experience of touch and the benefits of massage is the massage chair. Chair massage has provided a means of bringing massage out of the private studio and into more public awareness. A massage chair can be set up essentially anywhere and provide the wider public the opportunity to experience the relaxing benefits of massage in a safe, nonthreatening environment without needing to disrobe. Many times, a chair massage leads a potential client to make an appointment for full-body massages.

Developing Promotional Material

An important part of your promotional activity is having appropriate printed materials to distribute when you come in contact with potential customers. Printed materials include business cards, brochures, stationery, and newsletters. Your printed material should appeal to your target market and reflect your professionalism. Always include your name, business address, and phone number on every piece of promotional material.

Whenever you speak to a group or an individual about your services, be sure to leave a card or brochure. Even though you will not generally get a new client directly from your printed material, it serves as a reminder and contains information about how to contact you.

Internet

The Internet has created a new marketing possibility called the Web page. Anyone can have a Web site on the Internet. A Web site is an efficient and cost-effective way for the massage practitioner or business owner to communicate with clients or to market to new clients. The Web site can be used to advertise the business; provide educational information; describe services; list policies, procedures, and prices for services; and even book appointments. The Web site may contain articles on wellness, describe or show catalog products that are for sale, or contain links to other sites that might be of interest. The Web site can be used as a contact page for clients to download forms, ask questions, or make comments about services they receive and make or cancel appointments. The Web site may be a simple one-page site with all the necessary information for a client to contact your business, or it may contain several pages crammed with interesting and vital information.

Building a Web site requires some skill. There are products available that simplify the process, so it is possible for anyone with sufficient computer skills to build and maintain a site. However, to save time and possible frustration, hiring or trading for the services of an experienced Web designer and explaining what features you want to include might be the wiser thing to do.

The practitioner may also stay in contact with clients or send out occasional promotional offers via e-mail. The fact that most households in the United States now are connected to the Internet and use it to gain information and communicate makes it an important and effective means of marketing and communication.

Advertising

Advertising is generally the marketing activity that is done in return for direct payment. This includes magazine and newspaper ads and listings, signs, embossed pens and calendars, and the like.

Advertising is important to business success because it notifies the public about your services and how to contact you. When giving personal services such as massage, it is particularly important that your advertising not be misunderstood and that it creates a favorable impression to the public. Advertising should always reflect your professional status and the quality of your services. Keeping your name before the public will be important to building your business and reminding clients to use your services.

Plan your advertising budget. You must try to obtain the most effective media for the amount of money you have budgeted for advertising purposes. Newspaper advertising is generally the most economical way to reach the most people when you are opening a new business. By placing your ad in a specific section of the newspaper, such as the health or sports section, you can target the ad to the market you want to reach. The people in the advertising department of the paper will help you determine cost, size, and style of your ad.

A classified ad in the Yellow Pages of your local telephone directory is a fairly inexpensive and effective method of advertising for personal service businesses. Make sure to list your service under Massage—Therapeutic, with your credentials and association affiliations.

Direct mail is effective advertising for certain target markets. You may want to obtain a mailing list from a company that sells specifically targeted consumer lists.

Advertising consultants are expensive, but if you have a flexible advertising budget, you may find that a professional consultant can save you both time and money. A good consultant will be able to help you with creative ideas for logos, letterheads, and advertising that gets your message across in the most professional, tasteful, and dramatic way (Figure 19.7).

Public Relations

Some of the best advertising you can get is free. A feature article in a local newspaper is an excellent way to gain recognition in your community. News releases that announce classes you offer or awards and certifications you receive are also ways of promoting your business.

Offer to make personal appearances to give talks and demonstrations to various groups. You may offer to speak at social meetings, health clubs, sports events, schools, or as a guest on a radio or television talk show. You could act as guest instructor at a school or health facility where your type of personal services could be taught.

An essential aspect in developing good public relations is networking. Networking is developing personal and professional contacts for the purpose of giving and receiving support and sharing resources and information. Become involved in networking groups such as the chamber of commerce or other business groups. Participate in seminars or functions to meet others with whom you may develop networking relationships. Always keep business cards handy when attending these functions and freely distribute them. It is a good practice to give two or three cards at a time so that the recipient can pass one along to someone else. When you receive a business card from someone, make a note on the card as to what that person may provide for you. Keep a professional card file or a Rolodex® with those cards and refer to it when needs arise or when you are mailing out information.

Encouraging Referrals

One of the most effective and inexpensive methods of creating new business is through referrals. The two main sources of referrals are current clients and other health care professionals.

Satisfied customers are one of your most effective means of advertising. Remember, in word-of-mouth advertising, the most important mouth is yours. Encourage referrals. Let your clients know that you not only appreciate their business, but that if they appreciate what you do, they should tell others. Give them extra business cards and encourage them to tell their friends and associates about your service.

To promote referrals from other professionals, make yourself and what you do known to them. Explain how your services would benefit them and their clients. Write letters, and then follow up the letter with a phone call. Set up a personal meeting or take them to lunch. Give them a treatment so that they can experience first-hand what you have to offer. Always present yourself in a professional manner. When other health care professionals send referrals, confer with them to determine their reasons and goals for sending the client to you. Report back to them about the client's progress as a result of massage. A good working relationship between health care professionals will generate more referrals. It will also initiate more holistic client care by promoting interdisciplinary treatment plans.

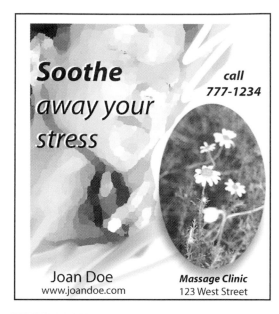

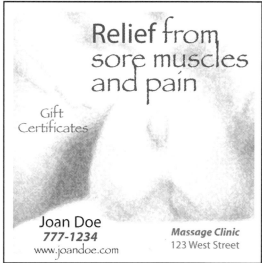

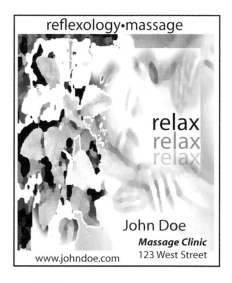

Figure 19.7
Effective advertising.

Whenever a new client comes in who has been referred, be sure to acknowledge the person who referred him with a thank-you note. Extend a special discount or even an occasional extra no-charge product or service to individuals who make multiple referrals.

When you do get referrals from someone, return the courtesy by referring people back or using the person's services yourself.

Remember the three R's of referrals: request, reward, and reciprocate. Request referrals from satisfied clients and professionals. Reward those who send you referrals with prompt thank-you cards or personal phone calls. Reciprocate by sending referrals or using the services of those who send you referrals.

Client Retention

Your clients are your most valuable asset. Clients who return on a regular basis are the mainstay of your practice. According to Cherie Sohnen-Moe *(Business Mastery, 1997)*, "On the average it costs six times as much money and takes three times the effort getting new clients as retaining current ones." Encourage clients to return for regular appointments. A weekly massage is a healthy investment. Before a client leaves your office, be sure that he has scheduled the next appointment.

Treat your clients with courtesy and respect. Give them the service for which they will want to return. It requires more than just being a skilled massage technician to retain clients. Beside giving a good massage, make sure that your client feels appreciated and cared for. Document each session, paying attention to the client's personal interests, likes, and dislikes. Refer to your records before each visit to remind you of their idiosyncrasies. Avoid their dislikes, discuss their interests, and do those special little things they like. Thank them for coming in.

Follow-up especially intense sessions with a phone call to ask how the client is. Send cards for important occasions such as birthdays and holidays. Always send thank-you notes when a client sends a referral. If a client is deserving, send a certificate for a free massage. Many personal service businesses offer gift certificates or special prices to loyal customers.

Keep your clientele on a mailing list, send them newsletters, periodic flyers, birthday or holiday greetings, or offer special discounts during slow times.

Remember, the clients are your reason for practicing, they are the source of your income, and they deserve the best service you can give.

BUSINESS LAW

In conducting business and employing help, it is necessary to comply with local, state, and federal laws and regulations. Federal laws cover social security, unemployment compensation or insurance, and tax payments on income as well as a number of other taxes. Income tax laws are covered by both the state and federal governments. State laws cover sales taxes, licenses, worker's compensation, employment regulations, and the like. Business owners and managers may hire a lawyer or a tax accountant, but they should also be familiar with these laws and regulations.

HIRING EMPLOYEES

Hiring employees increases your potential to provide services to more people. It also increases the employer's responsibility regarding recordkeeping and tax regulations. An employer is required to maintain separate payroll records for each employee, withhold state and federal taxes and social security, prepare quarterly payroll tax returns, pay the employer's portion of social security and unemployment taxes, and purchase worker's compensation insurance.

Many businesses will want to hire massage therapists as *contract labor*. When doing so, a person is an *independent contractor* and is hired on as her own boss for a per client fee or a percentage without taxes, worker's compensation, or social security being deducted from wages. An independent contractor is self-employed and is responsible for her own taxes. If you hire an independent contractor and pay her more than $600 in the course of a year, you are required to file tax forms 1099 and 1096. There are federal IRS guidelines that must be followed closely when dealing with contract labor. Be sure to check with the state employment office or the IRS for a copy of these guidelines before hiring contract labor.

If you are an employer, you are expected to be fair and honorable in dealing with employees, and you have a right to expect the same consideration from those you hire. Employees can make the difference between success and failure of a personal service business. Clients often return to a place of business because they like the people who serve them as much as, if not more than, the products and services. The following are important considerations when hiring someone to represent your place of business. The potential employee should:

1. Have the necessary licenses or other credentials required by law

2. Set a good example by having clean, healthy personal habits

3. Be profit conscious and willing to work hard to achieve business goals

4. Be courteous and professional when dealing with all clients

5. Obey all rules, regulations, and laws pertaining to the business

6. Be willing to learn new techniques and to grow both personally and professionally

7. Be self-motivated and industrious

8. Be honest and ethical

CHECKLIST

In summary, there is more to being successful in a massage business than being able to perform a good massage. A positive attitude, clear goals, and some understanding of business practices are essential for success.

The following is a checklist of important basics to consider before opening a business of your own. Use this checklist as a guide to important factors before opening a business.

- Capital
    - Amount available
    - Amount required
- Organization
    - Sole proprietor, partnership, corporation
- Banking
    - Opening a business account
    - Deposits, drawing checks
    - Monthly statements
    - Establishing credit
    - Business loans
- Selecting a location
    - Population
    - Transportation facilities
    - Quiet enough to induce relaxation
    - Space required
    - Zoning ordinances
    - Parking
    - Accessibility
    - Surrounding neighborhood
- Decorating and floor plan
    - Interior decorating
    - Installing telephones
    - Exterior decorating
- Bookkeeping system
    - Record of appointments
    - Receipts and disbursements
    - Petty cash
    - Profit and loss
    - Inventory
    - Client files
- Cost of operation
    - Supplies, depreciation
    - Rent, lights, utilities

- Cleaning service, laundry
- Salaries
- Products for services
- Telephone
- Taxes, insurance

● Management
- Methods of building goodwill
- Client courtesies, gifts
- Adjusting complaints
- Personnel relations
- Public relations
- Selling merchandise

● Equipment and supplies
- Selecting equipment
- Installation of equipment

● Advertising
- Planning
- Business cards and brochures
- Direct mail
- Internet
- Newspaper
- Radio
- Personal appearances

● Legal
- Lease, contracts
- Compliance with state, local, and government laws
- Licensing of business
- Licensing of managers and practitioners

● Ethics and professional growth
- Setting goals
- Courtesy
- Observation of professional practices
- Interaction with professional groups

● Insurance
- Public liability and malpractice
- Compensation, unemployment
- Automobile
- Fire and theft

● Methods of payment
- Cash

In advance

Open account

Time payments

Charge cards

QUESTIONS FOR DISCUSSION AND REVIEW

1. How do attitude and self-image relate to business success?

2. Explain the difference between a partnership, a corporation, and a sole proprietorship.

3. What start-up costs may you expect when beginning a massage business?

4. List five important considerations when choosing a location for a massage business.

5. List the various permits and licenses that may be required to operate a massage business.

6. List the types of insurance a massage business owner should carry to protect the business.

7. Why is keeping accurate records necessary in a successful business?

8. List the major ingredients of a basic bookkeeping system.

9. What is marketing?

10. What are the main marketing techniques used in the massage industry?

11. Define target market.

12. What are the three R's of referrals?

Bibliography

Aaland, Mikkel. *Sweat: The Illustrated History and Description of the Finnish Sauna, Russian Bania, Islamic Hammam, Japanese Mushi-Buro, Mexican Temescal, and American Sweat Lodge.* Santa Barbara, CA: Capra Press, 1978.

Barstow, Cedar. *Right Use of Power.* Boulder, CO: Many Relms Publishing, 2003.

Benjamin, Ben E.; Sohnen-Moe, Cherie. *The Ethics of Touch.* Tucson, AZ: Sohnen-Moe Associates, 2003.

Bowman, Michelle; Lawlis, G. Frank. *Complementary and Alternative Medicine Management.* Gaithersburg, MD: Aspen Publishers, 2001.

Callahan, Margery; Luther, David W. *The Medical Massage Office Manual,* 2nd ed. Steamboat Springs, CO: Author, 1999.

Calvert, Robert N. *The History of Massage.* Rochester, VT: Healing Arts Press, 2002.

Chaitow, Leon. *Positional Release Techniques,* 2nd ed. London: Churchill Livingston, Harcourt, 2002.

Chaitow, Leon. *Muscle Energy Techniques.* London: Churchill Livingston, Harcourt Brace, 1996.

Chaitow, Leon. *Soft Tissue Manipulation.* Rochester, VT: Healing Arts Press, 1988.

Chaitow, Leon; Walker Delany, Judith. *Clinical Application of Neuromuscular Techniques, Vol. 1.* London: Churchill Livingston, 2000.

Chapman, Cheryl; Kennedy, Eileen. Mastectomy Massage. *Massage Therapy Journal* 39(3), 91–99, Fall 2000.

Chilky, Bruno. *Silent Waves, Theory and Practice of Lymph Drainage Massage.* Scottsdale, AZ: International Health & Healing, 2002.

Clay, James H.; Pounds, David M. *Basic Clinical Massage Therapy.* Baltimore: Lippincott Williams & Wilkins, 2003.

Clemente, Carmine D. *Anatomy, A Regional Atlas of the Human Body,* 3rd ed. Baltimore: Urban & Schwarzenberg, 1987.

Consumer & Spa Trends Report. Presentation at 2004 Spa & Resort Expo and Conference by Spa Finder's, (212) 924-6800.

Curties, D. Cancer Treatments. *Massage Therapy Journal* 39(4), 80–85, Winter 2001.

Curties, Debra. *Massage Therapy and Cancer.* Moncton, New Brunswick, Canada: Curties-Overzet Publications, 1999.

Curties, Debra. Could Massage Therapy Promote Cancer Metastasis? *Massage Therapy Journal* 39(3), 83–88, Fall 2000.

Curties, Debra. Could Massage Therapy Promote Cancer Metastasis? *Journal of Soft Tissue Manipulation* 3–5, April/May 1994.

D'Ambrogio, K.; Roth, G. *Positional Release Therapy.* St. Louis: Mosby, 1997.

Denning, Ed. *The Medical Code Manual for Massage Practitioners.* Clinton, OH: Massage Therapy Associates, 2001.

Devereux, Charla. *The Aromatherapy Kit.* London: Eddison Sadd Editions, 1993.

Eisenberg, D.M.; Davis, R.B.; Etner, S.L.; Apple, S.; Wilke S.; Van Rompey, M.; Kessler, R.C. Trends in Alternative Medicine Prevalence and Costs 1990–1997: Results of a Follow-Up National Survey. *Journal of the American Medical Association 280,* 1569–1575, 1998.

Eisenberg, D.M.; Kessler, R.C.; Foster, C.; Norwalk, N.E.; Calkins D.R.; Delbanco, T.L. Unconventional Medicine in the United States: Prevalence, Costs and Patterns of Use. *New England Journal of Medicine* 328(4), 246–253, 1993.

Fong, Elizabeth; Ferris, Elvira B.; Skelley, Esther G. *Body Structures & Function,* 7th ed. Clifton Park, NY: Thomson Delmar Learning, 1989.

Fritz, Sandy. *Fundamentals of Therapeutic Massage,* 2nd ed. St. Louis: Mosby, 2000.

Fritz, Sandy. *Fundamentals of Therapeutic Massage.* St. Louis, MO: Mosby Year Book, 1995.

Hoppenfeld, Stanley. *Physical Examination of the Spine and Extremities.* New York: Appleton Century Crofts, 1976.

Hungerford, Dr. Myk. *Beyond Sports Medicine.* Costa Mesa, CA: Sports Massage Training Inst., 1991.

Hungerford, Dr. Myk. *The Professional's Guide to Massage Therapy.* Costa Mesa, CA: Sports Massage Training Inst., 1988.

International Spa Association (ISPA) 2004 Spa Industry Study. Prepared by Association Resource Centre, Inc. (Contact ISPA in Lexington, Kentucky, at (888) 651-4772 for copies.)

Jones, Lawrence, D.O. *Strain and Counterstrain.* Colorado Springs, CO: American Academy of Osteopathy, 1981.

Juhan, Deane. *Job's Body, A Handbook for Bodyworkers.* Barrington, NY: Station Hill Press, 1987.

Hart, Marcia. *Structural/Muscular Balancing.* Carson City, NV: Thoth, 1992.

Kamoroff, Bernard. *Small Time Operator.* Laytonville, CA: Bell Springs, 1987.

Kapit, Wynn and Elson. *The Anatomy Coloring Book.* New York: Harper & Row, 1977.

Kendall, Florence; McCreary, Elizabeth. *Muscles: Testing and Function,* 3rd ed. Baltimore: Williams & Wilkins, 1983.

Knapp, Joan E.; Antonucci, Eileen J. *A National Study of the Profession of Massage Therapy and Bodywork.* Princeton, NJ: Knapp & Associates, 1990.

Lillis, Carol A. *Brady's Introduction to Medical Terminology.* Bowie, MD: Robert J. Brady, 1983.

Lindner, Harold H. *Clinical Anatomy.* Norwalk, CT: Appleton & Lange, 1989.

Lowe, Whitney. *Functional Assessment for Massage Therapists,* 3rd ed. Bend, OR: Orthopedic Massage Education and Research Institute, 1997.

MacDonald, Gayle. How Cancer Spreads. *Massage Therapy Journal* 39(4), 74–78, Winter 2001.

MacDonald, Gayle. *Medicine Hands: Massage Therapy for People with Cancer.* Findhorn, Scotland: Findhorn Press, 1999.

Madison-Mahoney, Vivian. *Comprehensive Guide to Insurance Billing.* Gatlinburg, TN: Author, 2002.

Magee, David. *Orthopedic Physical Assessment.* Philadelphia: W. B. Saunders, 1987.

Malloy, Janice. Do the Benefits of Massage Outweigh the Risks? *Massage Therapy Journal* 39(4), 60–73, Winter 2001.

McIntosh, Nina. *The Educated Heart.* Memphis, TN: Decatur Bainbridge Press, 1999.

Memmler, Ruth L.; Wood, Dena Lin. *The Human Body in Health and Disease,* 5th ed. Philadelphia: J. B. Lippincott, 1983.

Michlovitz, Susan L.; Wolf, Steven L. *Thermal Agents in Rehabilitation.* Philadelphia: F. A. Davis Company, 1986.

Moody-French, Ramona. *Guide to Lymph Drainage Massage.* Clifton Park, NY: Milady/ Thomson Delmar Learning, 2004.

Moor, Fred B., Peterson, Stella C., Manwell, Ethel M., Noble, Mary C., Meunch, Gertrude. *Manual of Hydrotherapy and Massage.* Oshawa, Ontario, Canada: Pacific Press Publishing Assn., 1964.

Mulvihill, Mary Lou. *Human Diseases, A Systematic Approach,* 2nd ed. Norwalk, CT: Appleton & Lange, 1987.

Platzer, Werner. *Color Atlas and Textbook of Human Anatomy,* 3rd ed. Stuttgart, Germany: Georg Thieme Verlag, 1986.

Prudden, Bonnie. *Pain Erasure.* New York: M. Evans & Co., 1980.

Salvo, Susan. *Massage Therapy Principles and Practice.* Philadelphia: W. B. Saunders, 1999.

Sieg, Kay M.; Adams, Sandra P. *Illustrated Essentials of Musculoskeletal Anatomy.* Gainesville, FL: Megabooks, 1985.

Smith, Genevieve Love; Davis, Phyllis E. *Medical Terminology,* 4th ed. New York: John Wiley & Sons, 1981.

Smith, Irene. *Guidelines for the Massage of AIDS Patients.* San Francisco: Service Through Touch, 1992.

Sohnen-Moe, Cherie. *Business Mastery,* 3rd ed. Tucson, AZ: Sohnen-Moe Associates, 1997.

St. John, Paul. *St. John Neuromuscular Therapy Seminars Manuals 1 & 4.* Largo, FL: Author, 1990.

Tappan, Frances M. *Healing Massage Technique, Holistic, Classical and Emerging Methods.* Norwalk, CT: Appleton & Lange, 1988.

Tappan, Frances M.; Benjamin, Patricia J. *Tappan's Handbook of Healing Massage Techniques.* Stanford, CT: Appleton & Lange, 1998.

Taylor, Kylea. *The Ethics of Caring.* Santa Cruz, CA: Hartford Mead, 1995.

Thompson, A.; Skinner, A.; Piercy, J. *Tidy's Physiotherapy,* 12th ed. Oxford, England: Butterworth & Heinmann, 1990.

Thompson, Diana L. *Hands Heal: Documentation for Massage Therapy.* Seattle: Howling Moon Press, 1993.

Travell, Janet G., M.D.; Simons, David G., M.D. *Myofascial Pain and Dysfunction, The Trigger Point Manual.* Baltimore: Williams & Wilkins, 1983.

Turchaninov, Ross; Cox, Connie. *Medical Massage.* Scottsdale, AZ: Stress Less Publishing, 1998.

van Why, Richard. *The Bodywork Knowledgebase, Lectures on the History of Massage.* New York: Author, 1991.

Voss, Dorthy E.; Ionta, Marjorie K.; Myers, Beverly J. *Proprioceptive Neuromuscular Facilitation.* Philadelphia: Harper & Row, 1985.

Walton, Tracy. Clinical Thinking and Cancer. *Massage Therapy Journal* 39(3), 66–80, Fall 2000.

Williams, Donna. Touching Cancer Patients, Guidelines for Massage Therapists. *Massage Magazine* 84, 74–79, March/April 2000.

Williams, Ruth E. *The Road to Radiant Health.* College Place, WA: Color Press, 1977.

Wilson, Jacob. Muscle Fibers—An In-Depth Analysis. http://www.abcbodybuilding.com, 2004.

Wood, Elizabeth; Becker, Paul. *Beard's Massage,* 3rd ed. Philadelphia: W. B. Saunders, 1981.

Yates, John. *A Physician's Guide to Therapeutic Massage.* Vancouver, BC: Massage Therapists' Association of British Columbia, 1990.

Ylinen, Jari; Cash, Mel. *Sports Massage.* London: Stanley Paul, 1988.

Appendix I:
Basic Pharmacology for Massage Therapists
by Faye N. Schenkman

Massage therapists frequently see clients who are taking prescription medications, vitamins, minerals, nutraceuticals, or herbal remedies. Often a client's complaints are not the result of a disease process but a reflection of the side effects of medications or the interactions between different medications or medications and supplements, which clearly affect the progress of treatments. For example, if a client comes for treatment complaining of muscle aches and pains in the legs, and the massage therapist does not recognize that they are caused by the client's medication(s), the therapist may find that the treatments are ineffective because the symptoms will continue unabated as long as the client continues taking the medication. Conversely, massage therapists may find that because of the physiological effects of massage on the body, their treatments can enhance the effects of certain medications, sometimes not only by improving the circulation of the medication but also its absorption. For example, if a client is taking an antihypertensive medication, the massage treatment can potentiate the medication's effects through improved circulation and muscle relaxation. This is a demonstration of how massage therapy can act as an adjunct to allopathic medicine, and how it can sometimes assist clients in lowering the dosage of their medication or, in some cases, eliminating the need for drug therapy altogether. Of course such changes in medications must be conducted under the supervision of the clients' physician because this is not within the scope of the massage therapist's practice. It should be noted, however, that massage can be practiced on many different levels. Clearly, the skill of the massage therapist is paramount in these cases. Practitioners of Asian bodywork therapies, who practice on an energetic as well as a physical level, can also find that they can help their clients minimize a drug's side effects and in some cases reduce its dosage by balancing the clients' energy system.

A responsible therapist asks his clients what medications, supplements, or herbs they are taking so he can look up information about them. The therapist should check if the client's complaints are related to the medications and whether the client needs to consult with the physician or other health care practitioner. In addition, the therapist must be aware that physical signs, such as bruising, may also be caused by medication and must therefore be cognizant of when to refer clients to a doctor or other health care practitioner for further evaluation before continuing with treatments. The more informed the therapist is regarding this topic, the better he will be able to help his clients and ensure a happy outcome for all. Many laypeople are completely ignorant about their medications' effects on the body and are often unaware that the symptoms they may be experiencing are the direct result of those medications. Clients are frequently embarrassed or afraid to question their physician about the drugs they have been prescribed or are afraid to tell their physician that they are taking supplements and herbs or seeing an alternative practitioner. Often they feel more comfortable discussing their concerns with other health care providers, such as the massage therapist. Physicians often do not have the time to address their clients' questions, whereas massage therapists can provide a nurturing environment where clients feel free to talk about their concerns. The ability of the massage therapist to discuss these issues intelligently and knowledgeably with the client is a great asset to both the client and the therapist's practice. A well-educated therapist can become a valuable resource of drug information for family and friends as well and can refer clients as needed.

Because of the myriad drugs on the market, many physicians are also unaware of the side effects of the drugs they prescribe and are even more ignorant of the interactions of their drugs with those prescribed by other physicians. It is not uncommon for a client, particularly an elderly one, to be placed on numerous medications prescribed by a retinue of physicians with no one overseeing the interactions of all the medications. Sometimes a client may experience lesser known side effects, adverse reactions that are considered more "rare" for a particular medication, and, therefore, the client's complaints are not investigated properly. An informed massage therapist can recognize adverse effects and point out to clients the need to discuss the medications with their physician or encourage them to do so, in some instances acting as an advocate on their behalf.

When a new client presents for treatment, the therapist should have the client fill out a patient intake form. This form should include questions concerning drug use, dosage, frequency of use, and duration. A sample of such a form is shown in Figure A.1.

With some clients, such a list might prove to be quite extensive. The massage therapist must do his "homework," checking out each and every entry for possible side effects that may be influencing the client's complaints and symptoms or that may affect the course of the massage treatment. Every therapist should purchase a text that can give them the information they need to reference. (See the suggested texts list at the end of this appendix for helpful information sources.) Therapists should also have a network of health care professionals to whom they can refer clients, if needed, for further evaluation.

The purpose of this appendix is to provide massage therapists with the basic and necessary information on this subject and to give them a

List all medications, vitamins, minerals, supplements, and herbs.			
Name	Dosage-Strength (# per day)	Reason for Taking	Duration

Figure A.1

Sample Patient Intake Form.

framework within which to better assess and treat their clients. Although it is certainly not within their scope of practice to prescribe any drug or supplement, it is necessary for massage therapists to be totally aware of their clients' conditions in order to better be able to treat them and help them achieve an optimum state of wellness.

There are many different types of massage therapy. Within Asian bodywork alone there are numerous "forms" or "styles," each one having its own variation on assessment and treatment, although all are rooted in the concept of an energy-based system. In Western massage, there are also many different methods and levels of treating. This appendix certainly cannot address the different ways and levels that various forms of massage can affect the body. Each therapist must hone his palpatory skills, develop an awareness of the client as a "whole"—as a physical, emotional, mental, and energetic being. Therapists must be observant of their clients' skin, musculature, posture, and such, and ask appropriate questions, always checking to see that their techniques are not causing more harm than good and using wisdom in deciding how much pressure can and should be applied. As long as therapists treat with the correct "intention" and take the time to assess their clients properly, a favorable outcome will most often result.

WHAT IS PHARMACOLOGY?

Pharmacology is a science that studies the effects that substances have on living organisms, the nature of their chemical structure, how they act within the body, and how the body responds to them. The word "pharmacology" is derived from the Greek word *pharmakon,* which translates as "drug," and also involves its mechanism of action. Knowledge of pharmacology is essential for all health care practitioners who are involved in the treatment of disease in humans or animals.

WHAT IS A DRUG?

Since time immemorial, man has used plants, minerals, animals, insects, and other substances found in nature to treat disease. In modern times, drugs can be bioengineered or developed from gene therapy. According to the World Health Organization (WHO), 80 percent of the world's population continues to use herbs and other natural substances as their first line of defense against disease. However, in modern societies, synthetically produced chemicals are most often developed into drugs that are used in the treatment, prevention, cure, alleviation of, or diagnosis of illness. This avenue is the most actively pursued by major drug companies today because natural substances cannot be patented. Research is therefore focused on artificially developed compounds in the competitive and lucrative world of the pharmaceutical industry.

Using a very broad definition, the term *drug* can also include common over-the-counter substances such as nicotine, alcohol, and caffeine; illegal drugs such as cocaine, heroin, and marijuana; cosmetic substances; and even food additives or any substance that has an effect on the body.

Chemicals developed as drugs are often a double-edged sword. While intended to have a selective action in the body, these drugs often fall short of that goal, producing instead a number of adverse effects, sometimes mimicking the very symptoms they are intended to relieve. Whenever more than one medication is taken, it is very possible that the combination of drugs may affect the expected response of each individual drug. One medication may affect another to increase, decrease, or cancel out the effects of the other, or to cause a different effect altogether.

All drugs, no matter what their origin, have one feature in common: they will affect the body in some way, they will cause cellular changes to take place, which, in turn, will cause an effect on the body's physiology. Some drugs will affect the entire body and have a "systemic" effect. Other drugs are only for local use, limited to one area or aspect of the body.

Another factor that must be considered with medications is the client's age. For example, the geriatric population's ability to metabolize and excrete medications is much slower. Most drugs are eliminated through the kidneys, so if the drug is not excreted sufficiently and the client continues to take it, the drug can accumulate and build up in the body to toxic levels, which can become life threatening. This is particularly true in the elderly. Also elderly people are often subjected to multiple physicians and multiple medications. In such cases, it is helpful to refer clients to a physician who specializes in geriatric or iatrogenic medicine or to a nurse practitioner, someone who will have an overview of all of these clients' pathologies and medications.

Children are another example of a population in which age influences the dosage of medications. Children react to medications differently from adults. They require less amounts of medication and need to be monitored frequently. Many drugs have not been adequately tested on children, and often the effects of a medication can be unpredictable.

Weight is also a factor in drug administration—heavier people usually need larger doses of medication versus thinner people. Often the dosages of drugs are prescribed based on how much a client weighs. However, certain individuals may be particularly sensitive regardless of their weight.

Women, men, people of different races, or persons in a diseased state do not always respond the same way to the same medications, owing to differences in hormone levels and body metabolism. And drugs are generally contraindicated if a woman is pregnant or nursing.

HOW ARE DRUGS NAMED AND CLASSIFIED?

Unfortunately, there is no uniform method for naming and classifying drugs. There are no international standards in pharmacology; therefore, the same medication can have multiple names, depending on the manufacturer and the country where it is being sold. In addition, an individual drug can belong to a number of different classifications.

Generic names are the common names of drugs. They contain prefixes and suffixes that indicate the drug classification and provide some clues as to its use and functions. When a company creates a new drug for market, it gives it a generic name. Once the drug is approved by the Food and Drug Administration (FDA), the pharmaceutical company will give it a trade name, something "catchy" that the public will remember easily. Generic names are usually recognized by their lowercase spelling; that is, the initial letter of the name is never capitalized.

Trade names are copyrighted brand names that often do not reflect the actions of the medication but rather are chosen because they are easy to recognize and remember. The initial letter of the name is capitalized and the name is followed with the symbol "®," indicating that the name is a registered trademark. After 17 years, however, the pharmaceutical company loses the exclusive rights to that drug; once the patent has expired, other companies can start to market the same drug, giving it their own trade name. Hence, the same medication can have multiple names from multiple manufacturers. The generic name, however, remains the same.

The chemical name of a medication is based on the molecular construction of the compound. It is usually a long, complicated, and difficult name and of little consequence to the massage therapist.

The official name of the drug is the name as it appears in the official government reference book, the *United States Pharmacopeia/National Formulary* (USP/NF). This is usually the generic name.

For example, note the different names of the following drug:

Trade Name	Darvon
Drug Company	Eli Lilly
Generic Name	propoxyphene hydrochloride
Chemical Name	alpha-4 dimethylamino-3-methyl-1-2,2-diphenyl-2 butanol, proprionate hydrochloride

Thus, the naming of drugs is often based not simply on chemical composition but also on marketing and the drugs' effects in the body. It is therefore necessary for the massage therapist to be acquainted with the different names of the same medication. In the same way that facial tissues can be referred to as Kleenex, Scott's, or Puffs, antihyperlipidemic agents such as atorvastatin calcium, fluvastatin sodium, lovastatin, pravastatin sodium and simvastatin are known by their trade names Lipitor®, Lescol®, Altocor® or Mevacor®, Pravachol®, and Zocor®, respectively. In this appendix, we use the trade names as examples for each category because these are the names that are advertised to the public and that are most recognizable to the layperson and the massage therapist.

There are many different ways to classify drugs and these are not exclusive because a drug that has multiple therapeutic actions can be found under more than one classification. For example, aspirin can act as an analgesic (relieve pain), an antipyretic (reduce fevers), and as an anti-inflammatory (reduce inflammation). Therefore, it can be found under three classifications.

In addition, there are different systems of drug classifications, which can be confusing because they are not standardized. Generally, drugs are classified based on their therapeutic effect, their pharmacologic actions, their actions at the molecular level, their origin (chemical, botanical, or animal), or their generic names.

HOW DO I LOOK UP A DRUG?

A valuable reference guide for the massage therapist is the *PDR Nurse's Drug Handbook*. This book provides an easy format for understanding individual drug monographs. Here the therapist will find how to read and interpret the information for a multitude of commonly prescribed medications, including the generic names and how to pronounce them properly, the trade name, the classification, the pregnancy category, whether a drug is a controlled substance, a drug's approved therapeutic uses, the contraindications, the special concerns, the side effects, the interactions with other medications or herbs, how the drugs are supplied, and the appropriate dosages. The *Physicians' Desk Reference* (PDR) is also a valuable tool, but it is not as easy to navigate for the novice practitioner.

WHAT ARE SOME COMMON DRUG GROUPINGS?

Following are some common categories of drugs, the conditions they treat, some of their side effects and contraindications (conditions or circumstances that indicate that a drug should not be given), and significant information that pertains specifically to the massage therapist. This list is by no means exhaustive but rather a general summary. The massage therapist must utilize additional sources of information, such as texts and the Internet, when researching a medication and also in determining whether massage is necessary, warranted, or should be avoided.

DRUGS TO TREAT THE SKIN

The skin is an area of particular interest to the massage therapist. The massage therapist must always be aware of conditions that may be contraindicated for massage or for her own safety when touching other people who may have areas of concern.

Relevance for the Massage Therapist

Fungi, bacteria, and viruses can easily be transmitted through open cuts in the skin. Universal precautions should always be taken, and any massage techniques that can irritate the skin in clients who already have inflamed skin should be avoided. Universal precautions are infection control guidelines designed to protect health care practitioners from exposure to diseases spread by blood and certain body fluids. Universal precautions stress that all clients should be assumed infectious for blood-borne diseases such as AIDS and hepatitis B.

Treatment for skin problems is usually topical; however, some conditions may be systemic and require oral medication. It should be noted that many persons self-medicate in this area without proper instructions or precautions. If the client is able to use an over-the-counter product, the FDA feels that it is safe enough to use without a physician's supervision. Clients should be advised to discuss these problems with their physicians and, as with any medication, to read the instructions completely before embarking on a drug therapy.

Categories of Skin Medications

Antipruritics

These drugs are used to relieve allergic reactions that cause rashes and itching. They may contain local anesthetics, drying agents, or anti-inflammatory agents such as corticosteroids and antihistamines.

   Side Effects: Skin irritation, rashes, stinging and burning, allergic reactions, or sedation if antihistamines are included.
   Contraindications or Cautions: Open wounds or prolonged use of corticosteroids.
   Examples: Benadryl, Solarcaine, and Cortaid.

Corticosteroids

These drugs can be used locally or systemically to treat allergic skin reactions and inflammation. They are also used topically to treat psoriasis and dermatitis.

   Side Effects: Thinning of the skin with increased wounds and infections, increased fragility of blood vessels, irritations, ulcerations, slow healing, bruising, water retention, or edema.

Contraindications or Cautions: Bacterial, fungal, or systemic viral infections; open wounds; immunocompromised persons; children; pregnant or nursing women; acne.
Examples: Cortaid, Valisone, and Aristocort.

Emollients and Demulcents

These topicals are used to soothe or protect the skin.

Side Effects: Generally, there are no side effects although the potential for an allergic reaction always exists.
Contraindications or Cautions: Known allergies to ingredients.
Examples: Desitin and A and D ointment.

Keratolytics

These drugs are used to treat abnormal flaking of the skin such as dandruff and psoriasis, or to catalyze peeling of the skin in conditions such as acne, calluses, and corns. Many keratolytics contain salicylic acid.

Side Effects: Skin irritations, burning, photosensitivity, or systemic effects in highly allergic persons.
Contraindications or Cautions: Open wounds, children, pregnant and nursing women. Keratolytics should not to be used for any lengthy periods.
Examples: Tegrin, Neutrogena, and Clearasil.

Scabicides and Pediculicides

These drugs are used to treat scabies and lice, respectively. The infestation can be either on the head or body. The name of the infestation depends on where it is occurring. Both organisms can be easily transmitted from one person to another through direct contact or through contact with contaminated clothing.

Side Effects: Irritations or rashes.
Contraindications or Cautions: Open, raw, or oozing skin; caution in the use of Lindane, which can be absorbed into the body, includes avoiding its use during pregnancy and lactation, and with children and the elderly.
Examples: Lindane, Acticin, and Nix.

Antifungals

These drugs are used in the treatment of candidiasis (vaginal, intestinal, systemic), aphtha (thrush), ringworm, athlete's foot, and so on.

Side Effects: Skin irritation, itching, and burning.
Contraindications or Cautions: Some oral preparations can cause serious side effects and should only be used under a physician's supervision.

Examples: Lamisil, Lotrimin, Mycostatin, Monistat, Gyne-Lotrimin, and Tinactin.

Antivirals

These drugs are used in the treatment of herpes simplex (cold sores, genital herpes), herpes zoster (shingles), or varicella zoster (chickenpox). Treatments may be topical or oral.

Side Effects: Skin irritations.

Contraindications or Cautions: Hypersensitivity to formulation; use of the cream in the nose, eyes, or mouth; use to prevent recurrent herpes simplex viral infections.

Example: Zovirax (generally effective only on the first outbreak).

Anti-infectives

These drugs include antiseptics, used to inhibit the growth of bacteria, usually on the skin. The two major antiseptics currently used are Hibiclens (chlorhexidene) and Betadine (povidone-iodine).

Side Effects for Chlorhexidene: Skin irritation, allergic reactions, or photosensivity.

Side Effects for Povidone-Iodine: Skin irritations, allergic reactions, or temporary discoloring of the skin.

Contraindications or Cautions: Open wounds, eyes, ears, pregnant women, lactating women. Hands must be washed thoroughly after use.

Examples: Hibiclens and Betadine.

Antibacterials

There are three over-the-counter topical antibacterial medications. Those that have a systemic effect are available by prescription only and have the potential for serious side effects. Therapists should look up these medications for more information.

Side Effects: Inflammation, itching, rashes, superinfections, or pruritus.

Contraindications or Cautions: Known allergic sensitivity, use of topical products in or around the eyes, contact dermatitis, or conditions where systemic absorption is possible.

Examples: Neosporin, Bacitracin, Polysporin, Myciguent, Akne-Mycin, and Erygel.

MUSCULOSKELETAL AND ANTI-INFLAMMATORY DRUGS

Generally, prescription drugs that are used to treat these problems fall into three categories: muscle relaxants, nonsteroidal anti-inflammatory drugs (NSAIDs), and corticosteroids. There are also a number of over-the-counter medications that clients may fail to mention; therefore, they should specifically be asked about any self-medicating. It should be noted that in many cases over-the-counter medications are prescription agents in a lower dose.

Relevance for the Massage Therapist

Musculoskeletal conditions are among the most commonly seen by the massage therapist. Neck and back pain are frequent complaints, and, just as frequently, clients take some type of medication to ease their spasms, pain, and inflammation. Massage is excellent for helping clients overcome these problems, but care should be taken not to use any techniques that will exacerbate inflammation or bruise the body. Also clients on medications for pain and inflammation may show a false tolerance for pressure, so the massage therapist should exercise great caution when applying pressure techniques. Massage therapy can be of great benefit in helping clients reduce the amount of medication they need. Many of the prescription medications have serious side effects, which the therapist should be aware of when reviewing the clients' symptoms and complaints.

Categories of Musculoskeletal Medications

Skeletal Muscle Relaxants

These drugs are used to treat pain, spasms, muscle contractions, and restricted range of motion. Generally, acute back and neck problems are treated medically with a combination of muscle relaxants, bedrest, physical therapy, massage therapy, and analgesics. Muscle relaxants are for short-term use, until the pain subsides, and other adjunctive therapies such as massage and exercise can take over to strengthen and relax the muscles.

> **Side Effects:** Dizziness, drowsiness, tremor, headaches, nausea, vomiting, diarrhea or constipation, urinary problems, liver toxicity, difficulty breathing, or confusion.
>
> **Contraindications or Cautions:** Muscular dystrophy, myasthenia gravis, pregnant and nursing women, and children under 12. These drugs may enhance the effects of alcohol, analgesics, psychotropic medications, and antihistamines.
>
> **Examples:** Soma, Flexeril, Valium, and Robaxin.

Nonsteroidal Anti-inflammatory Drugs (NSAIDs)

These medications are used to treat inflammatory conditions such as arthritis, bursitis, gout, muscle strains and sprains, and spondylitis. Symptoms include inflammation, pain, swelling, heat, or limited range of motion. Often these drugs are used for prolonged periods of time in low doses as maintenance therapy, in contrast to the steroids, which should be used only for acute disorders. NSAIDs work by inhibiting the synthesis of prostaglandins, chemicals that create much of the inflammation and pain associated with rheumatism, aches and pains, sprains, and so forth. Note that elderly people are particularly sensitive to the side effects from these drugs, which are often stomach irritation and diarrhea, and should be advised to call their physician immediately if any of the negative symptoms should present.

COX-2 inhibitors are a newer class of NSAIDs that are supposed to pose less of a risk for gastrointestinal bleeding; however, recent studies have shown that they pose more of a risk for heart disease and stroke. Therefore, many of them have been recalled from the market by the FDA and drug manufacturers.

> **Side Effects:** Gastrointestinal (GI) bleeding and ulceration, which does not have to be preceded by any warning signs or symptoms; epigastric pain, nausea, heartburn, gastroesophageal reflux disease (GERD), constipation, tinnitus, headaches, dizziness, visual disturbances, hypersensitivity reactions, bronchospasm, or liver toxicity.
>
> **Contraindications or Cautions:** Asthma, cardiovascular disease, kidney disease, liver disease, history of ulcers or inflammatory bowel disease, clotting disorders, thyroid disease, GERD, the elderly, pregnant and nursing women, or children with viral infections.
>
> **Examples:** Voltaren, Motrin, Advil, Nuprin, Aleve, and Relafen.

Gout Agents

Colchicine is a medication used to treat gout. Gout is caused by a buildup of uric acid crystals in different joints, especially the big toe, ankle, knee, and elbow.

> **Side Effects:** Rashes, GI problems, diarrhea, and blood disorders.
>
> **Contraindications or Cautions:** Blood dyscrasias; serious GI problems; hepatic, cardiac, or renal disorders; lactation; children, and the elderly.
>
> **Example:** Colchicine.

Adrenal Corticosteroids

Corticosteroids are secreted by the adrenal glands, which are located next to the kidneys. The function of corticosteroids is to act on the immune system to suppress the body's response to infection or trauma. Corticosteroids relieve inflammation, reduce swelling, and suppress symptoms in acute conditions. They basically have two functions: either as replacement therapy when the adrenal glands or pituitary glands are deficient in secreting or for their anti-inflammatory and immunosuppressant qualities. Corticosteroids are not meant to cure a disease but rather are used as adjunctive therapy in conjunction with other medications. They are used to treat acute asthma attacks, acute skin conditions, acute rheumatism or arthritis attacks, acute attacks of colitis, cancer treatments, and so on. Because their side effects are potentially very serious, they should be given for a short time only and locally, wherever possible.

Side Effects: Nausea, vomiting, diarrhea, constipation, gastric ulceration or hemorrhage, headaches, vertigo, insomnia, psychosis, anxiety, easy bruising, skin thinning and tearing, fluid and electrolyte imbalance, edema, hypertension, congestive heart failure, increased chance of infections, delayed wound healing, or adrenocortical insufficiency.

Contraindications or Cautions: Long-term use, viral or bacterial infections, fungal infections, hypertension, congestive heart failure, psychosis or emotional instability, diabetes, children, pregnant or nursing women, history of seizures or immunosuppression, hypothyroidism, and cirrhosis.

Examples: Cortisone, Prednisone, Deltasone, Florinef, Decadron, Medrol, and Aristocort.

GASTROINTESTINAL MEDICATIONS

Gastrointestinal medications can be subdivided into eight categories based on their various actions in the body. Disturbances of the GI system are among the most common complaints of clients and it is one of the main areas where clients self-medicate. Also GI side effects are the most common among all medications. Therefore, if the client complains of GI problems, one of the first areas to be considered should be the client's medications.

Relevance for the Massage Therapist

Many of the gastrointestinal complaints are rooted in response to stress. Massage is most beneficial for helping clients relax and as supportive therapy in the treatment of constipation or diarrhea. One of the positive results of regular massage treatment can be the reduction in the need for medication once the client is able to achieve deepening levels of relaxation.

Categories of Gastrointestinal Medication

Antacids

Antacids neutralize gastric hydrochloric acid and are among the most widely purchased over-the-counter medications used to treat indigestion, heartburn, and sour stomach. They may also help in the treatment of gastric and duodenal ulcers. Because they interact with almost all other medications and have an impact on the effectiveness of other drugs, they should not be taken within 2 hours of other medications.

Side Effects: Constipation, diarrhea, electrolyte imbalance, urinary stones, osteoporosis, or flatulence.

Contraindications or Cautions: Kidney disease, liver cirrhosis, electrolyte imbalance, and congestive heart failure.

Examples: Tums, Maalox, Gelusil, Mylanta, and Amphojel.

Drugs to Treat Ulcers and Gastroesophageal Reflux Disease (GERD) (H₂ Blockers)

Some of these drugs reduce gastric acid secretion by acting as histamine$_2$ receptor antagonists. They treat duodenal and gastric ulcers and give short-term relief from GERD.

Side Effects: Diarrhea, dizziness, rash, or headaches.

Contraindications or Cautions: Kidney disease, liver disease, children, and pregnant and nursing women.

Examples: Tagamet, Zantac, Pepcid, Axid (the latter two are better tolerated in the elderly with fewer adverse reactions).

Cytotec (misoprostol)

This is a synthetic drug used to block gastric acid secretion and to protect the mucosa from the effects of other drugs such as NSAIDs. It is not used for the treatment of ulcers.

Side Effects: Diarrhea, nausea, abdominal pain, menstrual problems, or spontaneous abortion.

Contraindications or Cautions: Women of childbearing age, pregnant women, and children under age 12.

Example: Cytotec.

Proton Pump Inhibitors

Prilosec (omeprazole) is a drug that prevents gastric secretions. It is meant for short-term use in the treatment of GERD, ulcers, and erosive esophagitis.

Side Effects: Diarrhea, constipation, nausea, vomiting, abdominal pain, headaches, or dizziness.

Contraindications or Cautions: Lactating women, the elderly, and children.

Examples: Prilosec, Prevacid, Nexium, Aciphex, and Protonix.

Carafate (sucralfate)

This is a medication that inhibits pepsin, and it is used to treat ulcers in a local, rather than a systemic, way by forming a paste with hydrochloric acid that then covers the ulcer site, protecting it from further irritation.

Side Effects: Constipation (most common), diarrhea, indigestion, flatulence, dry mouth, gastric discomfort, urticaria, rash, insomnia, vertigo, angioedema, or facial swelling.

Contraindications or Cautions: Safety for use in children and during lactation has not been fully established.

Example: Carafate.

Antispasmodics/Anticholinergics

These medications work by decreasing motility in the GI tract.

> **Side Effects:** Urinary retention, constipation, confusion, dry mouth, or blurry vision.
> **Contraindications or Cautions:** Glaucoma, cardiovascular disease, myasthenia gravis, pregnancy, lactation, and obstructive GI disease.
> **Examples:** Cystospaz, Levsin, and Levsinex.

Drugs for Inflammatory Bowel Disease

These drugs act as anti-inflammatory agents in the GI tract and are used to treat ulcerative colitis.

> **Side Effects:** Nausea, vomiting, anorexia, headaches, dizziness, pruritis, or fever.
> **Contraindications or Cautions:** Use with caution during lactation, in persons with known drug hypersensitivity or related drug hypersensitivity, and children below 2 years of age.
> **Example:** Azulfidine.

Antidiarrhea Drugs

These medications have various modes of action in diminishing loose stools. Some act as adsorbents, whereas others slow intestinal motility.

> **Side Effects:** Constipation, nausea, vomiting, abdominal distention, or confusion.
> **Contraindications or Cautions:** Infants, the elderly (unless under medical supervision), and ulcerative colitis.
> **Examples:** Kaopectate, Lomotil (a controlled substance), Imodium, and Imodium A-D.

Antiflatulents

These drugs help break up gas in the GI tract.

> **Side Effects:** None.
> **Contraindications or Cautions:** None.
> **Example:** Simethicone.

Laxatives and Cathartics

These drugs help stimulate evacuation of the intestines. Laxatives have a more gentle action than cathartics or purgatives, which promote a rapid evacuation. There are numerous subdivisions of laxatives such as bulk-forming laxatives, stool softeners, mineral oil, saline laxatives, stimulant laxatives, and hyperosmotic laxatives. Each division should be investigated separately for more specific contraindications. Many clients self-medicate in this area. Massage can be very helpful in stimulating the movement of the clients' colonic contents.

Side Effects: Generally rare but may include diarrhea, anal irritation, or electrolyte imbalance.

Contraindications or Cautions: Acute abdominal pain, partial bowel obstruction, young children, debilitated individuals, prolonged use, and congestive heart failure.

Examples: Metamucil, Colace, Milk of Magnesia, Dulcolax, and glycerin suppositories.

Antiemetics

These medications are used to treat nausea, vomiting, and motion sickness. There are many different drugs on the market with different actions and means of administration.

Side Effects: Confusion, anxiety, drowsiness, vertigo, depression, blurry vision, or weakness.

Contraindications or Cautions: Children, pregnant and lactating women, geriatric or debilitated individuals, seizures, and cardiac arrhythmias.

Examples: Torecan, Compazine, Tigan, Phenergan, Zofran, Antivert, and Bonine.

RESPIRATORY SYSTEM MEDICATIONS AND ANTIHISTAMINES

The main classifications of respiratory system drugs are bronchodilators, corticosteroids, mycolytics, expectorants, and antitussives.

Relevance for the Massage Therapist

Massage can be very beneficial for relaxing the muscles of the chest and upper back, thereby helping the client take in more oxygen and breathe easier. However, some respiratory medications can induce drowsiness, and the increased relaxation from massage techniques may exacerbate this symptom. It is therefore imperative that the massage therapist be aware of the medications the client is taking. Conversely, some medications can induce anxiety states, and the client may be unable to relax on the table no matter what efforts the therapist puts forth. Because many of these drugs can cause dizziness, the therapist should check to see if the client gets dizzy when she sits up at the end of the treatment. If the client is dizzy, the therapist can press an acupuncture point directly under the client's nose in the center of the philtrum. The therapist can press the point with the tip of the index finger or instruct the client to do so. This is a very helpful technique for ameliorating dizziness. Also it should be noted that decreased sweating is sometimes a side effect of these medications and the body's temperature may increase with the use of hydroculators or other heat therapies. They should therefore be avoided in these cases.

Many clients self-medicate in this area with over-the-counter medications and it is important to get a complete list of the drugs the clients are taking before treatment begins.

Bronchodilators

These drugs act by alleviating bronchospasms and increasing the capacity of the lungs. These medications are used to treat acute respiratory conditions such as asthma and chronic obstructive pulmonary disease (COPD). There are three types of bronchodilators: sympathomimetics (adrenergics), parasympatholytics (anticholinergics), and xanthine derivatives. The therapist must research each category for more specific information regarding actions, side effects, and contraindications. General information is listed next.

> **Side Effects:** GI effects such as nausea, vomiting, nervousness, tremors, dizziness, cardiac irregularities, hypertension, drowsiness, dizziness, confusion, agitation, seizures, or palpitations.
>
> **Contraindications or Cautions:** Cardiovascular, kidney, pulmonary, or liver dysfunction; diabetes; children; the elderly; and pregnant and lactating women.
>
> **Examples:** Ventolin, Proventil, Primatene, Adrenalin, Alupent, Atrovent, and Theo-Dur.

Corticosteroids

These drugs are discussed under the section for musculoskeletal problems. For respiratory problems, corticosteroids can be administered orally, intravenously, or by inhaler or aerosol. Corticosteroids that are inhaled have less systemic effects than those that are taken orally or intravenously.

> **Side Effects:** Coughing, fungal infections, sore throat, or dry mouth.
>
> **Contraindications or Cautions:** Viral, bacterial, or fungal infections; hypertension; cardiac disease; diabetes; and kidney disease.
>
> **Examples:** Vanceril, Beconase, Pulmicort, Rhinocort, Flovent, AeroBid, Nasonex, and Nasacort.

Asthma Prophylaxis

These medications are used to prevent asthma attacks in clients who suffer from chronic asthma. They include antileukotrienes and cromolyn, which is usually listed separately because its action is different. Cromolyn can also be used in the prevention of exercise-induced asthma.

> **Side Effects:** Headaches, dizziness, nausea, pain, fatigue, or infections.
>
> **Contraindications or Cautions:** Liver toxicity, pregnant and lactating women, and children under 12.
>
> **Examples:** Accolate, Singulair, and Cromolyn.

Mucolytics and Expectorants

Mucolytics are drugs that liquefy pulmonary secretions, whereas expectorants increase secretions, reduce viscosity, and help expel sputum. Expectorants are often combined in cough syrups to help with coughs caused by upper respiratory infections, bronchitis, postnasal drip, and so on. However, a chronic cough may indicate a serious problem—any cough that lasts for more than a week or which recurs frequently needs the attention of a physician.

Side Effects: Drowsiness, nausea, vomiting, runny nose, or stomach upset.

Contraindications or Cautions: Cardiovascular disease, diabetes, pregnant and lactating women, and some clients with asthma.

Examples: Mucomyst, Humibid, Robitussin, Iophen, and Pima Syrup.

Antitussives

These are drugs used to prevent coughing in patients who have a nonproductive cough. Dry, persistent coughs can produce fatigue, prevent sleep, and sometimes cause pulled or strained muscles. Massage can help relieve the pain of muscle strain and sprain although narcotic antitussives are sometimes utilized. Codeine is often used but can become addictive with long-term use if not monitored properly by a physician. There a number of over-the-counter cough syrups that combine several drugs—antitussives, expectorants, antihistamines, and decongestants. Clients should be encouraged to consult with their physician, pharmacists, nurse practitioners, or medical assistants because some of these ingredients are contraindicated with specific medical conditions. For example, decongestants can produce negative effects in persons with cardiovascular disease or thyroid conditions.

Side Effects of Narcotic Antitussives: Constipation, urinary retention, drowsiness, dizziness, nausea, vomiting, or respiratory depression. Non-narcotic antitussives do not depress respiration or cause addiction and have few side effects.

Contraindications or Cautions: Clients prone to addictions, asthma, and COPD.

Examples of Narcotic Antitussives: Codeine, Robitussin A-C, Histussin, and Lorcet.

Examples of Non-Narcotic Antitussives: Robitussin and Tessalon Perles.

Antihistamines

These drugs provide relief from the symptoms of allergic reactions caused by histamine responses, such as inflammation, itching, and edema. They are also used to assist in treatment of anaphylactic shock after the acute stage has been treated with epinephrine and corticosteroids.

Antihistamines are often used to treat the symptoms of allergic rhinitis, although when they are used to reduce nasal secretions in persons suffering from the common cold, the subsequent thickening of bronchial secretions may result in further airway obstruction, especially in those with COPD and asthma. Some antihistamines are also used to treat motion sickness and vertigo.

> **Side Effects:** Dry eyes, ears, nose, and throat; drowsiness; dizziness; low blood pressure especially in the elderly; muscular weakness; urinary retention; constipation; visual disorders; insomnia; tremors; nausea; vomiting; or anorexia.
>
> **Contraindications or Cautions:** COPD, asthma, operating machinery or driving a car, the elderly, cardiovascular disease, infants, pregnant and lactating women, seizure disorders, and benign prostatic hypertophy (BPH).
>
> **Examples:** Zyrtec, Dimetapp, Chlor-Trimeton, Benadryl, Claritin, and Allegra.

Decongestants

Decongestants constrict the blood vessels in the respiratory tract, helping to shrink swollen mucous membranes, and open the nasal and sinus pathways. Also known as adrenergic drugs, these medications can be administered orally or nasally but should be used only on a short-term basis because they will cause rebound congestion after a few days. Many decongestants, often sold over the counter, are combined with antihistamines, analgesics, caffeine, or antitussives. Because of these combinations, the potential for negative side effects increases. Oral decongestants in particular, such as pseudoephedrine, can raise blood pressure; therefore, clients who already have high blood pressure should consult with their physician.

> **Side Effects:** Anxiety, nervousness, tremor, seizures, palpitations, hypertension, headaches, or electrolyte imbalance. Rhinitis medicamentosa may occur if a patient has taken Afrin for 3 continuous days. This is called a *rebound effect.*
>
> **Contraindications or Cautions:** Cardiovascular disease, diabetes, hyperthyroid, the elderly, and pregnant and lactating women.
>
> **Examples:** Afrin, Allerest, Neo-Synephrine, No-stril, and Sudafed.

Smoking Cessation Aids

These drugs are used in conjunction with behavior modification programs to help people stop smoking. Sometimes Zyban is also prescribed in smoking cessation.

> **Side Effects:** Lightheadedness, nausea, vomiting, throat and mouth irritation, or cardiac irritability.
>
> **Contraindications or Cautions:** Overdosage, pregnant and lactating women, and history of drug abuse or overdependence.
>
> **Examples:** Nicorette gum, Nicoderm patch, and Nicotrol inhaler.

CARDIOVASCULAR MEDICATIONS

These include drugs that affect the heart, the vascular system, and anti-coagulants. There are seven subcategories of medications; however, some of the drugs have multiple uses and overlap more than one category.

Relevance for the Massage Therapist

Massage therapy can help promote blood and lymph circulation through its vasodilatory effects and can augment the actions of certain medications. Also through its effects on lowering blood pressure, clients may find that the dosages of their medications can be lowered. Therapists should always be mindful that clients, whether on medication or not, may get dizzy when they sit up at the end of the treatment and should be encouraged to wait before getting off the table. Gently pressing an acupuncture point directly under the nose in the philtrum can alleviate the dizziness. Therapists should monitor the clients' heart rate as well as be on the lookout for any unusual responses. They should have their clients contact their physician if they think there is cause for concern.

Also it is important to note that clients who are on blood-thinning medication may be particularly sensitive to pressure. Massage therapists must use a light touch, avoid any techniques that have the potential for bruising, and be on the lookout for any bruising or irritations from treatment. If bruising should occur despite the therapist's best efforts to use only very light techniques, the client should be informed and the treatment should be terminated.

Cardiac Glycosides

These medications are also called cardiotonics because of their ability to strengthen the heartbeat. They are used mostly in the treatment of congestive heart failure in which the heart fails to pump properly and increases in size to compensate. In congestive heart failure, these medications increase the force of cardiac contractions without increasing oxygen consumption. Because the heart works more efficiently, it beats more slowly and decreases from its increased size, and the diuretic action decreases edema as well. Sometimes cardiac glycosides are also used with antiarrhythmic drugs to slow the heart rate in tachycardia, atrial fibrillation, or flutter. Lanoxin (digoxin) is the most commonly used drug in this category. Because there is a fine line between appropriate dosage and dangerous levels of toxicity, clients should be told to see their physician immediately if there are any side effects.

Side Effects: Anorexia, nausea, vomiting, diarrhea, abdominal bloating or cramping, headaches, fatigue, muscle weakness, vertigo, restlessness, irritability, tremors, seizures, blurry vision, cardiac arrhythmias, electrolyte imbalance, insomnia, and confusion, especially in the elderly. A symptom of toxicity is seeing a yellow-greenish-bluish halo.

Contraindications or Cautions: Elderly clients, pregnant and lactating women, hypothyroidism, pulmonary disease, acute heart disease, and kidney disease.

Examples: Digitalis and Lanoxin (digoxin).

Antiarrhythmic Drugs

These medications are used to treat atrial or ventricular tachycardia, atrial fibrillation or flutter, and arrhythmias that are the result of digitalis toxicity. Most of these medications can lower blood pressure and slow the heartbeat, which, if not monitored properly, could lead to hypotension, bradycardia, and cardiac arrest. These drugs have the potential to make existing arrhythmias worse or cause new ones, and they can also cause negative effects when interacting with other medications.

There are several groups of antiarrhythmic drugs that function with different mechanisms of action. For example, beta-adrenergic blockers such as Inderal work by inhibiting adrenergic (sympathetic) nerve receptors; calcium channel blockers such as Isoptin work by suppressing the action of calcium in contraction of the heart muscle; Norpace decreases myocardial excitability and inhibits conduction; Lidocaine is an anesthetic that stabilizes membranes; Pronestyl is used mostly as prophylactic therapy; and Quinaglute and Cardioquin decrease myocardial excitability. Extra caution for all these categories must be exercised in elderly clients. Therapists should check each drug for more specific side effects and contraindications.

Side Effects: Hypotension, bradycardia, dizziness, confusion, insomnia, weakness, fatigue, nausea, vomiting, diarrhea or constipation, or edema.

Contraindications or Cautions: Diabetes, kidney disease, asthma, bradycardia, heart failure, pregnant and lactating women, children, and liver disease.

Examples: Tenormin, Inderal, Isoptin, Xylocaine, Cordarone, Tonocard, Cardioquin, and Norpace.

Antihypertensives

These medications are also called *hypotensives*. There are numerous drugs in this category that lower blood pressure. Clients who suffer from mild hypertension can often regulate their pressure with a program that includes dietary changes (for example, reducing their salt intake), consistent massage therapy treatments, and appropriate exercise (e.g., walking, tai chi chuan). It goes without saying that if clients smoke, they should stop. Nutritional counseling can also be of benefit. Therapists may want to network with a nutritionist and help their clients establish a more wellness-oriented lifestyle. Note that antihypertensives do not cure high blood pressure; they simply manage the symptoms. Clients should never simply stop their medication on their own. Abruptly stopping can cause rebound hypertension. They should discuss their medication and concerns with their physician.

Hypertension is usually viewed as mild, moderate, or severe, and there are different drugs for each class. In addition, their actions are varied. Patient history is also a factor in determining what medication is chosen. It is often difficult to initially choose the right drug, and clients often have their dosages and medications changed or combined, causing different kinds of side effects. Thiazide diuretics are sometimes used by themselves to treat mild hypertension but are more frequently combined with other hypotensive medications to lower high blood pressure. The types of antihypertensives are listed in the next sections.

Beta-Adrenergic and Calcium Channel Blockers

Examples: Inderal, Tenormin, Cardizem, Procardia, Coreg, Corgard, and Verelan (previously discussed under "Antiarrhythmic Drugs").

Aldomet (methyldopa)

This drug treats moderate to severe hypertension and is usually given with a diuretic. It can be used in pregnancy because it is safe for the fetus, but it is rarely used.

Side Effects: Low blood pressure, drowsiness, anemia, nausea, vomiting, diarrhea, constipation, sore tongue, sexual dysfunction, liver problems, or nasal congestion.

Contraindications or Cautions: Liver disease, dialysis, and elderly clients.

Example: Aldomet.

Apresoline (hydralazine)

This drug is a peripheral vasodilator used in the treatment of moderate-to-severe hypertension, especially in clients with congestive heart failure. It is often administered with a diuretic and another hypotensive agent, for example, a beta blocker, but it is very rarely used today.

Side Effects: Tachycardia, palpitations, headache, flushing, orthostatic hypotension, nausea, vomiting, diarrhea and constipation, blood abnormalities, or allergic reactions.

Contraindications or Cautions: Kidney disease, coronary artery disease, pregnant women, and lupus.

Example: Apresoline.

ACE Inhibitors

These drugs are called angiotensin-converting enzymes, which work to lower mild-to-moderate blood pressure and also treat congestive heart failure by decreasing vasoconstriction. They can be used alone or with a diuretic. ACE inhibitors can interact negatively with a number of other medications, and the client needs to be made aware of the potential side effects from the interactions of these medications with other drugs.

Side Effects: Rash, photosensitivity, loss of taste, blood dyscrasias, renal disease, severe hypotension, cough, nasal congestion, or hyperkalemia.

Contraindications or Cautions: Renal disease, lupus, scleroderma, heart failure, pregnant and lactating women, and children.

Examples: Captopril, enalapril, Accupril, Monopril, Zestril, and Prinivil.

Angiotensin Receptor Blockers

These drugs are generally used in clients who cannot tolerate ACE inhibitors.

Side Effects: Lower chance of taste loss, rashes, or cough than those caused by ACE inhibitors.

Contraindications or Cautions: Renal disease, lupus, scleroderma, heart failure, pregnant and lactating women, and children.

Examples: Cozaar and Diovan.

Coronary Vasodilators

These medications are used to treat angina. Angina pectoris is pain in the chest as a result of ischemia, or decreased blood supply, to the heart muscle. When the coronary arteries are constricted or blocked, pain will result. Coronary vasodilators are used to dilate the blood vessels and stop an attack of angina pectoris, or they can be used preventatively to stop further attacks or at least reduce their frequency. The three subcategories of coronary vasodilators include nitrates, beta blockers, and calcium channel blockers.

Nitrates

Nitroglycerin comes in several different forms. These are administered for an acute attack, and if the attack is not halted after the first dose, additional doses can be given every 5 minutes, not to exceed three doses in 15 minutes. If three doses should fail to bring relief, a physician must be called immediately so as to avoid a myocardial infarction. Nitroglycerin is also available in timed-release capsules and tablets as well as IV solution. Persons using nitroglycerin preventatively over the long term often use a transdermal ointment or a patch—the location must be only on the upper arm or body and must be rotated to avoid irritating the skin. Therapists should avoid any areas of skin irritation or raw areas as well as the area of the patch itself.

Side Effects: Headaches, postural hypotension including dizziness, flushing, blurry vision, dry mouth, nausea, vomiting, diarrhea, cold sweats, tachycardia, or syncope.

Contraindications or Cautions: Glaucoma, anemia, and frequent bowel movements. Note that alcohol will interact with nitrates and exacerbate their effects.

Examples: Nitroglycerin, Isordil, and Sorbitrate.

Beta Blockers and Calcium Channel Blockers

These drugs are discussed under "Antiarrhythmic Drugs."

Antilipemic Drugs

These medications are among the most frequently prescribed drugs and are used to lower serum cholesterol and low-density lipoprotein (LDL), the "bad" cholesterol. Clients who have high cholesterol and high LDL (>130) are at a greater risk of myocardial infarction and atherosclerotic coronary disease. Dietary changes that include a low-fat and low-cholesterol diet as well as appropriate exercise, stopping smoking, and weight loss are all significant factors in lowering cholesterol; however, medications are added in this effort frequently. It should be noted that there are fairly new tests available that often provide better indications of coronary disease, such as reactive c-protein and homocysteine tests. Clients should be advised to discuss these additional tests with their physicians before ingesting hyperlipidemia agents. All hyperlipidemia medications have potentially serious side effects, and sometimes two or three of them are combined together. Types of hyperlipidemia agents include statins, niacin, and bile acid sequestrant.

> **Side Effects:** GI upset, GI bleeding, bleeding gums, constipation, flushing, liver damage, muscle cramps, muscle weakness, renal failure, eye problems, cataracts (with long-term use), headaches, dizziness, insomnia, or fatigue.
>
> **Contraindications or Cautions:** Liver, kidney, or gallbladder disease; diabetes, gout, allergies, alcoholism, ulcers, low blood pressure, pregnant and lactating women, and women of childbearing age.
>
> **Examples:** Questran, Nicobid, Mevacor, Lipitor, Zocar, Lopid, and Pravachol.

Anticoagulants and Antithrombolytics

These two classes of drugs include coumarin medications and heparins. Their mode of action is different—anticoagulants, such as Coumadin, prevent the blood from clotting and are referred to as blood thinners, while antithrombolytics, such as Heparin, dissolve clots that have already been formed to prevent a cerebrovascular accident. They are also used with postsurgery clients such as those who have had a bypass or hip or knee replacement. Particular caution must be exercised with elderly clients who are at higher risk for internal bleeding. Also, it is important to note that coumarin derivatives (warfarin) interact negatively with many drugs and herbal supplements. Some drugs increase the blood-thinning effect and greatly increase the potential for internal bleeding. These include aspirin and other NSAIDS.

> **Side Effects:** Major hemorrhage, minor bleeding, blood in the urine (hematuria) or stools (melena), or gums bleeding easily on brushing.

Contraindications or Cautions: GI problems, ulcers, liver or kidney disease, bood dyscrasias, pregnant women (heparin can be used with caution because it does not cross the placenta), and poststroke.

Examples of Anticoagulants: Coumadin and aspirin.

Examples of Antithrombolytics: Heparin and Lovenox.

Platelet Inhibitors

These medications are used prophylactically to decrease platelet clumping in clients with a history of recent stroke, recent myocardial infarction, or peripheral vascular disease.

Side Effects: Headache, dizziness, weakness, nausea, vomiting, diarrhea, flushing, rash, or bleeding.

Contraindications or Cautions: Elderly clients.

Examples: Aspirin, Plavix, and Ticlid.

URINARY SYSTEM MEDICATIONS

The most frequently used drugs in this category are diuretics, which are drugs that increase the excretion of urine.

Relevance for the Massage Therapist

Massage can help move fluids through the body, reduce edema, and can help these medications to work more effectively. The therapist should be cognizant that the client may need to urinate midway through the treatment.

Diuretics

There are four classes of diuretics, depending on their actions: thiazides, loop diuretics, potassium-sparing diuretics, and osmotic agents. The condition being treated will determine which type is used. These drugs also interact with a number of other medications and can have serious side effects. Because many of these drugs deplete potassium, potassium supplementation is often recommended.

Thiazides

These drugs are the most commonly used diuretic. They increase the excretion of water, sodium, chloride, and potassium. They are used to treat edema and hypertension and prevent stone formation in persons with hypercalciuria (too much calcium in the urine) and those suffering from electrolyte imbalance because of kidney disease.

Side Effects: Potassium deficiency, which can lead to cardiac arrhythmias; chloride deficiency, which can lead to alkalosis; muscle weakness or spasms, nausea, vomiting, diarrhea, cramping, low blood pressure, vertigo, headaches, fatigue, skin conditions, hyperglycemia, or increased uric acid.

Contraindications or Cautions: Diabetes, gout, kidney disease, liver disease, long-term use, and elderly clients.

Examples: Lozol, Esidrex, HydroDIURIL, and Zaroxolyn.

Loop Diuretics

These drugs act directly on the loop of Henle in the kidneys, and although not classified as thiazides, they have a similar action in that they increase the secretion of water, sodium, chloride, and potassium. Their action is quicker than thiazides. They are used to treat edema from pulmonary, renal, or hepatic disease; congestive heart failure; ascites; and hypertension.

Side Effects: Chest pain; electrolyte imbalance; potassium deficiency; vertigo; low blood pressure; GI effects including anorexia, nausea, vomiting, diarrhea, and abdominal pain; hyperglycemia; increased uric acid; blood dyscrasias; tinnitus; skin conditions; allergic reactions; headaches; muscle cramps; mental confusion; and dizziness.

Contraindications or Cautions: Liver disease, kidney disease, diabetes, gout, pregnant and lactating women, and children.

Examples: Edecrin, Lasix, Bumex, and Demadex.

Potassium-Sparing Diuretics

These are used when deficiency of potassium has reached a dangerous level.

Side Effects: Excess potassium that can lead to cardiac arrhythmias, dehydration, weakness; GI symptoms including nausea, vomiting, and diarrhea; fatigue; weight loss; and low blood pressure.

Contraindications or Cautions: Kidney disease, liver disease, and pregnant and lactating women.

Examples: Aldactone and Dyrenium.

Osmotic Drugs

These medications are most often used to reduce intracranial or intraocular pressure.

Side Effects: Fluid and electrolyte imbalance, headache, vertigo, mental confusion, nausea, tachycardia, hypertension, hypotension, allergic reactions, or severe pulmonary edema.

Contraindications or Cautions: Kidney and cardiovascular disease.

Examples: Osmitrol and Ureaphil.

Gout Medications

These drugs include uricosuric agents, which help with the urinary excretion of uric acid and which are used for chronic gout and gouty arthritis. The other type of medication used is allopurinol, which lowers uric acid levels. These drugs are not utilized in the treatment of acute gout attacks because they have no anti-inflammatory action nor do they relieve pain. Acute attacks are treated with medications in which colchicine, an anti-inflammatory, has been added.

Side Effects: Headaches, nausea and vomiting, kidney stones, rash, low blood pressure.

Contraindications or Cautions: History of kidney stones, history of peptic ulcer, nausea, vomiting, diarrhea, kidney disease, liver disease, and pregnant and lactating women.

Examples: Benemid and allopurinol.

Antispasmodics

These drugs are anticholinergic, meaning that they block parasympathetic nerve impulses, which, in turn, reduce spasms in the urinary bladder.

Side Effects: Dryness, dizziness, drowsiness, headaches, urinary retention, constipation, blurry vision, mental confusion (especially in the elderly), tachycardia, palpitations, nausea, vomiting, or skin reactions.

Contraindications or Cautions: Elderly clients, kidney or liver disease, GI obstruction, cardiovascular disease, prostatic hypertrophy, glaucoma, pregnant or nursing women, and children under 5 years of age.

Examples: Pro-Banth-ine, Detrol, Ditropan, and Cystospaz.

Cholinergics

In this case, cholinergics stimulate the parasympathetic nerves to help the urinary bladder contract.

Side Effects: Nausea, diarrhea, vomiting, sweating, headache, bronchial constriction, or urinary urgency.

Contraindications or Cautions: Obstruction of the urinary tract, hyperthyroidism, peptic ulcer, asthma, cardiovascular disease, parkinsonism, and pregnant and lactating women.

Example: Urecholine.

Analgesics

The main analgesic used is Pyridium. It is used in the treatment of the burning, pain, and urgency of cystitis, procedures that irritate the lower urinary tract, or trauma. It is not to be taken for more than 2 days. Pyridium treats only the symptoms, not the cause of the condition. Anti-infective drugs are necessary to treat urinary tract infections.

Side Effects: Headaches, vertigo, mild GI disturbances, or orange-red urine.

Contraindications or Cautions: Kidney dysfunction and hepatitis.

Examples: Pyridium and Azo-Standard.

Drugs to Treat Benign Prostatic Hypertrophy (BPH)

There are two classes of drugs to treat BPH: antiandrogens and alpha blockers.

Antiandrogens

The main drug is Proscar, which is used to reduce the size of the prostate and the symptoms of BPH—urgency, nocturia, and urinary hesitancy. This medication does not cure BPH; it only suppresses the symptoms, which return once the medication is stopped.

> **Side Effects:** Impotence, decreased libido or decreased volume of ejaculate, breast enlargement. Proscar may increase hair growth.
>
> **Contraindications or Cautions:** Infections, liver disease, prostate cancer, urinary tract disease, and any allergies. The drug can be absorbed through the skin. If the film coating of the tablet has been broken or the tablet crushed, it should not be handled by a woman who is pregnant or planning to become pregnant. Any contact with Proscar by a developing male fetus could result in abnormalities of the external sex organs. Proscar should not be used in women or children.
>
> **Example:** Proscar.

Alpha Blockers

The main drug is Flomax, which relaxes the smooth muscles of the bladder mouth and prostate, thus increasing the flow of urine and decreasing the symptoms of BPH. Other drugs such as Hytrin and Cardura treat hypertension as well as BPH.

> **Side Effects:** Dizziness, headaches, palpitations, or hypotension.
>
> **Contraindications or Cautions:** Hypertension and concurrent use with warfarin.
>
> **Examples:** Cardura, Flomax, and Hytrin.

ANTINEOPLASTIC DRUGS

Tumors are considered to be neoplastic (new growth) cells. There are both benign and malignant tumors. Tumors that are considered to be benign do not metastasize (spread) from their original location. Tumors that are malignant, also known as cancers, metastasize by one of three means: extending or spreading into the adjacent tissues, spreading via the lymphatic system, or spreading via the blood. The growth of a tumor or cancer is called carcinogenesis or tumorigenesis. Cancer cells follow the path of least resistance. Some cancers have a strong genetic link, that is, mutations in the DNA. Other cancers may develop from environmental exposure to toxins, viruses, stress, and so forth. Antineoplastic drugs stop the growth and spread of malignant cells. Generally, cancer is most successfully treated with combinations of therapies such as surgery, radiation, chemotherapy, medications, nutrition, and holistic therapies such as acupuncture, bodywork, imagery therapy, herbs, and supplements.

Chemotherapy involves using drugs, often in combination, to relieve the symptoms of cancer while attempting to kill the cancer cells. These drugs are called cytotoxic, meaning they destroy cells. They are aimed at the cells that are metastasizing or spreading rapidly; however, because they are so toxic, they affect the "good" cells as well, destroying healthy tissue and creating many negative side effects. Many of these medications also function to suppress the immune system because cancer is considered to be an autoimmune disease. By decreasing the production of antibodies and phagocytes, the "defenders" of our immunity, clients become more susceptible to infections, which can become, in and of themselves, life threatening.

Antineoplastic drugs are often given in very high doses on an intermittent schedule. After several weeks of chemotherapy, for example, a client may have a rest period before resuming treatments. The hope is that during this rest period, the client's good cells, tissues, and organs will have a chance to recover from the chemotherapy. These medications are so toxic that they require special handling by health care personnel. Direct skin contact can result in absorption of these toxic chemicals. Pregnant women, those who are breastfeeding, or those who are trying to conceive should not be caring for clients receiving chemotherapy.

Relevance to the Massage Therapist

Massage can be very beneficial to patients undergoing chemotherapy or radiation, or both, as well as drug therapies. Many clients with cancer suffer from extreme stress and anxiety, and massage can help alleviate these symptoms. In addition, massage can help the medications circulate within the body and be more effective as well as help alleviate some of the other symptoms such as constipation, weakness, fatigue, nausea, and vomiting. Treatments should be gentle and consistent. Care should be taken that the client does not get a chill or draft and that the client is not exposed to anyone with an infection. Also certain tests that the client may be undergoing, such as a PET scan, involve radioactive substances being injected into the client. Clients should not be receiving massage on the day that they have such tests.

There are seven classes of neoplastic drugs:

- Antimetabolites: Methotrexate is the most famous drug in this class. It is also used in the treatment of rheumatoid arthritis, psoriatic arthritis, and lupus. Other drugs in this category are fluorouracil and cytarabine.
- Alkylating drugs: Some examples of alkylating drugs are carmustine, cisplatin, and thiotepa.
- Plant alkaloids: Vinblastine and vincristine are examples of plant alkaloids.

- Paclitaxel (Taxol): Paclitaxel comes from the bark of the Pacific yew. It is often used as adjunct therapy in patients with metastatic breast or ovarian cancer.

- Antitumor antibiotics: Some examples include bleomycin, dactinomycin, and mitomycin.

- Hormone therapy: Hormone therapy consists of corticosteroids such as prednisone, antiestrogen drugs such as tamoxifen, and antiandrogen drugs such as Lupron Depot.

- Biological response modifiers: Interferon is the most commonly used drug in this category. It also has an antiviral action.

All of these classes of drugs have a multitude of side effects. The most commonly experienced side effects are nausea, vomiting, diarrhea, rash, alopecia, loss of the ability to reproduce, neurotoxicity including numbness, tingling, ataxia, footdrop, visual disturbances, pain in the jaw, severe constipation, oral or GI ulceration, peripheral neuropathy, bone marrow depression, pulmonary disease, fatigue, weakness, osteoporosis, hot flashes, and so on.

Another type of drug administered in cancer therapy is the radioactive isotope. Sometimes radioactive material is planted inside the body in the form of capsules, needles, or seeds. Clients receiving such treatment should not be massaged until they are no longer a danger to others around them as certified by their physician.

DRUGS THAT TREAT THE ENDOCRINE SYSTEM

The endocrine system regulates many important activities of the body. The term *endocrine* is a reference to a hormone, an internal secretion, which is produced by a ductless gland that secretes directly into the bloodstream. Hormones can be natural or synthetically produced. The four classes discussed here are pituitary hormones, adrenal corticosteroids, thyroid medications, and antidiabetic drugs. Hormones that affect the reproductive system are discussed under their own category.

Relevance for the Massage Therapist

Treatment for clients taking hormones vary, depending on the type of hormone therapy they are undergoing. Hormones can affect the entire body. Generally speaking, the massage therapist should be aware of thin skin and easy bruising and adjust pressure as needed, using more gentle techniques. For example, poor circulation and slow healing are some symptoms of type 2 diabetes (other symptoms can be excessive weight gain, excessive thirst and urination, weakness, and vision problems). Massage therapists should be aware of these symptoms and refer clients to their physicians for approval of treatment if they have not already consulted with them. Massage can be very helpful to diabetics, improving their circulation and helping them cope with stress more effectively. This, in turn, may help them lower the dosage of their medications under their physician's supervision. However, the therapist must pay particular attention to the level of pressure used or the use of heat therapies because many diabetics not only bruise easily but also have decreased sensation due to neuropathies.

Clients who are taking steroids may find that their skin is easily irritated or inflamed. Therapists should be careful to avoid any techniques that will exacerbate these symptoms and be careful not to pull and tear any tissue.

Clients who are taking estrogen, birth control pills, or who are on hormone replacement therapy can develop problems with blood clots. Therapists should be mindful of the signs and symptoms of blood clots and refer these clients to their physician immediately if they suspect a clot is present or if they notice excessive or unusual edema. Symptoms of a blood clot in the leg, when a clot obstructs blood flow and causes inflammation, may include swelling, gradual onset of pain, redness, warm to the touch, worsening leg pain when bending the foot, leg cramps (especially at night), and a bluish or whitish discoloration of the skin.

In general, massage can help reduce stress and help balance the entire system, improving circulation and helping medications to move more freely through the system, as well as reducing any stagnation of fluids and swellings.

The classes of hormones are discussed in the next sections.

Pituitary Hormones

The pituitary is called the "master gland" of the body because it regulates the functions of the other glands. It secretes four hormones: somatotropin, adrenocorticotropic hormone (ACTH), thyroid-stimulating hormone (TSH), and gonadotropic hormones (follicle-stimulating hormone [FSH], luteinizing hormone [LH], luteotropic hormone [LTH]). Abnormalities are treated by an endocrinologist. Two examples are Acthar and ACTH.

Adrenal Corticosteroids

Adrenal corticosteroids are secreted by the adrenal glands, which are located next to the kidneys. Their job is to suppress the body's response to infections or trauma. They are used for acute symptoms of inflammation, swelling, and where symptoms need to be suppressed. They are also used when secretions of the pituitary or adrenal glands are deficient. Corticosteriod therapy should be used on a short-term basis, and it can be used to treat conditions such as allergic reactions with rash or hives, flare-ups of rheumatoid arthritis, psoriasis, asthma, sarcoidosis, cancers, organ transplants, and ulcerative colitis. Long-term use of corticosteroids can suppress the pituitary gland and create atrophy so that the body no longer can produce its own hormones. Therefore, steroids should only be used on a short-term basis and withdrawal should always be gradual.

Side Effects: Adrenocortical insufficiency, delayed wound healing and increased susceptibility to infections, muscle pain or weakness, osteoporosis, stunting of growth in children, cataracts, nausea, vomiting or diarrhea, hemorrhage, or easy bruising.

Contraindications or Cautions: Long-term use, viral or bacterial infections, fungal infections, cirrhosis, hypothyroidism, hypertension, diabetes, glaucoma, children, pregnant and lactating women, and history of seizures.

Examples: Cortone, Decadron, Florinef, Medrol, prednisone, Deltasone, Aristocort, and Kenalog.

Thyroid Medications

These medications can be natural or synthetic. They are used as replacement therapy for hypothyroidism caused by deficient thyroid function. Hypothyroidism causes the metabolism to slow, with symptoms of fatigue, dry skin, weight gain, sensitivity to cold, and irregular menstruation. This condition is diagnosed by blood tests, and periodic lab monitoring is necessary to maintain the correct dosage.

Side Effects: Due to overdosage and can include palpitations, tachycardia, cardiac arrhythmias, increased blood pressure, nervousness, tremors, headache, insomnia, weight loss, diarrhea, intolerance to heat, or menstrual irregularities.

Contraindications or Cautions: Cardiovascular disease, elderly clients, and diabetes.

Examples: Synthroid, Levothroid, and Levoxyl.

Antithyroid Medications

These drugs are used to treat hyperthyroidism.

Side Effects: Rash, urticaria, pruritis, or blood dyscrasias.

Contraindications or Cautions: Long-term therapy, patients older than 40 years, pregnant and lactating women, and liver disease.

Examples: Tapazole and PTU.

Antidiabetic Drugs

These drugs are used to lower blood glucose levels in persons with impaired metabolism of carbohydrates, fats, and proteins. There are two main types of diabetes: type 1, or insulin-dependent (IDDM), and type 2, or non-insulin-dependent (NIDDM). Type 2 has also been called "adult onset" because in the past it was usually found in adults over 40 years old. However, in recent years it has been frequently discovered in children and young adults due to the increase in obesity in children. Diabetes can also occur in pregnancy and is then called gestational diabetes.

Insulin is used for type 1 diabetes when there is insufficient insulin production from the islets of Langerhans in the pancreas. It is also given to clients with type 2 diabetes who are unable to balance their blood glucose with diet and oral drugs. Traditionally, insulin was prepared from either beef or pork pancreas. Pork insulins are still used but other forms, such as biosynthetic insulin (Humulin) and semisynthetic insulins (Iletin II Purified), are available.

Hyperglycemia or elevated blood glucose may result from undiagnosed diabetes, not enough insulin, infections, emotional stress, trauma, pregnancy, or other endocrine disorders. Symptoms may include excessive thirst, dehydration, anorexia, unexplained weight loss, frequent urination, weakness, or vision problems.

Hypoglycemia or lowered blood glucose may result from an overdose of insulin, not eating enough (e.g., dieting), excessive exercise, or change in the type of insulin. Symptoms may include increased perspiration, irritability, confusion, tremors, headaches, tingling in the fingers, or blurry vision.

Persons who have type 2 diabetes sometimes are treated with dietary changes alone or with a combination of dietary changes and oral antidiabetic drugs. There are several classes of these drugs with differing modes of action, and often they are combined in treatment. They are called first-generation sulfonylureas, second-generation sulfonylureas, alpha-glucosidase inhibitors, biguanides, benzoic acid derivatives, and thiazolidinediones. It should be noted that many of these medications interact negatively with many other medications such as beta blockers, alcohol, NSAIDS, thyroid hormones, diuretics, steroids, oral contraceptives, and so on.

> **Side Effects:** GI distress, skin reactions, liver dysfunction, weakness, fatigue, headaches, or hypoglycemia.
> **Contraindications or Cautions:** Liver and kidney dysfunction, severe infections, debilitated or malnourished persons, pregnant and lactating women, and children.
> **Examples:** Amaryl, Glucotrol, Diabeta, Micronase, Glynase, Precose, Glyset, Glucophage, Prandin, Actos, and Avandia.

REPRODUCTIVE SYSTEM MEDICATIONS

There are four main classes of hormones that regulate the functions of the reproductive system: gonadotropic, androgens, estrogens, and progestins. The gonadotropic hormones include FSH, which catalyzes the development of ovarian follicles in the female and the production of sperm in the male testes; LH, which works with FSH to facilitate secretion of estrogen, ovulation, and development of the corpus luteum; and LTH, which stimulates the production of progesterone by the copus luteum and secretion of milk by the mammary glands.

Relevance for the Massage Therapist

Therapists should be aware that blood clots are a potential side effect of estrogen therapy. Therapists should be on the lookout for easy bruising and use more gentle techniques as needed. They should also know the signs of blood clotting. Clients should immediately be referred to their physician if the therapist suspects the presence of blood clots. Also increased fluid retention is possible when taking estrogens and progestins. Massage improves the movement of blood and fluids throughout the system and helps reduce edema. Any highly unusual signs should be noted and the client referred to a physician. Also, hormones can certainly affect emotions, and massage can be of great benefit in helping clients deal with stress, balance the emotional states, and maintain a greater sense of wellness.

When treating clients on thyroid medication, it should also be noted that the thyroid is greatly affected by increasing stress, which, in turn, can affect how much medication a person needs to take. Massage can help maintain emotional well-being, thus potentially reducing the need for higher dosages of medication.

Androgens—Male Hormones

Androgens stimulate the development of male characteristics and include testosterone and androsterone. Although these hormones are used in males who show deficiency symptoms, such as impotency, they are also used in women with advanced breast cancer, endometriosis, or fibrocystic breast disease. Use of anabolic steroids by athletes, especially teenagers, in order to build muscles and physique is illegal and potentially very dangerous. In addition to the side effects listed next, such drugs can produce psychosis, paranoia, depression, mania, and aggressive and violent behavior.

> **Side Effects:** Edema, acne, deficient sperm production, increased or decreased libido, anxiety, depression, or headache.
>
> **Contraindications or Cautions:** Cardiac, renal or hepatic disease; elderly men (may stimulate cancer), boys who have not yet reached puberty, and diabetics.
>
> **Examples:** Danocrine, Android, Deca-Durabolin, Depo-Testosterone, and Estratest.

Drugs for Impotency

The most popular drug in this category is Viagra, which treats male erectile dysfunction.

> **Side Effects:** Headaches, flushing, abnormal vision, dizziness, nasal congestion, dyspepsia, urinary tract infection, diarrhea, rash, angina, palpitations, or low blood pressure.
>
> **Contraindications or Cautions:** Cardiovascular disease, kidney or liver disease, pregnant and lactating women, or use in children. These drugs should not be taken by individuals taking nitrates.
>
> **Examples:** Viagra, Cialis, and Levitra.

Estrogens

Estrogens are the female sex hormones produced mainly by the ovaries and secondarily by the adrenal glands. These hormones produce female sexual characteristics such as breast size, and during the menstrual cycle they produce the proper environment for the fertilization, implantation, and growth of the embryo. They also affect the secretions of the hormones FSH and LH from the anterior pituitary gland, which can prevent lactation and stop ovulation. At one time, estrogen therapy was extremely common for women entering menopause; however, recent studies have shown that the health risks are great for women using these medications. The WHO now classifies estrogen as a known carcinogen.

Estrogen therapy is used in contraceptives, to treat menstrual problems, to treat menopausal symptoms, to prevent osteoporosis in postmenopausal women, to treat vaginal dryness, to inhibit lactation in nursing mothers, and in treatment for men with advanced prostate cancer.

Side Effects: Increased risk of stroke; myocardial infarction; thromboembolic problems; GI effects including vomiting, diarrhea, or constipation; weight gain; edema; skin discolorations; increased triglyceride levels; folic acid deficiency; liver disease; breakthrough vaginal bleeding; increased risk of cervical erosion and candidiasis; headaches; migraines; depression; visual problems; gallbladder disease; cancer of the uterus; endometrial cancer; or breast cancer.

Contraindications or Cautions: Thromboembolus, stroke, myocardial infarction, liver disease, gallbladder disease, cancer, migraines, shortness of breath, seizures, asthma, kidney disease, and pregnant women.

Examples: Estrace, Estraderm, Depo-Estradiol, Premarin, Estratab, Climara, and Vivelle.

Progesterone

Progesterone is a hormone secreted by the corpus luteum and adrenal glands. It is responsible for changes in the uterine endometrium in the second half of the menstrual cycle and is used to treat amenorrhea, abnormal uterine bleeding, and contraception. It is also used in postmenopausal therapy and as adjunctive therapy in the treatment of advanced endometrial or breast cancer. Synthetically produced progesterone drugs are called progestins.

Side Effects: Menstrual problems, breakthrough bleeding, spotting, edema, weight gain, nausea, breast tenderness, rash, headaches, depression, thromboembolic disorders, or decrease in bone density.

Contraindications or Cautions: History of depression, thromboembolic disorders, cardiovascular disease, liver disease, pregnant women, and cardiac or renal dysfunction.

Examples: Provera, Depo-Provera, Megace, and Cycrin.

Contraceptives

Contraceptives can be either estrogen-progestin combinations or progestin-only contraceptives. They are used to prevent pregnancy and to treat endometriosis, painful periods, heavy periods, irregular periods, acne, ovarian cysts, pelvic inflammatory disease, benign breast disease, and ectopic pregnancy.

> **Side Effects:** Nausea, edema, weight gain or loss, breakthrough bleeding, mood changes, libido changes, migraine headaches, severe depression, blurry vision, or loss of vision.
>
> **Contraindications or Cautions:** Thrombophlebitis or thromboembolic disorders, history of cerebrovascular accident, breast cancer or estrogen-dependent malignancy, pregnant and lactating women, liver disease, smoking, hypertension, diabetes, and gallbladder disease. They should not be prescribed to female clients over the age of 35.
>
> **Examples:** Ovral, Ovcon, Norinyl, Loestrin, Ortho-Novum, Tri-Norinyl, Depo-Provera, Norplant, and Progestasert.

Lupron and Depot

These are used as antineoplastic drugs to stop the growth of hormone-dependent tumors. They are used in the treatment of prostate and breast cancers. Sometimes they are combined with tamoxifen for the treatment of breast cancer.

> **Side Effects:** Hot flashes, headaches, insomnia, mood swings, nasal congestion, or weight gain or loss.
>
> **Contraindications or Cautions:** Not to be used as a contraceptive or during pregnancy or lactation.
>
> **Examples:** Lupron and Lupron Depot.

Fertility Medication

Clomid is a drug used for treatment of infertility.

> **Side Effects:** Nausea, vomiting, nervousness, insomnia, or multiple pregnancies.
>
> **Contraindications or Cautions:** Ovarian cysts, endometrial cancer, liver, thyroid, adrenal disease.
>
> **Example:** Clomid.

ANTI-INFECTIVE DRUGS

The most important first step in the treatment of infections is to identify the pathogen and then the specific medication to which it is sensitive. Often the physician will order a broad-spectrum antibiotic while waiting for the results of culture and sensitivity tests. This can sometimes cause additional problems if the organism is resistant to the antibiotic, or if it turns out that the pathogen is not bacterial but rather viral. Because antibiotics do not discriminate between good and bad bacteria, taking antibiotics when the infection is really a viral one can often compromise the immune system and inhibit the client's ability to heal from the organism. In addition, certain bacteria that are immune to specific antibiotics can pass that immunity to other types of bacteria. The result is that the antibiotics that are ineffective for one type of infection, for example, respiratory, may prove to be ineffective for another type of infection, such as a urinary tract infection.

Relevance to the Massage Therapist

Persons taking anti-infectives have a compromised immune system. Care must be taken by the massage therapist when treating immunocompromised clients so they are not exposed to any infections, colds, or drafts. If the therapist is sick, for example, with a cold, she should not be treating clients. Conversely, if the client is ill, it may be advisable to reschedule the appointment if the client is in the contagious stage of the disease, rather than expose the therapist and other clients to the pathogens. If the weather is inclement, the client should be instructed to reschedule rather than expose them to conditions that can exacerbate their illness. GI distress is a common side effect of these medications. Massage can be very helpful for treating constipation or diarrhea, nausea, and abdominal bloating as well as calming the client.

Of course, universal precautions should always be followed, especially when treating anyone suffering from pathogens.

Antibiotics

A major problem that has resulted from the overuse of antibiotics is the emergence of resistant strains of bacteria. Consequently, many antibiotics that at one time were in the forefront of the treatment of bacterial infections are no longer effective, and researchers are scrambling to discover new drugs so that organisms such as tuberculosis and *Staphylococcus aureus* can be kept under control. That is why antibiotics should never be used to treat the common cold, which is generally caused by a virus, even though the public may, in their ignorance, demand antibiotics from their physician.

Although there are numerous antibiotics, the side effects are generally of three types:

a. Allergic reactions resulting in rashes, hives, or low fevers. In such cases, medication should be terminated. Sometimes a severe reaction, like anaphylaxis, can follow a mild one and can be life threatening. Anaphylaxis is an allergic hypersensitivity reaction of the body to a foreign protein or drug. It can lead to anaphylactic shock, which can sometimes result in unconsciousness and death.

b. Damage to the tissues, hearing loss, kidney damage, liver damage, blood dyscrasias (abnormalities in blood components). Sometimes the damage may be permanent or it may reverse when the medication is discontinued.

c. Superinfections—a new infection with different resistant bacteria or fungi as a result of killing off the normal bacteria in the intestines or mucous membranes, particularly when broad-spectrum antibiotics are used. It is helpful to eat yogurt or take a broad-spectrum probiotic supplement to continually replenish the gut with good bacteria.

Other common side effects can include headaches, diarrhea, constipation, nausea, vomiting, or blurry vision.

Contraindications and cautions would certainly apply to the elderly, pregnant and lactating women, and anyone with a history of kidney or liver disease. Quinolones should not be prescribed to individuals under the age of 18, and tetracyclines should not be given to children under the age of 9.

The most common groupings of antibiotics are discussed in the next sections.

Aminoglycosides

These drugs are used to treat infections caused by gram-negative bacteria such as *Escherichia coli, Pseudomonas,* and *Salmonella,* as well as gram-positive bacteria such as *Staphylococcus aureus.* Aminoglycosides are used for short-term treatment of serious infections only when other less-toxic antibiotics have failed. These antibiotics are generally administered through an IV because they do not absorb well in the GI tract.

Side Effects: Kidney disease, hearing loss, vertigo, headaches, tremors, numbness, seizures, blurry vision, or rash.

Contraindications or Cautions: Tinnitus, vertigo, hearing loss, kidney dysfunction, pregnant or nursing women, infants, or the elderly.

Examples: Amikin, Garamycin, and Nebcin.

Cephalosporins

These drugs are semisynthetic antibiotics that are produced by a fungus. They are related to penicillin; therefore, clients who are allergic to penicillin may also be allergic to cephalosporins. They are broad spectrum and are active against many gram-positive and gram-negative bacteria.

Side Effects: Hypersensitivity, rash, edema, anaphylaxis (especially in those allergic to penicillin), blood dyscrasias, kidney disease, liver disease, nausea, vomiting, diarrhea, seizures, or respiratory distress.

Contraindications or Cautions: Renal disease, known allergies to penicillin, prolonged use leading to superinfections, severe colitis, pregnant or nursing women, and children.

Examples: Keflex, Ceftin, Suprax, Maxipime, Ceclor, and Rocephin.

Macrolides

These drugs are used to treat infections of the respiratory tract, skin (e.g., acne), and some sexually transmitted infections when the client is allergic to penicillin. Erythromycins are the best known antibiotic in this class and are considered to be the least toxic of all the antibiotics. They are chosen first if they are effective against an organism rather than use more toxic antibiotics and run the risk of serious side effects. Pregnant women and children, for example, would be good candidates for this class of drugs, if necessary. Unfortunately, there are now many erythromycin-resistant strains of bacteria. Erythromycin also has another effect unrelated to its antibacterial activity—it is used in certain mobility disorders of the GI tract because it stimulates gastric emptying.

Side Effects: Anorexia, nausea, vomiting, diarrhea, cramps, urticaria, and rash; superinfections.

Contraindications or Cautions: Liver dysfunction and alcoholism.

Examples: Biaxin, Zithromax, erythromycin, E.E.S., E-Mycin, ERYC, and Ilosone.

Penicillins

These drugs are created by a particular species of fungus and treat many strains of streptococci, staphylococcus, and meningococcal infections, including respiratory and intestinal infections. Penicillins are the preferred antibiotic for treating gonorrhea and syphilis. Amoxicillin has been used to treat *Helicobacter pylori* infections in ulcer disease. Some semisynthetic penicillins have a broad spectrum of activity and are called "extended-spectrum" penicillins. Augmentin and Timentin are examples. A number of pathogens have become resistant to many forms of penicillin.

Side Effects: Hypersensitivity reactions range from rash to anaphylaxis, superinfections, nausea, vomiting, diarrhea, blood dyscrasias, kidney and liver disease, confusion, anxiety, or seizures.

Contraindications or Cautions: History of allergy to any drugs, kidney dysfunction, and electrolyte imbalance.

Examples: Amoxil, Omnipen, Bycillin L-A, and Ampicillin.

Quinolones

These drugs, such as Cipro or Levaquin, are used to treat infections of the urinary tract, respiratory tract, GI tract, skin, bones, and joints. These medications have potentially severe side effects, especially in children and the elderly. Unfortunately, some pathogens have already demonstrated resistance to the quinolones; therefore, these drugs should be used only when other antibiotics have failed or the client is allergic to other antibiotics. These medications should not be used in children under the age of 18.

Side Effects: Nausea, vomiting, diarrhea, abdominal pain, colitis, headaches, dizziness, confusion, irritability, seizures, anxiety, superinfections, rash, or phototoxicity; may cause injury to tendons.

Contraindications or Cautions: Elderly clients, children, adolescents, pregnant and lactating women, severe kidney disease, seizure disorders, and cardiac disease.

Examples: Cipro, Levaquin, Noroxin, and Maxaquin.

Tetracylines

These drugs are broad-spectrum antibiotics used to treat infections caused by rickettsia, Chlamydia, or uncommon bacteria. Severe cases of acne, Rocky Mountain spotted fever, Lyme disease, and atypical pneumonia are treated with tetracycline, also called doxycycline. Unfortunately, the number of organisms resistant to tetracyclines is growing, so they should only be used after other antibiotics have failed.

> **Side Effects:** Nausea, vomiting, diarrhea, superinfections, photosensitivity, discolored teeth in the fetus or children, or vertigo.
>
> **Contraindications or Cautions:** Pregnant and lactating women, children under age 8, clients exposed to direct sunlight, liver or kidney disease, esophageal obstruction or dysfunction.
>
> **Examples:** Sumycin, Vibramycin, and Acromycin.

Sulfonamides

These are some of the oldest anti-infective drugs. Because of increasing resistance to them, they are now used mostly in combination with other medications.

> **Side Effects:** Rash, dermatitis, nausea, vomiting, diarrhea, high fever, headaches, stomatitis, conjunctivitis, blood dyscrasias, liver toxicity, kidney damage, or hypersensitivity reactions that can be fatal.
>
> **Contraindications or Cautions:** Impaired liver or kidney function, urinary obstruction, blood dyscrasias, severe allergies, asthma, and pregnant or lactating women.
>
> **Examples:** Azulfidine, Septra, and Bactrim.

Other Anti-infective Drugs

These include Cleocin, which is used to treat severe respiratory tract infections, severe pelvic infections, and certain bacteria associated with AIDS. Flagyl is a synthetic combination antibacterial and antiprotozoal drug useful in treating Crohn's disease and rosacea. Vancomycin (Vancocin) is the drug of last resort, which is used in the treatment of life-threatening infections when all other medications have failed. For example, it is the drug of choice for methicillin-resistant *Staphylococcus aureus*. Strains of pathogens, however, are becoming increasingly resistant.

Antifungals

These drugs are used to treat specific fungi, such as candidiasis or tinea. The medications used are very different in their actions. Some are administered intravenously for severe infections, while others are given orally and some are used topically. Common side effects are headaches, fatigue, nausea, vomiting, diarrhea, and rash.

> **Side Effects:** Headaches, chills, fever, hypotension, malaise, muscle and joint pain, weakness, anorexia, nausea, vomiting, cramps, anemia, or hypokalemia, which can lead to congestive heart failure.

Contraindications or Cautions: Children, pregnant and nursing women, and kidney or liver disease.

Examples: Diflucan, Grisactin, Abelcet, and Nystatin.

Antituberculosis Drugs

These drugs are used to treat tuberculosis (TB) if someone has been exposed to it, even though the person may not have symptoms, or if the TB test comes back positive, and, of course, if someone has an active case of the disease.

Side Effects: Nausea, vomiting, diarrhea, dizziness, blurry vision, headaches, fatigue, numbness, weakness, liver disease, or hypersensitivity reactions.

Contraindications or Cautions: Chronic liver disease, alcoholism, kidney dysfunction, diabetes, ocular defects, pregnant and lactating women, gout, and children.

Examples: INH, Myambutol, Rifadin, and Streptomycin.

Antivirals

These medications are used to treat a range of viruses and share common side effects.

- Acyclovir (Zovirax, Valtrex) is used to treat initial outbreaks of herpes simplex, herpes zoster (shingles), and chickenpox infections.

- Amantadine (Symmetrel) is used to treat influenza A virus strains.

- Neuraminidase inhibitors (Tamiflu, Relenza) are a new group of antivirals used to treat influenza A and B virus strains.

- Ribavirin (Virazole) is used to treat severe lower respiratory tract infections in children and in adults, hantavirus, hepatitis C.

- Interferons are used to treat AIDS-related Kaposi's sarcoma, chronic hepatitis B, and some cancers.

Side Effects: Nausea, vomiting, abdominal pain, diarrhea, rash, fatigue, or headaches.

Contraindications or Cautions: Children, pregnant women, and lactating women.

Drugs to Treat AIDS

These medications are called antiretrovirals and are classified by their mechanism of action. They include protease inhibitors, nucleoside reverse transcriptase inhibitors (NRTIs), and nonnucleoside reverse transcriptase inhibitors (NNRTIs). AIDS is often treated through a combination of drugs, called "cocktail therapy." Treatment does not eradicate the disease; instead it is aimed at attacking the virus at different stages in its evolution. All of these drugs potentially have the standard GI effects—nausea, vomiting, abdominal pain, and diarrhea, and can have much more severe adverse reactions, some having a high mortality rate.

Side Effects: Nausea, vomiting, diarrhea, hyperglycemia, exacerbation of existing diabetes, spontaneous bleeding, kidney stones, liver dysfunction, bone marrow suppression, pancreatitis, hypersensitivity reactions that can be fatal, severe rashes, dizziness, insomnia, confusion, hallucinations, or amnesia.

Contraindications or Cautions: Pregnant and lactating women, and children.

Examples: Viracept, Retrovir, Sustiva, Epivir, Videx, Combivir, Crixivan, Zerit, Hivid, Kaletra, Norvir, and Fortovase.

Antiurinary Drugs

Most of these drugs prevent the growth of bacteria rather than kill them. They are usually used for recurrent urinary tract infections.

Side Effects: Nausea, vomiting, diarrhea, numbness, weakness, headaches, dizziness, weak muscles, or anemia.

Contraindications or Cautions: Liver or kidney impairment, anemia, diabetes, electrolyte abnormalities, asthma, pregnant and lactating women, and infants under 1 month of age.

Examples: Macrodantin, Trimpex, and Macrobid.

ANALGESICS, SEDATIVES, AND HYPNOTICS

The purpose of analgesics is to relieve pain, that of sedatives is to calm, and hypnotics are to help the person sleep.

Relevance to the Massage Therapist

Massage therapy can be very helpful for pain reduction and also for relaxation and calming patients. With consistent massage therapy treatments, a client may be able to reduce the dosage of her medications. Massage therapists should work in conjunction with the client's physician in such matters. Some analgesics like aspirin thin the blood and produce the potential for bleeding and easy bruising. Therapists must be aware of such potentials and adjust their pressure accordingly. In addition, the client's ability to discern how much pressure can be applied in the treatment may be impaired because of the effects of the medication. Therapists must be mindful that due to the medications that the client is taking, she may not be in touch with her body to know whether the pressure is too much. Therefore, therapists should avoid using deep pressure techniques until they feel certain that they will not mistakenly injure the client. Many of these drugs are also constipating, and massage can certainly help with this problem.

Analgesics

Analgesics can be classified as opioid (narcotics), nonopioid (nonnarcotics), and adjuvant.

Opioid Analgesics

Opioid analgesics are a controlled substance and include natural opium alkaloids such as morphine and codeine as well as the synthetics such as Demerol and Darvon. Opioids tend to cause tolerance and dependence and can have severe withdrawal symptoms if the drug is abruptly discontinued. For individuals with bona fide pain, the likelihood of dependence is extremely slim. A massage therapist must have a clear understanding of dependence, tolerance, and addiction.

> **Side Effects:** Confusion, euphoria, restlessness, headaches, dizziness, nausea, vomiting, diarrhea, or physical and emotional dependence.
>
> **Contraindications or Cautions:** CNS depression, liver and kidney disease, hypothyroidism, COPD, addiction-prone personalities, the elderly, and pregnant and lactating women.
>
> **Examples:** Demerol, Darvon, Dilaudid, OxyContin, Morphine, Percocet, Tylenol with Codeine, and Vicodin.

Nonopioid Analgesics

Many nonopioid analgesics are available over-the counter and are heavily advertised and very popular. Nonopioids are used to relieve mild-to-moderate pain, fever, and anti-inflammatory conditions such as arthritis. They are also used with opioids to manage severe, acute, or chronic pain. The salicylates (aspirin, salsalate, choline magnesium trisalicylate) are used mostly for their analgesic, anti-inflammatory, and antipyretic qualities. Ibuprofen is also used as an analgesic. (NSAIDs are discussed elsewhere in this appendix.) Acetaminophen (Tylenol) has analgesic and antipyretic properties but has almost no effect on inflammation. Aspirin and acetaminophen are frequently combined to treat migraine headaches (Excedrin) and are combined with opioids for severe pain.

> **Side Effects of Salicylates:** Bleeding, frequent bruising, tinnitus, drowsiness, dizziness, depression, or rash.
>
> **Contraindications or Cautions:** GI bleeding, liver disease, asthma, kidney disease, pregnant and lactating women, and Hodgkin's disease.
>
> **Side Effects of Acetaminophen:** Severe liver toxicity, rash, renal insufficiency.
>
> **Examples:** Tylenol, Panadol, and Genapap Extra Strength.

Tramadol (Ultram)

Tramadol is a synthetic analgesic whose effect is similar to that of opioids; however, it is a nonopioid and it is not a controlled substance.

> **Side Effects:** Dizziness, headache, lethargy, nausea, constipation, anxiety, confusion, or rash.
>
> **Contraindications or Cautions:** Head injury, liver and kidney disease, seizures, pregnant or nursing women, and children under 16 years of age.
>
> **Example:** Tramadol.

Adjuvant Analgesics

These medications enhance the analgesic effect when used in conjunction with opioids and nonopioids. The two main classes of these drugs are anticonvulsants and tricyclic antidepressants. Anticonvulsants such as Dilantin and Tegretol are often used for the management of nerve pain from neuralgia, herpes, and cancer. Tricyclic antidepressants such as Elavil, Pamelor and Tofranil are used in the treatment of herpes, arthritis, diabetes, cancer, migraine or tension headaches, insomnia, and depression. Side effects of antidepressants may include dry mouth, urinary retention, constipation, sedation, arrhythmias. Side effects from anticonvulsants can also include dizziness, confusion, rash, nausea, vomiting, and diarrhea.

Sedatives and Hypnotics

These are controlled substances used in small doses to calm the client, and in larger doses to help the client sleep. There are two classes of sedative-hypnotics: barbiturates and nonbarbiturates. These drugs can foster psychological and physical dependence, so they should not be used for a long period of time except in the treatment of epilepsy. Prolonged use produces a severe rebound effect, resulting in nightmares and hallucinations. Gradual reduction of dosage is essential to avoid rebound insomnia.

Barbiturates

Barbiturates are sedatives that can be very dangerous. Many suicides and fatalities due to accidental overdose have been reported, especially when combined with central nervous system (CNS) depressants or alcohol. Children or elderly persons may manifest opposite behavior with these medications such as hyperactivity, confusion, or hallucinations. Because of slower metabolism, barbiturates remain in the system longer and pose a greater threat to the elderly or weakened patient.

Side Effects: Depression, headache, fatigue, nausea, vomiting, constipation, rash, confusion, coma, or fatal overdoses.

Contraindications or Cautions: Elderly clients, debilitated clients, pregnant and lactating women, children, liver disease, kidney disease, depressed, mentally unstable, suicidal persons, and addictive personalities.

Example: Luminal (phenobarbital—also used for seizures).

Nonbarbiturates

Even though these drugs are supposed to be safer than barbiturates, they have also been misused and have resulted in fatalities.

Side Effects: Nausea, vomiting, diarrhea, rash, or dizziness.

Contraindications or Cautions: Hypersensitivity, severe liver impairment, severe renal impairment, elderly, debilitated, addiction prone, depressed or mentally unstable, suicidal tendencies, pregnant and lactating women, children, COPD, and sleep apnea.

Examples: ProSom, Dalmane, Restoril, Halcion (rarely used), Ambien, and Sonata.

PSYCHOTROPIC MEDICATIONS, ALCOHOL, AND DRUG ABUSE

Psychotropic drugs are medications that have a therapeutic effect on a person's mind, emotions, and actions. There are a number of medications that have psychotropic effects as secondary to their main functions. For example, many analgesics and sedatives can affect mental and emotional behavior.

Relevance for the Massage Therapist

Massage therapy treatments can help clients relax and deal with stress in a more productive fashion and may also affect the dosage of medication being used. The therapist should be in communication with the client's psychiatrist or psychologist so that the client's best interests are served. If the massage therapist's clientele consists of clients who suffer from mental and emotional disorders, he should take additional courses in psychology and further study pharmacology to understand what clients are experiencing and find ways to make the massage treatments better serve them. The mind, body, and emotions are intricately connected in one bioenergy system, and the positive effects of massage therapy and regular treatments will assist clients in moving toward greater well-being. Massage can help energize a depressed client or calm an agitated one. The therapist must assess each client individually and adjust treatment based on his findings. Also, as with all clients, records that chart each treatment and the effects of the massage treatment should be kept.

The four classes of medications are CNS stimulants, antidepressants, anxiolytics, and antipsychotic.

CNS Stimulants

CNS stimulants are medications that affect the functioning of the CNS. One well-known drug in this class is caffeine citrate. Long-term use with high intake of caffeine in any form can result in tolerance, habituation, and psychological dependence. If stopped suddenly, symptoms such as nervousness, anxiety, headaches, and dizziness can result. Because caffeine can cross the placenta and also be present in the milk of nursing mothers, it is generally recommended that pregnant and nursing mothers do not ingest foods and beverages or any drugs, including over-the-counter medications, that contain caffeine.

Other CNS stimulants include amphetamines such as Adderall, Ritalin, Concerta, and Dexedrine, all of which are used to treat attention deficit disorder (ADD) syndrome in children over the age of 6 and narcolepsy. Prolonged use of CNS stimulants in children with ADD has been reported to temporarily suppress normal weight and height patterns and also produce or exacerbate motor and vocal tics. Children must be observed very carefully for adverse effects. The use of amphetamines to lose weight is not advised because tolerance develops very rapidly and a person can develop physical or psychological dependence quickly.

Side Effects: Nervousness, insomnia, irritability, seizures, psychosis, tachycardia, palpitations, hypertension, cardiac arrhythmias, dizziness, headaches, blurry vision, or GI distress.

Contraindications or Cautions: Treatment for obesity; patients suffering from anxiety; history of drug dependence, alcoholism, or eating disorders; hyperthyroidism; pregnant or nursing women; and abrupt withdrawal.

Examples: Cafcit, Adderall, Dexedrine, Ritalin, and Concerta.

Antidepressants

Antidepressants are also known as mood elevators and are used primarily to treat clients suffering from depression. Persons who are depressed may have a shortage of the neurotransmitters dopamine, serotonin, or norepinephrine. These substances, which are supposed to travel across the synapse between two neurons, sometimes fail to cross the synapse and instead get reabsorbed by one nerve ending; thus they are unable to perform their function. Clients who have this problem are said to suffer from a chemical imbalance, which medication seeks to rectify.

There are four classes of antidepressants: tricyclics, monamine oxidase inhibitors (MAOIs), selective serotonin reuptake inhibitors (SSRIs), and heterocyclic antidepressants.

Tricyclics

Tricyclics take between 2 and 4 weeks to reach their maximum effect. They have a mild sedative action and are generally taken many times during the day. They generally have many side effects. They are also used as adjuncts in pain control. Tricyclics can interact with other medications, producing more severe side effects.

Side Effects: Dry mouth, increased appetite and weight gain, dizziness, drowsiness, constipation, urinary retention, palpitations, confusion, cardiac arrhythmias, or blurry vision.

Contraindications or Cautions: Cardiac, liver, kidney, and GI disease; the elderly; glaucoma; obesity; seizures; pregnant and lactating women; use with MAOIs.

Examples: Elavil, Norpramin, Adapin, Tofranil, Pamelor, and Anafranil.

Monoamine Oxidase Inhibitors

MAO inhibitors are used rarely because of potential serious side effects and negative interactions with food and other drugs. Persons stopping tricyclics must wait 2 weeks before starting MAO inhibitors. These drugs are generally used for atypical depression, panic disorders, or phobias.

Side Effects: Nervousness, agitation, insomnia, headaches, stiff neck, hypertension, tachycardia, palpitations, chest pain, nausea, vomiting, diarrhea, or blurry vision. Interactions of the MAOIs with some drugs and food can cause a hypertensive crisis that can be fatal.

Foods containing tyramine, tryptamine, or tryptophan such as yogurt, sour cream, all cheeses, turkey, liver, figs, bananas, wines, and so on must be avoided.

Contraindications or Cautions: Clients with cerebrovascular and liver disease.

Examples: Marplan, Nardil, and Parnate.

Selective Serotonin Reuptake Inhibitors (SSRIs)

These are the first choice of drugs in the treatment of depression. They have fewer side effects and greater safety. Sometimes the client must be on the drug for 2 to 4 weeks before effects are seen. These drugs also may interact negatively with other medications such as anticoagulants and beta blockers as well as other CNS drugs.

Side Effects: Sexual dysfunction, nausea, anorexia, diarrhea, constipation, sweating, insomnia, anxiety, nervousness, tremors, fatigue, dizziness, or headaches.

Contraindications or Cautions: Liver or kidney disease, suicidal history, diabetes, bipolar disorders, eating disorders, pregnant and lactating women; never take with MAOIs.

Examples: Prozac, Paxil, Zoloft, Celexa, and Effexor.

Heterocyclic Antidepressants

These drugs are useful in treating severe depression and also in helping people stop smoking. Some are used to treat clients suffering from both anxiety and depression and also help with the treatment of fibromyalgia. Others are useful for treating the agitation that elderly clients can experience when suffering from dementia. Heterocyclic antidepressants should never be taken with MAOIs.

Side Effects: Sleepiness, insomnia, restlessness, agitation, anxiety, dry mouth, dizziness, confusion, or weight gain.

Contraindications or Cautions: Suicidal history, seizures, and cardiac or liver disease.

Examples: Wellbutrin, Remeron, Serzone, and Desyrel (should not be taken by young males).

Antimanic Medications

These drugs are used to treat bipolar (manic-depressive) disorders. Clients must be monitored carefully for signs of toxicity.

Side Effects: GI distress, cardiac arrhythmias, low blood pressure, tremors, thyroid problems, coma, or muscle weakness.

Contraindications or Cautions: Seizure disorders, parkinsonism, cardiovascular and kidney disease, the elderly, or thyroid disease. Blood levels of clients taking Lithium must be monitored.

Examples: Lithobid (lithium), Tegretol, and Depakote.

Anxiolytics

These are medications that treat anxiety and act as minor tranquilizers. They are used for short-term treatment of anxiety, neurosis, some psychosomatic disorders, insomnia, and nausea and vomiting. When given in small doses, these drugs can reduce anxiety without causing drowsiness. Larger doses at bedtime are used for insomnia. These drugs are for short-term use only because persons can become physically and psychologically dependent to them. Withdrawal must be gradual, otherwise severe side effects, such as seizures and psychosis, can develop. Many of the anxiolytics are controlled substances.

Side Effects: Depression, hallucinations, confusion, agitation, bizarre behavior, amnesia, drowsiness, lethargy, headache, rash, or itching.

Contraindications or Cautions: Mental depression, suicidal history, pregnant and lactating women, children, liver and kidney disease, elderly clients, and persons operating machinery.

Examples: Xanax, Librium, Valium, Ativan, BuSpar, and Atarax.

Antipsychotic Medications

These drugs are major tranquilizers and are also called neuroleptics. They are used to treat psychoses and severe neuroses, relieve nausea and vomiting, and are used as adjunctive therapy with analgesics. These drugs can interact negatively with a number of medications such as antihypertensives and anticonvulsants.

Side Effects: Insomnia, agitation, depression, headaches, seizures, dry mouth, blurry vision, fever, jaundice, rash, confusion, drowsiness, weakness, constipation, or anorexia; parkinsonian symptoms such as tremors, drooling; involuntary and often irreversible movements (tardive dyskinesia) such as tics; dystonic reactions (spasms of the head, neck or tongue—more frequent in children).

Contraindications or Cautions: Seizure disorders, Parkinson's disease, severe depression, and pregnant women.

Examples: Thorazine, Haldol, Compazine, Risperdal, Zyprexa, and Seroquel.

Anticonvulsants

These drugs are used to reduce the severity and frequency of seizures in persons suffering from epilepsy. Although the cause of epilepsy is often unknown, seizures can be associated with disorders such as head trauma, brain tumors, chemical imbalances, cerebrovascular disease, or high fever. Medications should never be stopped abruptly. Drugs can be used to treat petit mal, also known as "absence epilepsy"—a momentary loss of consciousness without falling—or grand mal seizures. Grand mal seizures and temporal lobe seizures are generally treated with Dilantin, which may be combined with other drugs. Another drug, Tegretol, is used mainly for partial seizures. Preventative treatment is difficult because the medications must be adjusted to prevent seizures without sedating the client too much.

Side Effects of Drugs for Petit Mal Seizures: Drowsiness, dizziness, irritability, anorexia, nausea, vomiting, diarrhea, rash, or leukopenia.

Contraindications or Cautions: Liver and kidney disease, and pregnant and lactating women.

Examples: Zarontin, Klonopin, Dapakene, Depakote, and Neurontin.

Side Effects of Drugs for Grand Mal and Partial Seizures: Sedation, dizziness, headaches, blurry vision, GI distress, or rash.

Contraindications or Cautions: Liver disease, kidney disease, diabetes, low blood pressure, blood diseases, and congestive heart failure.

Examples: Dilantin and Tegretol.

Antiparkinsonian Medications

These drugs are used to treat Parkinson's disease, a neurological disease with symptoms of muscle tremors, rigidity, and weakness of muscles. Medications are aimed at relieving symptoms. Sinemet is the main drug used for long-term treatment. Eldepryl is another drug used to treat Parkinson's disease. It is never used alone but is added to Sinemet when Sinemet becomes less potent or less effective. The dosage of Sinemet can be reduced to lessen the side effects. Use of Eldepryl is contraindicated with certain drugs when severe side effects can result, including death.

Side Effects: These are numerous and generally serious. They may include anorexia, nausea, vomiting, anxiety, confusion, depression, psychosis, agitation, dizziness, syncope, low blood pressure, or involuntary movements.

Contraindications or Cautions: Bronchial asthma, emphysema, heart disease, low blood pressure, diabetes, kidney disease, liver disease, glaucoma, psychoses, and pregnant and lactating women. Clients must be weaned off the medication.

Examples: Sinemet and Eldepryl.

Anticholinergic Drugs

These drugs can help with mild forms of the disease and for symptoms induced by drugs. They include Cogentin, Artane, Symmetrel (amantadine).

Side Effects: Dizziness, drowsiness, constipation, confusion, depression, nausea, tachycardia, dry mouth, urinary retention, headache, or insomnia.

Contraindications or Cautions: Elderly clients and benign prostate disease.

Examples: Cogentin, Artane, and Symmetrel.

Drugs to Treat Alzheimer's Disease

These medications do not cure the disease but are aimed at slowing down its progress. They include Cognex, Aricept, and Exelon. All of these drugs produce GI distress (nausea, vomiting, anorexia) and other side effects that can be severe.

Alcohol

Alcohol is perhaps the biggest drug problem in the United States today and can be considered a psychotropic drug and a CNS depressant. It is pharmacologically similar to ether and is rapidly absorbed from the GI tract into the bloodstream, causing excitement, sedation, and, finally, anesthesia. It decreases a person's ability to make decisions and impairs memory as well as mental and emotional functioning. Prolonged use affects most organs of the body, causing liver and pancreatic damage, malnutrition, cardiovascular effects, GI damage, and permanent CNS damage.

> **Side Effects of Chronic Alcoholism:** Frequent falls and accidents, blackouts, memory loss, neuritis, muscular weakness, tremors, irritability, gastroenteritis, or neglect of personal appearance and responsibilities.

Drug Abuse

Drug abuse is the use of drugs for recreation or for purposes other than therapeutic reasons, for example, weight loss or to improve athletic performance. Drug addiction means that the person has psychological dependence, physical dependence, tolerance, and withdrawal reactions with physiological effects. Sometimes clients can become addicted to medications, especially when pain relief is being sought. Some of the major drugs that are abused are discussed next.

Amphetamines

These are known as "uppers" and are sometimes illegally used for weight loss. Symptoms of chronic abuse are anorexia, mental confusion, social withdrawal, paranoia, or continuous teeth grinding.

Marijuana

This drug has both euphoriant, sedative, CNS depressant, and hallucinogenic properties. However, marijuana as a medication can be very helpful for nausea induced by chemotherapy, for treatment of glaucoma, and as an appetite stimulant for persons suffering from cancer or AIDS. It has also been reported to have beneficial effects for persons suffering from multiple sclerosis. Cannabis seeds have been used traditionally in Chinese herbal medicine, in conjunction with other herbs, for the treatment of constipation. Despite its potential benefits, the U.S. government considers marijuana illegal to possess even for medical purposes.

> **Side Effects:** Short-term memory loss, slowed reflexes, apathy, increased heart rate, or lung irritation.

Cocaine

This drug is a CNS stimulant that produces euphoria. Its only approved medical use is for topical application as a local anesthetic. Cocaine is highly addictive and a growing health problem in the United States. It can be sniffed or snorted, which will damage the mucous membranes of the nose; intravenous use can be fatal; and smoking "crack" causes the most rapid addiction, sometimes after only one use. Withdrawal is very difficult and lengthy and may lead to severe depression.

> **Side Effects:** Euphoria, agitation, excitation, cardiac arrhythmias or failure, tremors and seizures, hallucinations, or possible psychosis.

Hallucinogens

Lysergic acid (LSD) and phencyclidine (PCP) are hallucinogens that can produce bizarre behaviors and distortion of perceptions.

> **Side Effects:** Rise in blood pressure, increased heart rate and pulse, panic, paranoia, or psychotic episodes.

ANTICONVULSANT DRUGS, ANTIPARKINSONIAN DRUGS, AND DRUGS TO TREAT ALZHEIMER'S DISEASE

These drugs are becoming more common as the general population ages and lives longer than previous generations. Nervous system disorders can be helped by massage therapy.

Relevance for the Massage Therapist

Massage can potentiate or decrease the effects of medications; therefore, dosages of medications may need to be adjusted with consistent treatments. Therapists should observe their clients carefully during and after treatment to ascertain the effects of treatment with the medication and work together with the clients' physician as part of a total wellness program.

VITAMINS AND MINERALS

The term *vitamin* was created in 1912 by Casimir Funk, a Polish biochemist who theorized that inherent in foods were "vita-amines," compounds that were vital to life. Even though most vitamins were discovered in the early 1900s, 1920s, and 1930s, most medical doctors have held a rather dogmatic view that supplements are unnecessary if one ingests a balanced and healthy diet. The reality is that most people do not eat a highly varied, well-balanced diet that follows the government's guidelines on eating. The majority of the population do not choose foods that are very nutritious. On the contrary, obesity has reached alarming rates, and, at the same time, many people in this country are, in fact, undernourished. The average diet in the United States contains too much fat and not enough fruits and vegetables, whole grains, fiber, nuts and seeds, and legumes. People do not eat the same foods that their ancestors ate. Family members who were born before World War II were not exposed to pesticides, herbicides, fungicides, preservatives, artificial ingredients, and toxic chemicals that now infest our food supply. In addition, modern fruits and vegetables are generally picked before they ripen, so those foods are lacking in vital nutrients. If we look at a loaf of bread as an example, we can see the dramatic difference in the way bread is prepared. A hundred years ago bread was made using flour, water, butter, yeast, and sugar to help the yeast rise. Today more than 100 ingredients can be used to create a loaf of bread, many of them artificial chemical compounds that are added to the food as well as the chemicals that leach into the food from manufacturing and packaging.

According to the U.S. Department of Agriculture (USDA), the nutrients in our soil have been severely depleted over the past six decades due to chemical fertilization. As an example, USDA tests show that in 1948 a cup of spinach contained 158 milligrams of iron per 100 grams. Today, the content of iron per 100 grams is about 2.7 milligrams. You would have to eat approximately 60 portions of spinach to receive the same amount of iron that you would have received from 1 cup in 1948.

In recent years, there have been numerous clinical studies demonstrating the benefits of nutritional supplements. While skeptics may continue to claim that nutritional supplements pose a health risk, the facts are that 150,000 people die yearly from prescription medications, compared to the rare incidence of overdose of a nutritional supplement.

Linus Pauling, a two-time Nobel Prize winner and the founder of orthomolecular medicine (the use of vitamins and nutrients to treat disease), concluded that supplementation should be based not on deficiency of nutrients but on optimal intake. According to him, what needs to be emphasized is not the minimal requirements of nutrients but rather optimal nutrition, giving the body's cells the levels of vitamins, minerals, and supplements that help them perform at their best. Currently, the Recommended Dietary Allowances (RDA) are established by the National Academy of Sciences and the National Research Council of the Food and Nutrition Board. These recommendations are considered by many researchers to be overly conservative and antiquated. They do not address the nutritional needs of people who are eating chemically laden foods, denatured foods, or people who are ill or sick. In addition, biochemical individuality exists in each person and, while everyone needs nutrients, the amounts from one person to the next will be varied. For example, one person might need 100 milligrams of vitamin C and another might need 1,000 milligrams. Stereotyped RDA values do not provide good nutrient guidelines.

Currently, a major project is under way to replace the RDA with Dietary Reference Intakes (DRI). This project is a collaborative effort between the United States and Canada. Until this project is completed, the RDA will unfortunately stand as the guideline for nutrient values. It remains to be seen whether the DRI will be a significant improvement over the RDA.

Massage therapists have many clients who use vitamins on a daily basis. Most supplements are considered to be safe. A good multivitamin with minerals can provide health protection for about 10 cents a day. Multivitamins can help protect against certain kinds of cancers, lower the risk of cardiovascular disease, strengthen the eyes against degenerative conditions such as cataracts and macular degeneration, and lower the incidence of birth defects. They also help strengthen the immune system; reduce the number of sick days; and help aging people strengthen their bones, reducing the risk of osteoporosis. In addition, vitamins can help people who are nutrient deficient, for example, persons suffering from anorexia, alcoholism, or illness; persons suffering from GI diseases that result in leaky gut syndrome and loss of nutrients; pregnant and lactating women who require increased nutrients; children, adolescents, and menopausal women; and people who are nutrient deficient due to medications, for example, deficiency of potassium due to use of diuretics or deficiency of vitamin B_1 due to loop diuretics.

If clients are taking numerous vitamins on their own, they should be referred to a health practitioner or nutritionist who is skilled in assessing their condition and who can make the proper recommendations for supplementation. Many massage therapists further their studies in nutrition and enhance their practice in this way. In either case, each individual should be under the care of a knowledgeable health care practitioner who can assist in choosing the right supplements for the individual's health and well-being. Although there have been no studies on any possible interactions between massage therapy and vitamins and minerals, suffice to say that the massage therapist must be aware of all the supplements and medications a client is taking. In addition to referring the client to the appropriate health care practitioner, the massage therapist must always be vigilant for any potential interactions between the treatments and what each client is taking.

Table A.1 and Table A.2 provide a summary of the food sources, functions, and illnesses caused by deficiency or excess of the major vitamins and minerals.

Table A.1

Summary of Water and Fat-Soluble Vitamins

NAME	FOOD SOURCES	FUNCTIONS	DEFICIENCY/ TOXICITY
Vitamin A (retinol, beta carotene)	Animal 　Oily saltwater fish 　Whole milk, cream 　Butter, cheese 　Egg yolk 　Fish liver oils Plants 　Dark-green leafy 　　vegetables 　Deep yellow or 　　orange fruit 　　and vegetables 　Fortified margarine	Dim light vision Maintenance of mucous membranes Growth of development of bones Healing of wounds Resistance to infection Beta carotene is an antioxidant	**Deficiency** Retarded growth Faulty bone and tooth development Night blindness Decreased ability to resist infection Abnormal function of gastrointestinal, genitourinary, and respiratory tracts due to altered epthelial membrane Shriveled, thickened skin Xerophthalmia **Toxicity** Irritability, lethargy, headache Joint pain, myalgia Stunted growth, fetal malformations Jaundice, nausea, diarrhea Dry skin and hair
Vitamin D (cholecalciferol)	Animal 　Fish oils 　Salmon, herring, 　　mackerel, 　　sardines 　Eggs, butter, milk Plants Fortified cereals	Healthy bones and teeth Muscle function Enables absorption of calcium	**Deficiency** Rickets (in children) Osteomalacia (in adults) Poorly developed teeth Muscle spasms **Toxicity** (Hypercalcemia) Kidney stones, kidney damage Muscle/bone pain Nausea, anorexia

continues

Table A.1 (continued)

Summary of Water and Fat-Soluble Vitamins

NAME	FOOD SOURCES	FUNCTIONS	DEFICIENCY/ TOXICITY
Vitamin E (tocopherol)	Plants Vegetable oils Seeds, nuts Wheat germ, cereals	Antioxidant	**Deficiency** Destruction of RBCs, muscle weakness **Toxicity** Prolonged bleeding time
Vitamin K (phytonadione)	Animal Egg yolk, cheese Liver Plants Vegetable oil Green leafy vegetables Cabbage, broccoli	Blood clotting	**Deficiency** Prolonged blood clotting time **Toxicity** Jaundice in infants
Vitamin B_1 (thiamine)	Animal Pork, beef, liver Oysters Plants Yeast Whole and enriched grains, wheat germ Legumes, collard greens, nuts, asparagus Oranges	Coenzyme carbohydrate metabolism Normal nervous and cardiovascular systems	**Deficiency** GI upset Neuritis, mental disturbance Cardiovascular problems Muscle weakness, fatigue **Toxicity** None known
Vitamin B_2 (riboflavin)	Animal Milk Meat, liver Plants Green vegetables Cereals Enriched bread Yeast	Aids in energy metabolism of glucose, fats, and amino acids	**Deficiency** Cheilosis Glossitis Photophobia, vision problems, itching eyes Dermatitis, rough skin **Toxicity** None

Table A.1 (continued)

Summary of Water and Fat-Soluble Vitamins

NAME	FOOD SOURCES	FUNCTIONS	DEFICIENCY/ TOXICITY

Vitamin B$_6$ (pyridoxine)	Animal
	
	  Pork, beef, chicken, tuna, salmon
	
	Plants
	
	  Whole grain cereals, wheat germ
	  Legumes, peanuts, soybeans
	  Bananas
		Synthesis of amino acids
		
		Antibody production
		
		Maintenance of blood glucose level
			Deficiency
			
			Anorexia, nausea, vomiting
			
			Dermatitis
			
			Neuritis, depression
			
			Toxicity
			
			Seizures in newborn
			
			120 mg–Neuropathy

Vitamin B$_{12}$ (cyanocobalamin)	Animal
	
	  Seafood/shellfish
	  Meat, poultry, liver
	  Eggs
	  Milk, cheese
	
	Plants
	
	  None
		Synthesis of RBCs
		
		Maintenance of nervous system
			Deficiency
			
			Nerve, muscle, mental problems
			
			Pernicious anemia
			
			Toxicity
			
			None

Niacin (nicotinic acid)	Animal
	
	  Milk
	  Eggs
	  Fish
	  Poultry
	
	Plants
	
	  Legumes, nuts
		Lipid metabolism
		
		Nerve functioning
			Deficiency
			
			Pellagra
			
			Toxicity
			
			Vasodilation of blood vessels

Folacin (folic acid)	Animal
	
	  Organ meats
	
	Plants
	
	  Green leafy vegetables
	  Avocado, beets
	  Broccoli, kidney beans
	  Orange juice
		Synthesis of RBCs, leukocytes, DNA and RNA
		
		Needed for normal growth and reproduction
			Deficiency
			
			Increased risk of neural tube defects
			
			Macrocytic anemia
			
			Irritability, behavior disorders
			
			Toxicity
			
			None

continues

Table A.1 (continued)

Summary of Water and Fat-Soluble Vitamins

NAME	FOOD SOURCES	FUNCTIONS	DEFICIENCY/ TOXICITY
Vitamin C (ascorbic acid)	Fruits 　All citrus, cantaloupe Plants 　Broccoli 　Tomatoes 　Brussel sprouts 　Cabbage 　Green peppers	Prevention of scurvy Formation of collagen Healing of wounds Absorption of iron Antioxidant	**Deficiency** Scurvy Poor healing Muscle cramps/weakness Ulcerated gums/mouth Capillary fragility **Toxicity** Raise uric acid level GI distress Kidney stones Rebound scurvy in neonates

Table A.2

Summary of Major Minerals

NAME	FOOD SOURCES	FUNCTIONS	DEFICIENCY/ TOXICITY
Calcium (Ca)	Milk, cheese Sardines Salmon Green vegetables except spinach	Development of bones and teeth Permeability of cell membranes Transmission of nerve impulses Blood clotting	**Deficiency** Osteoporosis Osteomalacia Rickets (in children) **Toxicity** None known
Potassium (K)	Oranges, bananas Dried fruits Tomatoes	Contraction of muscles Transmission of nerve impulses Carbohydrate and protein metabolism Maintaining water balance	**Deficiency** Hypokalemia **Toxicity** Hyperkalemia
Sodium (Na)	Table salt Beef, eggs Milk, cheese	Maintaining fluid balance in blood Transmission of nerve impulses	**Deficiency** Hyponatremia **Toxicity** Increase in blood pressure

Table A.2 (continued)

Summary of Major Minerals

FOOD NAME	SOURCES	DEFICIENCY/ FUNCTIONS	TOXICITY
Chlorine (Cl)	Table salt	Gastric acidity Regulation of osmotic pressure Activation of salivary amylase	**Deficiency** Imbalance in gastric acidity Imbalance in blood pH **Toxicity** Diarrhea
Magnesium (Mg) (DRI 320–420 mg)	Green vegetables Whole grains	Synthesis of ATP (adenosine triphosphate) Transmission of nerve impulses Relaxation of skeletal muscles	**Deficiency (seldom)** Imbalance Weakness **Toxicity** Diarrhea
Iron (Fe)	Meat Liver Eggs Poultry Spinach Dried fruits Dried beans Prune juice	Hemoglobin formation Resistance to infection	**Deficiency (anemia)** Pale Weak Lethargy Vertigo Air hunger **Toxicity** Vomiting Diarrhea Erosion of GI tract
Iodine (I)	Freshwater shellfish and seafood Iodized salt	Major component of thyroid hormones Regulating rate of metabolism Growth, reproduction Nerve and muscle function Protein synthesis Skin and hair growth	**Deficiency** Goiter Hypothyroidism **Toxicity** "Iodine goiter" Hyperactive, enlarged goiter
Zinc (Zn)	Meat Liver Oysters Poultry Fish Whole-grain bread and cereal	Wound healing Mineralization of bone Insulin glucose regulation Normal taste Antioxidant	**Deficiency** Poor wound healing Reduced taste perception Alcohol/glucose intolerance **Toxicity** GI distress Copper deficiency with extended use of high levels of zinc

HERBS AND SUPPLEMENTS

Herbalism is one of the oldest healing arts with extensive roots in many cultures—Native American, Chinese, and Indian just to name a few. Herbs are defined in different ways, depending on the discipline in which they are used. To a gardener, herbs are plants that help decorate and beautify the land, whereas to a chef, herbs are used for culinary purposes. To a medical herbalist, however, herbs are defined as any plant material that can be used in medicine for healing. All parts of plants can be used in treatment—flowers, seeds, roots, stems, and fruit as well as non-flowering plants such as mosses, seaweed, ferns, and lichen. Chinese herbal medicine also includes nonbotanical substances such as minerals and entomological and zoological substances.

Throughout the world the use of botanicals to treat disease far exceeds the use of conventional synthetic drugs. According to the WHO, 80 percent of the world's population utilizes herbal therapy as their first line of defense against illness. In many European countries, such as Germany, herbal medicine, called phytotherapy, is not considered alternative but mainstream, and physicians prescribe herbs more frequently than they do prescription drugs.

Most people do not realize that herbs form the foundation for much of modern medicine. Many years of scientific research resulted in the extraction of the active ingredients of plants and the creation of potent drugs. For example, aspirin came from willow bark, digoxin for heart failure from the foxglove, and steroids from the wild yam. Currently about 25 percent of all prescription drugs are derived from botanical sources, whereas the other 75 percent of drugs are synthetically produced.

The United States has a long tradition of herbal medicine use, employing primarily native American plants and plants brought to our shores by early settlers. Back in the 1700s and 1800s, the *U.S. Pharmacopeia,* our official compendium of medicinal substances, primarily contained entries of natural substances, including herbal extracts and whole herbs. Herbs were traditionally prepared as teas, tinctures, liniments, ointments, tablets, washes, douches, and poultices, and many modern herbalists still concoct their herbal remedies in myriad ways, depending on the needs of the client.

Today, the *U.S. Pharmacopeia* contains far fewer herbal medicines and a far greater number of synthetic drugs. This change in the makeup of the compendium took place over a period of years, beginning with the introduction of reductionism and the scientific analysis of herbs, the discovery of antibiotics, and the subsequent growth of the pharmaceutical industry. This shift continued, resulting in a complete departure from our natural herbal tradition as the "active compounds" of herbs were isolated, extracted, and concentrated.

Pharmacognosy is the study of natural drugs and their constituents and plays a major role in modern drug development. Because a plant cannot be patented, plants are researched for their active constituents, which are then isolated. In the United States, if the constituent is powerful enough, the drug company will begin the process to get FDA approval. Because it typically takes 10 to 18 years at a cost of hundreds of millions of dollars to get approval and the lack of patent protection, the American pharmaceutical industry has done very little research on plant extracts as medicinal agents.

In contrast, European governments have made it economically possible for companies to research and develop herbs as drugs. In Germany, herbal products can be sold with drug claims if they have been proven to be safe and effective. The legal requirements for herbal products are the same for medications. Therefore, whether the herbal product is given by prescription or sold over the counter, it has met the requirements for safety and efficacy of use.

In Germany, a special expert commission called the German Commission E has developed a series of several hundred monographs (a treatise or detailed research article) on herbal products. This commission is composed of physicians, pharmacists, pharmacologists, toxicologists, representatives of the pharmaceutical industry, and laypersons. Its conclusions are independent of the German Federal Health Agency, the German counterpart of the FDA. Unlike the FDA, which relies on drug data compiled by the pharmaceutical manufacturers, the Commission E checks independent data from clinical trials, field studies, scientific literature, and traditional usage, including information from standard reference texts, and the expertise of medical persons. After completing its work, the commission issues a monograph with a positive or negative recommendation regarding medicinal use. A number of reputable American herbal companies utilize the monographs from the German Commission E in the preparation of their herbal supplements and follow the recommendations of the commission regarding dosage and potency.

The supplement industry continues to grow dramatically worldwide as more and more consumers seek natural methods of dealing with their health. In this country, many studies have shown that consumers buy dietary supplements for a number of reasons—to prevent disease, as therapeutic agents for the treatment of diseases, to maintain health, and as adjunctive therapy for persons also receiving allopathic treatment.

In 1994, due to public demand, Congress passed the Dietary Supplement Health and Education Act (DSHEA), which recognizes herbs or other botanicals, vitamins, and supplements as dietary supplements distinct from drugs. According to the DSHEA, manufacturers cannot make statements that these substances cure or treat a disease, but they can make "statements of nutritional support" or "structure and function" claims. For example, a company cannot say that glucosamine sulfate treats or cures arthritis, but it can say that it helps build and support joint cartilage. In order to make these claims, manufacturers must document and substantiate their statements. They must also state that their supplements are not drugs; their labels must say that they are "dietary supplements" and have a "supplement facts" panel on them.

The term *supplement* can cover a broad range of substances, including herbs and other botanicals, vitamins, minerals, antioxidants, enzymes, amino acids, metabolites, concentrates, constituents, extracts of natural substances, or combinations of these substances. The term *nutraceutical* is commonly used to describe supplements that combine a number of these substances together in a formulation. For example, a supplement for cardiovascular support might include:

Hawthorn berry—botanical

Ginger—botanical

Garlic—botanical

CoQ10—antioxidant

Vitamin C

Vitamin B$_{12}$

L-Carnitine—amino acid

Magnesium—mineral

Potassium—mineral

Consumers need to be educated about supplements and quality control. They must be on the lookout for fraudulent products. Products that are significantly cheaper than others; products that are not made by known, reputable companies; products that make claims of "cure" or "miracle"; or products whose claims are not backed by scientific studies should be avoided. Consumers who wish to utilize the growing market of supplementation would be wise to consult with a certified herbalist, nutritionist, or other health care provider who is knowledgeable in the field of supplementation. Special warnings should be given to clients who have diabetes or who are taking cardiac drugs, particularly anticoagulants, because of the increased risk of serious interactions and side effects. Knowledge of the interactions between dietary supplements and medications is in its infancy stage. Therefore, clients should consult not only with their physicians, who have limited information in this area, but also with qualified persons in the field of herbs and nutrition. Massage therapists should have such people involved as part of their network of health care professionals so that they can refer their clients to the best health care practitioner for their specific needs.

There are numerous herbal and nutraceutical remedies on the market today, and they are clearly beyond the scope of this appendix. Table A.3 lists some of the more popular ones with some information about their uses, cautions, and known interactions. Check the suggested reading list at the end of this appendix for additional sources of information.

Table A.3

Uses and Side Effects of Some Herbs and Supplements

HERBS OR SUPPLEMENTS	POSSIBLE USES	POSSIBLE SIDE EFFECTS/CAUTIONS
Aloe Vera	Topical use for minor burns, minor wounds, psoriasis, seborrhea, diabetes; laxative; antiulcer effects on the GI tract; immune enhancing and antiviral	Not to be used for deep surgical wounds
Black Cohosh	Phytoestrogen for premenstrual syndrome (PMS), menopausal symptoms	Not to be taken with estrogen or by clients with history of estrogen-dependent breast cancer; high doses can cause frontal headaches
Capsaicin	Topical pain relief, anti-inflammatory for arthritis	Local burning sensation, usually fades with time
Chamomile	Anti-inflammatory, antispasmodic for the digestive tract, mild sedative, antiulcer	Persons with a known sensitivity to members of the Compositae family of plants (such as ragweed, daisies, chrysanthemums), may be allergic
Coenzyme Q10	Improves blood circulation; increases tolerance to exercise; protects heart tissue from free-radical damage, congestive heart failure, hypertension, cardiomyopathy; periodontal disease; Parkinson's disease	Very safe, no serious side effects. Numerous drugs impair the synthesis of CoQ10 in the body (beta blockers, tricyclic antidepressants, etc.); therefore individuals taking these drugs will find it useful to supplement with CoQ10
Echinacea	Enhances resistance to infections, especially of the upper respiratory tract; assists in recovery from chemotherapy; anti-inflammatory	Side effects are rare; those allergic to the Compositae family of plants may be allergic. There are no data to suggest that long-term use of echinacea is harmful to immune function
Ephedra	Asthma, bronchitis, sinusitis (ephedrine was synthesized in 1927 and since then has been used extensively in over-the-counter cold and allergy medications)	Can raise blood pressure in persons who are hypertensive; palpitations, insomnia, anxiety
Evening Primrose Oil	Anti-inflammatory disorders, including rheumatoid arthritis, ulcerative colitis; diabetic neuropathy; hypotensive; PMS	Headaches, mild nausea; use caution in persons with a history of epilepsy
Feverfew	Migraine headaches, tension headaches, arthritis	Well tolerated; no serious side effects; those allergic to the Compositae family may be allergic. Possible allergic dermatitis

continues

Table A.3 (continued)

Uses and Side Effects of Some Herbs and Supplements

HERBS OR SUPPLEMENTS	POSSIBLE USES	POSSIBLE SIDE EFFECTS/CAUTIONS
Garlic	Lowers blood pressure, lowers cholesterol; antimicrobial against many types of bacteria, viruses, worms, and fungi; strengthens the immune system	Use with caution in patients on anticoagulants; can cause allergic contact dermatitis; irritation to the digestive tract
Ginger	Nausea, motion sickness, anti-inflammatory, antiplatelet, carminative; relaxes the intestinal tract; migraine headaches, arthritis	Contraindicated in persons with gallstones; not more than a daily dose of 2 g should be taken during pregnancy; possible heartburn at high doses
Gingko	Improves memory and cognitive function for ordinary memory loss, dementia, Alzheimer's; increases blood flow to the brain; tissue oxygenation and nutrition; improves peripheral circulation	Extremely small incidence of side effects; use caution in clients who are on anticoagulants or antiplatelets
Panax Ginseng (Chinese, Korean)	Adaptogenic; tonic; cardiotonic, cancer preventative; improves performance and well-being; antifatigue	Contraindicated in acute infections, hypertension, anxiety, insomnia, excessive menstruation or nosebleeds, signs of heat; avoid concurrent use of stimulants; may interact with anticoagulants
Glucosamine	Anti-inflammatory for osteoarthritis	May increase insulin resistance in diabetes; mild gastrointestinal distress
Green Tea	Cancer protective; may reduce heart cancer risk	Generally very safe—does contain some caffeine so it may cause nervousness or insomnia
Hawthorn	Congestive heart failure angina, antiarrhythmia; protects against myocardial damage; hypotensive	No contraindications; may act with hypotensive drugs and increase their actions; modification of drug dosage may be necessary
Licorice	Healing of peptic ulcers (deglycyrrhizinated licorice [DGL]); anti-inflammatory; antitussive; expectorant; menopausal symptoms	High doses can cause signs of pseudo-hyperaldosteronism—sodium retention and high blood pressure—use with caution in patients taking loop diuretics, thiazides, or digitalis
Melatonin	Insomnia, jet lag, cancer treatment—prevents some of the side effects of chemotherapy; helps to inhibit the growth of breast cancer cells	May cause sedation and affect balance; may help with withdrawal from benzodiazepine drugs

Table A.3 (continued)

Uses and Side Effects of Some Herbs and Supplements

HERBS OR SUPPLEMENTS	POSSIBLE USES	POSSIBLE SIDE EFFECTS/CAUTIONS
Milk Thistle	Enhances liver function; alcoholic liver disease; cirrhosis; viral hepatitis; protects against hepatotoxic chemicals; prevents cholelithiasis—increases bile flow	Very safe, no adverse effects even with long-term use and high-dose administration; safe in pregnancy and lactation.
Probiotics	Inflammatory bowel disease; antibiotic diarrhea; irritable bowel syndrome; eczema; vaginal candidiasis, traveler's diarrhea; acute infectious diarrhea in children—both prevention and treatment; prevents respiratory infection in children; prevents otitis media	No side effects or safety issues; no known drug interactions
Saw Palmetto	For treatment of benign prostatic hypertrophy (BPH); improves urinary tract symptoms in men	Very safe and well-tolerated

SUGGESTED READINGS

Bratman, S., & Girman, A. (Eds.). (2003). *Mosby's handbook of herbs and supplements and their therapeutic uses.* St. Louis, MO: Elsevier Science.

Harkness, R., & Bratman, S. (2003). *Mosby's handbook of drug-herb and drug-supplement interactions.* St. Louis, MO: Elsevier Science.

Mills, S., & Bone, K. (2000). *Principles and practice of phytotherapy—modern herbal medicine.* London: Churchill Livingstone.

Ottariano, S. G. (1999). *Medicinal herbal therapy—a pharmacist's viewpoint.* Portsmouth, NH: Nicolin Fields.

Spratto, G. R. & Woods, A. L. (2005). *PDR nurse's drug handbook.* Clifton Park, NY: Thomson Delmar Learning.

Woodrow, R. (2002). *Essentials of pharmacology for health occupations* (4th edition). Clifton Park, NY: Thomson Delmar Learning.

Appendix II:
Answers to Questions for Discussion and Review

Chapter 1 Historical Overview

1. Massage is the manual (use of hands) or mechanical (use of machines or apparatus) manipulation of a part of the body by rubbing, kneading, pressing, rolling, slapping, and like movements for the purpose of improving circulation of the blood, relaxation of muscles, and other benefits to body systems.

2. Various artifacts show evidence that ancient civilizations used massage and exercise in their social, personal, and religious practices.

3. Massage is said to be the most effective and most natural means of obtaining relief from pain or discomfort, because a person can use his hands to rub, touch, or exercise a part of the body to obtain immediate relief.

4. The Chinese called their massage system *anmo*. This method grew from various pressing and rubbing of parts of the body to produce therapeutic effects.

5. The Greeks and Romans were health and beauty conscious. Both men and women believed that exercise improved the body and the mind. Exercise and massage were utilized in the training and rehabilitation of gladiators. Both Greek and Roman physicians prescribed various kinds of exercise and massage movements as aids to the healing of diseases and wounds.

6. Hippocrates, the Greek physician, became known as the father of medicine and originator of the Hippocratic oath, which is still used as the ethical guide to the medical professions. The Hippocratic oath can be found in its entirety in most modern dictionaries.

7. The Middle Ages were called the Dark Ages because the arts and sciences were allowed to deteriorate, leading to the decline of learning.

8. As the Greco-Roman culture fell into the decay of the Middle Ages, many of the important teachings of the great physicians and philosophers were carried on by the Persians of the Arabic Empire. The Islamic Persian philosopher/physicians, Rhazes or Razi and Avicenna, who followed the teachings of Hippocrates and Galen, authored important books that eventually returned to the West by way of trade and conquest and paved the way for the Renaissance.

9. The Renaissance, meaning "rebirth," revived interest in the arts and sciences and renewed interest in health and personal hygiene practices.

10. The invention of the printing press in the latter part of the fifteenth century led to the publishing of more writings in the arts and sciences. This improved circulation of educational materials led to a better understanding of the value of massage and exercise as therapeutic aids.

11. Per Henrik Ling based the Swedish Movement Cure on the developing science of physiology applied to the treatment of disease. The system's primary focus was on gymnastics, which consisted of movements classified as active, duplicated, and passive.

12. In 1858, the brothers Charles Fayette Taylor and George Henry Taylor started an orthopedic practice in New York. They specialized in the Swedish movements.

13. There were several reasons for the decline of the scientific and medical use of massage at the turn of the twentieth century. An inquiry by the British Medical Association in 1894 revealed numerous abuses in the education and practice of massage practitioners, including unscrupulous recruitment practices, inadequate training, deceptive advertising, and false certification. Technical innovations, such as the invention of electricity and various electrical apparatuses (such as the vibrator) and intellectual advances in medicine that led to new treatment strategies based more on pharmacology and surgical procedures, also had a detrimental effect on massage.

14. Because there were more diseases and injuries during wartime, physicians employed therapeutic massage and exercise more often. The good results led to wider acceptance of massage and exercise as aids to healing.

15. Manual massage became a secondary treatment following World War II because new mechanical and electrical devices were designed to take over some of the manipulative movements.

16. The increased awareness of physical and mental fitness as well as the increasing cost of traditional medicine opened the way for viable alternatives in health care. The development of the wellness model, which placed more emphasis on prevention and recognized the importance of controlling stress, has caused a renewed interest in massage.

17. Passive exercise of muscles incorporates massage and is done by the practitioner on the client. Active exercise of muscles is movement done by the individual, as in sports or gymnastics.

18. The Japanese use a system called shiatsu (shi, fingers; atsu, pressure). It is the finger pressure method based on the Oriental concept that the body has a series of energy points. When pressure is properly applied to these points, circulation is improved and nerves are stimulated. This system is said to improve body metabolism and to relieve a number of physical disorders.

19. Athletes often have injuries and sore muscles that can be relieved by massage. Massage and proper exercise also help to prevent fatigue and contribute to the maintenance of optimum fitness.

20. A person contemplating a career in any important field should have some understanding of problems of the past and the progress that has been made over a period of time. Understanding the past helps us to measure our own progress in the development of the art and practice of therapeutic body massage.

21. The Swedish massage system is still the most widely used and is most frequently incorporated into other systems.

22. The points of stimulation in Japanese massage (tsubo) are much the same as points used in Chinese traditional medicine.

23. Sports massage is used in sports medicine as an aid to treating injuries that have occurred during sports activities. It is also used as a means of keeping the athlete's muscles supple and strong.

Chapter 2 Requirements for the Practice of Therapeutic Massage

1. The practitioner must be concerned about the laws, rules, regulations, and obligations concerning the practice of therapeutic body massage because the practitioner has a responsibility to the public and to individual clients. Massage is a personal, health-related service, and, as such, strict rules must be observed.

2. The scope of practice defines the rights and activities legally acceptable according

to the licenses of a particular practice or profession. Scope of practice is defined legally and determines the educational focus and requirements that become the national standards of a given profession.

3. Laws governing the practice of massage often differ because there are no national standards and some states have fewer complaints, or problems, whereas others have found it necessary to establish state boards and stringent guidelines for licensing practitioners, schools, and establishments.

4. Being licensed in one locality does not guarantee that the same license will be valid or recognized in another locality. Because laws and regulations vary greatly from state to state and city to city, a practitioner who has a license and wishes to practice in another city or state should contact the proper agency in the area where she wishes to practice, provide proof of ability to meet any requirements, and make any applications that are required.

5. The general educational requirements to practice massage vary depending on discipline or techniques and the licensing requirements of the city or state where the practice is located. Because there is not a national standard for massage therapy, licensing laws may contain no educational requirement or may require as much as 1,000 hours of training. The educational requirements to enroll in a program of instruction at a certificate-granting school or institute of massage may differ, but generally a high school diploma or equivalency diploma is required.

6. A person may receive a certificate in recognition of an accomplishment or achieving or maintaining some kind of standard. Certificates are awarded by schools and institutions to show the successful completion of a course of study and by professional organizations to indicate that the recipient has met the qualifications to become a member or in recognition of achievements in the recipient's chosen profession.

7. The grounds upon which the practitioner's license may be revoked, canceled, or suspended are the following:
   1. Practicing fraud or deceit in obtaining a license

   2. Being convicted of a felony
   3. Being engaged in any act of prostitution
   4. Practicing under a false or assumed name
   5. Being addicted to drugs, alcohol, or the like
   6. Being willfully negligent of the health of a client
   7. Prescribing drugs or medicine
   8. Being guilty of fraudulent or deceptive advertising.

Chapter 3 Professional Ethics for Massage Practitioners

1. It is important to have a code of ethics for your business in order to protect the public and your reputation.

2. A satisfied client is your best means of advertising because he will recommend you, your business, and your services.

3. Successful business managers know that employees who practice sound personal and professional ethics will help them to build their business and keep their customers.

4. Boundaries are the basis of ethics. By honoring personal and professional boundaries, ethical dilemmas are averted.

5. Personal boundaries define an individual's comfort zone and are either innate or developed beginning at a very early age that dictate how a person interacts with the world. Professional boundaries are the basis for operating a professional practice that protects the safety of the client and practitioner and are outlined in policy and procedure statements.

6. Some major areas to consider when establishing professional boundaries are location of service, interpersonal space, appearance, self-disclosure, language, touch, time, money, and sexual intimacy.

7. The power differential favors the person in the position of authority, usually the practitioner or therapist.

8. When a boundary is crossed, there is a feeling of discomfort.

9. The practitioner can reduce the risk of crossing a client's boundary by asking the client to articulate or speak up any time

the practitioner says or does anything that causes any discomfort to the client.

10. Transference is the unconscious tendency for the client to project onto the practitioner attributes of someone from a former relationship. Countertransference is when the practitioner personalizes the relationship with the client.

11. It is always the responsibility of the practitioner to manage transference, countertransference, and boundary issues.

12. A dual relationship is any situation that combines the therapeutic relationship with a secondary relationship that extends beyond the massage practitioner/client relationship. Examples might be when someone you know becomes a client, when services are bartered, or when a therapeutic relationship becomes a romantic relationship.

13. The appropriate response to sexual arousal depends on the circumstance. If there is discomfort on the part of either the client or the practitioner, immediate steps should be taken, such as massaging a less sensitive area of the client's body, opening a dialogue with the client or having the client, turn over. It is the practitioner's responsibility to act in a nonsexual manner, clarify to the client that there is no sexual intent or involvement in the relationship, and maintain the appropriate boundary.

14. Supervision is the practice of a professional counseling with another professional about difficult situations or conditions that may arise in a helping practice such as transference, countertransference, or sexual issues.

15. It is necessary for the massage practitioner to be concerned with personal hygiene and health habits because his own good health inspires confidence on the part of clients. Good health is also a form of protection for the practitioner and the client.

16. Professional projection in attitude and appearance means that the practitioner acts, speaks, and dresses to project a professional image.

17. Human relations is defined as the art of being able to work successfully with others and to give excellent service.

18. The practice of good human relations is important because it helps the practitioner interact successfully with different personalities.

19. When building your business image, pay attention to the use of appropriate wording in your business name and in advertising so that potential clients get the right message.

Chapter 4 Human Anatomy and Physiology Overview

1. Anatomy is defined as the study of the gross structure or morphology of the body or the study of an organism and the interrelations of its parts.

2. Physiology is the science and study of the vital processes, mechanisms, and functions performed by the various systems of the body.

3. Histology is the branch of biology concerned with the microscopic structure of tissues of a living organism.

4. Pathology is the study of the structural and functional changes caused by disease.

5. Disease is an abnormal and unhealthy state of all or part of the body wherein it is not capable of carrying on its normal function.

6. A symptom is caused by the disease and is perceived by the victim, such as dizziness, chills, nausea, or pain. A symptom is a clear message to the individual that something is wrong. Signs of a disease are observable indications such as abnormal pulse rate, fever, abnormal skin color, or physical irregularities.

7. Regardless of the source or nature of stress, the physiological reaction of the body is essentially the same. When we encounter high levels of stress, our bodies respond with the "fight or flight" reactions. The adrenal secretions, adrenaline and cortisol, give us a physical and mental boost that heightens our senses, sharpens our reflexes, and strengthens our muscles.

8. There are two responses to pain: psychological and physical. The physical response to pain is very similar to the body's response to stress. Blood pressure and pulse increase, blood flow is shifted from the intestines and brain to the muscles, and

mental alertness intensifies, readying the body for a fight or flight. The physical experience also informs us of the location, intensity, and duration of the pain.

9. The pain-spasm-pain cycle is associated with muscle spasms. The natural reflex reaction to the tissue damage and pain is a contraction of the muscles that surround the injury. Contracted muscles pinch the blood vessel and capillaries in the muscles, restricting blood flow and causing ischemia. Metabolic activity of the muscles increases as oxygen and nutrients are burned, producing increased amounts of metabolic wastes. Lactic acid and other toxins collect in the tissues, and soon ischemic pain appears. Reflex reactions to the ischemic pain mirror and perpetuate the reaction to the original injury to become a vicious cycle.

10. In the case of the pain-spasm-pain cycle wherein pain is intensified because of ischemia, skillfully applied massage therapy diverts some attention away from the acute intensity of the pain. By massaging the contracted ischemic tissues, chronic spasms can be relieved and circulation restored. As oxygen and nutrients flood the area and lactic acid and other irritants are removed, the pain disappears and mobility is restored.

11. Infection is the result of the invasion of the body by disease-producing microorganisms such as bacteria, viruses, fungi, or protozoa. If microorganisms enter the body in sufficient numbers to multiply and become harmful and are capable of destroying healthy tissue, the body reacts by developing an infection. Inflammation is a protective and healing response that happens when tissue is damaged. Blood vessels in the area of the damaged tissues dilate, increasing blood flow to the area; capillary walls become more permeable, allowing large quantities of blood plasma and white blood cells to enter the tissue spaces; and leukocytes flood the area to engulf and digest the invading organisms and the damaged tissue debris.

12. The four principal signs and symptoms of inflammation are swelling, redness, heat, and pain.

13. Fever is a warning sign that usually accompanies infectious diseases or infected burns and cuts. A disturbance of the body's heat-regulating system causes an elevated body temperature.

14. Extreme or prolonged fever may be dangerous or even fatal. Prolonged fever will cause dehydration, so fluids must be replaced. Fevers above 106° to 108°F may cause damage to the tissues of the kidneys, liver, or other organs or may cause irreparable brain damage, possibly resulting in death.

15. Medical terms are usually compound words constructed of root words, or stems, prefixes, and suffixes. Anatomical terms often include more than one word. Generally the first word acts as an adjective and will indicate the region or location of the structure. The second word is the noun and names the structure.

16. The stem, or root word, generally indicates the body part or structure involved. A prefix is added in front of the stem to further its meaning. Suffixes often denote a diagnosis, symptom, or surgical procedure or identify a word as a noun or adjective.

Chapter 5 Human Anatomy and Physiology

1. All living matter consists of various cells.

2. Nucleus, centrosome, cytoplasm, and the cell membrane or wall.

3. The nucleus and the centrosome control cell reproduction.

4. As long as the cell receives an adequate supply of food, oxygen, and water, eliminates waste products, and is surrounded by a favorable environment (proper temperature and the absence of waste products, toxins, and pressure), it will continue to grow and function. When these requirements are not provided, the cell will stop growing and will eventually die.

5. Cell reproduction in human tissue occurs by the process called mitosis, the indirect division of cells.

6. The five phases of mitosis are interphase, prophase, metaphase, anaphase, and telophase.

7. Catabolism and anabolism.

8. Anabolism is the process of building up of larger molecules from smaller ones.

9. Catabolism is the process of breaking down of larger molecules into smaller ones.

10. Enzymes are protein substances that act as organic catalysts to initiate, accelerate, or control specific chemical reactions in the metabolic process, while they themselves remain unchanged.

11. All tissues are composed of specialized cells.

12. The five main categories of tissues are epithelial, connective, muscular, nervous, and liquid tissue.

13. Endoderm, mesoderm, and ectoderm are the cell layers of the embryo that form the primary germ layers that, in turn, form all the tissues and organs of the body.

14. Epithelial tissues cover all surfaces of the body, both inside and out, and function in the process of absorption, excretion, secretion, and protection.

15. Two main types of membranes are epithelial and connective.

16. The main function of connective tissue is to bind structures, to create a framework, and to provide support.

17. The main function of areolar (loose) tissue is to bind the skin to underlying tissues and to fill spaces between the muscles.

18. Adipose tissue is areolar tissue with an abundance of fat-containing cells.

19. Three types of cartilage are fibrous, hyaline, and elastic.

20. Bone tissue is made hard by mineral salts, calcium phosphate, and calcium carbonate.

21. Dentine is the hard, dense, calcareous tissue that forms the body of a tooth beneath the enamel.

22. Three types of muscle tissue are skeletal, smooth, and cardiac muscle tissue.

23. Striated muscle tissue is made of cylindrical fibers, is found in voluntary muscles, and appears striated if observed under a microscope. Smooth muscle tissue fibers are not striated and are found in involuntary muscles.

24. Cardiac muscle tissue is found only in the heart.

25. The main function of nervous tissue proper is to initiate, control, and coordinate the body's adaptations to its surroundings and environment.

26. Liquid tissue is found in blood and lymph.

Chapter 5 The Anatomical Position of the Body

1. Anatomic position shows a person from the front standing upright with the palms of the hands facing forward.

2. The three imaginary planes are called the sagittal (vertical), the coronal (frontal), and the transverse (horizontal) planes.

3. When studying anatomy, it is important to know the anatomical position and the regions and planes of the human body to describe the position of a structure or to locate one structure in relation to another. Once you know the body planes, you will understand the location of body cavities and which organs are located in a particular cavity.

4. The subdivisions of the ventral cavity are the thoracic cavity, containing the heart and lungs; the abdominal cavity, containing the liver, stomach, spleen, pancreas, small and large intestines; and the pelvic cavity, containing the bladder, rectum, and some of the reproductive organs. The dorsal cavity is divided into the cranial cavity, containing the brain, and the spinal or vertebral cavity, containing the spinal cord.

5. The four main anatomic parts of the body are the head, consisting of the cranium and the face; the spine, including the vertebrae and the sacrum; the trunk, including the chest or thorax and the abdomen and the organs they contain; and the extremities—the upper extremities, including the shoulders, arms, and hands, and the extremeties—and the lower extremities, including the hips, legs, and feet.

6. The ten most important systems of the body are the integumentary (skin), skeletal, muscular, nervous, endocrine, circulatory (blood and lymph vascular), digestive, excretory, respiratory, and reproductive systems.

Answers to Matching I

1. g; 2. j; 3. i; 4. k; 5. h; 6. e; 7. c; 8. b; 9. d; 10. a; 11. f

Answers to Matching II

1. f; 2. c; 3. i; 4. g; 5. a; 6. d; 7. j; 8. b; 9. e; 10. h

System 1: The Skin

1. The skin (integumentary system) is the external covering and largest organ of the body.

2. The skin protects the parts of the body situated beneath its surface, regulates body temperature, and functions as an organ of secretion and excretion, absorption, and respiration.

3. The two main layers of the skin are the epidermis and the dermis.

4. The layers of the epidermis are the stratum corneum, lucidum, granulosum, and mucosum.

5. Keratin is both hard and soft. Soft keratin is found in the skin, and hard keratin is found in hair and nails.

6. Subcutaneous tissue is a layer of fatty tissue found below the dermis. It contains a network of arteries and a superficial and deep layer of lymphatics.

7. The color of the skin depends partly on the blood supply but more on melanin, the pigment or coloring matter deposited in the deepest layer of the epidermis and the superficial layer of the dermis.

8. The layers of the dermis are the papillary and the reticular layers.

9. A gland is an organ of either excretion or secretion, taking materials from the blood and forming new substances.

10. The two major glands in the skin are the sudoriferous glands, which excrete sweat, and the sebaceous glands, which secrete sebum.

11. Sebum is an oily substance of the sebaceous glands. A duct is a passage or canal for fluids.

12. Appendages of the skin include hair and nails. In addition, the oil and sweat glands are appendages.

13. A lesion is a structural change in tissues caused by injury or disease.

14. Contact dermatitis is a skin condition or reaction caused by some substance or exterior agent that causes a rash or irritation on contact with the skin.

15. The massage practitioner should observe the client's skin condition because the skin often gives clues as to whether massage would be beneficial or potentially harmful.

System 2: The Skeletal System

1. The skeletal system is composed of bones, cartilage, and ligaments.

2. The functions of the skeletal system are:
   1. To offer a framework that supports body structures and gives shape to the body
   2. To protect delicate internal organs and tissues
   3. To provide attachments for muscles and act as levers in conjunction with muscles to produce movement
   4. To manufacture blood cells in the red bone marrow
   5. To store minerals such as calcium phosphate, calcium carbonate, magnesium, and sodium

3. Organic matter of bones consists of bone cells, blood vessels, connective tissue, and marrow. Inorganic matter consists of calcium phosphate and calcium carbonate.

4. Two types of bone tissue are cancellous (spongy) tissue and dense (compact) tissue. Dense bone tissue is found on the outer portion of the bone just under the periosteum. Cancellous tissue is found on the interior of flat bones and in the ends of long bones.

5. The periosteum covers and protects bone.

6. Bones receive their nourishment through blood vessels that enter through the periosteum into the interior of the bone. Bone marrow also aids in the nutrition of the bone.

7. Flat bones, such as the skull; long bones, such as the legs; short bones, such as the fingers; and irregular bones, such as the vertebrae of the spine.

8. Yellow bone marrow is found in the medullary cavity of the long bones. Red bone marrow is located in the ends of the long bones and in flat bones. In infants and young children, red marrow also occupies the cavities of long bones.

9. Red bone marrow is the site of blood cell synthesis.

10. The main parts of the skeleton are the axial skeleton and the appendicular skeleton.

11. The three classifications of joints are synarthrotic joints such as those in the skull, which are immovable; amphiarthrotic joints, which have limited motion; and diarthrotic joints, which are freely movable.

12. Articular cartilage cushions bones at the joints.

13. Bones are supported at the joints by ligaments.

14. Joints are lubricated by synovial fluid or synovium.

15. There are approximately 206 bones in the adult human body.

16. The form or outline of the bones must be carefully followed and the limitations of the range of movements be considered when practicing massage therapy. Knowing the names of bones serves as a guide in recalling the names of related structures connected with the body part being massaged.

17. Pivot joints, as in the neck between the atlas and the axis. Hinge joints, as in the elbow, knees, and two distal joints of the fingers. Ball-and-socket joints, as in the hips and shoulders. Gliding joints, as in the spine or hand. Saddle joints, as in the wrist, thumb, and ankle.

18. A fracture is a break or rupture of a bone.

19. A sprain is an injury to a joint that results in the stretching or tearing of the ligaments. In a class I sprain, there is a stretch in the ligament, some discomfort, and minimal loss of function. In a class II sprain, the ligament is torn with some loss of function. In a class III sprain, the ligaments are torn, and there is internal bleeding and severe loss of function.

20. Arthritis is an inflammatory condition of the joints often accompanied by pain and changes of bone structure. The three most common types of arthritis are rheumatoid arthritis, osteoarthritis, and gouty arthritis.

21. Osteoporosis literally means porous bones and is a condition where minerals are drawn out of the bones, leaving them brittle and weak. When massaging a person with osteoporosis, the therapist must not use heavy pressure or forceful joint movements, either of which may fracture the weakened bones.

22. Three abnormal curves of the spine are as follows: Kyphosis is an exaggerated convex curve usually associated with the thoracic spine. Lordosis is an exaggerated concave curve usually associated with the lumbar spine. Scoliosis is an abnormal lateral curve of the spine.

Answers to Matching I

1. i; 2. g; 3. b; 4. e; 5. h; 6. f; 7. j; 8. c; 9. a; 10. d

Answers to True or False Test

1. F; 2. T; 3. T; 4. F; 5. F; 6. T; 7. T; 8. T; 9. T; 10. F

Answers to Matching II

1. c; 2. e; 3. h; 4. j; 5. b; 6. a; 7. d; 8. i; 9. f; 10. g

System 3: The Muscular System

Matching Test I	True or False Test I
1. c; 2. e; 3. a; 4. b; 5. d	1. F; 2. F; 3. T; 4. T; 5. F

Matching Test II	True or False Test II
1. c; 2. d; 3. b; 4. e; 5. a	1. T; 2. F; 3. F; 4. T; 5. T

Matching Test III	True or False Test III
1. b; 2. c; 3. d; 4. e; 5. a	1. T; 2. F; 3. T; 4. F; 5. T

Matching Test IV	True or False Test IV
1. e; 2. a; 3. d; 4. c; 5. b	1. F; 2. F; 3. T; 4. T; 5. T

Matching Test V	True or False Test V
1. b; 2. c; 3. d; 4. e; 5. a	1. T; 2. T; 3. F; 4. T; 5. F

1. Muscles are contractile fibrous tissue that produce various movements of the body.

2. There are approximately 600 muscles in the human body.

3. Voluntary (striated) muscle is found in the muscles that attach to the skeleton; involuntary (nonstriated) muscle is found in the hollow muscular organs such as the stomach, intestines, bladder, and blood vessels; heart (cardiac) muscle is found only in the heart.

4. Voluntary muscles can be controlled by the will; involuntary muscles are not controlled by the will and receive nerve stimulation from the autonomic nervous system.

5. The characteristics that enable muscles to produce movement are irritability, contractility, and elasticity.

6. Skeletal muscles are striated muscles attached to the bones of the skeleton.

7. The functional unit of skeletal muscle is the muscle cell or muscle fiber.

8. The striated appearance of voluntary muscle is due to the arrangement of the actin and myosin in the myofibrils.

9. Beside the muscle fibers, muscle contains a variety of connective tissue, blood and other fluids, blood and lymph vessels, and nerves.

10. Muscles are attached to bones, cartilage, ligaments, tendons, skin, and sometimes to each other.

11. Origin of a muscle refers to the more fixed attachments, such as muscles attached to bones, that act as anchors for movements.

12. Insertion of a muscle refers to the attachments that perform the action, such as muscles attached to skin, other muscles, or the more distal and movable attachment.

13. Tendon or sinew attaches muscles to the bone.

14. The function of fibrous connective tissue is to organize and support muscle tissue, blood vessels, and nerves. Connective tissue anchors the muscle fibers and connects them to the structures they act on.

15. Fascia is a delicate membrane of connective tissue covering muscles and separating their several layers or groups of layers.

16. Three layers of connective muscle are the epimysium that covers the muscle, the perimysium that separates the muscle bundles, and the endomysium that surrounds each muscle cell.

17. A motor unit is all the muscle fibers that are controlled by a single motor neuron.

18. Acetylcholine is a chemical neurotransmitter found at the myoneural junction. When a nerve impulse travels to the end of a motor neuron, acetylcholine is released and travels across the gap to excite the muscle cell to contract.

19. Muscles receive energy from the breaking down of adenosine triphosphate (ATP) into adenosine diphosphate (ADP).

20. Oxygen debt results from the muscles expending energy faster than the body can supply the oxygen needed to produce the energy. When oxygen debt becomes extreme, the muscles will stop functioning in a condition known as muscle fatigue.

21. A muscle has tone if it is firm and responds readily to stimulation.

22. A muscle lacks tone if it is flabby.

23. When massage practitioners understand how muscles function, they are better able to apply massage techniques that will relax tense muscles and rejuvenate tired muscles.

24. Extensibility is the ability of muscle fibers to lengthen and stretch.

25. An isometric muscle contraction is a static contraction wherein the distance between the ends of the muscle does not change, so there is no movement. With an isotonic muscle contraction, the distance between the ends of the muscle changes, and there is movement.

26. Eccentric and concentric muscle contractions are both isotonic contractions. In a concentric contraction, the ends of the contracting muscle are coming closer. In an eccentric contraction, the ends of the contracting muscle are moving farther apart.

27. Prime mover and agonist both refer to the primary muscle that is responsible for a specific movement.

28. When flexing the elbow, the triceps become the antagonist.

29. The three components of motion are flexion/extension, adduction/abduction, and rotation.

30. Diarthrotic joints are freely movable.

31. There are three degrees or grades of muscle strain. Grade I is an overstretching of a few of the muscle fibers with a minimal tearing of the fibers. Grade II involves a partial tear of between 10 and 50 percent of the muscle fibers. Grade III is the most severe injury with between 50 and 100 percent muscle tearing.

32. Muscle atrophy is a degenerative process due to muscle disuse. The muscle fibers reduce in size, blood supply is reduced, and the muscle weakens.

33. Ampiarthrotic joints have limited motion.

34. Synarthrotic joints, as in the skull, are immovable.

System 4: The Circulatory System

Matching Test I

1. b; 2. c; 3. d; 4. e;
5. a

True or False Test I

1. T; 2. F; 3. T; 4. F;
5. T

Matching Test II

1. d; 2. a; 3. e; 4. c;
5. b

True or False Test II

1. T; 2. F; 3. T; 4. F;
5. F

1. The heart, blood vessels (arteries, veins, and capillaries), lymph vessels, and the fluids that circulate through them are the main parts of the circulatory system.

2. The two divisions of the circulatory system are the blood-vascular system and the lymph-vascular system.

3. The heart is an efficient pump that keeps the blood moving in a steady stream through a closed system of blood vessels.

4. The pericardium is a protective sac surrounding and supporting the heart in position and at the same time allowing it to move frictionlessly as it continually pulsates.

5. The chambers of the heart are the right atrium (or auricle), the right ventricle, the left atrium, and the left ventricle.

6. Two sets of nerves, the vagus and sympathetic nerves, regulate the heartbeat.

7. The arteries carry blood away from the heart to the capillaries.

8. An arteriole is the microscopic final division of the arteries before the capillaries.

9. Movements of the arterial walls are controlled by vasomotor nerves from the autonomic nervous system consisting of the vasoconstrictor nerves and the vasodilator nerves.

10. The capillaries connect the smaller arteries with the veins. The permeable walls of the capillaries allow a two-way diffusion of substances between the blood and the tissue fluid, thereby bringing nourishment to the cells and removing waste products.

11. The veins carry blood from the various capillaries back toward the heart. Veins of general circulation carry waste-laden, oxygen-poor blood from the body, whereas pulmonary veins carry freshly oxygenated blood from the lungs.

12. A venule is the smallest vessel of the venous system that collects blood from the capillaries.

13. The purpose of the venous pump is to assist in moving the blood through the veins and toward the heart.

14. The main artery is the aorta.

15. Two portions of the blood-vascular system are the pulmonary circulatory system and the general or systemic circulatory system.

16. The pulmonary veins carry freshly oxygenated blood.

17. The constituents of blood include plasma, red corpuscles, white corpuscles, and platelets.

18. The red blood cells primarily carry oxygen from the lungs to the cells and carbon dioxide from the cells to the lungs.

19. The primary function of white blood cells is to protect the body against disease by combating different infectious and toxic agents that may invade the body.

20. Blood carries water, oxygen, food, and secretions to the body cells.

21. Blood carries carbon dioxide gas and metabolic waste products away from the body cells.

22. The blood protects the body against extreme heat or cold, harmful bacteria, and

the excessive loss of blood by forming an external clot.

23. Normal body temperature is 98.6°F (37°C).

24. The lymph system includes the lymph, lymphatics, lymph ducts, lymph nodes, glands, and lacteals. Also considered a part of the lymph system are the tonsils, the spleen, and the thymus gland.

25. The function of the lymph-vascular system is to collect excess tissue fluid, invading microorganisms, damaged cells, and protein molecules. The lymphoid tissue also produces lymphocytes, a white blood cell that is an important element of the body's immune system.

26. The lymph nodes filter harmful bacteria and toxic matter from the lymph and are the site of production of lymphocytes.

27. The parts of the body containing lymph nodes are the back of the head, around the neck muscles, under the armpit, under the pectoral muscles, along the blood vessels of the abdomen and pelvis, the back of the knees, and the groin.

28. Lymph is derived from interstitial or extracellular fluid.

29. Lymph returns to venous blood through the brachiocephalic veins.

30. Lymph drainage is draining of lymph fluids from various areas of the body.

31. The lacteals are lymphatic vessels that carry chyle from the small intestine to the thoracic duct.

32. Massage increases flow of lymph and prevents stagnation.

33. Lymphatics are named according to their location in the body.

34. The lymphatic pump is similar to the venous pump. A system of valves in the lymph vessels operates so that external pressure on the walls of the vessel force the movement of lymph through the vessel in one direction.

35. Tissue fluid becomes lymph when it enters through the wall of a lymph capillary. From there, lymph flows into larger lymphatics and into the first of possibly several lymph nodes. Eventually, the lymph flows out of the nodes, through another lymph vessel, and into either the right or thoracic lymph duct. From the lymph duct, lymph flows into the brachiocephalic vein.

System 5: The Nervous System

Matching Test I	*True or False Test I*
1. c; 2. d; 3. e; 4. b; 5. a	1. F; 2. T; 3. F; 4. T; 5. T

Matching Test II	*True or False Test II*
1. e; 2. d; 3. a; 4. c; 5. b	1. F; 2. T; 3. T; 4. F; 5. T

Matching Test III	*True or False Test III*
1. b; 2. e; 3. a; 4. c; 5. d	1. T; 2. F; 3. F; 4. T; 5. T

Matching Test IV	*True or False Test IV*
1. b; 2. e; 3. d; 4. c; 5. a	1. F; 2. T; 3. T; 4. F; 5. T

Matching Test V	*True or False Test V*
1. e; 2. c; 3. b; 4. a; 5. d	1. T; 2. F; 3. T; 4. F; 5. T

1. The nervous system controls and coordinates the functions of other systems of the body so that they work harmoniously and efficiently. The primary function of the nervous system is to collect a multitude of sensory information; process, interpret, and integrate that information; and initiate appropriate responses throughout the body.

2. The main parts of the nervous system include the brain, spinal cord, and the peripheral nerves.

3. A nerve cell is called a neuron and consists of a cell body, a single axon, and numerous dendrites.

4. Neurons have the ability to react to certain stimuli (irritability) and to transmit an impulse generated by that stimulus over a distance or to another neuron (conductability).

5. A synapse is the junction between two nerve cells where a nerve impulse is transmitted from one nerve cell to another.

6. A sensory neuron or afferent neuron carries impulses from the sense organs in the periphery of the body toward the central nervous system. A motor or efferent neuron carries impulses away from the central nervous system to the muscles or glands that they control. Interneurons, located in the spinal cord or brain, transmit impulses from one nerve cell to another.

7. A nerve is a bundle of nerve fibers held together by connective tissue that extends from the central nervous system to the tissue that the neurons innervate.

8. An efferent nerve or motor nerve is composed of motor neurons.

9. An afferent nerve or sensory nerve is composed of sensory neurons.

10. A mixed nerve is composed of both sensory and motor nerves. Most nerves in the body are mixed nerves.

11. The two divisions of the nervous system are the central nervous system (CNS) and the peripheral nervous system.

12. The central nervous system consists of the brain, which is located in the cranium, and the spinal cord, which is located in the vertebral canal of the spine.

13. The meninges is a fibrous connective tissue covering of the CNS consisting of the dura mater, the arachnoid mater, and the pia mater.

14. Cerebrospinal fluid is a clear fluid derived from the blood and secreted into the inner cavities or ventricles of the brain. Cerebrospinal fluid carries some nutrients to the nerve tissue and carries wastes away; however, its main function is to protect the CNS by acting as a shock absorber for the delicate tissue.

15. The main parts of the brain are the cerebrum, the cerebellum, and the brain stem consisting of the midbrain, the pons, and the medulla oblongata.

16. The peripheral nervous system consists of all the nerves that connect the central nervous system to the rest of the body and therefore is located throughout all the innervated tissues of the body.

17. The two divisions of the peripheral nervous system are the somatic nervous system and the autonomic nervous system.

18. There are 12 pairs of cranial nerves.

19. The 12 cranial nerves are the I olfactory nerve, II optic nerve, III oculomotor nerve, IV trochlear nerve, V trigeminal or trifacial nerve, VI abducent nerve, VII facial nerve, VIII acoustic or auditory nerve, IX glossopharyngeal nerve, X vagus or pneumogastric nerve, XI spinal accessory nerve, and XII hypoglossal nerve.

20. There are 31 pairs of spinal nerves.

21. The spinal nerves are numbered according to the vertebral level where they exit the spinal column. They are numbered as follows: cervical nerves—C1 through 8; thoracic nerves—T1 through 12; Lumbar nerves—L1 through 5; sacral nerves—S1 through 5; one pair of coccygeal nerves.

22. A nerve plexus is a network or gathering of nerves located outside of the CNS.

23. The important nerve plexuses are: The cervical plexus formed by the spinal nerves C 1–4, serving the structures in the region of the neck; the brachial plexus formed by the spinal nerves C5–T1, serving the shoulder, arm, and part of the chest; the lumbar plexus formed by the spinal nerves T12–L4, serving the muscles and organs of the abdomen, hip, and upper leg; the sacral plexus formed by the spinal nerves L4–S4, creating the sciatic nerve and serving the legs; the coccygeal plexus formed by part of S4 and S5, serving the area around the coccyx.

24. The autonomic nervous system regulates the action of glands, smooth muscles, and the heart.

25. The parasympathetic and sympathetic are the two divisions of the autonomic nervous system. The activity of the sympathetic system is primarily to prepare the organism for energy-expending, stressful, or emergency situations. Stimulation of the sympathetic nerves can bring about rapid responses, such as increased respiration, dilated pupils, and increased heart rate and cardiac output. Blood vessels dilate, the skin constricts, and the liver increases conversion of glycogen to glucose for more energy. There is increased mental activity

and production of adrenal hormones. The parasympathetic nervous system balances the action of the sympathetic system. The general function of the parasympathetic division is to conserve energy and reverse the action of the sympathetic division.

26. The involuntary muscles, heart, lungs, stomach, intestines, and blood vessels are supplied by the sympathetic nervous system. Also the adrenal and salivary glands, the bladder, and reproductive organs.

27. Reflex action is the involuntary response of a muscle to a stimulus.

28. Proprioception is a system of sensory and motor nerve activity that provides information as to the position and rate of movement of different body parts to the central nervous system. Proprioception provides information as to the state of contraction and position of the muscles.

29. Two categories of proprioceptors are spindle cells and Golgi tendon organs. Spindle cells located mostly in the belly of the muscle record changes in the length and stretch of the muscle as well as how far and fast the muscle is moving. The Golgi tendon organs are located in the tendon near its connection to the muscle and record the amount of tension produced in muscle cells that occurs as a result of the muscle stretching and contracting and the amount of force pulling on the bone to which the tendon attaches.

System 6: The Endocrine System

1. The endocrine system is composed of a group of glands whose functions are vital to the maintenance of health.

2. The major function of the endocrine system is to assist the nervous system in regulating body processes.

3. A duct gland possesses a duct or canal that carries its secretions to their destination, whereas a ductless gland has no duct and therefore must depend on the circulatory system to carry its secretions to various affected tissues.

4. The blood supplies the raw materials that glands use to produce secretions. The nerves control many of the functional activities of the glands.

5. Sebaceous glands are duct glands that provide sebum (oil) to lubricate the skin.

6. A ductless or endocrine gland has no duct but delivers its secretion directly into the bloodstream, affecting the growth, development, sexual activity, and health of the entire body, depending on the gland's target organs and the quality and quantity of its secretions.

7. The pancreas and sex glands (gonads) function as both duct and ductless glands.

8. The ductless or endocrine glands produce hormones.

9. Hormones are specialized to act on specific tissues (target organs) or influence certain processes in the body. Some have a profound effect on physical or sexual development. Others regulate metabolism or body chemistry. Some hormones stimulate or restrain the activity of another gland. The endocrine glands operate cooperatively with one another and the nervous system to maintain a state of homeostasis within the organism.

10. The important endocrine glands are the pituitary gland, thyroid gland, parathyroid glands, adrenal glands, sex glands (gonads), and pancreas. Other organs that have hormone-producing tissue include the pineal gland, the hypothalamus, the kidneys, the placenta, and intestinal mucosa.

11. Most diseases or dysfunctions of the endocrine system are the result of overactivity or underactivity of one or more glands. Overactive or hyperactive glands oversecrete hormones due to lack of regulation or glandular tumors. Underactive or hypoactive glands secrete insufficient amounts of their respective hormones.

12. The pituitary gland is often called the master gland because many of the hormones it secretes stimulate or regulate other endocrine glands.

13. The hormone-producing parts of the adrenal glands are the adrenal cortex and the medulla.

14. The male sex glands produce testosterone, and the female sex glands produce estrogen and progesterone.

Answers to Matching I

1. a; 2. f; 3. g; 4. a; 5. b; 6. i; 7. a; 8. e; 9. h; 10. e; 11. a; 12. g; 13. f; 14. c; 15. a

Answers to Matching II

1. j; 2. a; 3. h; 4. d; 5. g; 6. f; 7. b; 8. i; 9. e; 10. c

System 7: The Respiratory System

1. The major respiratory organs include the nose, nasal cavity, pharynx, larynx, trachea, bronchial tubes, and the lungs.

2. The respiratory system is responsible for the vital exchange of oxygen and carbon dioxide.

3. The lungs are two sacs composed of spongy tissue, blood vessels, connective tissue, and microscopic air sacs called alveoli.

4. The three levels of respiration are external respiration, internal respiration, and cellular respiration or oxidation. External respiration takes place in the lungs. Internal respiration takes place between the bloodstream and the cells of the body. Cellular respiration or oxidation takes place within the cells.

5. The alveoli are microscopic air sacs at the terminal ends of the bronchioles that are surrounded by the pulmonary capillaries, where the exchange of carbon dioxide for oxygen takes place.

6. Breathing or ventilation is the process of inhaling and exhaling air.

7. The natural rate of breathing is 14 to 20 breaths a minute.

8. The diaphragm is a muscular sheet separating the thorax from the abdominal cavity. It is the major muscle used in breathing.

System 8: The Digestive System

1. Structures of the digestive system include the alimentary canal and accessory digestive organs. The alimentary canal consists of the mouth, pharynx, esophagus, stomach, small intestine, and large intestine. The accessory organs include the teeth, tongue, salivary glands, pancreas, liver, and gallbladder.

2. The main functions of the digestive system are digestion and absorption. Digestion is the process of converting food into substances capable of being used by the cells for nourishment.

3. Absorption is the process in which the digested nutrients are transferred from the intestines to the blood or lymph vessels so that they can be transported to the cells.

4. The physical process of digestion involves the teeth, which tear and grind the food, and the action of the muscles, which churn and mix the food as well as push it through the digestive tract.

5. Enzymes aid digestion.

6. In the mouth, food is chewed and mixed with saliva, and carbohydrates begin to be digested to the sugar stage.

7. The alimentary canal is a muscular tube about 30 feet in length that extends from the mouth to the anus. The wall of the alimentary canal consists of four distinct layers: The mucosa or mucous membrane is made up of epithelial cells, connective tissue, and a variety of digestive glands. This layer protects the underlying tissues and carries on secretion and absorption. The submucosa consists of connective tissue, nerves, and blood and lymph vessels that serve to nourish the surrounding tissues and carry away the absorbed material. The muscular layer has two layers of smooth muscle that churn the contents and propel it through the canal. The serous layer is the outer covering of the tube.

8. Peristaltic action is a rhythmic, wavelike muscular action of the smooth muscles of the alimentary canal that propels and churns the food throughout the length of the canal.

9. In the stomach, food is mixed with gastric juice. Protein digestion begins.

10. The parts of the small intestine are the duodenum, the jejunum, and the ileum.

11. Digestive secretions in the small intestines are supplied by the liver, pancreas, and glands in the small intestine.

12. In the small intestine, food is completely digested.

13. The blood vessels and lacteals in villi in the walls of the small intestine absorb the end products of digestion.

14. The rectum of the large intestine eliminates undigested food waste from the body.

System 9: The Excretory System

1. The organs that comprise the excretory system are the lungs, kidneys, skin, liver, and large intestine.
2. The body will become poisoned by its own waste products.
3. The excretory system eliminates metabolic waste and undigested foods from the body.
4. The urinary system includes two kidneys, two ureters, the bladder, and a urethra.
5. The functional unit of the kidney is the nephron.
6. A urinalysis will indicate the presence of white blood cells, blood, glucose, or other chemicals in the urine that may be an indication of metabolic imbalance, infection, or numerous other conditions.
7. A change in the color of the urine, such as cloudiness or a reddish or brownish color, can indicate infection or other health problems.
8. The liver secretes bile.
9. The main excretory function of the liver is the production of urea, which is returned to the blood to be excreted by the kidneys. The liver also excretes bile into the small intestines.

System 10: The Reproductive System

1. The reproductive system is the generative apparatus necessary for organisms to reproduce organisms of the same kind or species.
2. Asexual reproduction, as in some one-celled organisms, means that no partner is needed to reproduce. In humans and animals, reproduction is sexual and requires a male and female to reproduce.
3. A gonad is a sex gland—the ovary in the female and the testes in the male.
4. A zygote is the fertilized ovum, the cell formed by the union of a spermatozoon (sperm) with the ovum (egg).
5. The reproductive system in males includes two testes, two vas deferens, two seminal vesicles, a prostate gland, the bulbourethral glands (Cowper's glands), and the penis.
6. The functions of the male reproductive system are the production of sperm, the production of the male hormones, and the performance of the sex act.
7. The reproductive system in females includes two ovaries, two fallopian tubes (oviducts), a uterus, a vagina, and the vulva or external genitalia.
8. The functions of the female reproductive system are to produce the ovum and female hormones, to receive the sperm during the sex act, and to carry the growing fetus during pregnancy.
9. From the beginning of conception until approximately the third month of pregnancy, the developing child is called an embryo. After that time, it is called a fetus.
10. Ovulation is the discharge of a mature egg cell from the follicle of the ovary.
11. Pregnancy lasts approximately 40 weeks or 280 days.

Chapter 6 Effects, Benefits, Indications, and Contraindications of Massage

1. The main physiological benefits of massage are stimulation of the muscular, vascular, and glandular activities of the body. Circulation is increased and soreness and stiffness of the muscles relieved.
2. The psychological benefits of massage result from the reduction of tension and relief from stress and anxiety. Massage can also promote a sense of renewed energy and well-being. Massage helps the client to feel healthier, invigorated, and more energetic.
3. Massage has direct mechanical effects and indirect reflex effects on the body.
4. Massage is beneficial to all body systems including the circulatory, nervous, skeletal, muscular, digestive, glandular, integumentary (skin), respiratory, and excretory systems.
5. Massage benefits the development of the muscular system by way of stimulation of its circulation, nerve supply, and cell activity. Massage is also an effective means of relaxing tense muscles and releasing muscle

spasms. Massage prevents and relieves stiffness and soreness of muscles. Muscle tissue that has suffered injury heals more quickly with less connective tissue buildup and scarring when therapeutic massage is applied regularly.

6. Nearly all massage movements enhance circulation; however, stroking, kneading, and compression most effectively promote circulation.

7. Massage relieves stiff, sore muscles by improving circulation of the blood through the body part. It helps in the removal of waste products and supplies the cells with oxygen and nourishment.

8. Cross-fiber friction and compression movements prevent the formation of adhesions and fibrosis in muscles.

9. The immediate effects of massage on the skin include increased circulation of the blood, which nourishes the skin, improves tone, and helps to normalize the functioning of the sebaceous (oil) glands.

10. Depending on the type of massage movement applied, the nervous system can be stimulated or toned.

11. Friction, vibration, and light percussion movements produce a stimulating effect on the nervous system.

12. Gentle stroking, light friction, and petrissage produce a sedative effect on the nervous system.

13. Massage affects the quality and rate of blood flowing through the circulatory system. Direct and reflex effects of massage increase circulation and stimulate the production of red and white blood cells.

14. Massage movements are directed toward the heart to facilitate the flow of blood and lymph back toward the heart.

15. Light stroking, deep stroking, light percussion, friction, petrissage, and compression are all useful in increasing the flow of blood and lymph.

16. Massage improves the circulation of the blood, which in turn supplies beneficial nutrients to the skin.

17. When the client has a condition that appears to be a contraindication to massage, massage should be avoided.

18. Contraindication means the expected treatment or process is inadvisable. In massage it refers to any condition in which massage is not advisable, as it would not be beneficial or may be dangerous.

19. It is important to take a client medical history to help determine potential indications and contraindications for the massage.

20. The practitioner should have a thermometer in order to take a client's temperature if a fever is suspected. Massage is not recommended when the client's temperature is abnormally high. An abnormally high temperature is an indication of illness or other health problems.

21. Massage should be avoided when there is a contraindication, such as a physical or mental condition that needs medical attention or when there is doubt of its benefits. The therapist should refer the client to an appropriate health professional.

22. The signs of inflammation are heat, swelling, pain, and redness.

23. In the case of local inflammation, massage must be avoided on the inflamed area and applied to the area of the body proximal to the inflammation in order to promote circulation toward and away from the area.

24. The practitioner will recognize varicose veins as bluish, protruding, thick, bulbous, distended superficial veins usually found in the lower legs.

25. A hematoma is a mass of blood trapped in some tissue or cavity of the body and is the result of internal bleeding. When the hematoma is in the acute phase, massage is contraindicated because of the risk of reinjuring the tissue. Once the bruise has changed colors, light massage will enhance circulation to the area and actually assist the healing.

26. Massage benefits a woman during a normal, healthy pregnancy by promoting relaxation, soothing nerves, relieving strained back and leg muscles, and instilling a sense of well-being.

27. Massage for the critically ill helps to control discomfort and pain; improves mobility; helps reduce disorientation and confusion by bringing the person back to a more positive body awareness; reduces iso-

lation and fear; helps to ease the emotional and physical discomfort of the individual.

28. The virus that causes AIDS is transmitted from person to person only through the exchange of body fluid that contains the virus.

29. Massage has been considered to be a contraindication when working with persons with cancer (PWC) because of the effects it has on blood and lymph circulation and the fear that massage may actually spread the cancer.

30. Some benefits of massage for people include the following: Pain relief or control; reduced nausea; better digestion and elimination; stress relief; relaxation; help for insomnia; reduced anxiety; relief from depression; relief from muscle tension and spasm; better flexibility; restored range of motion; improved lymph movement; reduced edema; increased body awareness; restored positive body image; enhanced self-esteem; improved outlook on life; improved quality of life; boosts to the healing process; health promotion; feeling good at a time where lots of things feel bad.

31. The practitioner can reduce promoting metastasis when massaging people with cancer by not massaging or putting pressure on the primary site of the cancer, avoiding infected lymph nodes, and not doing circulatory massage on possible secondary sites.

32. Stages of cancer are a classification of the growth or progress of the disease: Stage 1: Cancer is still small and contained in the original tumor; Stage 2: Cancer has grown and/or spread to nearby lymph nodes; Stage 3: Cancerous cells have spread to regional lymph nodes and/or other tissues in the area; Stage 4: Cancer is well developed and has spread to other tissues or organs in the body; Recurrent: Cancer has returned after being treated. It may come back at the original site or another part of the body.

33. The common treatments for cancer are: surgery; chemotherapy; radiation; bone marrow transplant; treatment with other drugs such as steroids, narcotics, and antidepressants; complementary and alternative therapies.

34. Important considerations when doing massage with people with cancer include the type and location of cancer; the stage of progression of the cancer; possible secondary sites of metastasis; the treatment type and stage; the condition of the immune system; the stamina of the person; the attitude of the person; the belief and desire of the person regarding massage; the purpose of the massage. Always work under supervision of the client's physician.

35. Massage seems to be more effective before chemotherapy and radiation treatments because it seems to improve the client's outlook and reduces anxiety. As a result, recovery from the treatment is quicker, and many of the side effects such as fatigue and nausea seem less drastic.

36. If the client fatigues easily or has a low energy level, adjust the massage by shortening the length of the session, lightening the pressure, and slowing the pace of the massage. How much adjustment is made in these areas depends on the client's condition and needs. It is better to do too little than to do too much.

37. Certain areas of the body warrant consideration while being massaged because of the underlying anatomical structure and the possibility of injury to the structure by certain massage manipulations.

Chapter 7 Equipment and Products

1. The massage practitioner should project a professional image of relaxed confidence.

2. A massage space should be comfortable, clean, and free of distractions and safety hazards.

3. A room that is 10 by 12 feet allows ample space for a massage table, desk, dressing area, and other equipment and supplies necessary to perform massage.

4. Equipment should be checked for safety and sanitation. Supplies must be checked to ensure an adequate supply and to see that they are clean and stored properly.

5. Preparation is essential to good service, and it shows that you are professional.

6. Lubricants, creams, and powders are products used for body massage.

7. The massage room is usually most comfortable for clients when the temperature is around 75°F.

8. The height of the massage table should be adjusted to give the practitioner more leverage to do the massage efficiently. Correct height also prevents the practitioner from becoming fatigued.

9. Soft, natural, indirect lighting is best in the massage room.

10. Some people find music distracting and prefer absolute quiet.

Chapter 8 Sanitary and Safety Practices

1. All states have laws pertaining to sanitation for the protection of the public. These laws protect both clients and practitioners.

2. The practitioner should practice the rules of sanitation because he is responsible for safeguarding the client's health as well as his own health.

3. The practitioner should have some knowledge of bacteria in order to understand the importance of preventing the spread of disease.

4. Pathogenic bacteria are harmful, whereas nonpathogenic bacteria are harmless and sometimes helpful.

5. The body produces antibodies to inhibit or destroy harmful bacteria.

6. Three forms of pathogenic (harmful) bacteria are cocci, bacilli, and spirilla.

7. The strict practice of sanitation is the best prevention against the spread of harmful bacteria.

8. Before using any disinfectant or antiseptic product, you should read the manufacturer's instructions and follow them.

9. Disinfectants are used in the practice of massage to keep all equipment and the premises in a clean, sanitary condition.

10. The best method for keeping the hands and nails clean is to scrub them with a brush in warm, soapy water; rinse with mild alcohol; and then pat them dry.

11. Suitable strengths for cresol and Lysol™ used to clean floors, sinks, and restrooms are 5 to 10 percent.

12. Sterilization is the procedure for making an object germ-free by destroying bacteria, both the harmful and harmless kinds.

13. Safety is an attitude put into practice that is concerned with the prevention of situations and elimination of conditions that may lead to injury of the massage practitioner or client.

14. Safety considerations in a massage practice need to focus on (1) the facility, (2) the equipment, (3) the massage practitioner, and (4) the client.

Chapter 9 The Consultation

1. The consultation is important to obtain certain data regarding the client's conditions and to determine the most effective treatments.

2. An assessment includes taking the client's medical history, observing the client's actions, and performing verbal and manipulative tests that may indicate the client's conditions.

3. A preliminary assessment is advisable when doing massage therapy because it clarifies the client's conditions, reveals indications and contraindications, determines whether referral to another health professional is advisable, and indicates which therapeutic techniques to use.

4. The treatment plan is an outline the practitioner can follow when giving massage treatments.

5. The treatment plan is formulated using information from the intake and medical history forms, the interview, and preliminary assessment to formulate session goals and choose massage techniques.

6. Informed consent is an educational and informative process that assures the client has received and understands the nature and extent of the massage services.

7. The practitioner will disclose adequate information regarding the practitioner's credentials, the services offered, policies and procedures used during the sessions, and will describe the massage techniques to be employed along with projected effects and outcomes, including benefits and possible side effects.

8. Accurate records are important to both the practitioner and client because special information may be needed for reference. Well-kept records also help the practitioner to determine and render the most effective treatments.

9. Information that is often found in a client file includes intake information (name, address, phone, etc.), medical information and history, treatment plan and recorded notes, and financial and billing information.

10. The client may not understand why premassage procedures are necessary or may feel uneasy and not know what is expected.

11. Being able to anticipate and answer questions the client may ask gives the practitioner more credibility.

Chapter 10 Classification of Massage Movements

1. The six basic classifications of movements are touch, stroking, kneading, friction, percussion, and joint movements.

2. The practitioner should regulate the intensity of pressure, direction of movement, and duration of each type of manipulation to meet the client's needs.

3. Light movements should be applied over thin tissues and bony parts.

4. Heavier movements should be applied over thick tissues and muscular parts.

5. Massage is generally applied in a centripetal direction, or toward the heart.

6. Massage strokes directed away from the heart should be light enough that they do not affect fluid flow.

7. The approximate duration of a full-body massage is about one hour.

8. When referring to massage technique, touch is the stationary contact of the practitioner's hand and the client's body.

9. Light or superficial touch is purposeful contact in which the natural and evenly distributed weight of the practitioner's finger, fingers, or hand is applied on a given area of the client's body. The main objective of light touch is to soothe and to provide a comforting connection that is calming and allows the powerful healing mechanisms of the body to function. Touch is effective in the reduction of pain, lowering of blood pressure, control of nervous irritability, or reassurance for a nervous, tense client.

10. Deep touch is performed with one finger, thumb, several fingers, or the entire hand. The heel of the hand, knuckles, or elbow can be used according to desired results. Deep touch is used when calming, anesthetizing, or stimulating effects are desired. Deep pressure is useful in soothing muscle spasms and relieving pain at reflex areas, stress points in tendons, and trigger points in muscle.

11. Aura stroking is done with long, smooth strokes where the practitioner's hands glide the length of the client's entire body or body part, coming very close to but not actually touching the body surface.

12. Another name for feather stroking is nerve strokes. These are usually used as the final stroke to the individual areas of the body.

13. Effleurage is a succession of strokes applied by gliding the hand over a somewhat extended portion of the body.

14. Superficial stroking is a kind of effleurage that requires the lightest possible touch.

15. Deep gliding strokes require firm pressure.

16. Superficial gliding strokes produce soothing effects and overcome tiredness or restlessness.

17. Deep gliding strokes have a stretching and broadening effect on muscle tissue and fascia. They also enhance and stimulate the venous and lymphatic flow.

18. Kneading movements are applied by grasping muscular tissue with one or both hands, then squeezing, rolling, or pinching with a firm pressure.

19. Kneading enhances the fluid movement in the superficial as well as the deeper tissues.

20. The classical term that means the same as kneading is petrissage.

21. Fulling is recommended for the muscular areas of the arms and legs.

22. Friction movements are applied to the body by moving more superficial layers of

flesh against the deeper tissues in order to flatten, broaden, or stretch the tissue.

23. Heat created during friction movements affects the connective tissues surrounding the muscles, making them more pliable so that they function more efficiently.

24. Cross-fiber friction uses short, deep strokes transverse to the direction of muscle, tendon, or ligament fibers. The fingers do not move over the skin but move the skin and superficial tissues across the target tissue.

25. Compression movements are rhythmic pressing movements directed into muscle tissue perpendicular to the body part by either the hand or fingers.

26. Compression movement invigorates the body, stimulates the flow of blood and lymph, and prevents muscular stiffness following exercise. Compression movements cause increased circulation and a lasting hyperemia in the tissue.

27. Vibratory movements are applied with a continuous shaking or trembling movement by means of the practitioner's hands or an electrical vibrator.

28. Vibration is safe at a rate of 5 to 10 times per second by hand, 10 to 100 times per second by electric vibrators.

29. The practitioner can control the effects of vibratory movements by controlling the rate of vibration, intensity of pressure, and duration of treatment.

30. Excessive vibration produces a numbing effect.

31. Percussion movements are applied with quick striking movements performed with both hands simultaneously or alternately.

32. Percussion movements are slapping, beating, hacking, cupping, and tapping.

33. Percussion movements tone the muscles and stimulate the nervous and circulatory systems.

34. Joint movements can be used to manipulate any joint in the body, including joints of the toes, knees, hips, arms, the vertebrae, or even the less movable joints of the pelvis and cranium.

35. Two types of joint movements are active joint movements and passive joint movements.

36. During an active assistive joint movement, the client is instructed to perform a motion at the same time the practitioner assists the movement. During an active resistive movement, the client is instructed to make a motion while the limb is held to resist movement.

37. Range of motion is the movement of a joint from one extreme of the articulation to the other.

38. End feel is the change in the quality of the feeling the therapist senses as the end of a joint movement is approached.

39. Pressure is regulated during a massage according to the technique used and according to the intended outcome. The rule is to begin with a light and sensitive touch, increase the pressure as you work into an area, and then gradually reduce pressure as you leave the area.

40. A person's pain threshold is the amount of discomfort or pain he can tolerate without adverse reactions. When the pain threshold is violated, the client will tense up and the massage work will become less effective or even be counterproductive.

Chapter 11 Application of Massage Technique

1. The massage practitioner must develop strong, flexible hands in order to deliver massage manipulations to the body over an extended period of time and to control the pressure and rhythm while working over the contours of the body.

2. Body mechanics is the observation of body postures in relation to safe and efficient movement in daily living activities.

3. Using good body mechanics increases the strength and power available in a movement while at the same time reducing the risk of potential injury to the individual.

4. To increase the power and strength in a movement and at the same time conserve energy, the practitioner must use the muscles in the legs and the movement of the whole body to deliver the strokes. Keeping the hands in good alignment and close to the practitioner's body and moving the

whole body conserves energy and increases the power and strength when performing massage.

5. Correct posture and stances aid balance; allow the delivery of firmer, more powerful massage strokes; conserve strength; and sustain energy when it is necessary to work long hours.

Chapter 12 Procedures for Complete Body Massages

1. The practitioner should wash hands before and after each treatment.

2. For reasons of safety and liability, it is advisable that the practitioner assist the client onto the table at the beginning of a massage and into a sitting position and off the table at the end of the massage.

3. Chilling of the client's body can be prevented by keeping the room warm and by using proper draping.

4. Two common methods of draping are: Top cover method, which uses a table covering and a separate sheet or towel to cover the client. Full sheet draping, which uses a double-size sheet to cover the table and wrap the client.

5. Besides draping, the therapist can ensure the client's warmth by keeping the room at a comfortable temperature or using an electric mattress pad or supplying extra coverings.

6. Scratching the client can be avoided by filing the nails short and smooth and removing jewelry.

7. Heavy pressure, rapid movement, or jarring contact cause fear and should be avoided.

8. It is better for the client to receive a massage before eating a meal.

9. The average duration of a massage is about an hour.

10. Massage should never be applied to an area where there is injury or abrasion of the skin, fever, inflammation of joints or veins, or when other contraindications are present.

11. Before a body massage, check facilities for readiness, obtain and arrange supplies, and check self for readiness. Obtain necessary information regarding client's needs and wishes, advise the client regarding preparation procedures and assist as necessary, record the client's pulse and body temperature when necessary.

12. The position the client assumes first for a massage depends on the treatment to be given and the preference of the therapist and the client; however, generally the massage begins with the client in supine (faceup) position.

13. The order of massage movements is determined by the purpose of the massage and the preference of the therapist. Movements should follow a logical sequence such as:

a. Begin with the hands and arms, left then right.

b. Proceed to front of the legs and feet, left then right.

c. Continue movements over chest, neck, and abdomen.

d. The client will turn over to assume a prone (facedown) position.

e. Begin with the back of the legs, right then left.

f. Finish the massage with the back of the body.

14. The final considerations of massage involve completing the client's record card, suggesting supplementary services, placing supplies in their proper places, discarding refuse, and arranging the massage table and bath for the next client.

15. Undesirable aftereffects may include a slight headache, upset stomach and nausea, or the feeling that comes with the onset of a cold. Such reactions are due to an increase in metabolic waste material in the circulatory system. This waste material puts an extra burden on the excretory system. If this waste is not flushed out of the system, it will be reabsorbed into the tissues. The particular symptom the client experiences depends on the organs that are being overtaxed.

16. The client should drink plenty of water to keep the system flushed out following a massage.

Chapter 13 Therapeutic Procedure

1. The four steps of the therapeutic procedure are assessment, planning, performance, and evaluation.

2. The purpose of assessment is to review any information available at the onset of the process in order to best understand the present conditions. During the planning stage, the information gained from the assessment is used to determine strategies and select therapeutic techniques to address specific conditions found during the assessment. The performance is the actual application of the selected techniques. The evaluation examines the outcome of the session in regard to the effectiveness of the selected procedure for the condition.

3. The therapeutic process can be implemented for long-range goal setting, covering several sessions, short-range planning, covering a single session, and during an actual massage session.

4. Five parts of the assessment are taking a client history, client interview, observation, palpation, and examination.

5. The pain scale is a subjective tool with which clients can describe the relative pain or discomfort they are experiencing on a scale of 1 to 10, where 1 is no pain and 10 is excruciating, unbearable pain. Clients are able to express the level of pain they are experiencing at the beginning of the session and again at the end to indicate any improvement. The therapist is able to determine the amount of pressure to use in certain interventions by asking for the client's feedback using the pain scale.

6. When testing range of motion, passive movement, active movement, and restricted movement are examined.

7. Soft tissue barriers represent the limits within which tissues are manipulated. The resistive barrier marks the first sense of tissue stretch. The physiologic barrier represents the extent of tissue stretch and easy, painless movement. The anatomic barrier represents the anatomical limit of a particular tissue. To move beyond the anatomical limit would result in tissue damage.

8. Soft tissues that can be palpated from superficial to deep include just above the surface of the skin, the skin surface, the superficial fascia including lymph nodes and blood vessels, muscles and related structures and textures, the musculotendinous junction, tendons, bones, ligaments, and joints.

9. According to Dr. James Cyriax, contractile tissues are the fibrous tissues that have tensions placed on them during muscular contractions and include muscle tissue, tendons, and the muscle attachments. Inert tissues are the tissues that are not contractile, such as bone, ligament, bursae, blood vessels, nerves, nerve coverings, cartilage, and the like. End feel refers to the quality of the sensation the therapist feels as he passively moves a joint to the full extent of its possible range.

10. Three classifications of normal end feel are hard end feel, soft end feel, and springy end feel.

11. Abnormal end feel is similar to normal end feel except that there is reduced movement or there is associated pain.

12. Acute and chronic are terms used to describe a condition, pain, or illness. Acute refers to a condition with a sudden onset and relatively short duration. Chronic refers to a lingering or ongoing condition.

13. The appropriate intervention in the initial stage of an acute soft tissue injury is rest, ice, compression, and elevation (RICE).

14. Information from the medical history, intake form, interview, observation, movement assessments, palpation, as well as the client's needs and concerns are used to develop a treatment or care plan.

15. Assessment findings and treatment plans are discussed with the client so that the client can actively participate in the therapy, better understand the condition and treatment, and give informed consent to proceed with the session.

16. A therapeutic massage is like an intense conversation in that the therapist listens, observes, and examines the client to get an idea of the condition. Then the therapist's hands listen to the client's body and re-

spond with manipulative touch. The body listens to the manipulations and responds. Hearing and feeling these responses, the therapist chooses the next delivery, and so on.

17. Three types of directional massage include gliding, J-strokes, and cross-fiber.

18. The evaluation is important because:
    - The client and therapist can gauge the effectiveness of the selected course of therapy according to the success in attaining the goals.
    - It provides a rationale for applying similar therapies for similar conditions in the future.
    - It is the grounds for altering portions or all of the process to better achieve desired results.
    - It helps determine whether goals have been met and whether referral to another professional is warranted.

Chapter 14 Hydrotherapy

1. Electrical apparatus should be used by qualified persons with proper training. The practitioner must have sound knowledge of procedures involving electrical equipment and its benefits as well as any contraindications of its use. Always follow manufacturer's instructions.

2. The application of heat causes an increase of circulation, pulse rate, and white blood cell count. A local application will cause local reddening, increased metabolism and leukocyte migration to the area, relaxation of local musculature, and a slight analgesia.

3. Cryotherapy is the application of ice for therapeutic purposes.

4. The local application of ice acts as an analgesic to reduce pain and causes vasoconstriction to limit swelling. It is beneficial on painful, inflamed, and swollen areas.

5. In the acronym RICE, R = rest, I = ice, C = compression, and E = elevation. RICE is the standard first-aid treatment when a soft tissue injury such as a sprain or strain occurs. It reduces swelling, pain, and the secondary tissue damage that results from excessive swelling.

6. A contrast bath is the alternating application of hot and cold baths to a portion of the body.

7. Contrast baths are one of the most effective methods of increasing local circulation by causing an alternating vasodilation and vasoconstriction of the blood vessels in an area.

8. Hydrotherapy is the application of water in any of its three forms (ice, water, vapor) to the body for therapeutic purposes.

9. Water treatments are controlled by regulating the temperature, pressure, and duration of the treatment.

10. The qualities of water that make it an effective therapeutic tool are that it is readily available, is relatively inexpensive to use, and has the ability to absorb and conduct heat.

11. The three classifications of effects of hydrotherapy on the body are thermal, mechanical, and chemical.

12. Water treatments that involve hot or cold applications should not be given when the client has cardiac impairment, diabetes, lung disease, kidney infection, extremely high or low blood pressure, or an infectious skin condition.

13. Cold applications are beneficial because they improve circulation, stimulate nerves, and increase the activity of body cells.

14. Cold applications are undesirable over prolonged periods as they may produce a depressing effect. If after a cold bath or shower the client comes out chilly, shivering, blue-lipped, or goosefleshed, it indicates that her body reaction is not good.

15. Hot water applications improve skin functions by promoting perspiration and by increasing the circulation of blood to the surface of the skin.

16. The skin can safely tolerate 115°F of hot water and approximately 140°F of steam vapor. Water at 110°F over a prolonged period of time would raise the body temperature to a dangerous level.

17. Two objectives of baths are external cleanliness and stimulation of bodily functions.

18. A warm bath is 95° to 100°F, equal to 35° to 37.7°C. A hot bath is 100° to 115°F, equal to 37.7° to 43.3°C.

19. The average duration of a cold bath, shower, or sitz bath is approximately 3 to 5 minutes.

20. The duration of a hot saline or sitz bath is approximately 10 to 20 minutes.

21. The purpose of a cabinet bath is to induce perspiration that contributes to a weight reduction and to induce relaxation. It is also considered to be a cleansing procedure.

22. Safety precautions to observe during the operation of a bath cabinet include following the manufacturer's instructions for use of the cabinet and observing the client's general reactions, state of health, and tolerance to temperature.

23. The main benefits of a whirlpool bath are increased blood circulation, the soothing of nerves, and relaxing of the muscles.

24. The Russian bath is a full-body steam bath for the purpose of causing perspiration. The primary benefits are cleansing, relaxation, and improved metabolism.

Chapter 15 Massage in a Spa Setting

1. The origins of the word spa come from a Latin acronym for *sanitas per aqua,* or "health through water." The term might also have derived from the Latin verb *spagere,* which means to sprinkle or flow, like a fountain or spring.

2. In Rome, early spas, or baths, were called *thermae.* In Turkey they were called *hammam,* and in Japan they were called *Onsen.*

3. In 2004, the U.S. spa market was a $11.2 billion industry with 12,102 locations and 136 million guest visits.

4. The major categories of spas are destination spas, hotel/resort spas, day spas, club spas, medical/dental spas, and mineral spring spas.

5. Some of the spa modalities in addition to massage that therapists might be required to perform include body wraps, body scrubs, foot treatments, back treatments, scalp treatments, face treatments, cellulite treatments, aromatherapy, parafango, clay/mud/seaweed treatments, specialized rituals and exotic services such as Ayurvedic and Indonesian treatments, herbal detoxification treatments, and hydrotherapy baths and showers.

6. The most important points to keep in mind while practicing massage in a spa setting are: scope of practice, intake procedures, optimal number of massages per day, timing of services, guest greetings, preparation, and cleanup.

7. The major challenges to consistently giving high-quality therapeutic massage in the spa setting are low expectations, time constraints, and inexperienced clients. In order to overcome them, therapists should pay special attention to the timing, transitions, and uniqueness of each massage.

8. No. The rules and laws vary widely state to state regarding what a massage therapist can and cannot do in the spa setting. In some states, the law requires massage therapists to perform body wraps and exfoliation treatments; in others, the law allows untrained spa technicians to perform these treatments.

9. A spa cellulite treatment features vigorous massage, wrapping, and special products (usually seaweed-based) to promote an improved appearance to affected areas. It often includes underwater massage in a hydrotherapy tub.

10. A spa parafango treatment uses a blend of paraffin wax and fango (mud from a volcanic source) that is smoothed onto a part of or the whole body while warm, then is wrapped.

11. In the spa industry, aromatherapy can be defined as the use of essential oils processed from herbs, flowers, fruits, spices, stems, bark, and roots in massage, inhalation, or other modalities to affect mood and improve health and well-being.

12. Some carrier oils commonly used for aromatherapy massage include apricot kernel, avocado, grapeseed, jojoba, sesame, sweet almond, and wheat germ.

13. Some distinctions that make an aromatherapy massage different from a Swedish massage include the following: Therapists should check for guests' sensi-

tivity to aromas and explain therapeutic outcomes prior to treatment. During the treatment, strokes are predominantly light and flowing, and time is allowed for the client to experience the aromas. Also, blankets and/or an infrared heating lamp should be in place if necessary to keep the client warm.

14. Spas offer body wraps for heating the body; detoxification; to relax and improve mood and well-being; to nourish, cleanse, and improve the superficial contour the skin; for purging and drawing impurities out through the pores, softening the skin, improving joint elasticity, remineralizing the skin and entire body, and less frequently for weight-loss or inch-loss.

15. The main benefits of exfoliation are that it assists the skin's own regenerative processes, aids in the absorption of spa products applied afterward, thoroughly cleanses and promotes overall hygiene, and creates a healthy glow and radiant shine to the skin.

16. The principle maneuver for all exfoliation techniques is a circular scrubbing action. This is to avoid stretching the delicate connective tissues of the skin too far in any one direction.

17. A spa's company policies cover time concerns, appearance, attitude, professional development, and physical attributes.

18. As a part of professional career management, the spa, in exchange for a percentage of the price of each treatment, offers therapists many benefits, including built-in clientele, marketing, advertising, appointment booking, billing, payroll, supplies, equipment, training, support staff, and a clean facility.

19. A Vichy shower is a multihead inline shower extending out over a treatment table under which clients recline on a wet table to receive spa services. It is primarily used for body wraps and exfoliation services, but it may also be used during specialty massages.

20. A wet table is a specially constructed waterproof treatment table with built-in drainage used in spas for exfoliation and body wrap services.

21. Customer service can be defined as the ability of an organization or individual to take care of the needs, wishes, questions, requests, and complaints of its clientele. Excellent customer service consists of doing these things consistently, to a very high standard of satisfaction, and in a largely transparent manner.

22. Most spas depend upon retail profits to keep the business operational. Without these profits, many spas would close, and many therapists would be out of work. It is therefore in spa therapists' best interests to help with retail sales, as long as these sales are executed with integrity, honesty, and skill.

23. The main teamwork skills required to work successfully in a spa are being able to follow direction, anticipate others' needs, present a united front, and pitch in toward a common goal, regardless of whether or not a particular task is in the therapist's job description.

24. Therapists should come to spa job interviews prepared to talk about how they chose massage as a career, past work situations, attitude toward clients, and how they would deal with problems on the job. In addition, they should have some knowledge of the spa where they are applying and be able to explain why they want to work at that particular facility.

25. Therapists considering opening a spa should start out slowly, honestly assess their own limitations, enlist valuable allies, and keep learning information from diverse fields such as bookkeeping, management, retail, housekeeping, human resources, equipment maintenance, customer relations, and, of course, hands-on skill.

Chapter 16 Athletic/Sports Massage

1. Athletic massage, also called sports massage, is the application of massage techniques that combine sound anatomical and physiological knowledge, an understanding of strength training and conditioning, and specific massage skills to enhance athletic performance.

2. Adaptive sports massage is sports massage for athletes with physical or mental

disabilities, given with special consideration for the specific disability the athlete may have.

3. The therapist must know the functions of the circulatory, skeletal, muscular, and nervous systems of the body.

4. The overload principle in conditioning refers to the necessity of applying stresses to the body greater than it is accustomed to in order to increase strength or endurance.

5. Negative effects of exercise include:
   - Increased metabolic waste buildup in the tissues
   - Strains in the muscle or connective tissue, which may range from microscopic microtrauma to major injury
   - Inflammation and associated fibrosis
   - Spasms and pain that restrict movement

6. Techniques commonly used in sports massage include those of Swedish massage plus compression, cross-fiber friction, deep pressure, and active joint movements.

7. The primary goal of compression is to create hyperemia in the muscle tissue.

8. In athletic massage, hyperemia refers to the increased amount of blood and other fluids in and moving through the muscle tissue.

9. In athletic massage, deep pressure is used to relieve stress points and deactivate trigger points.

10. Transverse friction massage was popularized by the British osteopath Dr. James Cyriax.

11. The objective of using cross-fiber friction in athletic massage is to reduce fibrosis, encourage the formation of strong, pliable scar tissue at the site of healing injuries, and prevent or soften adhesions in fibrous tissue.

12. The four basic applications for athletic massage are massage previous to an event, massage after an event, massage during training, and massage during injury rehabilitation.

13. The goal of pre-event massage is to increase circulation and flexibility in the areas of the body about to be used. The goal of post-event massage is to increase circulation to clear out metabolic wastes, reduce muscle tension and spasm, and quiet the nervous system. The goal of massage during training is to allow the athlete to train at a higher level of intensity, more consistently, with less chance of injury, and to maintain muscles in the best possible state of nutrition, flexibility, and vitality. The goal of massage during rehabilitation is to get the athlete back into full performance as soon as possible with less chance of reinjury.

14. Massage is considered to be most beneficial to the athlete as a regular part of his scheduled training.

15. Stress points are areas of chronic stress or the site of microtrauma that are generally located at the ends of muscles or in taut bands of muscle tissue.

16. The therapist must be sure to apply proper techniques in order to avoid aggravating a condition or causing permanent damage to the area.

17. The best way to treat an athletic injury is to prevent it.

18. Rehabilitative massage:
   - Shortens the time it takes for an injury to heal
   - Maintains or increases range of motion
   - Helps to reduce swelling and edema
   - Helps to form strong, pliable scar tissue
   - Eliminates splinting in associated muscle tissue
   - Locates and deactivates trigger points that form as a result of the trauma
   - Helps get the athlete back into training sooner with less chance of reinjury

19. Proper massage therapy improves circulation, enabling damaged tissue to be carried away while making rebuilding nutrients available so that healing time is reduced.

20. Massage for new or fresh injuries should only be given by properly trained therapists in conjunction with a physician's approval.

21. RICE is an acronym for rest, ice, compression, and elevation. This represents proper first aid for soft tissue injuries.

22. Acute injuries have a sudden and definite onset and are usually of relatively short duration. Chronic injuries have a gradual onset, tend to last for a long time, or recur often.

23. Massage is contraindicated at the site of fresh acute muscle injuries.

24. Strains involve the tearing of muscle tissue or tendons. Sprains involve ligaments.

25. Athletic massage is contraindicated in any abnormal condition, injury, illness, or disease except as advised by the athlete's physician.

Chapter 17 Massage in Medicine

1. Charles Fayette Taylor and George Henry Taylor were brothers who both traveled to Europe, one to Sweden and the other to England, to study the Swedish Movement Cure. They both returned to New York, where they practiced, taught, and wrote about the Cure until their deaths in 1899.

2. CAM is an acronym for complementary and alternative medicine.

3. Alternative medicine insinuates using unconventional medical practices instead of conventional allopathic medical practices. Complementary medicine insinuates using conventional allopathic methods along with unconventional practices to address a medical condition.

4. Integrative medicine combines conventional allopathic medicine with appropriate alternative and complementary practices to provide the best possible health benefits to the client/patient.

5. Massage is the most requested integrative medicine (IM) modality and the mainstay of many Integrative Medicine clinics. Several massage modalities are practiced in IM clinics, including Classical Swedish for stress and pain relief, NMT, trigger-point, manual lymph drainage, pre- and postnatal, and energy modalities to serve a variety of patient conditions.

6. For hospital-based massage, the patient must have a referral, prescription, or at least a release from the attending physician for massage. The massage will probably take place with the patient in her hospital bed, so the therapist must make certain adjustments such as working around medical equipment. The therapist must be aware of the client's condition, special precautions, contraindications, and

indications and work according to the physician's recommendations.

7. Warning signs of cancer include the following:
   - Any sore that has not healed normally
   - A mole, skin tag, or wart that is changing in color or size
   - Lumps underneath the arms or in the breasts
   - Persistent hoarseness, coughing, or sore throat
   - Abnormal functioning of any internal organ, such as changes in the bladder or bowels
   - Discharge or bleeding from any part of the body
   - Persistent indigestion or difficulty in swallowing

8. Medical massage can be defined as medically necessary massage performed with the intent of improving pathologies or conditions diagnosed by a physician.

9. A massage therapist should obtain verification from the insurance company to determine whether and to what extent massage services will be covered by the client's insurance policy. The therapist can also inquire as to the correct CPT codes to use; if there is a deductible, has the deductible been met; if there is a co-pay, how much it is.

10. The HCFA 1500 form is a standardized form created by the Health Care Financing Administration that is used throughout the health care and insurance industry for billing purposes.

11. ICD-9 codes are diagnostic codes used by doctors to aid in the uniform reporting of ailments. ICD-9 is an acronym for the document International Classification of Disease, 9th Edition, in which every human health condition is assigned a decimal number.

12. CPT is an acronym for current procedural terminology codes, which were developed by the American Medical Association to categorize and quantify medical services and create a common base of communication between physicians, therapists, patients, and insurance companies.

13. Documents that should be included in an initial insurance claim include the HCFA 1500 form, the physician's prescription

and/or referral, the client history, initial assessment, preliminary session notes, and the assignment of benefits form.

Chapter 18 Other Therapeutic Modalities

1. Properly applied, prenatal massage can aid relaxation, benefit circulation, and soothe the nerves.

2. Correct lymph massage helps to stimulate the flow of lymph, which rids the body of toxins and waste materials. Lymph massage promotes the balance of the body's internal chemistry, purifies and regenerates tissues, and helps to normalize the functions of all body organs and the immune system.

3. Lymphocytes (leukocytes) are white corpuscles found in lymphatic tissue, blood, and lymph. They are active in the immune responses of the body and play a major part in healing wounds and fighting infections.

4. Lymph is the portion of the interstitial fluid that is absorbed into the lymph capillaries. It consists of water, proteins, cellular debris, bacteria, viruses, and other inorganic materials.

5. Deep tissue massage refers to various regimens or massage styles that affect the deeper tissue structures of the body. Deep tissue massage techniques affect the various layers of fascia that support muscle tissues and loosen bonds between the layers of connective tissues.

6. Structural integration attempts to bring the physical structure of the body into balance and alignment around a central axis.

7. Neurophysiological therapies recognize the importance of neurological feedback between the central nervous system and the musculoskeletal system in maintaining proper tone and function. Alterations or disturbances in the neuromuscular relationship often result in dysfunction and pain. Neurophysiological therapies utilize methods of assessing tissues and soft tissue manipulative techniques to normalize the tissues and reprogram the neurological loop in order to reduce pain and improve function.

8. A trigger point is a hyperirritable spot that is painful when compressed. When stimulated, active trigger points refer pain and tenderness to another area of the body. Latent trigger points only exhibit pain when compressed and do not refer pain.

9. Myofascial trigger points are found in muscle tissue or its associated fascia. They are located in a taut band of muscle fibers.

10. Procedures for deactivating trigger points include injections, stretch and spray, active stretching, and ischemic compression.

11. Neuromuscular therapy was developed in England in the 1930s by Dr. Stanley Lief. It has been popularized in the United States through the teachings of Paul St. John.

12. Abnormal tissue signs that indicate neuromuscular lesions include:
    - Congestion in the tissues
    - Contracted tissue or taut, fibrous bands
    - Nodules or lumps
    - Trigger points
    - Restrictions between the skin and underlying tissues
    - Variations in temperature (warmer or cooler than surrounding tissues)
    - Swelling or edema
    - General tenderness

    Neuromuscular lesions are always hypersensitive to pressure and often associated with trigger points.

13. The primary treatment techniques used in neuromuscular therapy include gliding, ischemic compression, skin rolling, and stretching.

14. The two basic inhibitory reflexes produced during MET manipulations are post-isometric relaxation and reciprocal inhibition.

15. The three active joint movements used in MET are contract-relax or agonist-contract, antagonist-contract, and contract-relax-antagonist-contract.

16. Passive positioning techniques are perhaps the gentlest of soft tissue manipulations wherein joints associated with constricted muscles are passively placed into their preferred position of greatest comfort.

17. Three important considerations of passive positioning techniques are:

a. Gently moving a joint into its position of maximum comfort

b. Holding that position for an adequate period of time

c. Slowly and passively returning the joint to its neutral position

18. Strain-counterstrain was developed by Dr. Lawrence Jones.

19. In strain-counterstrain, the preferred position is determined by palpating and monitoring the sensitivity of the associated tender points while positioning the joint. When the client indicates that the pain in the point is reduced and there is a noticeable "letting go" in the palpated tissues, when the pain or discomfort in the joint is also reduced, and the client is in a comfortable position, the correct position has been established.

20. The primary techniques used in structural muscular balancing include precision muscle testing, passive positioning, directional massage, and deep pressure.

21. Precision muscle testing is a type of specialized kinesiology that is used to evaluate energetic imbalances in the body and determine exactly what remedies will work best for the individual at that particular time.

22. Acupuncture is said to have originated in China more than 5,000 years ago.

23. Yin and yang are the two parts that contrast or exist as opposites of the same phenomenon.

24. Acupressure techniques include rubbing, touching, and pressing of pressure points.

25. The Japanese word shiatsu (*shi*, finger; and *atsu*, pressure) means pressure of the fingers.

26. Doctors often recommend massage for the relief of tension, anxiety, and stress.

27. Reflexology is used to stimulate the body's own healing forces through the stimulation of reflex points on the hands, feet, or other areas of the body.

Chapter 19 Business Practices

1. A positive attitude and good self-image are reflected in the enthusiasm and quality exhibited in your work. They are the foundation for creating a good public image. A good public image along with good business practices breed success.

2. A sole proprietorship is a business owned and operated by an individual. In a partnership, two or more people combine resources to operate a business. In both a sole proprietorship and a partnership, the owners are responsible for the obligations and liabilities of the business and take the profits. A corporation is managed by a board of directors, the owners are not directly liable, and the profits are shared by the stockholders.

3. Start-up costs of a massage business may include rent or lease, equipment, supplies, furniture and decorating costs, printing and advertising, license, insurance, and other miscellaneous expenses.

4. The location for a massage business should accommodate your business needs, be pleasing to your clients, fit your image, be properly zoned, and be within your budget. The office location must be easy to locate, with the address clearly visible from the street. It should be easily accessible and relatively quiet. An ideal space would have one or more massage rooms, a reception/waiting area, an office, and bathroom facilities with a shower.

5. Permits and licenses necessary to operate a massage business may include fictitious name statement; business license; massage license, sales tax permit; planning and zoning permits; building safety permit; employer's identification number (EIN).

6. The types of insurance a massage business owner should carry to protect the business include liability insurance; malpractice liability insurance; automobile insurance; fire and theft insurance; medical health insurance; workers' compensation insurance.

7. Keeping accurate records is necessary in a successful business in that it records the progress of the business, especially the cost of doing business in relation to income. Business records are also necessary to meet the requirements of local, state, and federal laws pertaining to taxes and employees.

8. The major ingredients of a basic bookkeeping system are a checking account with an updated ledger; income and disbursement

ledgers; accounts receivable and accounts payable files; bank statements and reconciliations; filed business receipts; an inventory system; an assets and depreciation file; a mileage log.

9. Marketing is the business activity done to promote and increase your business. Marketing is an educational process of getting yourself and what you do known. It is the enticement that encourages people to seek your services.

10. Marketing activities commonly used in the massage industry include advertising, promotion, public relations, referrals, and client retention.

11. A target market is a segment of the population with certain characteristics that make them good prospective consumers of a particular product or service.

12. The three R's of referrals are:
   - Request: Request the referral.
   - Reward: Acknowledge and reward the person who sends the referral.
   - Reciprocate: Use the services of or send referrals back to those who send you referrals.

Glossary

A

Abdomen contains the stomach, intestines, liver, and kidneys.

Absorption is the process in which the digested nutrients are transferred from the intestines to the blood or lymph vessels.

Accessory digestive organs consist of the teeth, tongue, salivary glands, pancreas, liver, and gallbladder.

Acne is a chronic inflammatory disorder of the skin, usually related to hormonal changes.

Acquired immunity results from an encounter with a new substance, which triggers events that induce an immune response specific to that particular substance.

Acquired immunodeficiency syndrome (AIDS) is a condition caused by HIV infection whereby a portion of the immune system is destroyed, making it easy for the infected person to get life-threatening diseases.

Active joint movements are movements in which the client actively participates by contracting the muscles involved in the movement.

Active stretching refers to techniques that utilize neuromuscular reflexes to enhance the elongation of muscles that are stretched.

Acupressure is based on traditional Oriental medical principles for assessing and treating the physical and energetic body, stimulating acupuncture points to regulate *chi* (life force).

Acupuncture is a traditional Chinese medical practice in which the skin is punctured with needles at specific points for therapeutic purposes.

Acute refers to a condition with a sudden onset and relatively short duration.

Adipose tissue is areolar tissue with an abundance of fat cells.

Adrenal glands, situated on the top of each kidney, produce epinephrine, norepinephrine, and corticosteroids.

Adrenocorticotropic hormone (ACTH) stimulates the adrenal cortex.

Aerobic cellular respiration makes energy for reconstituting ADP in cell mitochondrion.

Aerobic exercise improves cardiorespiratory fitness.

Albinism is a congenital absence of melanin pigment in the skin, hair, and eyes.

Aldosterone regulates the sodium/potassium balance in the extracellular fluid and in the blood.

Alimentary canal consists of the mouth, pharynx, esophagus, stomach, and small and large intestines.

Allergy is a sensitivity to normally harmless substances.

Alternative medicine is a term that implies using services other than those usually accepted from allopathic physicians.

Alveoli are microscopic air sacs in the lungs.

Amitosis is a process of cell division.

Amphiarthrotic joints, such as the symphysis pubis, have limited motion.

Anabolism is the process of building up of larger molecules from smaller ones.

Anaerobic respiration is a process in which glucose is broken down in the absence of oxygen.

Anal canal is the distal part of the large intestine, which ends with the anus.

Anaphase is a stage in cell division.

Anatomical barrier refers to the anatomical limit of motion of particular tissue. To move beyond the anatomic barrier would cause injury and disruption of tissues and supportive structures.

Anatomy is the study of the gross structure of the body and the interrelations of its parts.

Anatripsis is the art of rubbing a body part upward.

Anemia refers to a number of conditions in which there is an inadequate production of red blood cells.

Aneurysm is a local distention or ballooning of an artery due to a weakening wall.

Angulus venosus is the juncture of the jugular and subclavian veins.

Ankylosing spondylitis is a chronic inflammatory disease of the spinal articulations and sacroiliac joint.

Anmo is a massage technique from China that finds the points on the body where various movements and manipulations are most effective.

Antagonist contraction technique takes advantage of reciprocal inhibition.

Antibodies are a class of proteins produced in the body in response to contact with antigens that immunize the body.

Antidiuretic hormone stimulates the kidneys to reabsorb more water, which reduces urine output.

Antigen is anything that can trigger an immune response.

Aorta is the main artery of the body.

Aortic semilunar valve of the heart permits the blood to be pumped from the left ventricle into the aorta.

Appendicular skeleton is made up of bones of the shoulder, upper extremities, hips, and lower extremities.

Arachnoid mater is the middle space of the meninges.

Areolar tissue is loose connective tissue that binds the skin to the underlying tissues and fills the spaces between the muscles.

Aromatherapy is the use of essential oils processed from herbs, flowers, fruits, stems, spices, and roots in massage, inhalation, or other modalities to affect mood and improve health and well-being.

Arteries are thick-walled muscular and elastic vessels that transport oxygenated blood from the heart.

Arteriosclerosis is a condition in which the walls of the arteries thicken and lose their elasticity.

Arthritis is an inflammatory condition of the joints.

Articular cartilage is a layer of hyaline cartilage covering the end surface of the epiphysis.

Ascete is a person who exercises body and mind.

Asexual reproduction is a method of reproduction of lower forms of life using nonsexual means.

Asteatosis is a dry, scaly skin condition.

Atherosclerosis is characterized by an accumulation of fatty deposits on the inner walls of the arteries.

Atoms are subatomic particles that all substances are composed of.

Atrophy is the result of muscle disuse and a condition in which the muscle wastes away.

Aura stroking is done with long, smooth strokes that do not actually touch the body surface but come close.

Autoimmune disease occurs when the immune system mistakes self for nonself and attacks itself.

Autonomic nervous system regulates the action of glands, smooth muscles, and the heart.

Axial skeleton is made up of bones of the skull, thorax, vertebral column, and the hyoid bone.

Axon conducts impulses away from the nerve cell body.

Ayurveda is an ancient system of Indian medicine and healing; it has been modified in recent years for use in spa treatments such as body scrubs, face treatments, and massages.

B

Bacteria are minute, unicellular organisms exhibiting both plant and animal characteristics and are classified as either harmless or harmful.

Balneotherapy uses water for its buoyancy, temperature, viscosity, and pressure as in hydrotherapy, with the added benefits of ingredients such as herbs, minerals, and gases (carbon dioxide, etc.).

Bania is a Russian-style communal steam bath.

Bartholen's glands are mucus-producing glands located near the vestibule of the vagina.

Basal cell carcinoma is a type of skin cancer.

Bath is a practice where the body is surrounded by water or vapor.

B-cells work by producing antibodies.

Beating is the heaviest and deepest form of percussion and is done over the denser areas of the body.

Bicuspid or mitral valve of the heart allows blood to flow from the left atrium into the left ventricle.

Bile is a bitter, alkaline, yellowish-brown fluid secreted by the liver that aids in fat digestion.

Blackheads (comedones) are small masses of hardened, discolored sebum that appear most frequently on the face, shoulders, chest, and back.

Bladder is an organ where the urine is stored.

Blood is the nutritive fluid circulating throughout the blood-vascular system.

Blood clot is a meshwork that entraps platelets and blood cells.

Blood platelets, or thrombocytes, are colorless, irregular bodies, much smaller than red corpuscles.

Blood-vascular system, or cardiovascular system, includes the blood, heart, and blood vessels.

Body mechanics is the observation of body posture in relation to safe and efficient movement in daily living activities.

Bone tissue is connective tissue in which the intercellular substance is rendered hard by mineral salts, chiefly calcium carbonate and calcium phosphate.

Boundaries are personal comfort zones that help an individual maintain a sense of comfort and safety. They can be professional, personal, physical, emotional, intellectual, and sexual.

Brachial plexus is composed of four lower cervical nerves and the first pair of thoracic nerves that control arm movements.

Brain is the principal nerve center and largest, most complex nerve tissue of the body.

Brain stem has three parts: the midbrain, the pons, and the medulla oblongata.

Breathing involves the act of inhaling and exhaling air.

Bruise is a superficial injury, caused by a blow, which does not break the skin but causes a reddish-blue or purple discoloration.

Bulla is a blister containing a watery fluid, similar to a vesicle but larger.

Bursae are fibrous sacks lined with synovial membrane and lubricated with synovial fluid, functioning as a cushion in areas of pressure.

Bursitis is inflammation resulting from injury to the bursae.

C

Calcitonin is a hormone that controls the level of calcium in the blood.

Cancer is the uncontrolled growth and spread of abnormal cells in the body.

Candida is a fungus found in the intestines, mouth, and vagina.

Capillaries are the smallest blood vessels and connect arterioles with the venules.

Capsular pattern refers to the proportional limitation of any joint that is controlled by muscular contractions.

Carbuncle is a mass of connected boils.

Cardiac muscle tissue occurs only in the heart and is responsible for pumping blood through the heart into the blood vessels.

Carpal tunnel syndrome is a compression of the median nerve as it passes through the wrist that causes pain and weakness in the fingers.

Carrier oil is massage lubricant into which essential oils are blended for aromatherapy applications.

Cartilage, or gristle, is a firm, tough, elastic substance that cushions the bones, prevents jarring between bones in motion, and gives shape to the nose and ears.

Cartilaginous joints are joints held together with cartilage with no joint cavity.

Catabolism is the metabolic breaking down of larger substances into smaller ones.

Cell membrane is the outer wall of the cell that permits soluble substances to enter and leave the protoplasm.

Cells are basic functional units of all living matter.

Centering is based on the concept that you have a geographical center in your body about 2 inches below the navel.

Central nervous system consists of the brain and spinal cord.

Cerebellum is the small part of the brain that controls muscular movement and balance.

Cerebrospinal fluid's main function is to act as a shock absorber for the brain and spinal cord and distribute nutrients.

Cerebrovascular accident, or stroke, is caused by a blood clot or ruptured blood vessel in or around the brain that subsequently destroys nerve tissue.

Cerebrum is the front and top of the brain and the center of mental activities, sensation, communication, memory, emotions, will, and reasoning.

Cervical plexus consists of the four upper cervical nerves that supply the skin and control the movement of the head, neck, and shoulders.

Chair massage takes place in a massage chair, which is a good choice for people not able to or not amenable to receive full-body massage on a table.

Chirugy is healing with the hands.

Chloasma is characterized by increased deposits of pigment in the skin; also called moth patches or liver spots.

Chronic refers to a lingering or ongoing condition.

Chucking involves the flesh being grasped firmly in one or both hands and moved up and down along the bone.

Chyle is a cloudy liquid, consisting mostly of fats, that passes from the small intestines, through the lacteals, and into the lymph system.

Chyme is a mixture of digestive juices, mucus, and food material.

Circular friction is movement in which the fingers or palm of the hand move the superficial tissues in a circular pattern over the deeper tissues.

Circulatory system is the network of vessels through which blood and lymph circulate.

Coccygeal plexus is formed from a portion of the fourth sacral nerves, the fifth sacral nerve, and the coccygeal nerve.

Compact bone tissue forms the hard bone found in the shafts of long bones and along the outside of flat bones.

Complementary medicine is the term that implies that the alternative practices can work along with more conventional medicine for the benefit of clients.

Compression is rhythmic pressing movements directed into muscle tissue by either the hand or fingers.

Concentric contraction occurs when the force of a contraction is greater than the resistance and the muscle shortens.

Connective tissue binds structures together, provides support and protection, and serves as a framework.

Connective tissue massage is massage directed toward the subcutaneous connective tissue believed to affect vascular and visceral reflexes related to a variety of pathologies and disabilities.

Contact dermatitis is abnormal skin conditions resulting from contact with chemicals or other exterior agents.

Contractile tissues are the fibrous tissues that have tensions placed on them during muscular contractions.

Contractility is the ability of a muscle to contract or shorten and thereby exert force.

Contract-relax technique incorporates postisometric relaxation theory that as soon as an isometric muscle contraction releases, the muscle relaxes.

Contracture occurs when joint mobility is reduced by decreased extensibility of muscle or other tissues crossing the joint.

Contraindication any physical, mental, or emotional condition a client may have that may cause a particular intervention or treatment to be unsafe.

Contrasting hot and cold causes alternating vasodilation and vasoconstriction in an area, which increases local circulation and relieves stiffness and pain and aids in healing.

Contusion, or bruise, is a common type of hematoma that is generally not too serious.

Corns are cone-shaped areas on or between the toes caused by pressure or friction.

Coronal plane divides the body into the front and back.

Corporation is a business setup subject to state regulation and taxation. A charter must be obtained from the state in which the corporation operates.

Corpus luteum is a yellowish endocrine body formed in the ruptured ovarian follicle that produces estrogen and progesterone.

Countertransference happens when a therapist or practitioner personalizes a therapeutic relationship by unconsciously projecting characteristics of someone from a former relationship onto a client. This is almost always detrimental to a therapeutic relationship.

Cowper's, or bulbourethral glands, produce mucus that lubricates the urethra.

Craniosacral therapy is a gentle, hands-on method of evaluating and enhancing the functioning of the craniosacral system.

Cretinism is caused by a lack of thyroxin during fetal development and results in a dwarfed stature and mental retardation.

Cross-fiber friction is applied in a transverse direction across the muscle, tendon, or ligament.

Crust is an accumulation of serum and pus, mixed perhaps with epidermal material.

Cryotherapy is the application of cold agents for therapeutic purposes.

Cryptococcal meningitis is caused by the fungus Cryptococcus neoformans.

Cupping is a technique used by respiratory therapists to help break up lung congestion.

Current procedural terminology (CPT) codes were developed and are maintained by the American Medical Association that categorize and quantify medical services and provide a common language and a base for communication between physicians, therapists, patients, and insurance companies.

Cushing's syndrome results from excess glucocorticoid production and is characterized by obesity, muscle weakness, elevated blood sugar, and hypertension.

D

Décolletage is the area of the upper chest above the breasts and onto the front of the neck.

Decubitus ulcers are bedsores.

Deep fascia refers to fibrous tissue sheaths that penetrate deep into the body, separating major muscle groups, and anchoring them to the bones.

Deep gliding indicates that the gliding manipulation uses enough pressure to have a mechanical effect.

Deep transverse friction massage is massage that broadens the fibrous tissues of muscles, tendons, or ligaments, breaking down unwanted adhesions and restoring mobility to muscles.

Dendrites connect with other neurons to receive information.

Dermatitis is an inflammatory condition of the skin.

Dermis is the deeper layer of the skin that extends to form the subcutaneous tissue.

Diabetes mellitus is caused by decreased output of insulin by the pancreas.

Diaphysis is the bone shaft between the epiphyses.

Diarthrotic joints are freely movable.

Diathermy is the application of oscillating electromagnetic fields to the tissue.

Differentiation is the repeated division of the ovum during early developmental stages, resulting in specialized cells that differ from one another.

Diffusers are devices using fans, heat, or steam dispersion to release the aromas of essential oils into a room for therapeutic and/or esthetic purposes.

Diffusion is a process in which substances move from an area of higher concentration to an area of lower concentration.

Digestion is the process of converting food into substances capable of being used by the cells for nourishment.

Digestive system consists of the mouth, stomach, intestines, salivary, and gastric glands.

Directional massage uses a short J-stroke on a specified body area or muscle.

Disease is an abnormal and unhealthy state of all or part of the body wherein it is not capable of carrying on its normal function.

Disinfection is the level of decontamination, nearly as effective as sterilization, but it does not kill bacterial spores.

Dislocation occurs when a bone is displaced within a joint.

Dopamine is a neurotransmitter that controls fine movement, emotional response, and the ability to experience pleasure and pain.

Draping is the process of using linens to keep a client covered while receiving a massage.

Dry room is a massage room used for spa treatments performed without the use of showers and baths.

Dr. Vodder's Manual Lymph Drainage is a method of gentle, rhythmical massage along the surface lymphatics that aids in lymphatic system functioning and treats chronic lymphedema.

Dura mater is the outer layer of the meninges covering the brain and spinal cord.

E

Ectoderm is the outermost layer of cells of the skin.

Eczema is an inflammation of the skin, usually a red, blistered, oozing area that itches painfully.

Edema is a condition of excess fluid in the interstitial spaces.

Effleurage is a succession of strokes applied by gliding the hand over an extended portion of the body.

Ejaculatory ducts enter the prostate gland and empty into the urethra.

Elasticity refers to the tissue's ability to return to normal resting length when a stress that has been placed on it is removed.

Embolus is a piece of a clot that loosens and floats in the blood.

Empty end feel is an abrupt restriction to a joint movement due to pain.

Emulsion is a uniform mixture of two or more liquids, such as an essential oil and a massage lotion.

Encephalitis refers to several related viral diseases that cause inflammation of the brain or the meninges.

End feel is the change in the quality of the movement as the end of a joint movement is achieved.

Endocardium is the thin, innermost layer of the heart.

Endocrine or ductless glands depend on the blood and lymph to carry their secretions to various affected tissues.

Endocrine system consists of a group of specialized glands that affect the growth, development, sexual activity, and health of the entire body.

Endoderm is the innermost layer of cells of the skin.

Endomysium is the delicate connective tissue covering of muscle fibers.

Endurance is the ability to carry on an activity over a prolonged period of time and resist fatigue.

Energetic manipulation makes use of techniques that detect imbalances in the flow of the force in the body and bring it back into balance.

Enzymes are proteins that act as catalysts for chemical reactions in metabolism while remaining unchanged themselves.

Epicardium is the protective outer layer of the heart.

Epidermis is the outermost layer of the skin.

Epididymis is located in the scrotum and receives sperm from the testes, which it stores until they become mature.

Epilepsy is a neurological condition in which there is an abnormal electrical activity in the CNS without apparent tissue abnormalities.

Epimysium is the layer of connective tissue that closely covers an individual muscle.

Epinephrine is the "fight or flight" hormone that prepares the body to respond to emergencies.

Epiphysis is an enlarged area on the ends of long bones that articulates with other bones.

Epithelial tissue is a protective layer that functions in the processes of absorption, excretion, secretion, and protection.

Esalen massage is a style of massage developed at Esalen Institute in northern California that features long, flowing strokes that connect all parts of the body into a whole.

Estrogen is a female hormone responsible for development of secondary sexual characteristics.

Ethereal body stroking is done with long, smooth strokes that do not actually touch the body surface but come close.

Ethics is a system or code of morals of an individual, a group, or a profession.

Excoriation is a skin sore or abrasion produced by scratching or scraping.

Excretory system includes the skin, kidneys, bladder, liver, lungs, and large intestines, which eliminate waste products from the body.

Exfoliation is any of a number of spa treatments whose primary purpose is to cleanse the body of dead skin cells, thus softening the skin, helping the body to eliminate better through the skin, and preparing the skin for better absorption of other therapeutic products.

Exocrine or duct glands possess tubes or ducts leading from the gland to a particular part of the body.

Extensibility is the ability of a muscle to stretch.

Exteroceptors record conscious sensations such as heat, cold, pain, and pressure throughout the body.

F

Fallopian tubes, or oviducts, are the egg-carrying tubes of the female reproductive system.

Fascia is the fibrous connective tissue between muscle bundles or between muscle fibers that supports nerves and blood vessels.

Fascicle is a bundle of muscle fibers.

Feather stroking requires very light pressure of the fingertips or hands with long flowing strokes.

Female reproductive system functions to produce the ovum and female hormones, to receive the sperm during the sex act, and to carry the fetus during pregnancy.

Fetus is the developing child from the third month of pregnancy until birth.

Fever is an elevated body temperature.

Fibrocartilage is found between the vertebrae and pubic symphysis.

Fibromyalgia is characterized by pain, fatigue, and stiffness in the connective tissue of the muscles, tendons, and ligaments.

Fibrosis refers to the formation of fibrous tissue.

Fibrous connective tissue is composed of collagen and elastic fibers that are closely arranged to form tendons and ligaments.

Fibrous joints have no space and are held together by fibrous connective tissue.

Filtration is a process in which blood pressure pushes fluids and substances through the capillary wall and into the tissue spaces.

Fissure is a crack in the skin penetrating into the derma.

Flat palpation is done with the fingertips or thumb either in line with or perpendicularly across the fibers of the muscle tissue.

Flexibility refers to the ability of a joint to move freely and painlessly through its range of motion.

Fracture is a break or rupture in a bone.

Freely flexible range of movement refers to the pliable and easily movable range of the tissue.

French and English massage employ many Swedish massage movements and facial massage and beauty therapy treatments.

Friction refers to a number of massage strokes designed to manipulate soft tissue so that one layer is moved over or against another.

Fulling is a kneading technique in which the tissue is grasped, gently lifted, and spread out.

Fungus (pl. fungi) is a diverse group of organisms potentially capable of causing disease that thrive or grow in wet or damp areas.

Furuncle is a boil caused by bacteria that enter the skin through the hair follicles.

G

Gait is a pattern or manner of walking.

Gait assessment is observing the manner in which a person walks to determine constrictions or related conditions.

Gamete is a reproductive cell that can unite with another gamete to form the cell that develops into a new individual.

Gate control theory maintains that the positive effects of relaxing massage interrupts the transmission of pain sensations of affected nociceptors from entering the central nervous system by stimulating other cutaneous receptors.

General or systemic circulation is the blood circulation from the left side of the heart throughout the body and back again to the heart.

German massage combines many of the Swedish movements and emphasizes the use of various kinds of therapeutic baths.

Glands are specialized organs that vary in size and function.

Gliding is the practice of gliding the hand over some portion of the client's body with varying amounts of pressure.

Glucagon, produced by the islets of Langerhans, increases the glucose level in the blood.

Glucocorticoids affect carbohydrate, protein, and fat metabolism.

Goals are specific, attainable, measurable accomplishments that you set and make a commitment to achieve.

Golgi tendon organs are multibranched sensory nerve endings located in tendons.

Gonad is a sex gland that produces the reproductive cell.

Gonadotropic hormones regulate the development and function of the reproductive systems in women and men.

Gonorrhea is a venereal disease characterized by a discharge and burning sensation when urinating.

Grounding is based on the concept that you have a connection with the client and that you function as a grounding apparatus in helping the client to release tension.

Gymnasium is a center where exercise and massage are combined to treat disease and promote health.

H

Hacking is a rapid striking movement that can be done with one or both hands.

Hammam (also spelled hamam) is a Turkish steam bath with elaborate cleansing, exfoliation, and massage rituals passed down for centuries, played an important role in Ottoman culture.

Hard end feel is a bone-against-bone feeling.

HCFA 1500 form is a standardized form created by the Health Care Financing Administration to be used by service providers when billing insurance for medical expenses.

Heart is a pump that keeps the blood circulating in a steady stream through a closed system of arteries, capillaries, and veins.

Heating pads are plastic-covered pads that contain electric heating elements.

Hematoma is a mass of blood trapped in some tissue or cavity of the body and is the result of internal bleeding.

Hemiplegia is unilateral paralysis caused by a stroke.

Hemophilia is characterized by extremely slow clotting of blood and excessive bleeding from slight cuts.

Herniated disc is a weakening of the intervertebral disc resulting in a protrusion into the vertebral canal, potentially compressing the spinal cord.

Herpes I is a virus that affects the mouth, skin, and other facial parts, commonly called cold sores and fever blisters.

High blood pressure refers to an elevated pressure of the blood against the artery walls.

Hippocratic oath is a code of ethics for physicians thought to have come from Hippocrates.

Histology is a branch of biology concerned with the microscopic structure of tissues of a living organism.

Holistic means to look at the whole picture.

Homeostasis is the internal balance of the body.

Hospitality industry is the combined hotel, resort, restaurant, and entertainment industries that rely especially upon customer service and professional hospitality for their success.

Hot tub is a tub with a heating device that may have jets and may or may not be large enough to accommodate several occupants.

Human immunodeficiency virus (HIV) is a virus that can multiply and destroy a portion of the immune system.

Hydrotherapy is the application of water in any of its three forms to the body for therapeutic purposes.

Hyperactive glands oversecrete hormones due to lack of regulation or glandular tumors.

Hyperadrenalism is the excessive release of adrenal hormones into the bloodstream.

Hyperemia is an increased amount of blood in the muscle.

Hyperparathyroidism causes loss of calcium from the bones and excessive excretion of calcium and phosphorus from the kidneys.

Hyperpituitarism is the production of excessive amounts of growth hormone.

Hyperthyroidism is excessive activity of the thyroid gland.

Hypertrophy is increased muscle bulk resulting from an increase in myofibril thickness in the muscle fiber and increased density of the muscle capillary bed.

Hypoadrenalism, or Addison's disease, is due to the failure of the adrenal cortex to produce aldosterone and cortisol.

Hypoparathyroidism results in low blood calcium.

Hypopituitarism results from inadequate stimulation from the hypothalamus or destruction of the pituitary gland.

Hypothyroidism is a condition of deficient thyroid activity.

I

ICD-9 codes are a system of decimal numbers that correspond to medical conditions diagnosed by doctors. ICD-9 is an acronym for International Classification of Disease, 9th Revision, and is published annually by the U.S. Health Services and Health Care Financing Administration.

Ice massage is a local application of cold achieved by massaging a cube of ice over a small area such as a bursa, tendon, or small muscle.

Ice packs are used for the local application of ice on a specific body part.

Immersion bath involves submersion of a body part in water.

Immune-deficiency diseases occur when one or more parts of the immune system are deficient or missing.

Immune system helps keep people safe from foreign invaders and diseases.

Immunity refers to all the physiological mechanisms used by the body as protection against foreign substances.

Impetigo is a highly infectious bacterial skin infection common in children.

Independent contractor determines own work schedule, provides own supplies, gets paid a flat fee, and is responsible for own taxes.

Inert tissues are the tissues that are not contractile such as bone, ligament, nerves.

Inflammation is a protective tissue response characterized by swelling, redness, heat, and pain.

Informed consent is a client's written authorization for professional services based on adequate information from the massage therapist about the massage, including expectations, potential benefits, possible undesirable effects, and professional and ethical responsibility.

Infrared radiation may be produced from a bulb or an element. Heat results in increased superficial circulation and sedation of nerve endings.

Innate immunity is present from before birth.

Insertion of a muscle is the more mobile attachment of a muscle to bone.

Insulin regulates the movement of glucose across the cell membrane and plays a role in protein and fat transport and metabolism.

Intake specialists, also known as hospitality coordinators, spa concierges, and other titles, are spa employees who focus on pairing guests with appropriate treatments, therapists, services, and lifestyle choices during their stay at the spa.

Integrative medicine combines complementary and alternative medicine with allopathic medicine.

Integumentary system is composed of the skin, hair, and nails. *See also* Skin.

International Spa Association (ISPA) is a professional organization consisting of member spas, owners, directors, technicians, consultants, writers, marketers, and suppliers of products and equipment who meet at conventions and roundtables to create standards, share information, and chart directions for the development of the spa industry worldwide (ISPA, 2365 Harrodsburg Road, Suite A325, Lexington, KY 40504, (888) 651-4772, www.experienceispa.com).

Interneuron carries impulses from one neuron to another.

Interphase is a stage in cell division.

Irritability, or excitability, is the capacity of muscles to receive and react to stimuli.

Ischemia is localized tissue anemia due to obstruction of the inflow of blood.

Ischemic compression involves digital pressure directly into a trigger point.

Islets of Langerhans, found in the pancreas, produce insulin and glucagon.

Isometric contraction occurs when a muscle contracts and the ends of the muscle do not move.

Isotonic contraction occurs when a muscle contracts and the distance between the ends of the muscle changes.

J

Jacuzzi is a tub equipped with multiple jets that cause the water to move in multiple directions.

Joint movements are the passive or active movement of the joints or the articulations of the client.

Joints connect the bones of the skeleton.

Jostling involves grasping the entire muscle, lifting it slightly away from its position, and shaking it quickly across its axis.

K

Kaposi's sarcoma is a form of cancer of the cells that line certain blood vessels.

Keratoma, or callus, is a superficial, thickened patch of epidermis.

Kidneys are bean-shaped organs that filter the blood.

Kinesiology is the scientific study of muscular activity and the anatomy, physiology, and mechanics of body movement.

Kiva is an underground chamber used by the Pueblo tribe of Indians for ceremonial sweats and other rituals.

Kneading lifts, squeezes, and presses the tissues.

Kyphosis is an abnormally exaggerated convex curve of the spine.

L

Labia majora are the outer lips of the vulva.

Labia minora are the small, inner lips of the vulva.

Lacteals are lymphatic capillaries located in the villi of the small intestine.

Large intestine, or colon, stores, forms, and excretes waste products of digestion and regulates water balance in the body.

Lentigines, or freckles, are small, yellowish to brownish color spots on parts exposed to sunlight and air.

Lesion is a structural change in the tissues caused by injury or disease.

Leucoderma are abnormal light patches of skin, due to congenital defective pigmentation.

Leukemia is a form of cancer in which there is an uncontrolled production of white blood cells.

Ligaments are bands of fibrous tissue that connect bones to bones.

Limited Liability Companies are a form of legal entity, something between a partnership and a corporation.

Liquid tissue is represented by blood and lymph.

Liver, the largest gland of the body, performs the body's chemical functions.

Local infection is invading organisms confined to a small area of the body.

Lordosis is concave curvature of the spine.

Lulur, a pre-wedding ritual originally practiced by Balinese royalty that is now incorporated as an advanced spa modality, includes massage, bath, and exfoliation with exotic tropical ingredients.

Lumbar plexus is formed from the first four lumbar nerves.

Lupus erythematosus is a chronic inflammatory autoimmune disease of the connective tissue.

Luteinizing hormone from the pituitary gland transforms the ovarian follicle into the corpus luteum.

Lymphedema is an accumulation of interstitual fluid, or swelling, in the soft tissues due to inflammation, blockage, or removal of the lymph channels.

Lymph nodes contain a large concentration of lymphocytes and serve to filter and neutralize bacteria and toxins collected in the lymph.

Lymph-vascular system consists of lymph, lymph nodes, and lymphatics through which the lymph circulates.

M

Macule is a small, discolored spot or patch on the surface of the skin, neither raised nor sunken.

Male reproductive system functions include sperm production, male hormone production, and performance of the sex act.

Malignant melanoma is a serious type of skin cancer.

Marrow is the connective tissue filling in the cavities of bones that forms red and white blood cells.

Massage is the systematic manual or mechanical manipulations of the soft tissues of the body for therapeutic purposes.

Medical gymnastics, gymnastics applied to the treatment of disease, consists of active, duplicated, and passive movements.

Medullary cavity is a hollow chamber formed in the shaft of long bones that is filled with yellow bone marrow.

Meningitis is an acute inflammation of the pia mater and arachnoid mater around the brain and spinal cord.

Menopause is the physiological cessation of the menstrual cycle.

Menstrual cycle is the periodically recurring series of changes that take place in the ovaries, uterus, and related structures in the female.

Menstruation is the cyclic, physiologic uterine bleeding that occurs at about four-week intervals during the reproductive period of the female.

Mesoderm is the middle layer of cells of the skin.

Metabolic wastes are products formed from cell metabolism.

Metabolism is the process taking place in living organisms whereby the cells are nourished and carry out their activities.

Metaphase is a stage in cell division.

Metastasis is the spread of cancer from one site to another location in the body.

Mission statement is a short, general statement of the main focus of the business.

Mitosis is the process of cell division.

Mixed nerves contain both sensory and motor fibers.

Moist heat packs are chemical gel packs that are heated in a water bath, wrapped in a terry cover, and placed on the body.

Molecules are specific arrangements of atoms.

Morphology is the structure of an organism or body.

Motor nerves, or efferent nerves, carry impulses from the brain or spinal cord to the muscles or glands.

Motor neuron carries nerve impulses from the brain to the effectors.

Motor unit consists of a motor neuron and all the muscle fibers it controls.

Multiple sclerosis occurs in young adults and results from the breakdown of the myelin sheath.

Muscle energy technique (MET), or PNF stretching, uses neurophysiological muscle reflexes to improve functional mobility of the joints.

Muscle fatigue is a condition in which the muscle ceases to respond due to oxygen debt from rapid or prolonged muscle contractions.

Muscle fiber is the functional contractile unit of muscle tissue.

Muscle spasm is a sudden involuntary contraction of a muscle.

Muscle strain is the most common injury to muscle.

Muscle tone is a type of muscle contraction present in healthy muscles even when at rest.

Muscular dystrophy is a group of related diseases in which the contractile fibers of the muscles are replaced by fat and connective tissue, rendering the muscles useless.

Muscular system is made up of voluntary and involuntary muscles that are necessary for movement.

Muslin is a thin plain-weave cotton fabric used to make herbal sheets for use in herbal wraps and other spa treatments. It is prized for its absorptive powers and natural, unbleached texture.

Myocardial infarction, or heart attack, is the result of a reduced blood flow in the coronary arteries supplying the heart muscle.

Myocardium is the cardiac muscle.

Myofibrosis is the process where muscle tissue is replaced by fibrous connective tissue.

N

Naevus, or birthmark, is a discoloration of the skin due to pigmentation or dilated capillaries, present on the skin at birth.

Neat refers to the application of an essential oil at its full, undiluted strength.

Nephron is the functional unit of the kidney.

Nerves are bundles of signal-carrying fibers held together by connective tissue that originate in the brain and spinal cord and distribute branches all over the body.

Nervous system controls and coordinates all the body systems and includes the nerves, spinal cord, and the brain.

Nervous tissue is composed of neurons and initiates, controls, and coordinates the body's adaptation to its surroundings.

Neuralgia is the pain associated with neuritis.

Neuritis is an inflammation of a nerve.

Neurological pathway is the route that a nerve impulse travels through the nervous system.

Neuromuscular junction is the site where the muscle fiber and nerve fiber meet.

Neuromuscular therapy is a system of soft tissue assessment and manipulation that was developed in the 1930s in England by Stanley Lief and Boris Chaitow and popularized in the United States by Paul St. John and Judith DeLany.

Neuron is the structural unit of the nervous system.

Neurophysiological therapies use soft tissue manipulation to reprogram the neurological loop to reduce pain and improve function.

Nonverbal communication, also known as body language, is how an individual's posturing, gestures, and facial expressions provide information about his mental, emotional, or physical condition.

Norepinephrine is the "fight or flight" hormone that prepares the body to respond to emergencies.

O

Onsen are Japanese hot springs at the site of natural volcanic springwater, usually with massage and other relaxing therapies available.

Opportunistic infection is caused by organisms commonly found in the environment and our bodies that become deadly when the body's immune system is weakened.

Oral cavity, or mouth, prepares food for entrance into the stomach.

Organ system is a number of organs working together to perform a bodily function.

Origin of a muscle is the point where the end of a muscle is anchored to an immovable section of the skeleton.

Orthobionomy is a healing system based on the body's self-correcting reflexes.

Osteoarthritis is a chronic disease that affects joints worn down by trauma or age.

Osteoporosis is a condition in which increased reabsorption of calcium into the blood causes a thinning of bone tissue, leaving it prone to fracture.

Ovaries are glandular organs in the pelvis that produce the ovum and female sex hormones.

Ovulation is the discharge of a mature ovum from the follicle of the ovary.

Ovum is the egg cell capable of being fertilized by a spermatozoon and developing into a new life.

Oxytocin causes the uterus to contract and causes the letdown of breast milk.

P

Pain has a primarily protective function in that it warns of tissue damage or destruction somewhere in the body. It is the result of stimulation of specialized nerve ends in the body.

Palmar compression is done with the whole hand or heel of the hand over a large area of the body.

Palpation is a skill and an art developed by the therapist that is a primary assessment tool allowing the therapist to listen to the client's body through the therapist's hands.

Pancreas is located behind the stomach and produces digestive enzymes and the hormones insulin and glucagon.

Papule is a small, elevated pimple in the skin, containing fluid, but which may develop pus.

Parafango is a combination of paraffin wax and fango mud used in spa wraps and localized applications to soften, moisten, and purify the skin while warming and relaxing the muscles.

Paraplegia is paralysis of the legs usually caused by spinal cord injury or disease.

Parasite is an organism that may potentially cause disease that exists and functions at the expense of a host organism without contributing to the survival of the host.

Parasympathetic nervous system functions to conserve energy and reverse the action of the sympathetic division.

Parathormone regulates the blood level of calcium.

Parathyroid glands come in two pairs situated on each lobe of and behind the thyroid and produce parathormone.

Parkinson's disease occurs as a result of the degeneration of certain nerve tissues that regulate body movements.

Partnership is a business setup in which two or more partners share responsibilities and benefits of running the business.

Passive joint movements stretch the fibrous tissue and move the joint through its range of motion.

Passive positioning involves the gentle, passive movement of a joint into a position of maximum comfort, holding it, and slowly returning it to its normal position.

Passive stretching moves body segments beyond their free ROM while the muscles that act on that segment remain as relaxed as possible.

Pathology is the study of the structural and functional changes caused by disease.

Penis is the male organ of copulation.

Percussion is a rapid, striking motion of the hands against the surface of the client's body, using varying amounts of force and hand positions.

Pericardial cavity is a space within the pericardium that contains a serous fluid that cushions the heart.

Pericardium is a double-layered membrane that encloses the heart.

Perichondrium is the membrane covering cartilage.

Perimysium separates the muscle into bundles of muscle fibers.

Periosteum is a fibrous membrane that functions to protect the bone and serves as an attachment of tendons and ligaments.

Peripheral nervous system consists of all the nerves that connect the CNS to the rest of the body.

Peristalsis is the wavelike muscular action of the alimentary canal.

Petrissage lifts, squeezes, and presses the tissues.

Petty cash fund is maintained to pay small disbursements for incidentals.

Phagocytosis is a process in which leukocytes engulf and digest harmful bacteria and other tissue debris.

Phlebitis is an inflammation of a vein accompanied by pain and swelling.

Physiologic barrier represents the extent of easy movement allowed during passive or active joint movements.

Physiology is the science and study of the vital processes, mechanisms, and functions of an organ or system.

Physiopathological reflex arc is a self-perpetuating dysfunctional neurological circuit.

Pia mater is the innermost layer of the meninges surrounding the brain and spinal cord.

Pincer palpation is employed in areas where the muscle tissue can be picked up between the thumb and fingers of the same hand (e.g., sternocleidomastoid muscle) where the belly of the muscle is rolled between the thumb and fingers to identify dysfunctional tissue.

Pituitary gland is a small gland, often called the master gland, because the hormones it secretes stimulate or regulate other glands.

Plasma is the fluid part of the blood.

Plastic body wrap is a thin, transparent, disposable plastic sheet used to wrap directly around the client's skin during mud, clay, and seaweed body wraps.

Plasticity refers to the tissue's ability to adapt to ongoing stresses and conditions.

Pneumocystis carinii pneumonia is caused by a protozoan commonly found in the lungs.

Polarity therapy uses massage manipulations derived from Eastern and Western practices.

Poliomyelitis is a crippling disease that affects the motor neurons of the medulla and spinal cord, resulting in paralysis.

Position release is a method of passively moving the body or body part toward the body's preference and away from pain, seeking the tissue's preferred position. Movements are toward ease and away from bind, away from any restrictive barrier and toward comfort.

Post-event massage is given the first hour or two after participating in an event to clear out metabolic wastes, reduce muscle tension, increase circulation, and quiet the nervous system.

Postisometric relaxation means that following an isometric contraction, there is a period of relaxation during which muscle impulses are inhibited.

Precision muscle testing utilizes a specialized kinesiology to evaluate energetic imbalances in the body.

Pre-eclampsia is a condition of pregnancy related to increased blood pressure in the mother that affects the placenta; can also affect the mother's kidney, liver, and brain.

Pre-event massage is given 15 to 45 minutes prior to an event and prepares the body for intense activity.

Pregnancy, or gestation, is the physiological condition that occurs from the time an ovum is fertilized until childbirth.

Prolactin stimulates the production of milk in a woman's breast.

Prophase is a stage in cell division.

Proprioception is a system of sensory and motor nerve activity that provides information on the position and rate of movement of body parts to the CNS.

Proprioceptors are nerve fibers that sense where the body is and how it moves.

Prostate gland secretes an alkaline fluid that enhances the sperm's motility.

Protoplasm is a colorless, jelly-like substance within the cell in which food elements, such as protein, fats, carbohydrates, mineral salts, and water, are present.

Psoriasis is a chronic, inflammatory disease usually found on the scalp, elbows, knees, chest, and lower back.

Pulmonary circulation is the blood circulation from the heart to the lungs and back again to the heart.

Pulmonary semilunar valve of the heart directs blood from the right ventricle into the pulmonary arteries.

Pulsating shower is a means of combining moist heat and mild compression, which calms sensory nerves and increases peripheral circulation.

Pustule is an elevation of the skin having an inflamed base, containing pus.

Q

Quadriplegia is paralysis of the arms and legs caused by a stroke or spinal cord injury.

R

Range of motion is the movement of a joint from one extreme of the articulation to the other.

Rasul is a special tiled steam chamber in which spa guests recline with multicolored therapeutic muds applied to the body then have it washed away with built-in rain showers.

Reciprocal inhibition occurs when a muscle acting on a joint contracts and the opposing muscle is reflexively inhibited.

Red corpuscles, or erythrocytes, are cells in the blood that carry oxygen from the lungs to the body cells and transport carbon dioxide from the cells to the lungs.

Reflex is the simplest form of nervous activity, which includes a sensory and motor nerve.

Reflex arc is the nerve pathway of a reflex.

Reflexology stimulates particular points on the surface of the body, which in turn affects other areas or organs of the body.

Rehabilitative massage focuses on restoration of tissue function following injury.

Reproductive system is the generative apparatus that functions to ensure continuance of the species.

Resistive barrier, also known as the pathological barrier, is the first sign of resistance to a movement as tissue is moved and manipulated through its range of motion.

Respiration is the exchange of carbon dioxide and oxygen that takes place in the lungs, between the blood and cells, and within the cell.

Respiratory system includes the lungs, air passages, nose, mouth, pharynx, trachea, and bronchial tubes.

Reticular layer of the skin contains fat cells, blood and lymph vessels, sweat and oil glands, hair follicles, and nerve endings.

Reticular tissue is composed of fibers that form the framework of the liver and lymphoid organs.

Rheumatoid arthritis, a chronic, systemic, autoimmune inflammatory disease, is the most serious type of arthritis.

Rocking is a push-and-release movement applied to the client's body in either a side-to-side or an up-and-down direction.

Rolfing aligns the major body segments through manipulation of the fascia or the connective tissue.

Rolling is a rapid back-and-forth movement with the hands, in which the flesh is shaken and rolled around the axis of the body part.

Rosacea is associated with excessive oiliness of the skin and a chronic inflammatory condition of the cheeks and nose.

S

Sacral plexus is formed from the fourth and fifth lumbar nerves, and the first four sacral nerves.

Sagittal plane divides the body into left and right parts.

Saliva contains enzymes that begin to digest carbohydrates.

Salt rub is a frictional application of wet salt over the client's body.

Sanitation is the third level of decontamination practiced in the massage studio and is done with soaps or detergents and water.

Sarcolemma is the cell wall of the muscle cell.

Sarcoplasmic reticulum is a network of membranous channels within the muscle cell.

Sauna baths use dry heat and have temperatures of 180° to 190°F.

Scale is an accumulation of epidermal flakes, dry or greasy.

Scar may form after the healing of an injury or skin condition.

Sciatica is neuralgia caused by injury or pressure on the sciatic nerve.

Sciatic nerve is the largest and longest nerve in the body.

Scoliosis is lateral curvature of the spine.

Scope of practice defines the rights and activities legally acceptable according to the licenses of a particular occupation or profession.

Seborrhea is a skin condition caused by overactivity of the sebaceous glands.

Semen is excreted from the body during ejaculation.

Seminal fluid forms the majority of the semen when ejaculated.

Seminal vesicles are two glandular tubes located on each side of the prostate that produce a nutritious fluid that is excreted into the ejaculatory ducts at the time of emission.

Sensory nerves, or afferent nerves, carry sensory impulses toward the brain or spinal cord.

Sensory neuron carries impulses from sense organs to the brain.

Septum is the wall that separates the heart's chambers.

Sequence refers to the pattern or design of a massage.

Serotonin is a neurotransmitter that helps regulate nerve impulses and influences mood, behavior, appetite, blood pressure, temperature regulation, memory, and learning ability.

Sex glands manufacture the reproductive cells and sex hormones needed for fertility and reproduction.

Shaking allows for the release of tension by gently shaking a relaxed body part so that the flesh flops around the bone.

Shampoo is a cleansing measure accomplished with water and soap.

Shiatsu is a massage technique from Japan in which points of stimulation are pressed to effect the circulation of fluids and *ki* (life force energy).

Shingles is an acute inflammation of a nerve trunk by the herpes varicella-zoster virus.

Sign (of disease) is an observable indication of disease of bodily disorder.

Skeletal membrane covers bone and cartilage.

Skeletal muscles are attached to bone by tendons and are responsible for moving the limbs, facial expression, speaking, and other voluntary movements.

Skeletal system is the bony framework of the body, composed of bones, cartilage, and ligaments.

Skin the largest organ of the body with functions that include protection, heat regulation, secretion and excretion, sensation, absorption, and respiration.

Skin brushing a light, brisk brushing using a dry vegetable bristle bath brush.

Skin rolling is a variation of kneading in which only the skin and subcutaneous tissue is picked up between the thumbs and fingers and rolled.

Slapping uses a rhythmical, glancing contact of the palm of the hand with the body.

Small intestine, the largest part of the alimentary canal, consists of the duodenum, jejunum, and ileum.

Smooth muscle tissue lacks striations and cannot be stimulated to contract by conscious effort.

Soft end feel is a cushioned limitation where soft tissue prevents further movement, such as knee flexion.

Soft tissue barriers are notable physiological changes in the quality of movement in soft tissue that represent the limits within which the tissues can be effectively manipulated.

Sole proprietor is an individual business owner responsible for all expenses, obligations, liabilities, and assets.

Somatotropic or growth hormone stimulates the growth of bones, muscles, and organs.

Spa massage is any massage given by a therapist within the structure and limitations of the spa setting, usually referring to the spa's basic Swedish massage, but also applicable to advanced modalities given in the spa.

Spa technicians are employees who assist therapists and estheticians in setting up treatment areas, keeping areas clean, preparing treatments, and in some cases performing certain modalities such as wraps and body scrubs.

Special water treatments use compresses, packs, and fomentations.

Spermatozoa are tiny detached male reproductive cells, egg-shaped, and equipped with a tail that enables them to swim.

Spinal cord functions as a conduction pathway for nerve impulses to and from the brain.

Spinal cord injury results in paralysis of the parts of the body controlled by the spinal nerves that exit the spinal cord below the injury site.

Spindle cells located in the belly of muscle, alert the CNS as to the length and stretch and speed of the muscle contraction.

Sponging is the application of a liquid to the body by means of a sponge, cloth, or the hand.

Spongy bone, located inside long bones, consists of irregularly shaped spaces defined by thin, bony plates.

Sports massage is a method of massage designed to prepare an athlete for an upcoming event. It is achieved through specialized manipulations that stimulate circulation of the blood and lymph.

Sprain is an injury to a joint resulting in stretching or tearing of the ligaments.

Sprays are the projection of one or more streams of water against the body.

Springy end feel is the most common end feel, and limitation is due to the stretch of fibrous tissue as the joint reaches the extent of its range of motion.

Squamous cell carcinoma is a type of skin cancer.

Stains are abnormal brown skin patches, having circular and irregular shape.

Steam baths use a steam generator as a heat source and have temperatures of 120° to 130°F.

Steatoma is a subcutaneous tumor of the sebaceous glands.

Sterilization is the most complete cleansing process that destroys all living organisms, including bacterial spores.

Strain involves the tearing of muscle tissue or tendons.

Stress is any psychological or physical situation or condition that causes tension or strain.

Stretching is passive and active stretching of muscle and connective tissue to achieve normal resting length.

Strigil is a curved, usually metallic, instrument used in ancient Greece and Rome to scrape dead skin cells, oil, and dirt from bathers' skin.

Structural integration attempts to bring the physical structure of the body into alignment around a central axis.

Structural/muscular balancing works with a client's self-knowledge to locate and release constricted tissues that cause pain and rigidity.

Subcutaneous tissue is regarded as a continuation of the dermis.

Sudoriferous glands are the sweat glands located in the dermis layer of skin.

Superficial fascia refers to the connecting layer between the skin and those structures underlying the skin.

Superficial gliding is when the practitioner's hand conforms to client's body contours so that equal gentle pressure is applied to the body from every part of the hand as the practitioner's hand glides over a portion of the client's body.

Sustained stretching uses slow, gradual movement to gently challenge the limitations at the edge of the ROM.

Sweat lodge is a Native American enclosure for sweating, cleansing, and purification, in which participants pour water over heated stones in ceremonial fashion to create heat while praying and chanting.

Swedish massage employs traditional manipulations of effleurage, petrissage, vibration, friction, and tapotement.

Sympathetic nervous system supplies the glands, involuntary muscles of internal organs, and walls of blood vessels with nerves.

Symptom is subjective evidence of disease or bodily disorder.

Synarthrotic joints, such as those of the skull, are immovable.

Synovial fluid lubricates the surfaces of joints.

Synovial joints have a joint cavity surrounded by an articular capsule.

Synovial membrane is a connective tissue membrane lining cavities and capsules in and around joints.

Syphilis is a serious disease that is transmitted by sexual contact with an infected person.

Systemic infection is invading organisms that have spread throughout the body.

T

Tapotement movements include tapping, slapping, hacking, cupping, and beating.

Tapping is the lightest, most superficial of the percussion techniques.

T-cells coordinate immune defenses and kill organisms in cells on contact.

Telophase is a stage in cell division.

Tendonitis is an inflammation of the tendon.

Tendons are bands that attach muscle to bone.

Testes are two small, egg-shaped glands that produce the spermatozoa.

Testosterone is a male hormone responsible for development of secondary sexual characteristics.

Thereapeutic procedure is the process of acquiring a concise medical history, assessment procedures to determine constricted and painful conditions, developing treatment plans, performing appropriate treatment practices to more specifically address the conditions, and evaluating the results.

Thermae are hot springs or baths, especially the baths of ancient Rome.

Thermal blanket, also known as a space blanket. This thin polyethylene and metallic-coated sheet retains heat during spa body wraps and aromatherapy.

Thoracic outlet syndrome is pain, numbness, or weakness in the shoulder, neck, and arm caused by a compression or entrapment of the brachial plexus.

Thorax (chest) is the upper part of the trunk containing the ribs, lungs, heart, esophagus, and trachea.

Thrombophlebitis is the inflammation of veins due to blood clots.

Thymus is located behind the sternum and above the heart and stimulates lymphoid tissue to produce lymphocytes.

Thyroid gland is situated on either side of the trachea and produces thyroxin, triiodothyronine, and calcitonin.

Thyroid-stimulating hormone (TSH) regulates the thyroid gland.

Thyroxin stimulates the metabolic rate of the body.

Tissues are collections of similar cells that carry out specific bodily functions.

Tonic friction is the application of friction to the body with cold water so as to produce a stimulating effect.

Touch refers to the stationary contact of the practitioner's hand and the client's body.

Touch for Health is a simplified form of applied kinesiology that involves techniques from both Eastern and Western origins.

Toxoplasmosis comes from a protozoan found in raw or undercooked meat.

Trager method uses movement exercises called mentastics along with massage-like, gentle shaking of different parts of the body to eliminate tension.

Transference happens when a client personalizes, either negatively or positively, a therapeutic relationship by unconsciously projecting characteristics of someone from a former relationship onto a therapist or practitioner.

Transverse plane divides the body horizontally into an upper and lower portion.

Transverse tubules are narrow tubes that are continuous with the sarcolemma of the muscle cell and extend into the sarcoplasm at right angles to the cell surface. Filled with extracellular fluid, they conduct electrical impulses that are the triggers for muscle fiber contraction.

Tricuspid valve of the heart allows blood to flow from the right atrium into the right ventricle.

Trigger point is a hyperirritable nodule associated with dysfunctional contractile tissue that illicits a pain response when digital pressure is applied.

Triiodothyronine stimulates the metabolic rate of the body.

Tschanpua is a Hindu technique of massage in the bath.

Tsubo are points on the body that are sensitive to pressure applied during shiatsu.

Tubercle is a solid lump larger than a papule, projecting above the surface or lying within or under the skin.

Tumor is an abnormal growth of swollen tissue that can be located on any part of the body.

U

Ulcer is an open lesion on the skin or mucous membrane.

Universal precautions is a system of infection control that protects persons from exposure to blood and bloody bodily fluids.

Urethra conveys urine from the bladder and carries reproductive cells and secretions out of the body.

Urinalysis is a chemical examination of the urine, usually part of a routine examination.

Urinary system includes two kidneys, two ureters, the bladder, and a urethra.

Urticaria are red, raised lesions or wheals that itch severely and are caused by an allergic or emotional reaction.

Uterus is a pear-shaped, muscular female organ that expands during pregnancy to accommodate the fetus.

V

Vaccine contains microorganisms that are either dead, weakened, or altered forms of a live infectious organism that stimulates an immune response without causing an illness.

Vagina is a muscular tube leading from the vulva to the cervix and is the lower part of the birth canal.

Vapocoolant sprays when sprayed on the skin, evaporate quickly, causing rapid cooling of the skin.

Varicose veins are protruding, bulbous, distended superficial veins, particularly in the lower legs.

Vasoconstriction is the contraction of the arterial walls.

Vasodilation is the relaxation and enlargement of the arterial walls.

Veins are thinner-walled blood vessels that carry deoxygenated blood and waste-laden blood from capillaries back to the heart.

Venereal diseases are associated with the sexual organs and are characterized by sores and rashes on the skin.

Venules are microscopic vessels that continue from the capillaries and merge to form veins.

Vesicle is a blister with clear fluid in it, lying within or just beneath the epidermis.

Vibration is a continuous trembling or shaking movement delivered either by the practitioner or an electrical apparatus.

Vichy shower is a multihead inline shower extending out over a treatment table under which clients recline on a wet table to receive spa services.

Villi are small, fingerlike projections.

Virus is any class of submicroscopic pathogenic agents that transmit disease.

Vitiligo is characterized by light patches of skin due to defective pigmentation.

Vulva forms the external part of the female reproductive system.

W

Warts are caused by the papilloma virus and are classified as common, plantar, and venereal.

Watershed is the separation lines of lymph into different drainage territories.

Wellness is behaviors and habits that have a positive influence on health.

Wet room is a tiled treatment room with plumbing that contains one or more of the following: wet table, shower, Vichy shower, hydrotherapy tub, Swiss shower.

Wet table is a specially constructed waterproof treatment table with built-in drainage used in spas for exfoliation and body wrap services.

Wet sanitizer is any receptacle large enough to hold a disinfectant solution in which the objects to be sanitized can be completely immersed.

Wheal is an itchy, swollen lesion that lasts only a few hours.

Whirlpool is a tub equipped with a powerful jet that causes the water to swirl around the occupant.

White corpuscles, or leukocytes, protect the body against disease by combating infections and toxins that invade the body.

Wringing is a back-and-forth movement in which both hands are placed a short distance apart on either side of the limb and work in opposing directions.

Y

Yoga is a form of exercise that combines mental concentration, muscular control, breathing, and relaxation.

Z

Zygote is a fertilized ovum.

Index

Notes

Notes

Notes

Notes

Notes

Notes

Notes

Notes

Notes

Notes

Notes